DIFFERENT VIEWS OF ANXIETY DISORDERS

Edited by **Salih Selek**

Different Views of Anxiety Disorders
Edited by Salih Selek

Published by InTech
Janeza Trdine 9, 51000 Rijeka, Croatia

Publishing Process Manager Ana Pantar

Technical Editor Teodora Smiljanic

Cover Designer InTech Design Team

Additional hard copies can be obtained from orders@intechopen.com

Different Views of Anxiety Disorders, Edited by Salih Selek
p. cm.
ISBN 978-953-307-560-0

For EU product safety concerns:
IN TECH d.o.o., Prolaz Marije Krucifikse Kozulić 3, 51000 Rijeka, Croatia,
info@intechopen.com or visit our website at intechopen.com.

Meet the editor

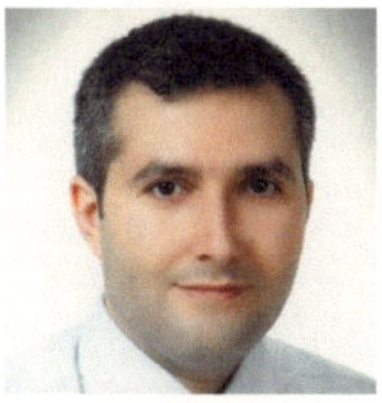

Dr. Salih Selek is an assistant professor of psychiatry at the Harran University Medical School, Turkey. His main interest is the biological basis of psychiatric disorders. He has written more than 40 papers most of which are published internationally. He participates as editor, associate editor, editorial board member and reviewer in several SCI-E/ Pubmed indexed international journals. He received 10 national and international awards and he also has international experience as a clinician in Germany and as a researcher in the U.S.A.

Contents

Preface XI

Part 1 Nosology and Defining Anxiety Disorders 1

Chapter 1 **Anxiety and Its Nosographic and Psychopathologic Place in German Psychiatry: A Historical Perspective 3**
Marc Géraud

Chapter 2 **Social Anxiety Disorder 23**
Nesrin Dilbaz, Aslı Enez and Serçin Yalçın Çavuş

Chapter 3 **Obsessive-Compulsive Disorders or Not: Differential Diagnosis of Repetitive Behaviors Among Individuals with Intellectual and Developmental Disorders 37**
Jarrett Barnhill

Chapter 4 **Reasoning in Anxiety, OCD and Related Disorders: Can Formal Reasoning Theories Inform Us About Psychopathology? 69**
Kieron P. O'Connor and Marie-Claude Pélissier

Part 2 Neuroscience 93

Chapter 5 **Animal Models of Anxiety Vulnerability - The Wistar Kyoto Rat 95**
X. Jiao, K.D. Beck, K.C.H. Pang and R.J. Servatius

Chapter 6 **Influence of Trait-Anxiety on Inhibition Function: Evidence from ERP Studies 121**
Yue-jia Luo, Ruolei Gu and Yu-xia Huang

Chapter 7 **Zebrafish, a Potential Novel Research Tool for the Analysis and Modeling of Anxiety 137**
Robert Gerlai

Chapter 8 **Acute Stress in Patients with Panic Disorder Produces Effects on Salivary Amylase and Cortisol 159**
Jotaro Akiyoshi,Yoshihiro Tanaka, Koichi Isogawa, Yoshinobu Ishitobi, JusenTsuru, Tomoko Ando, Aimi Kawano, Shizuko Okamoto, Masayuki Kanehisa, Yoshihiro Maruyama, Haruka Higuma, Taiga Ninomiya, Hiroaki Hanada and Kensuke Kodama

Part 3 Assessment 167

Chapter 9 **Measuring States of Anxiety with Clinician-Rated and Patient-Rated Scales 169**
Per Bech

Chapter 10 **Social Anxiety Disorder, Fear of Public Speaking, and the use of Assessment Instruments 185**
Flávia de Lima Osório, José Alexandre S Crippa, Jaime Eduardo C. Hallak and Sonia R.Loureiro

Chapter 11 **The Measurement of Health-Related Quality of Life in a Population with Generalized Anxiety Disorder – Findings from the QUEST Study 199**
Neesha Harnam, Kathleen W. Wyrwich, Dennis Revicki, Julie C. Locklear and Jean Endicott

Part 4 Treatment: Dealing with Resistance 217

Chapter 12 **Treatment Resistant Generalized Anxiety Disorder 219**
Nesrin Dilbaz, Serçin Yalcın Cavus and Aslı Enez Darcin

Chapter 13 **The Treatment of Obsessive-Compulsive Disorder and the Approaches to Treatment Resistance 233**
Stefano Pallanti, Giacomo Grassi and Andrea Cantisani

Chapter 14 **A Review of Interventions for Treatment-Resistant Posttraumatic Stress Disorder 251**
Cara Katz, Murray Stein, J. Don Richardson, Soraya Seedat and Jitender Sareen

Part 5 Treatment: Alternative Approaches 271

Chapter 15 **Herbal Remedies to Treat Anxiety Disorders 273**
Bhagya Venkanna Rao, Bettadapura N. Srikumar and Byrathnahalli S. Shankaranarayana Rao

Chapter 16 **A Context-Aware System for Anxiety Disorders 293**
Theodor Panagiotakopoulos, Maria-Anna Fengou, Panagiotis Malliaris and Dimitrios Lymberopoulos

Part 6 Anxiety in Children 311

Chapter 17 **Separation Anxiety in Children and Adolescents 313**
Malgorzata Dabkowska, Aleksander Araszkiewicz, Agnieszka Dabkowska and Monika Wilkosc

Chapter 18 **Using Stories to Prevent Anxiety Disorders in a School Context: Dominique's Handy Tricks Program 339**
Jean Gervais, Stéphane Bouchard and Nadia Gagnier

Chapter 19 **Rational-Emotive and Cognitive-Behavioral Interventions for Children with Anxiety Disorders: A Group Counseling Curriculum 355**
Jerry Wilde

Preface

Anxiety, whether an illness or emotion, is a term with historical roots even in the Bible, but it was not popular until the modern age. If we speak of anxiety as an disorder, advances in psychiatry in the last decades have revealed some biological as well as psychosocial basis of the phenomenon. On the other hand, advances in neuroscience have not yet found the "real cause" of anxiety. Today, we can group, diagnose and treat several anxiety disorders to an extent, but the assessment of symptoms and severity, dealing with resistant conditions, new treatment modalities and specific patient population, such as children, are still the challenging aspects of anxiety disorders.

This book intends to present anxiety disorders from a different view and discusses several issues. The first part begins with historical perspective of the nosology of disorder in German lexicon and continues with new definitions or issues in anxiety disorders. You can find the clues of "the invasion of the anxiety phenomenon" and close relation of repetitive behaviors and anxiety in the chapters. Part two, reports innovative animal and human studies of molecular and electrophysiological origin that may stimulate further research in neuroscientific field. In the third part, the authors focus on various assessment tools, which may provide useful information for mental health professionals. The topic of the following two parts is treatment. Treatment resistant conditions and new treatment approaches are mentioned in the chapters. The readers may be particularly interested in herbal remedies. The final part focuses on a specific population- children.

Finally, this book is neither a classically designed textbook nor a collection of reviews. It is a mixture of traditional and novel knowledge discussing a wide variety of anxiety topics from a multidimensional approach. The book addresses not only psychiatrists but also a broad range of specialists, including psychologists, neuroscientists and other mental health professionals with open access choice.

Salih Selek, M.D.
Psychiatry Department, Harran University Medical School, Sanliurfa, Turkey

This book is for information only and should not be used for diagnosis and treatment. Consult a doctor or other health care professional for the diagnosis and treatment of medical conditions.

Part 1

Nosology and Defining Anxiety Disorders

1

Anxiety and Its Nosographic and Psychopathologic Place in German Psychiatry: A Historical Perspective

Géraud, Marc
Centre Hospitalier Charles Perrens
France

1. Introduction

The Germans use the term "*Angst*" more often than we do. The preposition which goes with it is "vor" (in front (of)): you can have "Angst vor…" (a storm, certain animals, etc.). It implies some imprecision with regard to the subject; when the subject is specified, the expression is *Furcht* (fear). It is etymologically derived, in the sense of tightness, oppression, from the Indo-European word group *eng*. Latin *angustus,* narrow, *angustiae* : narrowness, compression, difficulty.

2. Recognition

Anxiety was acknowledged only relatively late on; although it is mentioned in one of the first German works on psychiatry, Reil's *Rhapsodies*, it does not begin to acquire a status more or less independent from melancholia until Krafft-Ebing, where it is linked in such a way as to become visible. The second moment of conception for anxiety disorders was the introduction of the term agoraphobia by Westphal (1872). But the real bombshell was the direct attack by Freud on neurasthenia, which left only a small group of symptoms remaining, opposed to anxiety neurosis, a new, independent entity considered, however, from the outset as often intertwined or associated with the other "important neuroses," hysteria and obsessional neurosis.

3. Anxiety in limbo

3.1 Reil

In one of the first works in German psychiatry, the *Rhapsodien über die Anwendung der psychischen Curmethode auf Geisteszerrütungen* (Rhapsodies on the Use of Psychological Therapies for the Mentally Disturbed) (1803) by Johann Christian Reil, the word Angst, along with its derivatives (ängstich, beängstigen), is indeed used, but anxiety is not described as such. The term is very often employed in association with other names for a series of emotions, such as: "It is in our power to produce a great number of illnesses and, through them, pathological feelings of the most diverse type: disgust, itching, tickling, pain, anxiety etc. which, as symptoms of these disorders, are inseparable from them." It can occur during the course of an illness: a propos of one woman who had visions: "One day, she was pacing backwards and forwards, in despair, in her room and someone who was trying to stop her placed a hand on one of her eyes by accident. Instantly, all the apparitions disappeared, and with them, her anxiety." Or again: "... If (certain organs) suffer from dynamic or organic illnesses, mood changes without external cause. The patient is dispirited, bad tempered, fixes on things of secondary importance concerning, in particular, his own body, swings between bravery and discouragement, fear and hope. The imagination fixes on obsessions, images of anxiety, and gives birth to the most curious monsters." "An elderly bachelor who had offended another, more courageous, feared his revenge. He left his home and bought a property in the country, several leagues away. But the inner anxiety persisted ..." "Professor Moritz was ill and so full of anxiety because of the uncertainty of his recovery that his fever was continually fuelled." And this wonderful sentence: "Melancholia is an anxiety plunged in a single thought and remains fixed there, with no fever." "In the beginning the fixed delusion is no doubt based on a physical or moral anxiety, which ends up by leading to a total confusion of understanding." These little clinical observations show us clearly that anxiety had been spotted, but that it only ranked as a symptom, certainly not as an illness.

Anxiety is taken into greater consideration in the fourth volume of his work on Fevers (on nervous disorders) (1812). Here we find the series (hunger, thirst, craving, fatigue, distaste, cold and hot, anxiety, etc., p. 49). Certain pathological pictures are observed early on (phobia: "Many people can't stand cats; their presence, even if they can't be seen, causes anxiety and fainting.").

3.2 Autenrieth

Ferdinand Autenrieth, who was not a specialist in psychiatry but wrote a text in 1807 concerning the installations he had had put in for the insane in Tübingen (*Über die im Clinicum in Tübingen getroffene Einrichtungen für Wahnsinnige*), very rarely mentions the word anxiety, whether in *Versuche für die praktische Heilkunde aus den clinischen Anstalten von Tübingen* (1808), in *Über den Menschen und seine Hoffnung einer Fortdauer vom Standpunkte des Naturforschers aus* (1825) or in *Ansichten über Natur- und Seelenleben* (1836). It is always presented in the form of an adjective (*ängstlich*) in the *Versuche,* generally in connection with respiration, except in one case where it is a question of a "really debilitating" anxiety (*Angst*) (Autenrieth, 1808, p. 421). Autenrieth also mentions the anxious movement of the hands and the feet of the newborn ("The infant suffers much during birth, the violent passage into a new world (the second for him); his first act is to cry and anxiously agitate his hands and feet."'Autenrieth, 1836, p. 86). Precognition of birth trauma? Autenrieth treated Hölderlin before placing him by the carpenter Zimmer. His "intern" was Justinus Kerner.

There was more regard for anxiety in the fourth volume of his work on Fevers (on nervous illnesses) (Authenrieth, 1812). Here too there are these series (hunger, thirst, craving, fatigue, disgust, cold and hot,Autenrieth anxiety, etc.). (ibid., p. 49). Some embryonic pathological pictures are noted (phobia: "Many people cannot endure cats; their presence, even if they can't be seen, causes anxiety and fainting fits.").

3.3 Heinroth

Heinroth is the dominant personality in psychiatry at the beginning of this century and era. The layout of his treatises is very systemized (it should be noted that the treatise on *Seelenstörungen* (Heinroth, 1818), psychological disorders, is subtitled: "outlined from a rational point of view"): section, chapter, segment, etc., they are cast in a mould. Heinroth describes himself as a doctor: *seelischer Artzt,* doctor of the soul . For him, psychiatry (Heinroth uses this term), compared to symptomatological psychology, takes the form of anthropology. It seems to be based on a unique ontological assumption: "The mind is like all other phenomena in nature, a force which can be excited by stimuli". This is the reason why it was said that Heinroth was a romantic. Heinroth considered life in moral depravity to be pathogenic. Health is freedom, and reason.

Heinroth's terminology is very idiosyncratic: for him the symptoms of melancholia are *Gemütsdepression* (depression of affectivity), *Insichversunkenheit* (being immersed in oneself), *Lossgerissenheit* (detachment) in relation to the world without replacement by something better. These two elements, putting forward *Gemüt* (affectivity) and erecting a concept of religious man, seem to us to be characteristic of Heinroth's psychiatry. The name chosen and developed by Heinroth for mental illnesses was *Seelenstörung,* literally "disorders of the soul." Pathological states appear in all regions of the mind, the common denominator being the stamp of non-freedom, and which, in addition, diverge individually.

The plan of divine creation in man is disrupted through the latter's fault. "Prey to passions, delusions and vice, the creative work of culture is in him often inhibited, interrupted and repressed; and thus, by considering a process of organisation of development towards a perfect life, that is free, we obtain the concept of a disorder of the life of the soul or, more briefly, soul disorder." (1818, p. 34-35).

From this point of view, any state of disease could be called a psychological disorder. It is therefore necessary to define more precisely the concept of mental disorder, as total stagnation, complete stop, inversion of the tendency to self-improvement, self-annihilation, and where these symptoms are the most marked, psychological disorders. And it is these states in which willpower has completely collapsed and in its place there is a total restraint, a total absence of idea, a perfect, persistent, non-freedom which is commonly called disturbance of the mind, obtuseness of intelligence, delusion, mood disorder, mental disorder in general. Not only freedom but the faculty of freedom has collapsed. Following the upsurge of natural necessity, internal and external (these patients) are not even animals directed by a healthy instinct, but machines.

Mental disorders are precisely the interaction between *Seelenstimmung* (psychological mood) and the stimulus (*Reiz*). "The mother is the psychological mood; the father is the stimulus." The latter is always evil.

It has to be said that Heinroth does not say much about anxiety, which shows the precariousness of this notion in psychiatric terms. But this negative result does have a positive side to it: Heinroth does not mention anxiety because his work is anthropological: he speaks of man from a holistic or global point of view and not as a series of fragmentary symptoms. We should therefore recognize that man may indeed enter freely into the life of consciousness, but with a freedom already tarnished, so that he brings with him into the world what is called the original sin (1918, 25). The following passage: If free self-determination is the root of virtue, of any worthy existence, then this unfortunate dissociation in relation to it is a blasphemy against our expectation of a saintly existence, a veneration of sin; because to be a servant of singular things and beings, that is the sin (1818, 95).

3.4 Ideler

In *Grundriss der Seelenheilkunde* (Elements of mental medicine) (1835-38), Ideler chooses the word *Furcht* as the leader in his series of pathological disorders: *Furcht, Angst, Verzweiflung* (fear, anxiety, despair), sometimes including the word *Schreck* (terror). Ideler introduces a theory based on the initial concept of reflex, of reaction: "Avoiding an unnecessary danger is a duty." ("Consciousness of an insurmountable danger arouses, through fear, the natural tendency to flee from it, which makes it a necessary affect when faced with the destructive violence of nature."; "In fear, the depressing agent of danger provokes the tendency to escape by flight.")

4. The premise of a theory for anxiety: March toward of an anxiety disorder

4.1 Flemming

Flemming (1859) showed that psychological doctrine had run out of steam. His aim was to create a "biological psychiatry." Previous science had only led to "a confusion, at which we have only glanced superficially, to make plain the vanity of efforts made to disentangle this mixture of impressions, memories, combinations of past and present, true and false, and to bring to light from this point of view the sterility of psychical symptomatology." It had been established that alongside the normal physiological functioning of mental activities, there are two deviations of this functioning: Error and Delusion. It is not possible to say how these two deviations differ from each other, nor how they are distinguished from the correct path. The difficulty in attributing a symptom to a given faculty or to a given mental element is similar to that of a carpet expert who has to say whether a defect is due to the carpet maker, the shuttle, the spindle or what. Whatever we try to do, there is mixing, vagueness, change everywhere. If we take disorders contemporary with the beginning of mental life, there are two types: either innate, or evolving with growth. In addition there is a much larger group of disorders which attack the already constituted, healthy mind; there are two types: one which resolves once more into a healthy mental life, one which becomes permanent until death. There is a third group: the case of a normal mental life but with certain particularities and striking deviances or coinciding with the nature of the mental disorder which follows: they bear the germ of a mental disorder (*Anlage*, disposition). Either the disorders are due to intelligence (errors of thought, delusion) and then attack the *Gemüt*; or the disorders develop the other way round: a clearer and clearer disharmony in the sphere of tangible feeling. There is thus a group of mental disorders which are accompanied by considerable prostration, a lack of courage, anxiety and an immutable concern. Everything that the sick person thinks and imagines is tinged with bleakness, nocturnal; everything that concerns them, concerns them deeply.

Flemming then comes to a symptom which must be placed amongst the most difficult for the patient, and be ranked amongst those which arouse to the highest degree the compassion of the entourage and the interest of the doctor: precordial anxiety. It appears preferably in states of depression, but it can also be added to states of elation. Even this feeling of anxiety is often taken to be a purely mental symptom, i.e. that it was considered to be a simple effect of the delusional idea, which the patient is occupied with. This is totally inaccurate. These delusional ideas, these distorted representations, about which the patient seems to be anxious, are rather as a general rule caused by feelings of anxiety. In other cases, the anxiety becomes associated with delusional ideas and accompanies them - either the patient places them both in relation with each other, side by side, or they survive beside each other without any relation. This relationship may even take place in the complication of precordial anxiety by hallucinations. For the fear and anxiety provoked by and following sensorial illusions must be clearly distinguished from precordial anxiety. In other cases, there may even be no distorted idea and yet the patient is affected for weeks and months by a great imprecise anxiety. Another fact shows the close relationship of this pathological manifestation with the essence of psychoses: it is that precordial anxiety is frequently the symptom occuring first of all, and remains that way for a long time. Whereas the patient feels correctly, thinks logically, carries out his duties and professional tasks, he confesses under the oath of secrecy, that he is accompanied by an unnameable anxiety. These disorders often afflict young adolescents and may last months before disappearing. In melancholy, it is the prevalent psychological symptom which, so to speak, carries all the others. Treatment is totally lacking.

4.2 Griesinger

Preceded by Jacobi, he was the reformer of a psychiatry in movement: mental disorders were brain disorders. In the field of mental life, Griesinger introduced the notion of psychic pain, likely to present degrees: "but there is in the sensation and the representation of these states a much more general, more vague feeling of discomfort (…) Thus bodily states of general malaise, bodily impediment, etc., with no localized pain, such as in the representation of feelings, for no reason, of oppression, of fear, etc." (Griesinger, 1861, p. 34). "States of psychic pain, anxiety, dread, sadness, chagrin, etc., can be motivated internally or externally, they have for the rest of the body exactly the same consequences as sensitivity to pain. Sleep does not come easily, nutrition suffers, weight loss, and general exhaustion take hold. Psychic pain sometimes alternates with sensory neuralgias." (ibid., p. 37). Anomalies in feelings (*Gemüt*) can trigger a great number of mental disorders. Feelings of concern are frequent; these feelings of anxiety sometimes reach an unbearable level, a despair that often transforms itself into rage. Anxiety of the soul (*Seelenangst*) sometimes makes the patient think that he has caused a crime. In melancholia attonita, anxiety is also expressed by physical agitation.

4.3 Krafft-Ebing's melancholic dysthymia with precordial anxiety

Certain patients with melancholic dysphoria complained of tormented states of anxiety, felt in the epigastric region, which were associated with distressing feelings of pressure and tightening in the precordial region (*Präcordiale Angst*, precordial anxiety). These disorders are not given much explanation. Even in physiological life, anxiety is a well known phenomenon. A danger, work where the result is uncertain, produce a distressing affect of expectation which is also associated with anxiety and with troublesome sensations in the epigastric region. What relationship do these precordial sensations have with the conscious state of anxiety that cannot be analyzed in more detail?

- Are they the expression of excitation of sensitive peripheral nerves, where the state of excitation is led right to the seat of consciousness, generates anxiety there, to be felt, projected eccentric in their place of generation? In this case, these paresthetic and paralgic feelings (sensitive nervous excitations, state of excitation sent to the seat of consciousness, generating *Angst* there, or Lust, projected towards the place of generation) would be the cause of *Präcordialangst*.
- Or are they, like anxiety, the expression of a central excitation of certain nerve paths serving the transmission of coenesthesic feelings to the peripheral terminal of the transmission channel? In this case, they would be simple co-sensations triggered centrally but felt peripherally, in the field of certain sensitive nerves.

In these two cases, it is a question of occasioning factors, not of the initial cause of the phenomenon. Precordial anxiety can be found in nicotine poisoning, hydrophobia, epilepsy, hysteria, hypochondria, melancholia, certain neuralgias of internal organs (angina pectoris, cardialgia, colic).

The circumstances in which precordial anxiety is observed are multiple. But precordial anxiety occurs during excitation of a sensitive nerve of internal organs and not in the spine. It is observed at best in angina pectoris. Even the vague nature, which does not permit location, is in favour of its formation in sensitive paths in internal organs.

Everything seems to indicate that the place where precordial anxiety arises is probably the cardiac plexus. Its constant location in the heart region, the fact that it generally appears in neuroses of the cardiac *plexus nervosus* (angina pectoris), that it is preferentially caused by nicotine, that other disorders occur at the same time as precordial anxiety (palpitations, disorders in regularity of heart beat, anomalies of pulse, etc.). all this indicated that the peripheral cause of precordial anxiety should be sought in the cardiac *plexus nervosus*. This nerve plexus consists of 1) the stimulating nerve fibres of the sympathetic, 2) the inhibiting nerve fibres of the vagus, 3) the autonomic cardiac nervous system. What one can suppose is that *Präcordialsangst* is probably a vasomotor neurosis of the heart. Angina pectoris, or eventually precordial anxiety, may be the expression of a vascular constriction striking the arterial vessels of the heart. However, in certain cases of stenocardia, there are no anatomical discoveries: these could be nervous forms.

The dependence of anxiety on these mental excitations can be easily explained. It is triggered by:

1. Mental stimuli (representations and frightening apperceptions, affects) conveyed through the paths of the vagus or the sympathetic towards the cardiac plexus. Predisposition consists in the increase of excitability and the lability of equilibrium (hysteria, epilepsy, melancholia, etc.).
2. By irradiation of internal organ neuralgia (cardialgia, colic) on the cardiac nervous system by sympathetic paths, which would explain the frequency of precordial anxiety during these neuralgia of internal organs.

So, precordial anxiety appears when a stimulus-representation, or the transfer of a state of excitation in the nervous paths of internal organs (sympathetic), place the *vasomotor* nerves of the heart muscle in a state of high excitation, which causes a vascular constriction in the heart muscle. The thus disrupted function of the autonomic ganglions of the heart muscle is transmitted to the seat of consciousness and causes the feeling of anxiety which is projected eccentric on the site of its origin.

Frequently these feelings of precordial anxiety are added to the pathological picture of *melancholia sine delirio*: it is a complication (*melancholia epigastrica, dysthymia epigastrica*).

This additional content of distressing consciousness has a much deeper significance because of the feelings of anxiety of the other mental functions. The depressive mood increases with anxiety and results in the affect of *Verzweiflung* (despair), which is also expressed by mimics and gesticulations. Apperception lead to a complete mental anaesthesia dolorosa, consciousness suffering from emptiness and desertification, because faced with this powerful internal state, external stimuli are no longer taken into account which often leads to temporary suppression of apperception and to the obscure representation of universal non-existence. The *Vorstellen* (ideation) sustains feedback because of the confusion in the unfolding of the course of representations, which is completely suspended and where the indeterminate confused representation of anxiety constitutes the content of consciousness, or by the filling of the representational field of a confused disorder of representations which are no longer dominated and no longer able to be associated and leads necessarily to confusion. At the highest point of the anxiety attack, there can even be momentary suspension of self-awareness. Anxiety always has effects on the motor response (importance in medico-legal psychiatry).

The motor agitation intended to resolve the mental tension may result, to a certain degree, in murder and suicide, in fires, destruction of everything which stands in the way of the patient. Analgesia which condition is mental and which belong to the upper degrees of anxiety attacks leads to the most appalling self-mutilation. In rare cases, precordial anxiety occurs as psychoneurosis (sic) fully acute, transitory, independent, elementary (*Raptus melancholicus*).

The course of melancholia with precordial anxiety is chronic or subacute. Prognosis is reasonably favourable.

5. The first anxiety disorder: Westphal's agoraphobia

Carl Westphal begins by remarking that for a number of years, repetitively, patients came to him with one particular complaint: that it was not possible for them to venture into open places or into certain streets, and that the fear inspired by these journeys hindered them in their freedom of movement. The patients were afraid that they would be made fun of, or that they would be considered to be mad. "This fear of crossing open spaces or eventually of going into streets represented the main phenomenon so clearly that, although it was related to some other situations and that the designation chosen – for I thought it necessary to do so – is not completely exhaustive, I believed I should construct the word agoraphobia (agora), fear of open spaces." (Westphal, 1872, p. 138)

It is impossible for the patient to walk in empty open places. If he tries to do so, he is immediately overcome by a feeling of anxiety, and when questioned, he situates this feeling more in the head than in the region of the heart, even though he often has palpitations. The feeling appears when he obliged to walk alongside a wall and alongside buildings or to go into streets when the shops are shut. To protect himself, he will follow a passer-by or walk with a demi-mondaine, or look for the red lanterns of cabarets.

In all these cases, the feeling of anxiety is perfectly unmotivated, the patient does not know why he is different from other men, and even "he cannot understand how others can walk across an open space." He has no idea what anxiety is, it is, so to speak, *Angst vor der Angst* (fear of fear itself) 'ibid.,p. 141.

At the history taking interview, the patient says he has *Flimmern* (flicker of light, luminous curtain) before his eyes.

From observation of his patients Westphal draws the following principles:

- The patients can find no reason for the anxiety which assails them.
- As if it were an integral element of the feeling of anxiety in the registers of the representation, the idea comes to the patient that he cannot cross the open space and he represents to himself (perceives ?) that it is monstrously large.
- Secondary idea that something might happen to them.
- The patient can only indicate the external circumstances in which this state occurs, and can say no more, apart from that the anxiety and the thought are suddenly there, psychologically perfectly unmotivated.
- The external circumstances are the same: the emptier the open space, the easier it is for the state to occur; even hugging the façades, sometimes just the simple fact of passing in uninhabited or empty streets, at worst just going a short distance along a known route, has the same effect.

- The state is eased or even disappears when there is an escort, when a carriage goes by, when the patient sees an open door in one of the houses in an empty street. But the ingestion of alcohol, by the excitation it causes, enables the patient to overcome the state.
- This state differs from the *Schwindel* (vertigo) of Benedict and Griesinger: "Right from the outset is it not vertigo, but a feeling of anxiety."
- It is manifestly cerebral (in the mind) and has little analogy with the normal psychological processes, it is also just as impossible to be understood by them, as with other pathological states, affects, directions of representations and wilful impulses.
- Appearance of the affect (fear, anxiety) under certain circumstances and conditions, disappearance when these are removed.
- The patients are not "mad."
- The absence of any resemblance to mental illnesses means it should be called "neuropathic." The name "mental illness" is not justified.

6. Definition of anxiety disorder: Freud's anxiety neurosis

In 1894, in an article entitled '*On the Grounds for Detaching a Particular Syndrome from Neurasthenia under the Name "anxiety neurosis"* ' Freud proposes to separate from neurasthenia neurotic syndromes more solidly related to each other than to the typical neurasthenic symptoms (pressure in the head; spinal irritation; dyspepsia with flatulence and constipation) and differing in their aetiological mechanism. The pseudoneurasthenias (nasal reflex neurosis, nervous symptoms of cachexia and of arteriosclerosis, preliminary stages of progressive paralysis and numerous psychoses), are finally separated from neurasthenia, as well as some *status nervosi* of hereditary degeneration, and the many neuroses of an intermittent nature which have to be classified in melancholia. It remains a complex whose symptoms are very close to each other (often appearing together or replacing each other) and whose aetiology and mechanism are fundamentally different from neurasthenia.

It is called *Angstneurose* (anxiety neurosis) because all the elements are grouped around the cardinal symptom of anxiety for each is connected with anxiety. Freud mentions Hecker[1] at the beginning of his article.

6.1 Clinical symptomatology of anxiety neurosis

It sometimes constitutes a *gemischte Neurose* (mixed neurosis with complex symptomatology). The clinical picture is as follows:

6.1.1 General excitability

As is, this is common to several neuroses. It is constant, corresponding to an accumulation of absolute or relative stimuli. There is an auditory hyperesthesia. It is often the cause of insomnia.

---

1 Hecker, 1893 « *Über larvierte und abortive Angstzustände bei Neurasthenie* ». For Hecker, more than half of neurasthenics have anxiety states. But Hecker emphasized a surprising fact, that is that the nature of the feeling which dominates the patient does not always come into consciousness as anxiety (*larvierte Angst* = masked anxiety), but is interpreted otherwise by them until someone enlightens them. In addition, it is sometimes one or other of the corporal markers of anxiety which occurs in very isolated and marked fashion: abortive or incomplete access.

6.1.2 Anxious expectation.

This includes "anxiety and pessimism." It often takes the form of a compulsion. When it concerns health, it leads to hypochondria (it then requires the presence, in addition, of paresthesias and distressing bodily sensations). In the most morally sensitive, it is expressed by *Gewissenangst* (anxiety of moral conscience), scrupulousness and meticulousness, which can even turn to *Zweifelsucht* ("folie du doute", doubting mania). It is the core symptom of neurosis. There is a *freely floating quantum of anxiety*, which dominates while awaiting the choice of representations and it is always ready to associate itself with a representation.

6.1.3 Anxiety attack

This is not the only way for anxiety, generally latent to consciousness but constantly on the watch, to express itself. Its sudden penetration into consciousness is the anxiety attack. Either the anxiety is by itself, or it is accompanied by a representation (annihilation, fit, threat of madness), or disorders of other functions (heart attack, respiratory distress, sweating, craving) and, in the words of the patient, anxiety remains hidden behind, or can only be described as "feeling faint" " feeling discomfort," etc.

6.1.4 Rudimentary anxiety attack and equivalents

- Disorders of cardiac activity (palpitations, etc.)
- Respiratory disorders
- Sweating
- Attacks of trembling and shaking
- Attacks of craving
- Acute diarrhoea
- Locomotor vertigo attacks
- Congestion attacks
- Paresthetic attacks

6.1.5 Pavor nocturnus

Variation on anxiety attack: frightened awakening at night, often with dread, dyspnea, sweating; it leads to a second form of insomnia.

6.1.6 Anxiety and vertigo

Schwindel (vertigo) differs from anxiety.

6.1.7 Phobias

Based on chronic *Ängstlichkeit* (anxiety) (anxious expectation) and a tendency to anxiety vertigo attacks, two typical groups of phobias develop:

- Anxiety in the face of universal physiological threat: snakes, storms, darkness, vermin, typical moral hyper probity (*Zweifelsucht*, doubting mania); the anxiety available is only used to reinforce instinctive repugnance. A compulsive phobia is generally only formed when there is a reminiscence during which anxiety was expressed. These events only remain intense in those with anxious expectations (*ängstliche Erwartung)* (these cases should not be explained by the persistence of strong impressions).
- The other group is that of locomotion which includes agoraphobia and all its variations. It is often preceded by a vertigo attack, but this is not an obligatory postulate.

The connection between these phobias and the phobias of obsessional neurosis is as follows: the displacement applies to both types of phobia (a representation becomes obsessional by connection with an available affect). But in the phobias of anxiety neurosis: 1) The affect is monotonous anxiety) but, 2) there is no substitution (it does not come from a repressed representation, it is invincible). But the substitution can be secondary, takes hold of protective measures: rumination for example, which initially serves to combat doubts concerning the faculty of reasonable thought. Doubting mania and other manifestations belong to anxiety neurosis.

6.1.8 Digestive activity

There is a few symptoms but they are characteristic. Nausea, craving, tendency to diarrhoea.

6.1.9 Sensitivity disorder

Paresthesias; increase in sensitivity to pain, tendency to hallucinations that cannot be interpreted as hysteria.

6.1.10 Chronicity

The symptoms which accompany anxiety attacks or its replacement also appear to be chronic.

6.2 Appearance and aetiology of anxiety neurosis.

There is often no recognized aetiology.

If the neurosis is acquired, there are a series of troubles and influence in sexual life that a careful, controlled examination will reveal.

6.2.1 In women

a. Virginal anxiety, anxiety of adolescents: first encounter with a sexual problem, such as a sudden disclosure of that which was previously hidden. It is typically combined with hysteria.
b. Anxiety of young brides.
c. Anxiety of women whose husband suffers from premature ejaculation or
d. Who practice *coitus interruptus or reservatus.*
e. Anxiety of widows and intentional practitioners of abstinence. This is often accompanied by an obsessional neurosis.
f. Climacteric/menopausal anxiety

6.2.2 In men

a. Abstinence, often with symptoms of defence (obsessional representation, hysteria).
b. *Frustrane Erregung* (frustrated excitation) (case of persons who are satisfied with touching)
c. Coitus interruptus,
d. In the *Senium* (old age):

α Neurasthenics following masturbation who fall into anxiety neurosis in the case of abstinence: they have become unable to tolerate abstinence.

β Overwork.

6.3 Outline of a theory of anxiety neurosis

- It must be an accumulation of excitation which does not allow a psychical derivation of anxiety.
- There is no trauma (which would lead to hysteria or accident neurosis).
- In certain cases, there is a decrease in sexual libido, of psychical pleasure.

Therefore: the mechanism of anxiety neurosis must be sought in the derivation of sexual excitation from the somatic to the mental and the abnormal use thus caused by this excitation.

The physiological functioning is the accumulation of somatic sexual excitation; at a certain level of accumulation, it becomes a *Reiz* (stimulus) for mental life, resulting in a psychic state of libidinal tension.

Discharge is only possible thanks to adequate, specific action.

When the action of discharge is not a specific action (masturbation) neurasthenia appears.

All the factors which prevent the psychic elaboration of somatic excitation lead to anxiety neurosis.

Example of a voluntary abstinent. Abstinence consists of the privation of the specific action, which otherwise follows the libido. This privation will have two consequences: accumulation of somatic excitation and dispatch towards routes where discharge is more possible than on the psychic route. Libido will end up by decreasing and the excitation will be expressed subcortically in the form of anxiety. Abstinence is also an effective element in the aetiological group of frustrated abstinence. In the case of *coitus reservatus* without consideration, libido disappears progressively, what follows is equal to the case of abstinence. In *senium*, there is such an increase in the production of somatic excitation that the psyche is relatively inadequate to control it.

In women, in the case of virginal anxiety, the representational groups to which somatic sexual excitation must be linked are not sufficiently developed. In the anaesthetic bride, anxiety only occurs when the first periods of cohabitation arouse a sufficient quantity of somatic excitation; where the local symptoms are lacking, anxiety does not appear. The case of premature ejaculation, of *coitus interruptus* has the same explanation as in men: libido disappears psychically for the act while the excitation aroused is discharged at the subcortical level. The case of widowhood and of intentional abstinence as well as that of the climacteric/menopause is resolved as for men.

Anxiety neurosis is therefore a neurosis which certainly does not have a sexual aetiology, but does have a sexual mechanism.

The symptoms are, so to speak, a surrogate for specific action.

Why does psychic failure to control sexual excitation lead to a neurosis? "The mind provides an *affect* of anxiety when it feels incapable of settling a task coming from outside (danger) by a corresponding reaction"; it arrives at anxiety neurosis when it sees it is incapable of counterbalancing the (sexual) excitation produced *endogenously*. It behaves as if it projected this excitation towards the exterior. The affect is a reaction to an exogenous excitation, neurosis to a similar endogenous reaction. The affect is a state which passes quickly (sudden); a neurosis is chronic (persistent). *In neurosis, the nervous system reacts against an internal source of excitation, whereas the affect corresponds to the reaction against a similar external source.*

6.4 Connection with other neuroses

Where a mixed neurosis exists, evidence can be found of a combination of several specific aetiologies. Comorbidity may be fortuitous, or indicate an even closer connection between symptoms since the same aetiological condition will regularly and simultaneously cause both neuroses.

7. Loewenstein

Loewenstein wrote a large volume on obsessional disorders in which there are some interesting notes concerning anxiety. He thus defines the anxiety state: "We call feelings of anxiety the specific emotional elements having a harmful significance for our person or for any person belonging to our sphere of interest which are attached to an imminent event or to one that has already occurred." The feeling of anxiety (*Angstgefühl*) corresponds to a psychological state characterised by the presence of feelings of anxiety, by an affect of anxiety, an anxious state in which the most intense feelings of anxiety are contained.
The pathological nature resides in the compulsive aspect, unable to be influenced by counter-representations; the phobias are insensitive to logical considerations and unable to be influenced by willpower.

7.1 Symptomatology of the state of anxiety

Loewenstein meticulously studied the psychic and somatic symptomatology of states of anxiety that we cannot detail for lack of space.
His analysis of any affect of anxiety arising from a representation shows that feelings of anxiety are a sort of feeling of displeasure which has no demonstrated location and should be considered to be a subjective accompanying manifestation of a general cortical state. We don't know where anxiety gets its special hue from. "Alongside cortical primary anxiety, a bulbar anxiety can be distinguished." (p. 316). Bulbar anxiety is distinguished by its disproportion; minimum stimulus, with disproportionate symptomatology. There are often inaugural organic symptoms. (Auras)

7.1.1 Abnormal predisposition to anxiety

Ängstlichkeit: abnormally increased tendency to anxious states, which appear on occasions that would cause no anxiety for the average person, and, on occasions that give rise to a trite fear, they react with an anxiety with extraordinary intensity. According to Freud, *ängstliche Erwartung* is the core symptom of anxiety neurosis. It may occur in a normal personality under harmful influence, weakening the nerves, but in general it is innate or inherited, developed and completed by toxic influences. It runs from pessimism or timorous tendencies through a series of nuances up to constant, irrational expectation of the worst misfortunes (Beard's pantophobia). General anxiety: fear at the slightest possibility of a drawback.

- Hypochondriac anxiety, in particular with regard to the state of health. It is innate or acquired.
- Moral anxiety seizing the slightest moral or religious scruple. A subspecies is the fear with regard to maintaining good manners in the world. Immense fear of a breach of courtesy or of morality leading to pedantry (exaggerated precision).
- Abnormal anxiety with regard to the state of health of relatives.
- Abnormal anxiety with regard to one's fortune and professional affairs. *Schwarzseher* (those who see everything on the black side), pessimists.

With regard to the organic foundation of abnormal predisposition to anxiety, one should first of all mention hyperexcitability of the cardiovascular system, innate or acquired. This means that emotional processes of a distressing nature and leading to a circulatory influence give rise to organic feelings which are attached preferably to representations of misfortune

(*Erwartungen*, expectations). Neurasthenia (lowering of performance of the nervous system) also encourages the development of an anxious disposition because it diminishes self-confidence and snatches from consciousness the ability to avoid certain dangers or to overcome them.

7.1.2 Simple anxious states, without content

They do not proceed from the representation of a danger. Their duration is variable (from one minute to several months). They are variable in intensity. Very frequently tied in secondarily to representations of a threatening danger explaining the anxiety.
Frequency varies a lot.
They are frequently incorrectly interpreted or designated: nervousness, excitation. Choice of an accompanying bodily manifestation (heart palpitations).

7.1.3 Chronic anxious states

These differ from the preceding not only in time, but also in the intensity of feelings of anxiety and in the influence thus produced on the general psychological state. Here it is not a question of duration of attack, but a remittent behaviour, sometimes even sporadic. Sometimes, the states of anxiety are reduced to a minimum for more or less limited periods of time and sometimes they disappear completely. By durable states of anxiety we mean those for whom, for a fairly long period of time, there are daily anxiety attacks and in general the free intervals give way to intervals more or less occupied by anxiety. Their intensity is low to moderate. There are sometimes developments of more intense anxiety, completely excessive.

7.2 Phobias

These are anxious states with particular triggering factors, or at least originating from certain representations. Some authors place them in the category of obsessional neuroses; they have been separated from the latter by Thomsen, Krafft-Ebing (changing opinion).
In fact, phobias are complex processes. There are three types of phobias:

- Phobias with constant representational content. The representation to which the anxiety becomes attached, the object of the fear, is that which occurs primarily in nature, it is a type of *Zwang* (compulsion), and has a well determined content (nosophobia, contact phobia, mysophobia, zoophobia, active and passive kleptomania).
- Phobias with floating representational content. The typical example is agoraphobia or *Platzangst* (fear of open spaces). These phobias change between individuals and even in the same individual (falling, vertigo, collapse, accident involving heart or brain, strange apparition or something quite indefinable, bad).
  The anxious state is the constant, prevalent factor here, whereas the related representations change. It differs in several phobias. Secondarily, obsessions can become intertwined between phobia and anxious state.
- In a third group of phobias, anxiety becomes attached to certain representations which do not have the character of obsession because it is simply perceptions that are involved; anxiety here is not conditioned by the content of problematical representations either, but is in fact empty. Certain zoophobias, fear of insects (spiders, cockroaches) of mice, necrophobias: the affected person does not know what it is they

are frightened of. Pathological increase in certain aversions situated in the realm of the psychological.

Only the first type of phobia can be classified in the obsessions.

7.2.1 Phobias with floating representational content (p. 332)

There are a large number of triggering factors. The characteristic of them all is that they offer no reason to be afraid, at least for the index cases, and that the patient knows it but cannot refrain from being subjected to it. There is no predisposition. They develop all by themselves in anxious, hesitant natures but many do not appear in those with anxiety disorders.

- Phobias of locomotion: a state of anxiety relating to locomotive acts, such as in agoraphobia. There are several degrees and nuances.
  - The more mild cases: occur often in the middle of the journey, in the form of discomfort or of an anxiety which makes continuation difficult, but not impossible, all the more so if the patient is following a person or a car.
  - Intermediate cases, crossing open spaces is impossible; great difficulty in crossing bridges and main road junctions.
  - The most serious cases: the patient can only go out into the street accompanied by another adult.

These nuances can be seen with the same patient.

- Phobias of situation: agoraphobia is only one type of obsessional representation that can be called topophobia. It is often accompanied by claustrophobia. The patient is not very clear about the nature of the disorder. Attacks can be repeated (theatre, Church) leading to *Zwangsbefürchtungen* (obsessional fears) that these will be repeated in the same place, or by a malaise that will encourage them to leave, or the obsessional idea that is impossible to remain. 1) Either the patients continue to frequent the places in question, taking a seat near to the exit or go with an escort. Or 2) they abandon the idea of going out - claustrophobia. Anthropophobia - the simple fact of being with another person, in some cases, can cause states of anxiety. In more mild cases, there is a certain aversion in relation to society (for there is a risk of discomfort, embarrassment). In the most serious cases, relationships with people are always accompanied by anxiety attacks, which drives the patient to abandon their work and give up all dealings with other human beings. Gynecophobia can occur in male neurasthenics with sexual hyperesthesia. Basically it is a fear of sexual excitation, caused by the sexual act or upon the sight of women. The fear of women amounts to the fear that they may cause states of anxiety (phobophobia). Solitude can trigger states of anxiety.

7.2.2 Functional phobias

These are anxiety states occuring during professional activity (previously carried out with no emotional excitation), following fortuitous circumstances. First of all, these anxiety attacks need to have developed during the work activity in question or when a disorder reoccurs in the given field,to the extent that itmore or less with its accomplishment. The patient develops the obsessional idea that during their work, the anxiety attack or a related disorder might reoccur, or that the level of performance required is impossible for them. Some continue the action, others do not. The energy of willpower, the pressure of external circumstances, the need to earn money, all play a very important role along with the intensity of the attack. Attacks occur in the clergy, more rarely in teachers, lawyers while pleading at the bar, musicians and singers. There are traumatic phobias so intense that the patient has to give up work. For topophobes, anxiety attacks can occur on a train or tram. An escort is necessary. Fear of heights (hypsophobia), vertigo.

7.2.3 Anxiety phobia without content

Necrophobia, morbid fear of blood, (haemophobia), fear of storms (astrophobia).
The triggering factors are very variable.
There are 4 types of case:

1. Sudden and spontaneous appearance, for example when crossing a bridge, of an intense anxiety with its somatic consequences. It can be without content or drag along with it the representation of a possible danger or accident if the same situation is maintained or continued.
2. Physical malaise, nausea, weakness and dizziness awaken the representation of helplessness in an accident, the possibility of a fall, of not being able to continue, or of arousing curiosity, where its representations are mixed with more or less intense feelings of anxiety.
3. In the rarest cases and in individuals who are anxious, there appears a representation of the possibility of an attack accompanied by helplessness, and this representation is associated with corresponding feelings of anxiety.
4. A first attack following a fright (accidents) (traumatic phobia). The same effect in the street or in public places with the appearance of serious medical conditions, in particular epileptic. The phobia can then develop after eviction of the stimulus.

7.3 Latent and incomplete attacks of anxiety (equivalent of anxiety attack)

Hecker drew attention to anxiety attacks without anxiety: masked, incomplete or abortive. For Freud (*Über die Berechtigung…*): any accompanying symptom can constitute the attack, such as anxiety.
There are three types of masked attacks:

a. Anxiety replaced by one of its preliminary stages (emotional elements).
b. Erroneous interpretation of anxiety as being a change in psychological state (*Verstimmung*, etc.)
c. Anxiety interpreted as being a purely physical disorder (asthma, nausea, palpitations, craving, etc.). In this case diagnosis is difficult. Attacks of dizziness in cerebrasthenics only became associated with feelings of anxiety later on. For Freud, dizziness differs from vertigo (*Drehschwindel*) and from Ménières disease.

7.4 Aetiology

The data indicates that anxiety affects men twice as much as women (2 to 1). The most affected being those between the ages of 30 and 40 years. It is rare in children but there are adults who have suffered since childhood. It is certain that hereditary is involved in 80% of cases. There is little connection between content and intensity. Sometimes there is a hereditary content with little or no neuropathic predisposition: there is a special predisposition to anxiety disorders. There is an influential sexual aetiology before the start in only 75% of cases (all disorders considered). There is no specific factor there. The importance varies greatly in individual cases. Do not support Freud's theory: 1) cases

without accumulation of somatic sexual excitation. 2) cases with accumulation, but lack of mental derivation. For Freud the symptom is abstinence or the disappearance of libido. In the case of Loewenstein with sexual abstinence, libido was as often increased as reduced. Sexual aetiology lacks in some cases such as phobias: agoraphobia with anxiety attacks.
The merit of Freud is in having drawn attention to the importance of toxic sexual agents in the origin of anxiety states. Mechanism: toxic chemical cause, nervous cause; nervous exhaustion. (Loewenstein, 1904, p. 473) "As we have seen, toxic sexual agents figure relatively rarely as the exclusive source in anxiety states." (ibid.) Phobia anxiety is habitual. It is triggered by psychical processes, in part subconscious. The subconscious processes often come from anxiety states with no content and masked.
Conclusion: 1) the hereditary component is most certainly not constant, but in a great majority of cases it operates in adults, although only rarely as exclusive cause; its role is restricted to raising the pathogenic action of other causal factors = main causes. 2) The main causes are etiological factors which are generally necessary to induce an anxiety state, and sometimes sufficient when they are fairly intense, we have met a series of somatic and mental disorders. Somatic: sexuality; mental: emotional toxicity. No specific cause, i.e. equal and constant etiological factor in all cases. In addition, we have found: 3) subordinate causes and 4) triggering factors.

8. Kraepelin

8.1 Anxiety as a morbid disposition

When the pathological emphasis of displeasure is accompanied by feelings of inner tension, the mental state is stamped with the seal of anxiety (*Ängstlichkeit*) (vol. I, p. 344) source of obsessional representations, phobias (*Zwangsbefürchtungen*) and expectation neurosis.
"The form broadly the most frequent of disagreeable pathological emotions is anxiety, that we can perhaps consider as an association of displeasure with inner tension. It is generally without object. It occurs in general by attacks, the most frequently in depressive states of circular madness." (I, p. 348).
"A clinical group of particular anxiety states, very extensive, is finally made up of disorders that it is customary to call *Zwangsbefürchtungen* (obsessive fears) or phobias. There are phobias of situation, and phobias of function." (p. 350). Particularly frequent is the fear of introducing needles or splinters of glass into food and to thus kill others. The thought of seeing the gaze of strangers directed towards oneself produces when there is a pathological predisposition a distressing feelings: this is the phobia of the stare." The best known example of phobia is *Platzangst,* or agoraphobia, the feeling of inability to walk in an empty open space, in a deserted street. With cathisophobia, the affected person is afraid of remaining still. Very often, progressively, it is not the original occasion for anxiety that the person dreads, but the anxious tension itself; there then develops an *Angst vor der Angst,* a fear of fear itself, or phobophobia. (355) Displeasure can be accompanied by inhibition or excitation (attack or transitional state).
We will first of all look at disorders arising from activity and related to it; since these are a question of very mild disorder, I will call them activity neurosis (ponopathies). They contain nervous exhaustion, acquired neurasthenia, which is formed from a durable tension, exaggerated, of a willingness to work. Attached to this is expectation neurosis, anxious discomfort of simple gestures through sombre memories of previous disorders.

8.2 Expectation neurosis

Expectation neurosis (Kraepelin, p. 1416) includes nervous disorders which develop on the common basis of anxiety expectation. Definition: "By expectation neurosis, I would place here a group of nervous disorders which develop on the common basis of anxiety expectation." Through healthy experience, we know that the expectation of any event gives rise to a progressively rising internal tension. If the imminent event is disagreeable, initial feelings can be extremely distressing and even painful. At the same time, the assurance of action is affected very noticeably.

Expectation neurosis offers a similar image, except that it is pathologically increased and coloured. The pathological development is brought about here because the distressing disorders do not occur on a single unique occasion, but follow processes which are unceasingly repeated every day. They do not take place in the usual manner, freely, but are uneasy and distorted by the interference of dysesthesias, feelings of displeasure and impulse unrelated to the goal. As these difficulties are repeated unceasingly and, in the processes influenced by it, expectation anxiety becomes more and more intense and thus reinforces the disorders.

The processes concerned are: (p. 1416-17) processes which in the healthy person occur with no particular intervention of a conscious mental activity, but occur fairly mechanically: walking, standing up, swallowing, falling asleep, reading, writing, speaking, micturition, sexual act, along with abilities such as the playing of the violin or the piano. As Möbius puts it, the disorder is conditioned by the memory of illnesses. (1417)

8.3 Symbantopathies

With blows of fate (ta symbanta) situation psychoses, or fate psychoses (symbantopathy) can appear. Terror neurosis and accident neurosis should be mentioned here.

Traumatic neurosis was defined in 1889 by Oppenheim. The main causes are in the region of the emotions. The role of legislation on accidents in 1884 was accused of generating and maintaining this battle for compensation. When injury and traumatic hysteria are eliminated, two scenarios remain: *Schreckneurose* (terror neurosis) and *Rentenkämpfer* (who seek compensation).

- For the first group, the designation "terror neurosis" seems the most appropriate because in these cases of terror, a misfortune which suddenly surfaces is the true pathological cause. It presents itself to us as an increase and pathological persistence of the effects that a violent emotional shock exerts on the mental and physical behaviour of humans. In essence, a rapidly installed disorder of consciousness is observed with general excitation of willpower, more rarely inhibition of willpower. The symptoms are those of confusion with impulsive excitation. The cause triggering terror neurosis is constituted by all the events producing violent emotional shocks whether there is physical injury or not. Anxiety also plays a role in the face of a grave danger, and the despair caused by personal misfortune and the misfortune of others.
- Traumatic neurosis (ibid., p. 1457): depressive or sulking dysthymia with moaning, lack of will power/difficulty making decisions and all kinds of symptoms in part generally nervous, in part local. The disorder only develops after a period of time. Months sometimes pass before the disorder is manifest. Patients sometimes go back to work but they have to abandon it again after a more or less lengthy period. Patient symptoms are

as follows: abnormal apprehension, dysaesthesia, mnemic disorders, mood generally dejected, whining, anxious; they have a "melancholic outlook." Very often they are emotional and sensitive. But what is at the centre of this picture is the inability to work. The tests show a susceptibility to fatigue.

8.4 Obsessional neurosis

"Faced with all these somewhat impersonal forms of compulsive thought, there is the bulk of observations where it is immediately a question of the relationship of the patient to life and to their entourage. We can group them under the general name of *Zwangsbefürchtungen* or phobias." (p. 1882)

The true obsession (impersonal) (p. 1832) is *Zwangsbefürchtung* (obsessive fear) or pathological fear. (p. 1840). Phobias are divided into: 1) *Unglücksangst* (vicissitude anxiety) or symbantopathies or symbantopathy; 2) anxiety of responsibility; 3) relational anxiety or homilophobias (phobia of contact with other human beings). The general disorder which is the basis of all declared obsessional processes is anxiety (p. 1863). "I believe that obsessional representations only become pathological manifestations and therefore symptoms of obsessional neurosis when they have become an integral part of *Zwangtsbefürchtung*, when the anxiety that they might return takes hold." (p. 1865). Obsessional neurosis is not a disorder of representation but of *Gemütsleben* (emotional life). But the causes of neurosis should be sought in the abnormal psychological constitution (p. 1881). This is what Kraepelin says of Freud: *völlig wilkürliche Annahme* (perfectly arbitrary assumption) (p. 1883-84).

9. Conclusion

"*Ihr habt Angst in der Welt,*" says John, 16,33 in the Bible in Luther's translation. Anxiety is one of the most awful companions that there are. It seems to belong more to the realm of good luck and bad luck than of illness. We have seen that the psychiatrists all mention it, more or less, without giving it any real status, without making it an illness, the core of a given illness, or even a symptom: it is an emotion, "*Gemüthsbewegung*." It is sometimes even considered to be a causal factor (pathogenic effect of affects). In short, it is not given any particular pathological or nosological importance. We have seen that it begins to assert itself as part of dysthymia with precordial anxiety (*Präkordialangst*), the authors seem divided between a number of solutions: turn it into an illness, a complication or a symptom. The first to define what is today called an anxiety disorder, Westphal, gives an admirable description of agoraphobia. It should be noted that it is the possibility of access to psychiatrists, for non severe patients who remain in the community, that enabled the description of "neurotic" disorders" (Westphal also provides the fullest description of obsessional representation). To a certain degree it is the structure of health care facilities (relative relationships between health care facilities and residential care facilities, consultations for outpatients, polyclinics), which has enabled this advance in diagnostics. But anxiety bursts into the open with Freud. In his 23rd conference, Wernicke did indeed describe a psychosis of anxiety, but it does not seem to have left any trace, notably because of its close proximity to anxiety neurosis and delusional depression, and the off-putting effect of Wernicke's idiosyncratic terminology. We have also seen that with German authors, the separation between anxiety, phobia and obsession is not very marked: phobia and obsessions are practically intermingled and anxiety is common to all of them; Freud's anxiety neurosis involves phobias. However, anxiety states are mentioned in Loewenstein's book on obsessional neurosis. What perspectives are open to this history which we have volontarily restricted to the 19th century? In the evening of his life, Freud takes up the problem of anxiety again and resuscitates at the same time the old term *Abwehr* (psychoneuroses of defence). Anxiety becomes *Realangst*, anxiety in the face of something real. It is a signal of the appearance of a danger. It is the archaic precipitate, *Erinnerunsgsymbol* (mnesic symbol) of a great trauma: the trauma of birth. Anxiety is no longer libido transformed, but a signal of the occurrence of a danger. Freudian theory becomes more and more complex; it will develop towards a study of the mechanisms of defence of the ego against anxiety, whereas originally with Freud they are a defence against drive. Another path is opened up, blazed in Germany mainly by a brilliant author, Viktor Emil Freiherr von Gebsattel. The vocabulary and discriminations of the established authors are smashed to pieces. Gebsattel's texts are extremely complex, it is impossible to summarize them. Let us say that Gebsattel moves away from the proliferation of anxiety (Gebsattel worked in consulting rooms for a long time and therefore with neuroses, terminology which he retains). He attributes it to a nihilistic tendency of society. For existential philosophy, which inspired Gebsattel, anxiety is "the fundamental position which places [one] before nothingness" (Heidegger). This theory is that "anxiety manifests nothingness." The nothingness that man meets with in anxiety is his own nothingness. In the Psychopathology *of Phobia,* he emphasizes the aspect of psychoasthenic weakness that through its hanging back prevents man from coming to grips with a world which fills him with anxiety. Gebsattel talks of *Aufdringlichkeit des Angsphänomens* (irruptivity and extension of the anxiety phenomenon). The extent of the "phenomenon" is measured, for example, in the quantity of psychotropic drugs taken. We have not mentioned here the differences between neurotic and psychotic anxiety (these two nosological vehicles which collapse), nor the "content" of the anxiety (death, castration, solitude, fragmentation) which exceeds our strictly clinical framework. Between anthropology, nothingness and synapse, anxiety is still searching for its place.

10. References

Autenrieth JCF (1807) *Über die im Clinicum in Tübingen getroffene Einrichtungen für Wahnsinnige.*

Autenrieth, JCF. (1808) *Versuche für die praktische Heilkunde aus den clinischen Anstalten von Tübingen.*

Autenrieth, JCF. (1825) *Über den Menschen und seine Hoffnung einer Fortdauer vom Standpunkte des Naturforschers aus* (Cotta) Tübingen

Autenrieth, JCF. (1836) *Ansichten über Natur- und Seelenleben* (Cotta) Stuttgart & Augsburg

Flemming, C. F. (1859) *Pathologie und Therapie der Psychosen.* Berlin

Freud, S. (1895) *Über die Berichtigung, von der Neurasthenie einen bestimmten Symptomenkomplex als « Angstneurose » abzutrennen,* in Studien Ausgabe, vol 6, Hysterie und Angst.

Freud, S. (1926) *Hemmung, Symptom und Angst,* Wien, 1926.

Gebsattel, V. E. Freiherr von (1951a) Die phobische Fehlhandlung, In : *Grundzüge der Neurosenlehre in 2 Bänden,* Urban & Schwarzenberg, München Berlin Wien 1972, pp. 57-81.

Gebsattel, V. E. Freiherr von (1951b) Zur Psychopathologie der Phobien, In : *Prolegomena einer medizinischen Anthropologie*, Springer Verlag 1954, pp 47-74

Griesinger, W (1861) *Die Pathologie und Therapie der psychischen Krankheiten*, Stuttgart.

Hecker, E. (1893) *Über larvirte und abortive Angstzustände bei Neurasthenie*. Zentbl. Nervenheilk. 16, pp. 565-572.

Heinroth, J. C. A. (1818) *Lehrbuch der Störungen des Seelenlebens oder der Seelenstörungen und ihrerBehandlung*, Vol I & II, Vogel, Leipzig

Heinroth, J. C. A. (1823) *Lehrbuch der Seelengesundheit*, Leipzig.

Ideler, K. W. (1835) *Grundriss der Seelenheilkunde*, Berlin.

Ideler, K. W. (1841), *Biographien Geisteskranker in ihrer psychologischen Entwickelung*. E.H. Schröder, Berlin.

Kraepelin, E. *Psychiatrie*. 8th Edition. 1915.

Krafft-Ebing R von. (1874) *Die Melancholie, eine klinische Studie*, Erlangen.

Loewenstein, L. (1904) *Die psychischen Zwangserscheinungen ; auf klinischer Grundlage dargestellet*. Wiesbaden.

Reil J. C. H. (1803) *Rhapsodien über die Anwendung der psychischen Curmethode auf Geisteszerrütungen*. Halle.

Reil, JC (1812) Besondere Fieberlehre, Nervenkrankheiten. In : *Über die Erkenntnis und Cur der Fieber*, vol. 4. Wien.

Schneider K (1946), *Klinische Psychopathologie*, 14ème éd., Thieme, Stuttgart New York, 1992.

Wernicke, Carl *Grundriss der Psychiatrie in klinischen Vorlesungen*. Leipzig: G. Thieme 1900. 23ème Conférence.

Westphal, C. (1872) *Die Agoraphobie, eine neuropathische Erscheinung*, Archiv für Psychiatrie und Nervenkrankheiten, vol III, Berlin.

2

Social Anxiety Disorder

Nesrin Dilbaz, Aslı Enez and Serçin Yalçın Çavuş
Ankara Numune Research and Training Hospital
Turkey

1. Introduction

1.1 Epidemiology of social anxiety disorder (SAD)

SAD, also known as social phobia, is characterised by excessive fear of embarrassment or humiliation in social situations, which in turn leads to marked distress or avoidance of these situations and functional impairment as described in DSM-IV-TR.

It is a common disorder with early onset, significant comorbidity and functional impairment (Meron Ruscia et al., 2008).

SAD has been ranked as one of the top ten chronic disorders - mental or physical - in terms of its effects on objective outcomes, such as days of work lost and reduced health-related quality of life (Alonso, 2004). According to the National Comorbidity Survey, SAD is the most reported anxiety disorder and has a lifetime prevalence of 12% (Kessler et al., 2005), with considerable coexisting psychiatric disorders, such as depression, anxiety, and substance-related disorders.Lifetime prevalence of social anxiety disorder among Turkish university students was 23% (Dilbaz 2006). Co-occurring SAD and depression carry a substantial risk of suicide, which further complicates treatment (Beesdo et al., 2007; Thase, 2007). SAD symptoms normally emerge during early adolescence and continue throughout adulthood; they affect women more often than men (Fehm et al., 2005).In clinical samples the ratio of male and female changes in the favour of males. (Dilbaz and Güz 2002). Trials suggest that social anxiety even below the diagnostic threshold is clearly associated with adverse outcomes like elevated risk for comorbid disorders and associated with impairment in diverse areas of life.

Despite the growing understanding of this condition, information is lacking on key aspects of the disorder and many individuals, including doctors, psychiatrists and patients, unaware about this condition.

1.2 Children and adolescents

SAD, which so often begins in childhood, precedes other comorbid disorders and may be a direct or indirect risk factor for other disorders, such as depression and substance abuse. Epidemiologic findings show that in the pediatric primary healthcare setting anxiety disorders are very common ranging from 1% to 10% (Briggs-Gowan et al., 2000; Busch et al., 2002; Costello, 1989), but are unrecognized and under-treated (Chavira et al., 2004; Wren et al., 2003). In community settings, rates of SAD in youth range from 0.5% to 4% (Essau et al., 1999; Wittchen et al., 1998) and from 3% to 6.8% in primary care settings (Busch et al., 2002; Costello, 1989; Chavira et al., 2004). Recent research suggest that lifetime prevalence rates in adolescents in the US and Germany are between 5% and 15% (Heimberg et al., 2000;

Lewinsohn et al., 1993). Although the age of onset is usually in the early teens with a mean age of onset of 15.5 years (Schneider et al., 1993) children as young as 8 years old have been diagnosed with the disorder (Beidel & Turner, 1998).

Shyness, behavioral inhibition and selective mutism can be considered in spectrum of social anxiety disorder in childhood. Children who are rated by their parents as having a shy temperament in infancy or in early childhood had an approximately 2 or 3 times increased probability of having an anxiety disorder in adolescence (Prior et al, 2000). In a five year longitudinal study, researchers found that behavioral inhibition-which can be described as a tendency to demonstrate fearfulness or resistance when faced with an unfamiliar stimuli, in pre-school children appeared to be a predictor for social anxiety in middle school (Hirshfeld-Becker et al., 2007). Selective mutism can be considered an extreme form of social anxiety including features of shyness and behavioral inhibition, where the most prominent feature is the inhibition of speech in select situations. Comorbidity rates between selective mutism and social anxiety disorder range from 70–95% (Dummit et al., 1997; Black & Uhde, 1995) and characteristics such as shyness, anxiousness, withdrawal and seriousness are used to describe both selective mutism and social anxiety alike (Steinhausen & Juzi, 1996; Kumpulainen et al., 1998).

Studies have shown that in children aged 7–13 years with SAD, 60% had an additional psychiatric diagnosis, of whom 36% had an anxiety disorder as follows: generalized anxiety disorder 10%; attention deficit hyperactivity disorder 10%; specific phobia 10%; and selective mutism 8% (Biedel et al., 1999). Those individuals who develop comorbid disorders will also have an increased risk of suicidal ideation and suicide attempts.

In treatment of social anxiety disorders in childhood and adolecence, most practitioners advise the initial use of psychological interventions followed by pharmacotherapy when necessary. Specific treatments have employed cognitive-behavioral group therapy for SAD in adolescents, social effectiveness therapy for children (Beidel et al., 2000) and 'coping cat' child behavior therapy (Flannery-Schroeder et al., 2000). Overall, most clinical researchers now believe that CBT is the treatment of choice for youth with internalizing disorders including SAD (March et al., 2003).

There are very few pharmacotherapy trials in general and even fewer randomized, double-blind, placebo-controlled trials in childhood anxiety disorders. Studies with both open-label and double blind placebo control groups have shown promising results ranging from 36–100% success rates (Compton et al., 2001; Mancini et al., 1999). Selective serotonin reuptake inhibitors (SSRI) and serotonin norepinephrine reuptake inhibitors (SNRI) are defined as first line pharmacotherapy for social anxiety disorders in youth with a careful assessessment of suicidal ideation before starting these antidepressants.

The development of comorbid mental disorders such as depression and substance abuse, children and adolescents with this illness are at risk for educational or occupational under-achievement, and failure to achieve financial and emotional independence. The challenge of preventing the consequences of SAD lies in early diagnosis.

2. Organic etiology of SAD

Although the etiology of SAD is poorly understood, emerging evidence indicates multidimensional causes. It is a distinct psychiatric disorder with genetic underpinnings and is associated with neurobiological and environmental mechanisms.

Over the past two decades, numerous neurobiological methods have been used in studies of SAD including structural, functional and receptor brain imaging, pharmacological trials, candidate gene investigations and studies of psychophysiological, endocrine, biochemical and behavioral responses to stressful challenges. It has been hypothesized that affect regulation is compromised in individuals with SAD, either due to hyperactivity in emotion triggering areas like the amygdala and insula, or hypoactivity in modulatory regions like the anterior cingulate and prefrontal cortices. It also has been hypothesized that SAD patients would show exaggerated amygdala responses to angry or threatening faces in comparison to healthy control subjects and that amygdala hyperresponsivity is associated with enhanced fear conditionability in SAD (Furmark, 2009).

A range of neurotransmitters may be important in SAD including the monoamines, glutamate, GABA, and several neuropeptides, but to date, the serotonergic and dopaminergic transmission systems have received most of the attention.

Serotonin has been implicated in animal models of fear and anxiety (Graeff, 2002) and the therapeutic efficacy of SSRIs (Ipser et al., 2008) strongly suggests that serotonin has a crucial role in SAD. Allelic variation in serotonin-related genes modulate amygdala responsivity both in healthy volunteers (Hariri & Holmes, 2006) and in patients with SAD (Furmark et al., 2004). Lanzenberger et al. demonstrated a significantly lower serotonin-1A receptor binding potential in SAD patients relative to controls in the amygdala, anterior cingulate cortex, insula, and dorsal raphe nuclei in their PET study (Lanzenberger et al., 2007). Serotonergic involvement is also supported by neuroendocrine challenges studies (Tancer, 1993).

Dopamine is known to play a central role in motivation and reward-seeking behaviors and several lines of evidence point to a dysfunction of this transmitter system in SAD like patients with Parkinson's Disease, which is associated with dopamine hypofunction, appear to have enhanced risk for developing SAD (Richard et al., 1996). Abnormal central dopaminergic neurotransmission has also been reported in animal trials relevant to SAD, such as studies of social subordination in primates (Grant et al., 1998). Two independent SPECT studies also point directly to an altered dopamine system activity in SAD. Tiihonen et al. reported that the striatal dopamine reuptake site density was markedly lower in patients with SAD than controls, presumably reflecting a smaller number of dopaminergic synapses and neurons in the basal ganglia (Tiihonen et al., 1997). Schneier et al. also observed that striatal dopamine D2 receptor binding was significantly lower in subjects with SAD than in comparison subjects (Schneier et al., 2000).

Genetically-oriented studies of SAD and related constructs such as behavioral inhibition, neuroticism, introversion and harm-avoidance suggest that genetic factors play at least a moderate role in the etiology of excessive social anxiety (Stein et al., 1994). The short (s) allele of the promoter polymorphism of the human serotonin transporter gene (the 5-HTT-linked polymorphic region; 5-HTTLPR) has been associated with anxiety-related personality traits, increased fear conditionability, and life-stress-induced aff ective disorder (Serretti et al., 2006). Several other genotypes influence amygdala responsivity and could thus be considered in future studies of SAD, for example the tryptophan hydroxylase-2 gene (G-703T polymorphism) (Brown et al., 2005) and the catechol-Omethyltransferase gene (COMT Val158Met) (Smolka et al., 2005).

3. Diagnosis and assessment of SAD

The first challenge in the treatment of SAD is making a correct diagnosis. There is evidence that SAD is under-diagnosed and under-treated in primary care and specialist settings alike

(Katzelnick & Greist, 2001). Possible reasons for this may be lack of diagnostic awareness, lack of diagnostic threshold clarity or the presence of co-morbid disorders. Moreover, as consultation with a clinician may be perceived as social interaction, the nature of the disorder may cause patients to delay seeking help, and when they eventually do, it is often with physical complaints or psychiatric comorbidity.

During the initial evaluation it is important to find out severity of symptoms as well as the degree of avoidance and functional impairment present. Rating scales such as the Liebowitz social anxiety scale that is translated and validated to Turkish also, may be helpful in assessing both feared situations and avoidance and can be used to monitor the patient's treatment progress (Liebowitz 1987, Dilbaz and Guz). A range of other SAD scales are also available, like the Brief Social Phobia Scale (clinician rated) and the Social Phobia Inventory (patient rated) (Davidson et al., 1997; Conner et al., 2000).

4. Co-morbidity

Significant comorbidity of social anxiety and mood disorders have been consistently shown in the literature (Kessler et al., 1999; Lecrubier & Weiller, 1997; Pini et al. 1997). Social anxiety has also been linked to severity (Merikangas & Angst, 1995) and persistence (Alpert et al. 1997) of mood disorders. Also comorbid mood disorders have worsen social anxiety symptoms and result in greater impairment in patients with SAD (Erwin et al., 2002). A significant number of patients presenting with social anxiety will have a secondary anxiety disorder, particularly panic disorder with agoraphobia and generalized anxiety disorder (Mennin et al. 2000, Schneier et al., 1992). Comorbid depressive or anxiety disorders complicate SAD, the severity of symptoms and suicidality should be assessed and hospitalisation considered if indicated. In such cases, the treatment of choice should ideally target both the mood and the anxiety components.

Social phobia and avoidant personality disorder were introduced in the DSM classification system nearly 30 years ago. Since then it has been shown that these two disorders can be found highly comorbid in patients, in some trials as high as 89% (Schneier et al., 1991). Some researchers have interpreted this high rate of overlap to mean that social phobia and avoidant personality disorder reflect a spectrum of social anxiety (Tillfors & Ekselius, 2009).

Social anxiety disorder is associated with high rates of alcohol use disorders (Morris et al., 2005). Almost half of the patients with lifetime SAD meet criteria for lifetime prevalence of an alcohol use disorder (Grant et al.,2005) and it is a significantly high rate when compared to general population. Among the anxiety disorders, SAD shows a particularly problematic risk profile for comorbid alcohol use disorders, as SAD is associated with higher rates of alcohol use disorders relative to most other anxiety disorders (Kessler et al.,1997).

Recently, researchers have identified that individuals with SAD appear particularly vulnerable to marijuana-related problems too. Data from the National Comorbidity Study suggest that individuals with SAD are 7 times more likely to experience marijuana dependence relative to the general population (Agosti et al, 2002) and undergraduates with higher social anxiety appear to be particularly vulnerable to marijuana use problems (Buckner et al, 2007; Buckner et al., 2008a). In a study, adolescents with SAD were nearly 5 times more likely to develop marijuana dependence as young adults compared to adolescents without SAD (Buckner et al., 2008b).

5. Treatment of SAD

Current recommended treatment options for social anxiety disorder include pharmacotherapy and cognitive behavioural therapy (CBT). (Dilbaz 2005) Although several randomised controlled trials (RCTs) have failed to show efficacy for β-adrenoceptor antagonists in generalised SAD, it has been suggested that these agents may be useful in non-generalised SAD, patients with performance anxiety only. Efficacy in the treatment of generalised SAD has been demonstrated for a number of interventions, (Stein, 2003; Blanco et al., 2003) including SSRIs, high potency benzodiazepines (e.g. clonazepam), MAOIs (e.g. phenelzine), reversible inhibitors of monoamine oxidase A (MAO-A) [RIMAs, e.g. moclobemide], certain antiepileptics (e.g. gabapentin, pregabalin), serotonin-noradrenaline reuptake inhibitors (venlafaxine) and CBT (Zaider & Heimberg 2003).

5.1 Nonpharmacological treatments

These treatments include exposure, cognitive re-structuring, relaxation techniques and social skills training, often used in combination. Literature have concluded that cognitive behavioral therapy (CBT) is often effective for treating social anxiety disorder. The goal of cognitive behavioral therapy (CBT) is to provide techniques and practice to patients with social anxiety disorder, so they can learn to change how they think about and behave in situations that terrify them. CBT may be offered individually or as part of group therapy. There is continued interest in the question of whether group or individual treatment is more effective. Early studies suggested some superiority for group treatment (Wlazlo et al., 1990), and arguments were raised that the group setting would provide a richness of exposure experiences not easily replicated in individual treatment; by the late 1990s the weight of evidence suggested that there was no clear superiority between group and individual treatment (Gould et al., 1997).

Meta-analyses of the efficacy of CBT for SAD that have compared various types of CBT with each other and with control conditions have yielded the highest effect sizes for exposure-based interventions (Federof & Taylor, 2001; Hope et al.,1995). In exposure therapy, the type of CBT most often used and studied for social anxiety disorder, therapists gradually expose patients to the dreaded situation and suggest ways to manage fear. The exposure-based extinction of fear is now thought to involve new learning that actively inhibits the fear reaction to a given cue (Davis et al., 2006). In other variations of CBT— not as well studied as exposure therapy— patients learn and practice social skills and relaxation techniques.

5.2 Pharmacological treatments

SSRIs; evidence from RCTs supports that the efficacy and tolerability of almost all SSRIs (escitalopram (Stein et al.,2005), fluvoxamine, (Van Vliet et al.,1994; Stein et al., 1999) paroxetine, (Liebowitz et al., 2002; Baldwin et al., 1999; Stein et al., 1998) sertraline (Katzelnicket al., 1995; Liebowitz et al., 2003), fluoxetin (Black et al., 1992), citalopram (Bouwer & Stein, 1998) in the treatment of SAD, so SSRIs can be regarded as first-line treatment in SAD. These agents have the additional benefit of treating comorbid conditions commonly seen with SAD (Van Ameringen et al., 2004). Fluoxetine, fluvoxamine and sertraline have been the most studied SSRIs in socially phobic children and adolescents and have shown good efficacy and tolerability in this group (Robinson & Hood, 2007).

Venlafaxine; has shown promising results in open-label and controlled trials in the treatment of SAD. Venlafaxine is an effective treatment option for generalised social anxiety disorder but has no superiority from paroxetine in clinical trials (Allgulander et al., 2004; Liebowitz et al., 2005). While venlafaxine is an effective treatment, this may be related to its serotonergic profile, and the authors are unimpressed with response to the specific noradrenergic agent reboxetine from both the literature and clinical experience. Venlafaxine is associated with significant side effects and discontinuation syndrome and described as second-line treatments of social anxiety in most settings (Robinson & Hood, 2007).

MAOIs; Phenelzine was one of the first established treatments for SAD with several early double-blind, placebo-controlled trials demonstrating efficacy in this disorder (Versiani et al., 1992; Gelernter et al., 1991). In light of their adverse effect profiles and the dietary restrictions associated with use of these agents, together with the availability of alternative treatments, MAOIs are currently not considered to be a first-line treatment for SAD.

RIMAs; reversible inhibitors of monoamine oxidase A, appears inferior to that of phenelzine in efficacy but the main advantages of moclobemide over phenelzine are superior tolerability and no concern about dietary restrictions at the standart dosage of 600 mg/day moclobemide. This may be a particularly important consideration in the long-term treatment of SAD (Stein et al., 2002).

Benzodizepines, despite the positive results, the adverse effect profile, the potential for dependence, the possibility of rebound anxiety, the possible negative consequences of state-dependent learning and their ineffectiveness in the treatment of depression shows that these agents should not be considered as first-line monotherapy for SAD (Jackson 1995; Keith et al., 2003).

Beta Blockers; Beta-blockers are effective at blocking peripheral autonomic symptoms such as tachycardia, tremor, sweating, blushing and dry mouth and thus have a potential role as anxiolytics. They are effectively used in the treatment of performance anxiety but there is substantial evidence that beta-blockers are not effective in social phobia (Liebowitz et al., 1992; Turner et al., 1994) and that better options are available. A limited role in performance anxiety is indicated.

Gabapentine, Pregabalin and Levetirasetam; Some anticonvulsants trials suggest that gabapentin, pregabalin and levetirasetam could be alternative agents for patients who are nonresponsive to SSRIs and SNRIs (Pande et al., 1999; Pande et al., 2004; Zhang et al., 2005). However these agents need further studies about the safety and efficacy in SAD.

Other pharmacological agents for treatment of SAD; *Tricyclic antidepressants* have been used but failed to be an effective treatment choice for social anxiety disorder (Emmanuel et al., 1997; Simpson et al., 1998). There are trials with *buspirone* in literature but these trials have both negative and positive outcomes in social anxiety disorder. So that buspirone may be a useful agent for augmentation in social anxiety disorder (Robinson & Hood, 2007). There is a little evidence for *bupropion* efficacy in social phobia (Emmanuel et al., 2000). There are trials that have found *mirtazapine* as an effective treatment option for social anxiety disorder (Mrakotsky et al., 2007; Mörtberg, 2006). However in a recent study mirtazapine showed no superiority to placebo for treatment of SAD (Shutters et al., 2010).

Atypical antipsychotics have been shown to have anxioloytic properties in the literature (Depping et al., 2010; Vulink et al., 2011). Olanzapine (Barnett et al., 2002) and quetiapine (Vaishavi et al., 2007) have been found effective as monotherapy in the treatment of SAD. In another study switchover to aripiprazole effectively improved social anxiety in patiets with schizophrenia (Stern et al., 2009).

5.3 Inadequate response to pharmacotherapy and augmentation strategies

Criteria for remission of SAD proposed by Ballenger (Ballenger, 2001) include absence of core symptoms of SAD, no or minimal anxiety (e.g. in anticipation of social interaction) as rated by rating scales such as the Hamilton Rating Scale for Anxiety, no functional impairment (the Sheehan Disability Scale may be used to evaluate this), (Sheehan et al., 1996) and remission of course of action when first-line treatment with a co-morbid depression as reflected by the Hamilton Rating Scale for Depression. It should, however, be noted that the mean reduction in Liebowitz Social Anxiety Scale scores was <50% in a review of 19 double-blind, placebo-controlled trials involving patients with SAD. Switching to another SSRIs, venlafaxine or MAOIs has been suggested in non responders or patients with adverse event. Augmentation strategies that may prove useful in partial treatment responders include buspirone, clonazepam, gabapentin, bupropion or new generation antipsychotics, although empirical data are lacking (Barnett et al., 2002; Schutters et al., 2005; Pallanti et al., 1999).

In case of comorbidity moclobemide was found to be effective and well-tolerated in the SAD patients with anxiety disorders as well as SSRIs. In the presence of co-morbid alcohol abuse, MAOIs and benzodiazepines can complicate the treatment, SSRIs have usefulness in reducing the alcohol consumption (Naranjo & Knoke, 2001). CBT may be the treatment of choice during pregnancy and lactation.

6. Conclusion

SAD is a prevalent and disabling disorder that often remains undetected unless the clinicaian takes a careful history. Present consensus supports that SSRIs can currently be regarded as first-line treatment in SAD because of their proven efficacy, tolerability and bility to treat co-morbid conditions such as depression or other anxiety disorders (Stein, 2003; Blanco et al., 2003; Ballenger et al., 1998). There is a recent evidence venlafaxine XR may also be considered in the first-line. Second-line treatments include MAOIs (e.g. phenelzine) and RIMAs (e.g.moclobemide).

The combination of CBT and an SSRI is often espoused as best practice, unfortunately there is little hard evidence supporting this (despite considerable face validity). Future studies taking a good look at combination therapies of this type are encouraged and also future research should focus on complicated and treatment refractory SAD and treatment strategies in special populations (e.g.children and adolescents).

7. References

Agosti V, Nunes E, Levin F. Rates of psychiatric comorbidity among U.S. residents with lifetime cannabis dependence. Am J Drug Alcohol Abuse 2002;28:643–652.

Allgulander C, Mangano R, Zhang J, et al. Efficacy of Venlafaxine ER in patients with social anxiety disorder: a double-blind, placebo-controlled, parallel group comparison with paroxetine. Hum Psychopharmacol 2004; 19: 387-396.

Alonso J, Angermeyer MC, Bernert S, Bruff aerts R, Brugha TS, Bryson H, de Girolamo G, Graaf R, Demyttenaere K, Gasquet I, Haro JM, Katz SJ, Kessler RC, Kovess V, Lepine JP, Ormel J, Polidori G, Russo LJ, Vilagut G, Almansa J, Arbabzadeh-Bouchez S, Autonell J, Bernal M, Buist-Bouwman MA, Codony M, Domingo-

Salvany A, Ferrer M, Joo SS, et al. Disability and quality of life impact of mental disorders in Europe. Acta Psychiatr Scand Suppl 2004;420:38–46.

Alpert JE, Uebelacker LA, McLean NE, Nierenberg AA, Pava JA, Worthington JJ III, Tedlow JR, Rosenbaum JF & Fava M. Social phobia, avoidant personality disorder and atypical depression: co-occurrence and clinical implications. Psychological Medicine 1997;27: 627-633.

Baldwin D, Bobes J, Stein DJ, et al. Paroxetine in social phobia- social anxiety disorder: randomised, double blind, placebo-controlled study. Br J Psychiatry 1999; 175: 120-6.

Ballenger JC, Davidson JA, Lecrubier Y, et al. Consensus statement on social anxiety disorder from the international consensus group on depression and anxiety. J Clin Psychiatry 1998; 59 (8 Suppl.): 54S-60S.

Ballenger JC. Treatment of anxiety disorders to remission. J Clin Psychiatry 2001; 62 Suppl. 12: 5S-9S.

Barnett SD, Kramer ML, Casat CD, Connor KM, Davidson JR. Efficacy of olanzapine in social anxiety disorder: A pilot study. J Psychopharmacol 2002;16:365–368.

Beesdo, K., Bittner, A., Pine, D. S., Stein, M. B., Höfler, M., Lieb, R., et al. Incidence of social anxiety disorder and the consistent risk for secondary depression in the first three decades of life. Archives of General Psychiatry 2007;64, 903–912.

Beidel DC, Turner SM, Morris TL. Behavioral treatment of childhood social phobia. J Consult Clin Psychol 2000; 68: 1072-80

Beidel DC, Turner SM, Morris TL. Psychopathology of childhood social phobia. J Am Acad Child Adolesc Psychiatry 1999; 38 Suppl. 6: 643-50

Beidel DC, Turner SM. Shy children, phobic adults: nature and treatment of social phobia. Washington, DC: American Psychological Association, 1998

Black B, Uhde TW, Tancer ME. Fluoxetine for the treatment of social phobia. J Clin Psychopharmacol 1992; 12: 293-5.

Black B, Uhde TW. Psychiatric characteristics of children with selective mutism: a pilot study. J Am Acad Child Adolesc Psychiatry 1995;34:847–856.

Blanco C, Schineider FR, Schmidt A, et al. Pharmacological treatment of social anxiety disorder:a meta-analysis. Depress Anxiety 2003;18(1):29-40.

Bouwer C, Stein DJ. Use of the selective serotonin reuptake and inhibitor citalopram in the treatment of generalized social phobia. J Affect Disord 1998; 49: 79-82.

Briggs-Gowan MJ, Horwitz SM, Schwab-Stone M, et al. Mental health in pediatric settings: distribution of disorders and factors related to service use. J Am Acad Child Adolesc Psychiatry 2000; 39: 841-9

Brown SM, Peet E, Manuck SB, Williamson DE, Dahl RE, Ferrell RE, Hariri AR. A regulatory variant of the human tryptophan hydroxylase-2 gene biases amygdala reactivity. Mol Psychiatry 2005;10:884–888.

Buckner JD, Bonn-Miller MO, Zvolensky MJ et al. Marijuana use motives and social anxiety among marijuana-using young adults. Addict Behav 2007;32:2238–2252.

Buckner JD, Schmidt NB, Lang AR et al. Specificity of social anxiety disorder as a risk factor for alcohol and cannabis dependence. J Psychiatr Res 2008a;42:230–239.

Buckner JD, Schmidt NB. Marijuana effect expectancies: relations to social anxiety and marijuana use problems. Addict Behav 2008b;33:1477–1483.

Busch B, Biederman J, Cohen L, et al. Correlates of ADHD among children in pediatric and psychiatric clinics. Psychiatr Serv 2002; 53: 1103-11

Chavira DA, Stein MB, Bailey K, et al. Child anxiety in primary care: prevalent but untreated.Depress Anxiety 2004; 20: 155-64

Compton SN, Grant PJ, Chrisman AK, Gammon PJ, Brown VL, March JS. Sertraline in children and adolescents with social anxiety disorder: An open trial. J Am Acad Child Adolesc Psychiatry 2001;40(5):564–571.

Connor KM, Davidson JRT, Churchill LE, et al. Psychometric properties of the Social Phobia Inventory (SPIN): new self-rating scale. Br J Psychiatry 2000; 176: 379-86

Costello EJ. Child psychiatric disorders and their correlates: a primary care pediatric sample. J Am Acad Child Adolesc Psychiatry 1989; 28: 851-5

Davidson JR, Miner CM, De Veaugh-Geiss J, et al. The Brief Social Phobia Scale: a psychometric evaluation. Psychol Med 1997; 27 (1): 161-6

Davis M, Myers KM, Chhatwal J, Ressler KJ. Pharmacological treatments that facilitate extinction of fear: relevance to psychotherapy. NeuroRx 2006; 3:82_96.

Depping AM, Komossa K, Kissling W, Leucht S. Second-generation antipsychotics for anxiety disorders. Cochrane Database Syst Rev. 2010;(12):CD008120.

Dummit ESI, Klein RG, Tancer NK, et al. Systematic assessment of 50 children with selective mutism. J Am Acad Child Adolesc Psychiatry 1997;36:653–660.

Dilbaz N, Güz H. Liebowitz Social Anxiety Rating Scale: Turkish reliability and Validity. 37. National Psychiatry Congress, İstanbul, 2-6 October 2001.

Dilbaz N. The prevelance of social phobia among the Turkish university students. XII. World Congress of Psychiatry, Yokohama, August 24-29, 2002.

Dilbaz N, Güz H. The gender differences in Social Phobia. (Sosyal kaygı bozukluğunda cinsiyet farklılıkları. Nöropsikiyatri Arşivi) Neuropsychiatry Archives 2002; 39: 79-86. (Turkish)

Dilbaz N. Treatment of Social Anxiety Disorders. Dilbaz N (ed.) Recent Advances in Anxiety Disorders . Ankara; Pozitif Matbaacılık, 2005. (Turkish)

Emmanuel N, Johnson M, Villareal G, *et al*. Imipramine in the Treatment of Social Phobia, A Double-Blind Study. Presented at the 36th Annual Meeting of the American College of Neuropsychopharmacology. 8-12-1997. Kohala Coast, Hawaii.

Emmanuel NP, Brawman-Mintzer O, Morton WA, Book SW, Johnson MR, Lorberbaum JP, Ballenger JC, Lydiard RB. Bupropion-SR in treatment of social phobia. Depress Anxiety. 2000;12(2):111-3.

Erwin BA, Heimberg RG, Juster H, Mindlin M. Comorbid anxiety and mood disorders among persons with social anxiety disorder Behaviour Research and Therapy 2002;40: 19–35.

Essau CA, Conradt J, Petermann F. Frequency and comorbidity of social phobia and social fears in adolescents. Behav Res 1999; 37: 831-43

Federoff IC, Taylor S. Psychological and pharmacological treatments of social phobia: a meta-analysis. J Clin Psychopharmacol 2001; 21: 311-24

Fehm, L., Pelissolo, A., Furmark, T., & Wittchen, H. U. Size and burden of social phobia in Europe. European Neuropsychopharmacology 2005; 15, 453–462.

Flannery-Schroeder EC, Kendall P. Group and individual cognitive-behavioral treatments for youth with anxiety disorders: a randomized clinical trial. Cognit Ther Res 2000; 24: 251-78

Furmark T, Tillfors M, Garpenstrand H, Marteinsdottir I, Langstrom B, Oreland L, Fredrikson M. Serotonin transporter polymorphism related to amygdala excitability and symptom severity in patients with social phobia. Neurosci Lett 2004;362:189–192.

Furmark T. Neurobiological aspects of social anxiety disorder. Isr J Psychiatry Relat Sci. 2009;46(1):5-12.

Gelernter CS, Uhde TW, Cimbolic P, et al. Cognitive behavioural and pharmacological treatment of social phobia: a controlled study. Arch Gen Psychiatry 1991; 48: 938-45.

Gould R, Otto M, Pollack M, Yap L. Cognitive-behavioral and pharmacological treatment for social phobia: a metaanalysis. Clin Psychol Sci Pract 1997; 4:291_306.

Graeff FG. On serotonin and experimental anxiety. Psychopharmacology 2002;163:467–476.

Grant BF, Hasin DS, Blanco C, et al. The epidemiology of social anxiety disorder in the United States: results from the National Epidemiologic Survey on alcohol and related conditions. J Clin Psychiatry 2005;66:1351–1361.

Grant KA, Shively CA, Nader MA, Ehrenkaufer RL, Line SW, Morton TE, Gage HD, Mach RH. Effect of social status on striatal dopamine D2 receptor binding characteristics in cynomolgus monkeys assessed with positron emission tomography. Synapse 1998;29:80–83.

Hariri AR, Holmes A. Genetics of emotional regulation: Th e role of the serotonin transporter in neural function. Trends Cogn Sci 2006;10:182–191.

Heimberg RG, Stein MB, Hiripi E, et al. Trends in the prevalence of social phobia in the United States: a synthetic cohort analysis of changes over four decades.Eur Psychiatry 2000; 15: 29-37.

Hirshfeld-Becker DR, Biederman J, Henin A, Faraone SV, Davis S, Harrington K, Rosenbaum JF. Behavioral Inhibition in Preschool Children At Risk Is a Specific Predictor of Middle Childhood Social Anxiety: A Five year Follow-up. J Dev Behav Pediatr 2007;28:225–233.

Hope DA, Heimberg RG, Bruch MA. Dismantling cognitive behavioral group therapy for social phobia. Behav Res Ther 1995; 33: 637-50

Ipser JC, Kariuki CM, Stein DJ. Pharmacotherapy for social anxiety disorder: A systematic review. Expert Rev Neurother 2008;8:235–257.

Jackson A. State-dependent effects of atypical benzodiazepine receptor agonists. Psychopharmacology 1995; 119 (4): 399-404.

Katzelnick DJ, Greist JH. Social anxiety disorder: an unrecognized problem in primary care. J Clin Psychiatry 2001; 62 (1 Suppl.): 11-6

Katzelnick DJ, Kobak KA, Greist JH, et al. Sertraline for social phobia: a double-blind, placebo-controlled crossover study. Am J Psychiatry 1995; 152: 1368-71 64.

Keith JR, Pitts RC, Pezzuit T, et al. Effects of positive GABA (A) modulators on a multiple-component, repeated-acquisition test of spatial learning. Behav Pharmacol 2003; 14 (1): 67-75.

Kessler RC, Crum RM, Warner LA, Nelson CB, Schulenberg J, Anthony JC. Lifetime co-occurrence of DSM-III-R alcohol abuse and dependence with other psychiatric disorders in the National Comorbidity Survey. Arch Gen Psychiatry 1997;54: 313–321.

Kessler RC, Stang P, Wittchen HU, Stein M, Walters EE. Lifetime co-morbidities between social phobia and mood disorders in the US National Comorbidity Survey. Psychological Medicine 1999; 29: 555-567.

Kessler, R. C., Berglund, P., Demler, O., Jin, R., Merikangas, K. R., & Walters, E. E. Lifetime prevalence and age-of-onset distributions of DSM-IV disorders in the National Comorbidity Survey Replication. Archives of General Psychiatry 2005; 6, 593–602.

Kumpulainen K, Rasanen E, Raaska H, Somppi V. Selective mutism among second-graders in elementary school. Eur Child Adolesc Psychiatry 1998;7:24–29.

Lanzenberger RR, Mitterhauser M, Spindelegger C, Wadsak W, Klein N, Mien LK, Holik A, Attarbaschi T, Mossaheb N, Sacher J, Geiss-Granadia T, Kletter K, Kasper S, Tauscher J. Reduced serotonin-1A receptor binding in social anxiety disorder. Biol Psychiatry 2007;61:1081–1089.

Lecrubier Y. & Weiller E. Comorbidities in social phobia. International Clinical Psychopharmacology 12 (suppl. 6) 1997;17-21.

Lewinsohn PM, Hops H, Roberts RE, et al. Adolescent psychopathology: I. Prevalence and incidence of depression and other DSM-III-R disorders in high school students. J Abnorm Psych 1993; 102: 133-44

Liebowitz MR, DeMartinis NA, Weihs K, et al. Efficacy of sertraline in severe generalized social anxiety disorder: results of a double-blind, placebo-controlled study. J Clin Psychiatry 2003; 64 (7): 785-92.

Liebowitz MR, Gelenberg AJ, Munjack D. Venlafaxine extended release vs placebo and paroxetine in social anxiety disorder. Arch Gen Psychiatry 2005; 62: 190-198.

Liebowitz MR, Schneier F, Campeas R, *et al.* Phenelzine vs atenolol in social phobia. A placebo-controlled comparison. Arch Gen Psychiatry 1992; 49: 290-300.

Liebowitz MR, Stein MB, Tancer M, et al. A randomised, double-blind, fixed-dose comparison of paroxetine and placebo in the treatment of generalized social anxiety disorder. J Clin Psychiatry 2002; 63: 66-74.

Liebowitz MR. Social phobia. Mod Probl Pharmacopsychiatry 1987; 22: 141-73

Mancini C, Van Ameringen M, Oakman JM, Farvolden P. Serotonergic agents in the treatment of social phobia in children and adolescents: a case series. Depress Anxiety 1999;10:33–39.

March J, Wells K. Combining medication and psychotherapy. In: Martin A, Scahill L, Charney DS, et al., editors. Pediatric psychopharmacology: principles and practice. New York: Oxford University Press, 2003: 426-46

Mennin DS, Heimberg RG, Jack MS.Comorbid generalized anxiety disorder in primary social phobia: symptom severity, functional impairment, and treatment response. J Anxiety Disord. 2000;14(4):325-43.

Merikangas KR & Angst J. Comorbidity and social phobia: evidence from clinical, epidemiologic and genetic studies. Archives of Psychiatry and Clinical Neuroscience 1995; 244,:297-303.

Meron Ruscio A, Brown TA, Chiu WT, Sareen J, Stein MB, Kessler RC. Social fears and social phobia in theUnited States: Results from the National Comorbidity Survey Replication. Psychol Med 2008;38:15–28.

Morris EP, Stewart SH, Ham LS. The relationship between social anxiety disorder and alcohol use disorders: a critical review. Clin Psychol Rev 2005;25:734–760.

Mörtberg E. Mirtazapine reduces social anxiety and improves quality of life in women with social phobia. Evid Based Ment Health. 2006;9(3):75.

Mrakotsky C, Masek B, Biederman J, Raches D, Hsin O, Forbes P, de Moor C, DeMaso DR, Gonzalez-Heydrich J. Prospective open-label pilot trial of mirtazapine in children and adolescents with social phobia. J Anxiety Disord. 2008;22(1):88-97.

Naranjo CA, Knoke DM. The role of selective serotonin- reuptake inhibitors in reducing alcohol consumption. J Clin Psychiatry 2001; 62 (20 Suppl.): 18S-25S.

Pallanti S, Querciolo L, Rossi A, et al. The emergence of social phobia during clozapine treatment and its response to fluoxetine augmentation. J Clin Psychiatry 1999; 60: 819-23.

Pande AC, Davidson JR, Jeff erson JW, et al. Treatment of social phobia with gabapentin: A placebo-controlled study. J Clin Psychopharmacol 1999;19:341–348.

Pande AC, Feltner DE, Jeff erson JW, et al. Efficacy of the novel anxiolytic pregabalin in social anxiety disorder: A placebo-controlled, multicenter study. J Clin Psychopharmacol 2004;24:141–149.

Pini S, Cassano GB, Simonini E, Savino M, Russo A & Montgomery SA. Prevalence of anxiety disorders comorbidity in bipolar depression, unipolar depression and dysthymia. Journal of Affective Disorders 1997;4,:145-153.

Prior M, Smart D, Sanson A, et al. Does shy-inhibited temperament in childhood lead to anxiety problems in adolescence? J Am Acad Child Adolesc Psychiatry 2000;39:461–468.

Richard IH, Schiff er RB, Kurlan R. Anxiety and Parkinson's disease. J Neuropsychiatry Clin Neurosci 1996;8:383–392.

Robinson HM, Hood SD. A review of Pharmacological treatments. Curr Psychiatry Reviews 2007;3:95-122

Schneier FR, Johnson J, Hornig CD, et al. Social phobia: comorbidity and morbidity in an epidemiologic sample. Arch Gen Psychiatry 1992; 49: 282-8

Schneier FR, Liebowitz MR, Abi-Dargham A, Zea- Ponce Y, Lin S-H, Laruelle M. Low dopamine D2 receptor binding potential in social phobia. Am J Psychiatry 2000;157:457–459.

Schneier FR, Spitzer RL, Gibbon M, Fyer AJ, Liebowitz MR. The relationship of social phobia subtypes and avoidant personality disorder. Compr Psychiatry 1991;32:496–502.

Schutters SI, Van Megen HJ, Van Veen JF, Denys DA, Westenberg HG. Mirtazapine in generalized social anxiety disorder: a randomized, double-blind, placebo-controlled study. Int Clin Psychopharmacol. 2010;25(5):302-4.

Schutters SI, van Megen HJ, Westenberg HG. Efficacy of quetiapine in generalized social anxiety disorder: Results from an open-label study. J Clin Psychiatry 2005;66:540–542.

Serretti A, Calati R, Mandelli L, De Ronchi D. Serotonin transporter gene variants and behavior: A comprehensive review. Curr Drug Targets 2006;7:1659–1669.

Sheehan DV, Harnett-Sheehan K, Raj BA. The measurement of disability. Int Clin Psychopharmacol 1996; 11 Suppl. 3: 89S-95S.

Simpson HB, Schneier FR, Campeas RB, *et al*. Imipramine in the treatment of social phobia. J Clin Psychopharmacol 1998; 18: 132-135.

Smolka MN, Schumann G, Wrase J, Grusser SM, Flor H, Mann K, Braus DF, Goldman D, Buchel C, Heinz A. Catechol-O-methyltransferase val158met genotype affects

processing of emotional stimuli in the amygdala and prefrontal cortex. J Neurosci 2005;25:836–842.
Stein DJ, Cameron A, Amrein R, et al. Moclobemide is effective and well tolerated in the long-term pharmacotherapy of social anxiety disorder with or without comorbid anxiety disorder. Int Clin Psychopharmacol 2002 Jul; 17 (4): 161-70.
Stein DJ, Kasper S, Andersen EW, et al. Escitalopram in the treatment of social anxiety disorder: analysis of efficacy for different clinical subgroups and symptom dimensions. Depress Anxiety 2005; 20 (4): 175-81.
Stein DJ. Algorithm for the pharmacotherapy of anxiety disorders. Curr Psychiatry Rep 2003:5:282-8.
Stein MB, Fyer AJ, Davidson JRT, et al. Fluvoxamine treatment of social phobia (social anxiety disorder): a double blind placebo-controlled study. Am J Psychiatry 1999; 156: 756-60.
Stein MB, Gelernter J, Smoller JW. Genetics of social anxiety disorder and related traits. In: Bandelow B, Stein DJ, editors. Social anxiety disorder. New York: Marcel Dekker, 1994: pp. 197–214.
Stein MB, Liebowitz MR, Lydiard RB, et al. Paroxetine in the treatment of generalized social phobia (social anxiety disorder): a randomised, double-blind, placebo-controlled study JAMA 1998; 280: 708-13.
Steinhausen HC, Juzi C. Selective mutism: an analysis of 100 cases. J Am Acad Child Adolesc Psychiatry 1996;35:606–14.
Stern RG, Petti TA, Bopp K, Tobia A. Aripiprazole for the treatment of schizophrenia with co-occurring social anxiety: an open-label cross-taper study. J Clin Psychopharmacol. 2009;29(3):206-9.
Tancer ME. Neurobiology of social phobia. J Clin Psychiatry 1993;54 suppl 12:26–30.
Thase, M. E. Recognition and diagnosis of atypical depression. Journal of Clinical Psychiatry 2007; 68 (Suppl . 8), 11–16.
Tiihonen J, Kuikka J, Bergstrom K, Lepola U, Koponen H, Leinonen E. Dopamine reuptake site densities in patients with social phobia. Am J Psychiatry 1997;154:239–242.
Tillfors M, Ekselius L. Social Phobia and Avoidant Personality Disorder: Are They Separate Diagnostic Entities or Do They Reflect a Spectrum of Social Anxiety? Isr J Psychiatry Relat Sci 2009; 46: 25–33
Turner SM, Beidel DC, Jacob RG. Social phobia: a comparison of behavior therapy and atenolol. J Consult Clin Psychol 1994; 62: 350-358.
Vaishnavi S, Alamy S, Zhang W, Connor KM, Davidson JR. Quetiapine as monotherapy for social anxiety disorder: a placebo-controlled study. Prog Neuropsychopharmacol Biol Psychiatry. 2007;31(7):1464-9.
Van Ameringen M, Mancini C, Pipe B, Bennett M. Optimizing treatment in social phobia: A review of treatment resistance. CNS Spectr 2004;9:753–762.
Van Ameringen MA, Lane RM, Walker JR, et al. Sertraline treatment of generalized social phobia: a 20-week, double- blind, placebo-controlled study. Am J Psychiatry 2001; 158: 275-81.
Van Vliet IM, den Boer JA, Westenberg HGM. Psycho-pharmacological treatment of social phobia: a double-blind, placebo.controlled study with fluvoxamine. Psychopharmacology (Berl) 1994; 115: 128-34.

Versiani M, Nardi AE, Mundim FD, et al. Pharmacotherapy of social phobia: a controlled study with moclobemide and phenelzine. Br J Psychiatry 1992; 161: 353-60 .

Vulink NC, Figee M, Denys D. Review of atypical antipsychotics in anxiety. Eur Neuropsychopharmacol. 2011 Feb 21. [Epub ahead of print]

Wittchen HU, Nelson CB, Lachner G. Prevalence of mental disorders and psychosocial impairments in adolescents and young adults. Psychol Med 1998; 28: 109-26

Wlazlo Z, Schroeder-Hartwig K, Hand I, Kaiser G, Munchau N. Exposure in vivo vs social skills training for social phobia: long-term outcome and differential effects. Behav Res Ther 1990; 28:181_193.

Wren FJ, Scholle SH, Heo J, et al. Pediatric mood and anxiety syndromes in primary care: who gets identified. Int J Psychiatry Med 2003; 33: 1-16

Zaider TI, Heimberg RG. Non-pharmacologic treatments for social anxiety disorder. Acta Psychiatr Scand Suppl 2003; 108 (417): 72S-84S

Zhang W, Connor KM, Davidson JR. Levetiracetam in social phobia: A placebo controlled pilot study. J Psychopharmacol 2005;19:551–553.

3

Obsessive-Compulsive Disorders or Not: Differential Diagnosis of Repetitive Behaviors Among Individuals with Intellectual and Developmental Disorders

Jarrett Barnhill
Department of Psychiatry
University of North Carolina School of Medicine
USA

1. Introduction

This chapter focuses on the complex psychobiology of Obsessive-Compulsive Disorder (OCD) among individuals with Intellectual and Developmental Disabilities (IDD). It begins with OCD as an anxiety-driven psychiatric disorder characterized by intrusive thoughts and images (obsessions) and a tendency to engage in a select group of escape behaviors (compulsions) of sufficient severity to interfere with daily life. Using these criteria to diagnose OCD in persons with IDD frequently results in a heterogeneous disorder that overlaps other forms as repetitive behaviors (Baldwin et al 2008; Pallanti et al 2008). Resolving the heterogeneity issue requires that we differentiate OCD from related stereotypies, ritualistic behaviors, self-injurious behaviors (Flavell, 1982), and OC-related behaviors associated with Autistic Spectrum Disorders(ASD),Tourette's Disorder (TD) and other movement disorders (Barnhill, 2008). To accomplish this task we will move beyond the descriptive criteria for OCD and anxiety disorders found in the Diagnostic and Statistical Manual- IV-TR (APA, 2000) and the Diagnostic Manual-Intellectual Disability (Fletcher et al, 2007). By the end of this review it will be readily apparent to the reader that OCD like other anxiety disorders represents a convergence of many functional abnormalities spread out across several neuro-anatomically distinct but functionally overlapping pathways. To reach this conclusion, we will come to understand that the symptomatic diversity of this group of disorders of repetitive thoughts and behaviors depends in large part on regional malfunctioning within a pathway or network rather than on any single "lesion" (Davis, 2002, Barnhill, 2008).

We will begin this exploration by examining fear, fear conditioning and their role in anxiety disorders. To do this requires an analysis of new findings in the neurosciences, especially gene-environmental interactions, temperament, physiological responses to stressful environmental events and the mode of anxiety-related behavioral responses (Feinstein et al 2007; De Mathis et al 2006) . Later, we will shift to an ethological model that uses reciprocal social, ritualized and attachment behaviours to describe subtypes of anxiety. This approach can be a useful tool can be useful tool for classifying OC related behaviors among nonverbal patients with severe- profound IDD. The remainder of the chapter will address the relationship between OCD, Obsessive-Compulsive Spectrum Disorder (OCSD) and repetitive behaviors in other neurodevelopmental disorders -including intellectual disability (IDD) (Parsons et al, 1985; Ruedrich et al 1985; Pallanti et al, 2008) .

2. Neurobiology of fear and anxiety

Fear is a state of cognitive, emotional and physiological arousal that is triggered by the presence of a direct threat or danger (Costello et al, 2005; Mobbs et al, 2008). Fear responses are characterized by increased arousal and vigilance, increased sympathetic output, changes in perception and cognitive appraisal of events, and flight-fight responses (Britton et al, 2010). The cognitive-emotional components of the fear response result from increased autonomic activation (sympathetic nervous system), neuro-endocrine changes represented by an increased CRF and hypothalamic-pituitary adrenal activity (Charney et al, 2002)) and activity in the peri-aqueductal gray region involved in motor activity and pain perception (Mobbs et al, 2007). These physiological reactions generate flight, fight or freezing responses may vary depending on the imminence of the danger, context (ecological factors), proximity of the threat, presence of others, availability of behavioral responses (including defensive aggression), age and temperamental variability in the threshold and intensity of approach/avoidance behaviors. Several of these variables also play a key role of vulnerability factors for anxiety and anxiety disorders (Davis 1997, Stein et al 2002, Neumeister et al 2003). Freezing responses are not included in this review. But we cannot overlook this physiological response among pre-adults, especially as it relates to catatonic and dissociative behaviours among adults under extreme duress. (Harris et al, 1997; Stein et al, 2002; Lee, 2007; Britton et al, 2010).

Fear conditioning is a form of associative conditioning in which the state of arousal is linked to an external threat. Under these conditions, this physiological state is associated activation of the amygdala and related hypothalamic /sympathetic circuitry serves as the unconditioned stimulus. (Mobbs et la 2007; Stahl et al 2008). Activation of this system leads to increases in autonomic and neuro-endocrine activity that results in an automatic or unconditioned response that consists of flight-fight and freezing behaviors (Zohar et al, 1991). Current research also points to the amygdala as a critical component of in fear conditioning (Mobbs et al, 2007). Fear conditioning is due to a pairing of an unconditioned stimulus (an approaching hungry tiger) and conditioned stimuli (setting or specific environmental cues) and an unconditioned response (intense fear and flight or fight activation). In time, some specific features of the encounter or its environmental context can activate the fear responses and associated avoidance or escape behaviors. Fear conditioned experiences are also subject to generalization so that additional neutral or previously nonthreatening stimuli (secondary conditioned stimuli), such as returning to similar conditions or experiencing less intense affective states of arousal, can now trigger the cascade of avoidance behaviors. With repeated exposure and avoidance the behaviors may occur without clearly re-experiencing of the originating stimuli or context. These stimulus-response trains can expand to include more generalized avoidance behaviours. These permit the individual to not only escape, but also evoke protective responses from significant others. At this point, operant or response conditioning also comes into play.By eliciting family or peer support, this social contact can also reinforce avoidance behaviours (Sturmey et al 2002, Joy et la, 2003, Britton et al 2010).

Although operant conditioning plays a key role in maintaining avoidance or protection seeking, generalization usually involves a blending of reinforcement types. The conditioning experiences also reflect reconfiguring long term potentiation (LTM) and changes in neuronal-synaptic interconnections and communication (Hades, 1985). Repeated exposure can solidify learned associations by a process of sensitization that can eventually contribute to the automazation of these stimulus response chains into pre-potent responses. This consolidation of these conditioned event-response chains is the result of reconfiguring synaptic and dendritic connections that facilitate the recruitment of additional resources from other neuronal systems. This process serves as the foundation for generalization of fear-response chains and underlies the transformation to more generalized responses to vague or diffuse threats. This process is much like kindling in epilepsy, mood disorders and substance abuse. The end result of these transformations is increased resistance to extinction (Post, 2007; Hefner, 2008; Gorman et al, 2010).

In contrast to fear, anxiety is a state-related affective change that remains disproportionate to the reality of internal or external threats (Neumiester et al 2003). Anxiety-mediated behaviors represent the metamorphosis of a fear/flight-fight or freeze responses. In this respect, anxiety is the neurobiological analog to widely generalized fear conditioning that is now recruiting from a much wider neuronal field (Heilman, 1997). In time this field includes linkages between the extended amygdala, hippocampus, and brainstem nuclei for multiple neurotransmitter systems, hypothalamic connections including the sympathetic adrenal-medullary and hypothalamic-adrenal axes (Stahl et al 2008), insular, orbitofrontal, striatal, medial prefrontal, cingulate and other associational or heteromodal cortices (Cherney et al 2002; Kada et al 2003; Fudge et al 2003; Millhelm et al 2005). The complexity of these interactions suggests that although related to fear, anxiety involves higher levels of integration between nominally compartmentalized networks devoted to perception, more nuanced forms of affective expression, cognitions and motor responses (Davis 2002). Anxiety is experienced through extensive recruitment and cross-communication between these systems. To achieve this level of integration requires extensive interaction between prefrontal and associational cortices; highly processed sensory input; limbic and motor circuits; and complex memory functions (Northoff et al 2002; Britton et al 2010).

Recent data suggests that obsessions and compulsive behaviors are the result of dysfunctional gating mechanisms- dysregulation of limbic input.Recruitment of other cognitive and memory sources and compromised top down regulation from the hippocampus, prefrontal and other heteromodal cortices (Harmon-Jones et al, 2007). This imbalance permits threat and conflict mediated sensory input intrude upon ongoing cognitive activity and release an automatic, but restricted group of stereotyped behavioral responses. These compulsions temporarily reduce the need to respond to the perceived threat but often at the expense of more adaptive behavioral responses. As we shall discuss later, the ethological model suggests that some forms of OCD may arise from the release of selected ritualistic behavior as a means of resolving similar conflict-mediated responses. In either case these escape or ritualized responses are enhanced by operant factors, especially negative reinforcement (Sturmey et al 2002). These conditioned links are also subject to sensitization and evolving resistance to reversal learning and extinction (Post et al 1998).

Yet even though these learning experiences are universal, most people do not develop PTSD (Stein et al 2002; King 12010), panic disorder-agoraphobia (Stein et al 2008; Koh et al 2010), generalized anxiety (Schienle, 2011; Turk et al 2011) or OCD (Atamura et al 2007; Stein 2008) or OCD. Later in this chapter we will address the underlying neurobiology of individual vulnerability to anxiety disorders but for now we will shift our attention to a group with significant deficits in adaptive and problem solving skills (fluid intelligence) as well as top down regulation of conditioned limbic subcortical responses.(Northoff, 2002; Stevens et al ,2007). This group includes individuals with IDD and autism (ASD). Individuals with severe IDD/ASD are also constrained by reductions in communication and problem solving skills as well as co-occurring brain disorders such as CP and epilepsy (Barnhill, 2000; Harris et al, 2009). These ADD: neurodevelopmental deficits also impact early attachment as well as interpersonal and emotional development (Althoff et al 2010). In addition, challenging experiences such as maternal depression, marital and/or family dysfunction, and extra-familial, psychosocial stress can overwhelm the individual's adaptive and problem solving skill (Hiem et al 2002;Haley et al 2003; Feldman et al, 2009) . Chronic stress can derail the neuro-endocrine regulatory organization and expression of stress responses while also adversely affecting new learning and more effective coping skills (Rueda et al 2007; Gunnar et al 2007).

Anxiety disorders are mental disorders characterized by negative affective experiences; specific patterns of responding to these state related changes; persistence; waxing and waning course and sufficient intensity to interfere with daily functioning (Costello et al 2005). Panic disorder (Nedstadt et al 2010) and OCD (Cooper et al 2007) appears more highly heritable than PTSD (Perez-Edgar et al 2005) or generalized anxiety disorders (Schienle et al 2011). Other anxiety disorders represent a more complex interaction between temperamental factors such as behavioral inhibition or high levels of neuroticism and life experiences (Merikanaga et al , 2009)). For these temperament-life experience dominated forms of anxiety, the major contributing factors may be less obviously genetic in origin and more the result of ongoing transactions between affective reactivity, negative emotional reactions to many environmental and social interactions; patterns of avoidance behaviors and life experiences. Another key factor is related to their high rates of comorbidity with other mental disorders (Perez-Edgar, 2005; Kagan et al 2007). But this is by no means a rigid asymmetry in gene-environment interactions. For example, until recently PTSD and other severe stress mediated conditions were considered as reactive disorders that occurred in response to overwhelming stress of aberrant social/emotional nurturing (Hiem et al 2002). Reality is not so simple. As we shall see later genetic factors associated with serotonin transporter protein activity (Sugden et al 2010), epigenetic changes affecting corticotrophin releasing factor receptors production and sensitivity and threshold of sympathetic arousal all play key roles in individual vulnerability to these stress reactions (Gunnar et al, 2007; Stahl et la 2008). These same forces are also operating in persons with IDD and ASD in which compromised adaptive and problem solving skills contribute to increased vulnerability and the high prevalence rates for anxiety related mental disorders in this population (Witwater et al 2008; Lunsky et al 2009).

3. Neuro-ethology and anxiety, anxiety disorders

Ethological analyses are useful tools for exploring the social-behavioural underpinnings of anxiety disorders. Their value is due in large part to the integration of neurobiology and social behaviour. This union provides into problems of social communication, reciprocity in interpersonal relationships and species-specific patterns of responding to perceived conflict. In this brief section we will apply ethological principles to subdividing anxiety based on its relationship to threat and threat perception, patterns of ritualized behaviors during conflicted social encounters with social dominance, disapproval, territoriality and group synchrony. Included also are attachment and attachment-proximity-seeking behaviors (Harris, 1996; Barnhill, 2000b). This approach is of limited utility for understanding panic attacks per se but may be useful in analyzing separation anxiety (attachment)), patterns of avoidance and co-morbidity of OCD and Panic disorder. The following demonstrate a few of these ethological concepts:

3.1 Panic-defensive aggression

Panic disorder, PTSD phobias and social anxiety disorders display a pattern of exaggerated fear response, increased hypothalamic-pituitary-adrenal drive and activation of the sympathetic nervous system in response to selected stimuli (Charney et al 2002). Aside from some rituals seen among individuals with performance anxiety, most affected individuals try to escape or submerge their anxiety (Neurmeister et al 2002). Fear conditioning is a major factor in PTSD and panic disorders and escape or avoidance behaviors that can perpetuate symptoms (Stein, 2002; Cooper et al 2007). Panic and phobic responses are less likely to be associated with rituals but do appear analogous to some flight behaviors (Barnhill 2000a, b). As a result, some forms of defensive aggression may occur during panic attacks (escape routes blocked) or during a flashback or other intrusive experiences in PTSD. In addition less intense forms of defensive aggressive may function as ritualized displacement behaviors (Harris 1996; Barnhill, 2000b). Agoraphobia can lead to chronic social isolation and anticipatory and context-dependent anxiety about the occurrence of rare panic attacks. A curious aspect of agoraphobia involves an individual's ability to use key people to compensate for avoidance behaviors (Gorman et al 2002; Chavira et al 2005). In this circumstance, ritualized proximity seeking (attachment behaviors) can mobilize group "protective behaviors", but over time may reinforce avoidance behaviors.

3.2 Social anxiety, dominance hierarchies and appeasement gestures

Generalized social anxiety represents a pattern of avoidance behaviors in response to social exposure and fears of being humiliated (Chavira et al, 2005). Many of these behaviors are analogous to problems associated with dominance conflicts and defeat-related (Swedo, 1989; Harris, 1996; Barnhill, 2000). In this paradigm, social anxiety represents an over activation of threat perception (disapproval, ostracism or attack) coupled with a lower threshold for behavioral inhibition (temperamental trait); reduced habituation to repeated exposure and resistance to extinction. There is an interplay between behavioural inhibition and over-reactive adrenergic responses to perceived threat or disapproval. Both temperamental and neurophysiological responses are related to misinterpreting neutral or ambiguous facial expressions (Alfano et la 2009). These state and trait patterns of affective response may explain the extensive comorbidity of social anxiety with several other internalizing disorders (mood, social anxiety and some forms of separation anxiety) and OCD. In addition, among nonhuman primates defeat contributes to submissive postures and increased grooming dominant members of the group. These behaviours also have analogues in social anxiety disorder and OCD (Feinstein et al, 2007; Baldwin et al, 2008). For example, cleaning/grooming may have its origins in conflicts over social dominance that predate our modern pre-occupation with germs. Ritual impurity or failing to live up to social group norms most likely predates contamination/cleaning rituals and checking rituals (Seuss et al 1989; Zohar et al 1991). OC Spectrum disorders like BDD and other disorders of excessive grooming may have similar origins. The need to escape such situations may play a more significant role in OCD than in the approach-mediated behaviors associated with some OCSDs.

3.3 Attachment- proximity seeking

Disrupted attachment and exaggerated proximity seeking behaviors create long term risks for psychopathology. Genetic risk factors for mood/anxiety disorders influence the transition from compromised attachment to psychiatric disorders (Koda et al, 2003; Barnhill 2007a; Ursano et al 2007). Lacking this genetic vulnerability, children with ambivalent and disorganized patterns of attachment remain at risk for both internalizing and externalizing disorders. Current social neuroscience research suggests that ongoing parental non-responsiveness, asynchronous reactions to infant signals, as well as abuse and neglect influence gene activation and modulation of stress response pathways (Gunnar et al 2007). These epigenetic events are critical to shaping the organization, intensity and threshold for neuroendocrine and sympathetic nervous system responses to later separation (Koda et al 2009). In the long term, these events result in an increased risk for deficits in stress and anxiety tolerance (Reiss, 2002), exploratory behaviors (Matthews et la 2008), threat perception and mastery of demands and new learning (Gunnar et al, 2007) . They can also influence exploratory behaviors, novelty seeking and involvement in key social learning experiences. Exaggerated sensitivity to danger or threat cues from parents and proximity-seeking attachment behaviors can be shaped by operant farces (social reinforcement). . These events influence the development of reactive attachment disorder (Barnhill 2007b), separation anxiety (Suveg et al 2005; Stahl et al 2010) , panic disorder/agoraphobia and later developing personality disorders (Hiem et al 2003; Feldman, 2009; Posnin et al, 2009; Knapp et al, 2011).

3.4 Rituals- compulsions

Ritualization in ethological terms represents a pattern of repetitive species-specific behaviors that can defuse ambiguous social confrontations, decrease the likelihood of attack, and convey social information about dominance (Harris 1996; Barnhill 2000 a and b). Ritualization in this sense lies on a continuum between obsessive and selected repetitive behaviours. As we shall see, transient rituals occur during normal development (Leonard, 1989). Dysfunctional rituals are more likely to occur in individuals with anomalous brain development (prefrontal injuries and perseveration); territorial and dominance challenges (social space and status issues); genetic risks for OCD; ASD and severe IDD (Pauls et al 2002; Bucan et al 2008); and degenerative disorders affecting fronto-striatal regulatory pathways (Mataix et al 2008). These behaviors are analogous to fixed action patterns (ritualized display behaviors) triggered by innate releasing mechanisms (social threat and conflict) (Swedo 1989, Harris 1996, Barnhill 2000b). Problems with excessive grooming behaviours are also driven by working memory deficits, difficulty disengaging from ongoing behaviors (checking behaviors) and worries about violating social taboos or cultural norms. These neuropsychological deficits play a role in contamination and cleaning rituals- especially in societies lacking our concerns with sanitation and cleanliness (Seuss et al 1989). This ethological/social acceptability subgroup also provides insights into BDD, anorexia nervosa, hypochondriasis and trichotillomania (Barnhill 2007; Fineberg et al 2006).

An ethological focus is of greatest value for clinicians dealing with nonverbal persons with severe-profound IDD. It is quite helpful to have a good working knowledge of ethology as a means of understanding nonverbal communication as it relates to aggression, SIB or stereotypies (Flavell, 1982). An ethological focus can also be useful in integrating information about challenging behaviors drawn from functional behavioral analyses-especially behaviors that appear mediated by social attention, or as a means of communicating pain or distress (Hall et al, 1992; Petty et al 2009). Self-injurious behaviors evolve during childhood from nonverbal forms of proto-imperative communication of immediate needs. In vulnerable children, these "distress" behaviors can morph over time from escape or avoidance behaviors into severe SIB. This transformation suggests roles for both associatively conditioned automatic responses and those operant learning experiences that serve to maintain by negative reinforcement. The missing piece is what forces shape this transformation in some individuals and not others (Flavell et al, 1982; Hall et al 1992; Hall et al 2001; Gardner , 2002; , Oliver et al 2005).

An ethological model also segues into integrating social responsiveness and communication, generalization of earlier learning experiences and sensitization/interactive specialization (changes in the molecular dynamics of gene, neuronal, and neurotransmitter adaptations). Ethological data can also provide a useful starting point for defining endophenotypes of ritualistic/anxiety mediated behaviors among individual with OCD, ASD, and SPID.

4. Developmental sources of anxiety and repetitive behaviors

Repetitive behaviors are common throughout much of childhood. Developmentally appropriate magical thinking and rituals help young children cope with normal childhood fears and anxieties. Later in childhood these rituals are incorporated into games, or "harmless habits" or superstitions (rabbit's feet, whistling past graveyards, salt over the shoulder). By late latency hero myths and fairy tales permit unconscious reworking of earlier anxieties. They allow the child to join the hero as he or she masters new concerns about family, academic performance in industrialized societies, and learning gender specific social roles, adult occupational skills and the intricacies of ritual life in non-industrialized settings (Leonard, 1989; Vaccarino et al, 2003; Barnhill, 2008b).

Later in childhood, rapidly developing cognitive-reasoning skills and approaching puberty signal another transformation. The ascendency of concrete and later formal operational thought permit future planning and worries, growing independence from the family of origin and emergence of issues related to status In the social hierarchy. By late childhood and early adolescence peer disapproval replaces perceptions of parental disapproval as a source of social anxiety (Gunnar et al 2007). In addition, cognitive maturation further insulates the child from the re-experiencing these childhood fears and magical thinking by binding them to more complex cognitions and defense mechanisms. In industrialized societies, these cognitive changes set the stage for an increasing reliance on scientific-rational causality. As a result magic devolves into entertainment as scientific modes of thought replace supernatural causality. Discordant or idiosyncratic religious beliefs can also foster anxieties about meeting the demands of religious communities. Among persons vulnerable to OCD these uncertainties are transformed into pre-occupations and ruminations (Suess et al 1989; Leonard et al, 2005; Barnhill, 2008).

Collective forms of fantasy and imagination are represented in magic and supernatural beliefs about causality (Seuss et al, 1989). For older children make-believe is replaced by shared social rituals and some devaluation of earlier modes of coping with of childhood fears. Yet even though reality is distinguished from earlier modes of thought and emotional expressiveness, these boundaries remain semi-permeable. During periods of stress or in creative play the boundary between ritual and realization is crossed by superstitions such the odd dressing and on field behaviors of some athletes, attempts to avoid stepping on cracks in the side walk, knocking on wood etc (Ursano et al, 2009).

During late childhood, and on into adolescence there is a growing divergence between adaptive fantasy and rituals of neuro-typical and those found in persons with IDD. For children with IDD, these earlier modes of fantasy-ritual expression may continue, leaving clinicians in limbo regarding whether these residual expressions are the result of developmental delays or "fixations" relative to developmental age- e.g. playing with toys or building blocks after coming home from high school or watching the same cartoon as a younger sibling (Leonard 1989). Children with ASD on the other hand, may have limited interest in play or social fantasy and prefer instead to line up toys or "play" alone. In a similar vein children who are genetically at risk for OCD are already expressing worries and rituals of at risk children differ from those of "normal children" (Black et al 2008; Baldwin et al 2008). For vulnerable children, magical beliefs, superstitions and rituals do not resolve but morph into patterns that are consistent with sub-clinical or full syndrome OCD. Not all children who reach this sub-clinical stage however will progress to full-blown OCD (Black et al 2008).

These changing patterns of magical beliefs, reasoning and ritualistic play do not occur in a vacuum but in the context of expanding social interests and desire to fit in. Successful transitions facilitate resilience in the face of complex endocrine andneurobiological changes. For example, social and learning experiences are shaped by temperamental factors (e.g. behavioural inhibition and high harm avoidance); deficits in language, social and cognitive skills; imaginative play and anxiety-mediated limits on exploratory behaviours and experiences with toys and enriching environments (Barnhill, 2008). By mid-adolescence there is a surge in the expression of genetic risk for specific disorders such as mood disorders, social anxiety and OCD. This is also a time when genetic vulnerability (positive family history), sexual maturation and yearning for novel experiences, an emerging developmental imbalance between heightened sensitivity to potential rewarding stimuli and need for external events to maintain positive affective states and maturation of top down regulation play increasingly critical roles in neuro-typically developing youth (McClure et al 2007; Kiddle et al, 2011).

This transformation overlaps the emergence of social anxiety, panic, OCD, major depressive disorder, OCSD/addictions in at risk children (Crews et al, 2007; Beesdo et a; 2009; Franc et al, 2010). These changes are also occurring among individuals with IDD and ASD (Joy et al 2003;. Cooray et al,2007). These some children with mild IDD face an additional problem- the growing realization that they are different and alienated from their peers. For adolescents with ASD/IDD uncertainty, limited ability to intuit social cues and impaired language pragmatics create increasing levels of stress and escalation in worries, and regression to modes of ritualistic behaviors (Barnhill, 2008; Jacob et al, 2009; Balemans et al 2010; Smith et al, 2010).

5. The problem of dimensional variability of OCD among individuals with IDD

OCD is an anxiety disorder characterized by intrusive thoughts and repetitive behaviors actions that interfere with a variety of daily activities and routines. Current data suggest that the prevalence rates for OCD range between 1 -2% of the population (Costello et al, 2005; King et al 2007;). The prevalence rates triple if we expand to include at risk individuals or those with subsyndromal OCD (failure to meet full criteria for OCD (Mataix e al 2008; Siminoff et al, 2008). Longitudinal studies also suggest that nearly 50% of this group will develop full syndrome OCD in time. Those converters are characterized by an early age of onset, positive family history of OCD and additional comorbid anxiety disorders (Murphy et al 2003; Black et al, 2008; Ginsberg et al 2008).

In behavioral terms OCD is a response to distress created by disturbing cognitions, images, urges (obsessions). These experiences trigger a restricted set of avoidance behaviors (cleaning, checking etc). These behaviors provide temporarily relief from the dysphoria and anxiety associated with obsessions these experiences. This pattern is best characterized as an escape from aversive cognitions (negative reinforcement). Over time these escape behaviors become increasingly ingrained and resistant to nonsystematic approaches to extinction (Noll et al, 2002; Prado et al, 2008; Sukhedalsky et al 2010).

Recent factor analytic studies report four major subgroups of obsessive and compulsive symptoms. These are pure obsessions, obsessions with compulsions such as anxiety about contamination leading to cleaning rituals; uncertainties about the completeness of actions contributing to doubting and checking; increased urge to arrange and order, organize and seeking balance in symmetry of thought and action; and hoarding (DeMathis et al , 2006; Mataix-Cols et al, 2008; Saxena, 2008). In addition to OCD, there are two subsets of OC-like symptoms, hoarding, and arranging, symmetry, counting and ordering rituals that are currently classified as Obsessive-compulsive Spectrum Disorder (OCSD). OCSD is further characterized by compliance with premonitory urges that differ from avoidance or escape from adverse emotional experiences or resulting behaviours (obsessions and compulsions). In addition, this group of patients also display higher rates of impulse control disorders and a propensity to react with anger or aggression when these repetitive behaviours are restricted(Fineberg et al 2007; Barnhill 2008; Pallanti et al, 2008). People with OCSD also differ from those with OCD in terms of high novelty seeking (impulsive risk taking) rather than behavioral inhibition/harm avoidance, and findings from neuropsychological testing, neuropharmacological trials and neuroimaging studies (Barnhill, 2008). These studies also note the relationship between intrusive aggressive, sexual or asocial urges and impulses and tic disorders. These studies also link hoarding with tic disorders and ASD (Kana et al 2007; Pallanti et al 2008, Saxena, 2008)).

Many individuals with IDD/ASD and severe sensory abnormalities also engage in stereotypic behaviors that function as an escape from overstimulation (Sayers et al, 2011). A similar pattern of escape-mediated, repetitive behaviors is also associated with psychophysiological distress secondary to pain, medical disorders, medication side effects and other environmental factors. In addition, individuals with IDD frequent display lower levels of stress tolerance, display exaggerated emotional, cognitive and behavioral reactions to environmental or interpersonal disruptions. Regressive behaviors in response to such stressors can also serve an escape function. Although not classified as OCD or OCSD these behaviors are likely to persist (negatively reinforced behavior), generalize and become increasingly resistant to extinction. It is noteworthy that the function and pattern of reinforcement for these behaviors is similar to that seen in obsession-triggered compulsive behaviors observed in OCD. Typologically, they differ in terms of a more diverse repertoire of repetitive behaviors than associated with OCD (contamination/washing-cleaning and doubting checking). These subtle differences pose problems with the differential diagnosis of OCD in persons with SPID (Noll et al 2002; Hoch et al, 2002; Barnhill 2008; Petty et al, 2009) .

We can also expand the 4-factor model of OCD by including food seeking and hoarding; impulsive-compulsive behaviors associated with compulsive computer use, stealing, shopping; pre-occupation with and compulsive attempts to correct quasi-delusional beliefs about dysmorphic appearance or disturbed body image (body dysmorphic disorder and anorexia nervosa) (Barnhill, 2007); self-grooming behaviors (skin picking, trichotillomania) and hypersensitivity to body sensations and uncertainties about health (hypochondriasis) (deMathis et al 2006; Stewart et al, 2008). Many of these OCSD symptoms are accompanied by comorbid anxiety/mood disorders, unstable negative affective responses associated with personality disorders (Borderline Personality Disorder) (Niedstadt et al, 2011); impulse control disorders including ADHD (Rifkin et al 2007; Farrone et al, 2010), other disruptive behavior disorders and addictions(Stevens et al 2007; Barnhill, 2010), delusional disorders, psychosis and schizophrenia; fronto-temporal dementias and other neurodegenerative disorders (Barnhill, 2008).

6. Autism, obsessive-compulsive behavior, and intellectual and developmental disabilities

Autism is a neurodevelopmental syndrome characterized by behavioral deficits in social functioning, language acquisition and usage, overly restrictive cognitive and inflexible behaviors and interests (Joy et al, 2003; Novotny et al 2003). Once considered a rare disorder, current data suggest that the actual prevalence rates for autism and related disorders (ASD) may be as high as 1:150 to 160 children (Ronald et al 2001; Jacob et al, 2009). The most likely reasons for this surge in prevalence rates include: changes in diagnostic criteria that widen the net for children at the mild end of the spectrum; heightened awareness among parents, classroom teachers, primary care physicians and mental health professional; better diagnostic tools; recognition of milder forms of ASD (Welschew, 2007), especially those not associated with intellectual disability; and the increasing potential impact of environmental toxins (Gunnar, 2007; Johnson et al, 2007; Siminoff et al 2008). In recent years there is an increasing emphasis on earlier recognition and implementation of aggressive behavioral interventions. This drive is in part related to data supporting more dramatic improvements from highly focused and intensive treatments during toddlerhood. The long term goal is to alter the developmental trajectory of children with ASD and IDD (Myers, 2007; Schaer et al 2007; Howlin et al, 2008)

These prevalence studies also point out several features not addressed in the diagnostic criteria. One major finding is the strong gender dimorphism in which males are at least 4-5 times more likely to express ASD (Avramopoulus 2010; Grafodotskaya et al, 2010; El-Fishaway et al, 2011). This degree of dimorphism is most dramatic among male probands in families with more than one affected child (multiplex families); increased frequency of ASD among first degree relatives; and in families in which one or both parents express subsyndromal impairments in social communication and cognitive/behavioral inflexibility (expanded behavioral phenotype) (Travis et al, 1998; Novotny et al 2003; Lunsky et la 2009). These findings dovetail into the ongoing genetic research that argues for the role of polygenic inheritance of rare alleles is responsible for heritability rates approaching 90% for ASD. But heritability studies run into a roadblock in singleton families in which only one child in the sibship is affected. ASD in these families is most likely linked to with known IDD, chromosomal and genetic/metabolic syndromes. Examples include conditions such a tuberous sclerosis, Rett's syndrome, phenylketonuria, Angelman's syndrome, FRAXA and nearly 40 other syndromes. Singleton families who chose not to have additional children can create similar uncertainties in the heritability data (Betancur et al, 2010; El-Fishaway et al 2010; Ronald et al 2011).

Neuroimaging studies of probands with ASD provide strong evidence for aberrant early brain development that includes neurogenesis, cell migration, white matter and structural organization of the brain regions such as the cerebral cortex, cerebellum and greater amygdala (Schaer et al 2000; Leckman et al 2003) . Microscopic analysis reveals problems with dendritic and synaptic integrity and stability, arborization and cellular maturation (Novotny et al, 2003). When combined, these findings reinforce the heterogeneity of ASD as well as support the final common pathway hypothesis (Betancur et al 2010) . Support for the idea of a final common pathway also comes from studies of primary and secondary ASD, and indirectly, from studies involving discordant monozygotic twins; and symptomatic diversity among multiple probands in multiplex families. From this data we can conclude that ASD is the result of multiple genes that influence and are influenced by complex gene-environmental and brain-behavior interactions (Ramocki et al 2009; Balemans et al, 2010; Ronald et al 2011)..

There are higher rate of comorbid psychiatric, neurocognitive (limited interests), language based learning disabilities and communication disorders (deficits in communication pragmatics and stereotyped speech) among families with ASD probands (Tavis et al, 1998; Smith et al 2010). The presence of OC-like symptoms lends further support the polygenic inheritance and the degree of overlap with OCD, Tic Disorders and ADHD (Barnhill, 2005). This data also reveals that the risk for ASD drops off rapidly when investigators focused on more distant relatives. These findings also suggest an answer to the clinical observation that many patients with treatment resistant OCD (Jacobs et al, 2009), and OC Personality Disorder (Baldwin et al, 2008) may in fact present with undiagnosed ASD. A downside to this argument is that when OCD and ASD co-occur, it is the ASD that exerts the more profound effects on both treatment response and clinical outcome. Both ASD and OCD are syndromes characterized by high heritability but different patterns of brain neurodevelopmental anomalies (Volpe, 2000; Joy et al, 2003; Knapp et al, 2009). With caution, there are differences can be useful for defining endophenotypes of OC behaviors and designing neuroscientific and neuropharmacological research (Hounie et al 2006; Jacob et al, 2009).

7. Behavioral phenotypes, ASD, OC behaviors

There are several behavioral phenotypes that are useful in teasing out and defining genetic subtypes of OCD among persons with IDD and ASD (Feinstein et al 2007; Levitas et al 2007). For example, Fragile X syndrome (FRAXA) is an X-linked form of IDD associated with a behavioral phenotype characterized by gaze aversion, speech dysfluency, social anxiety and avoidance behaviors, repetitive behaviors and increased risk for complex partial seizures and paroxysmal episodes or panic-like symptoms. Males with the full syndrome are frequently diagnosed with ASD (Joy et al 2003; Lambroso et al 2008). On closer inspection, many affected individuals present with anxiety that appears more closely related to social anxiety and exaggerated avoidance behaviors than compromised social communication observed in ASD. Among both pre-mutational as well as full-syndrome females, there are increased problems with neurocognitive deficits, difficulties with social relatedness, and language development. In both groups, the preservation of social relationships in familiar settings become useful tools in the differentiating ASD from FRAXA without ASD (Barnhill 2000a and b).

Prader-Willi/Angleman's, Cornelia de Lange, Rett's (Ghidoni et al, 2007; Cahro et al, 2010), Velocardiofacial (Gothelf, 2007) and Chromosome Xq15.13 duplication are associated with ASD, OC related repetitive behaviors, IDD, and social communication deficits. A substantial minority of individuals with 15q11-13 duplications present with ASD based on impairments in cognition, social relatedness and behavior. Many affected individuals also present with increased rates of anxiety/OC spectrum disorders (El-Fishaway, et al 2010). For most, the typology of OC behaviors does not meet the criteria for OCD but instead present with hoarding, SIB, skin picking, aligning, arranging and other rituals (Levitas et al, 2007). Under these circumstances the diagnosis of OCD may not be appropriate and are best classified as Stereotypic Movement Disorder (Barnhill, 2006; Barnhill et, al 2007).

8. Obsessive-compulsive disorder, repetitive behaviors, and abnormal movements

The co-occurrence of repetitive behaviors, intellectual disability, and underlying movement disorders provides a viable test case for investigating a hypothesized linkage between repetitive behaviors, tics and abnormal movements, fronto-striatal dysfunction and psychopathology (Welschew et al, 2005; Barnhill, 2005a; Joostin et al, 2010). Aside from neurodegenerative syndromes, most movement disorders are characterized by waxing/waning and topographically variable patterns of repetitive movements. Most are also associated with cognitive, emotional and behavioral symptoms that are associated with dysfunctional fronto-striatal-limbic and ventral basal ganglia systems (Robertson et al, 1996; Barnhill, 2007b). In Tourette's Disorder, most affected children present with simple motor and vocal tics. But 5-10% may progress to more complicated movements. This group may also develop prodromal urges or sensations to move. Ticqueing can temporarily satisfy this state of heightened motivation. A feeling that things are "just right" frequently terminates these apparently voluntary motor actions. In addition these behaviors also permit the individual to escape from the unpleasant or annoying sensation (Leckman et al 2003; Prado et al 2008; de Mathis et al 2010). There is considerable overlap between neuronal circuits involved with these escape functions and negative reinforcement, OC behaviors and abnormal movements. Upon closer analysis however, the abnormal movements are neither voluntary nor involuntary but appear related to urges rather than anxiety. These responses represent a mixture of voluntary, repetitive motor responses to involuntary urges to think or act. Although this mixture of motivational states is also characteristic of OC spectrum disorders (OCSD) additional research is needed to differentiate these behaviors from complex sensory tics (Robertson et al 1996; Nedstadt et al 2010).

The onset of OCD in males under 5 is associated with the emergence of tics within three to five years of onset. These boys belong to families with loading for both Tourette's disorder and OCD. Young girls share different ages of onset, clinical symptomatology and clinical outcomes. For affected females are genetically at risk and far are more likely to develop obsessive-compulsive disorder. This observation suggests a gender bias towards obsessive-compulsive symptoms rather than motor or phonic tics (Nedstadt et al 2010; Grados et al, 2010). There are also phenomenological differences between obsessive-compulsive symptoms associated with tics and those without. For example, contamination/cleaning and doubting/checking rituals are less common among individuals with tics (Rasmussen et al 2002). The group presenting with tic disorder is more likely to develop arranging, organizing, need for symmetry, and various impulsive-compulsive symptoms (Leckman et al, 2003). Even though obsessions are less likely, intrusive images or aggressive sexual or religious preoccupations are more likely (Suess et al 1989; Pallinta et al, 2008; Jacob etc al, 2009). Obsessions in tic disorders appear analogous to mental tics or perhaps intrusive symptoms observed in PTSD (King et al, 2010). As noted above, premonitory urges present as a building tension that frequently precedes complex tics among individuals with tic disorders (Leckman et al 2003; Prado et al, 2008). In general, attempts to inhibit these urges do not generate anxiety, but instead contributes to an increasing intensity. This contrasts with the usual anxiety/obsession-driven, ego alien behaviors commonly associated with OCD.

Among individualswith ASD these difference can be more difficult to appreciate (Barnhill, 2007b; King et al, 2007). These distinctions are even more difficult to make among individuals with co-occurring SPID. In this population it is difficult to differentiate these more ambiguous repetitive behaviours from complex tics and stereotypies/ritualistic behaviors. For example, self-injurious behavior is also associated with severe tic disorders with IDD/ASD (Barnhill, 2005a). In affected individuals SIB presents in at least three forms. One presents as the consequence of a low intensity/high frequency pattern of repetitive behaviors that eventually result in tissue damage. Cuticle and other forms of skin picking, nail biting and trichotillomania are examples (Leckman et al 2003; De Mathis et al, 2006) . These "aberrant grooming behaviors" frequently occur during "down time" or reduced environmental stimulation. Severe SIB on the other hand can occur in "binges" of high frequency/high intensity repetitious hitting, nail pulling, and eye poking, touching hot objects and other driven-behaviors. These usually terminate when the individuals reports that things now "feel right." Another group is triggered by prodromal sensations, pain and discomfort. Their SIB is directed at the affected body part. There appears to be some overlap between this form of SIB and Lesch-Nyhan syndrome (Levitas et al, 2007), neuro-acanthocytosis and other neurogenetic behavioral phenotypes (Barnhill, 2003; 2010). Two characteristics are especially striking: persistence of SIB in spite of intact pain perception and the frequent use of self-restraint to interrupt the compulsive drive to self-injury (Barnhill 2003a, 2005b; 2010).

The treatment of OC behaviors in individuals with Tourette's disorder also differs from commonly used treatment interventions for patients with OCD. For example, habit reversal therapies appear more effective for tic/OC behaviors than exposure-response prevention, and cognitive-behavioral training (Roblek et al 2005; Howlin et al, 2009). One explanation is that tic-related OC behaviors are less likely to have associated obsession or premonitory urges that signal the individual to initiate the program. A second but not exclusionary explanation involves differences in the underlying neurobiology of tics/OC behaviors- e.g. differences in pre-movement potentials, caudate activation and medial prefrontal activation that render repetitive behaviors as habits rather than anxiety-driven behaviors. These differences may also explain why individuals with tic disorders and co-occurring obsessive-compulsive behaviors respond better to habit reversal than exposure-response prevention programs while being less sensitive to SSRIs to the point of frequently requiring a combination of SSRIs and neuroleptic drugs (Myers et al, 2007; Pallanti et al 2008; Stein 2008; Leckman et al 2003).

9. IDD, ASD and anxiety as developmental phenomena

IDD and ASD are the result of ongoing gene-environment interactions beginning during prenatal development. Many genetic disorders associated with IDD display considerable variability in terms of severity, dysmorphology, age of recognition and rapidity of psychomotor regression (Vacarrino et al, 2003; Barnhill, 2004; Bagot, et al 2010). The natural course of many of late-onset genetic disorders displays periods of autism-like behaviours. These transient "autisms" can be confusing to clinicians, especially for children with milder forms of the neuro-metabolic disorders. This pattern can also be seen in children with ASD but without IDD Bagot et al 2010, Betancur, 2010). Many parents of probands with ASD report that "something isn't right" with their infant. Unfortunately many describe a vague sense of emotional disengagement or disinterest in reciprocal parent-infant verbal and imitative "play". Other parents report "normal development" until 18-24 months of age followed by a regression in language about the time the child begins combining words into "sentences". A third group described dramatic regression to autistic like behaviors Beginning around 4 years of age, many of these children regress neurologically at highly individualized rates of decline. This subgroup is currently classified as Childhood Disintegrative Disorder (Novotny et al 2003).

Recent infant research describe early aberrant social interaction, lack of consistent response to their name and shared attention beginning between 9-18 months of age. In neuro-typical infants this period is associated with increasingly sophisticated reciprocal interaction, emergence of joint attention as both emotional engagement and early "learning" about the environment (Knap et al, 2009) . Social neuroscientists suggest that this emotional dance is involved in priming and entraining the language cortex (interactive specialization) (Fries et al 2007). In children at risk for ASD, this is also a time of a rapid expansion of head circumference and maturational disturbances in facial processing, emotional memory, and a preference for inanimate objects over human faces (Volpe, 2000, De Haan et al, 2009). Behaviorally these changes include emotional and social detachment, impaired locking onto speech and communication, emotional play, joint attention and pleasurable sharing with others (Knutson et al 2007; Dawson et al, 2009).

In general, the developmental impact of this impairment is related to the severity of ASD plus IDD. In contrast, infants with IDD only display attenuated but largely functional interests in social interaction, rudimentary communication and emotional attunement to parents (Fries et al 2007; Grey et al 2010). The presence of severe neurodevelopmental disorders also increases the probability of temperamental differences such as increased irritability, negative affective reactions to novelty or change, poor affect regulation and behavioral inhibition. During toddlerhood, behavioral inhibition is a risk factor for mood and anxiety disorders (including syndromal and subsyndromal OCD) later in life. Toddlers with high levels of motor activity, irritability, impulsivity and poor affect regulation are more at risk for high rates of repetitive behaviors and externalizing behaviors (Kagan et al,

2007). This group may be at greater risk for ADHD and in some cases disruptive behaviour disorders, addictions and some forms of OC spectrum disorders (Feinstein et al, 2007; Jacob et al, 2009).

This brief portrait of early development suggests a complex transaction between the infant, parent and the psychosocial environment. In addition to IDD and ASD, neglect and abuse can also have a profound effect on emotional attachment and sense of basic trust (Knapp et al, 2009). Maternal depression may also be equally distressing. The infant cannot elicit maternal responsiveness and will try valiantly to engage the affected parent. The chronic lack of intuitive nurturance and emotional responsiveness to the infant can result in the dysregulation of both the hypothalamic- pituitary- adrenal and sympathetic adrenal medullary pathways (Skuse et al 2003; Feldman et al 2009). At a behavioral level these changes compromise cognitive development and increase the risk of persistent high levels of emotional and neuroendocrine over responsiveness. Neurophysiological changes also impede novelty learning, exploratory behaviors and increase the levels of ritualistic and repetitive behaviors (Stahl et al, 2005; Romocki et al 2009; Joosten et al, 2010).

10. Genes, ASD, OCD, tic disorders and repetitive behaviors: A synthesis

For OCD, it is difficult to isolate a single gene, precise neuroanatomical lesion or single neurotransmitter system responsible for this syndrome (Murphy et al, 2003; Lehman et al, 2010). Functional neuro-imaging studies point to disequilibrium between the prefrontal-caudate, striatal and anterior cingulate prefrontal regulation (Pauls et al, 2002; Schaer et al 2007)). Neuropsychological studies point to problems with set shifting and regulation of sensory- motor responses, manipulation of social cues and decision-making. These findings support dysfunction in the fronto-striatal, limbic anterior cingulate, ventral striatum and multi-modal sensory cortices (Anderson et al, 2004; Mataix-Cols et al 2008)). Neuro-ethological studies describe regulatory deficits in terms of a"breakthrough" of grooming, territorial and conflict mediated ritualized behaviors (Harris, 1996; Barnhill, 2000b). Neuro-pharmacologically, there are both similarities and major differences between serotonin, dopamine, glutamate, opiate and other peptides and GABA systems. Many of these studies also reveal neurobiological differences between OCD and related OC behaviors (Pauls et al, 2002; Reinblatt et al, 2006; Waslick, 2006). These observationsmay explain the contributions made by overlapping but dysfunctional neurobiological mechanisms that underlie OCD and OCSD- the disruption in the convergence of social-emotional perceptual processing and the cross-talk between multiple neuronal networks involved in integrating and responding to this input. In this sense, OCD is but one possible expression of a dysfunctional pathway that can no longer efficiently reglate multiple interconnected systems of neurons.

The qualitative difference between the degree of impairment in social communication and cognitive/behavioural inflexibility are useful tools in the differential diagnosis of ASD from OCD among individuals with IDD (Barnhill, 2005a; Jacob et al, 2009; Ronald et al, 2011) . Persons with ASD but without IDD still display high levels of executive deficits, compromised coherence, language pragmatics and higher modes of social-emotional information processing. These differences also suggest fundamental differences in the timing of the "insults"- for ASD and IDD during embryological and early developmental; OCD somewhat later during maturation of regulatory pathways Barnhill, 2004; Northoff et al, 2006; Hofvander et al, 2009) For autism and schizophrenia the expression of these aberrant gene-environment interactions impact embryological events associated with neuro-genesis, cell migration, differentiation/maturation and stabilization of dendritic pathways (Betancur, 2010; Gorman et al 2010). At the other end of the gene-environment dimension, PTSD was once considered to result from overwhelming external stress (Stahl, 2010; Sugden et al 2010; Qureshi et al, 2011). Genetic risk factors or gene-environmental interactions were considered to be bystanders. This assumption proved premature. It also appeared that the neurodevelopmental events associated with OCD, mood and anxiety disorders fell somewhere in between. Full expression of these disorders provides more room for epigenetic effects- the phenotype for many late onset mental disorders require a second or third "hit". For example, the second hit for OCD may be the presence of tic disorders/basal ganglia disorders, gender effects, and in some cases, an additional developmental or acquired insults for full expression include PANDAS (Asbhar et al, 2005; McNally et al 2008),traumatic brain injury (Vasa et al, 2004; Max et al, 2011); onset of depression and neurodegenerative disorders (Barnhill, 2008b).

Genetic studies thus far reveal more than 100 separate alleles of interest associated with ASD (El-Fishaway et al, 2011). Many involve promoter or regulatory genes, histone chromatin and gene activation/deactivation during critical periods of embryological and postnatal brain development; localized protein production; aberrancies in several key neurotransmitter and intracellular pathways and disruption of signals for neuronal differentiation, dendritic activity, pruning and myelination (Gorman et al, 2002; Bird et al, 2008; Lombroso et al 2008). Each of these gene- environment interactions impact brain-behavior interactions that underlie the core symptoms of ASD. Many also play key roles in learning/memory; challenging behaviors and behavioral phenotypes among individuals with IDD; temperament/emotional processing/affect regulation, language development, social reciprocity and mental disorders (Kana et al, 2007; Vicarrino et al, 2008).

Data from multiplex families suggest a "critical mass" of rare genes is needed for the expression of full syndrome autism. Yet the gender –risk for ASD is substantially higher in males. In addition, recent studies also suggest that neither the severity nor gender of the affected probands predict the risk for ASD in other siblings and first degree relatives (Jacob et al, 2009; Mosconi et al , 2010). This observation suggests that at least for males the vulnerability to ASD may not be determined solely by quantitative threshold effects. This imply a model in which a threshold effect (sufficient number or alleles) or an or epigenetic effects on "Y" or genomically imprinted "X" chromosomes- contributing to gender biases in epidemiological data. This hypothesis also leaves room for the actions of mitochondrial genes, and chromosomal abnormalities such as copy number variants (deletions or duplications) or single nucleotide polymorphisms. These mechanisms point to sources of genetic variability among individuals with ASD. This diversity also provides a mechanism for how some individuals with atypical forms of OCD (including those probands with IDD) may lie on a continuum with the expanded phenotype of ASD (Avramopoulos, 2010; El-Fishaway et al 2011, Ronald et al,2011).

ASD brings several additional developmental issues to the table. Reduced coherence, facial processing deficits and early problems with synchrony and reciprocity of emotional and social communication suggest that ASD differs from OCD and tic disorders in terms of brain structure and function. These differences arise from the regulation of key genes during early brain development and maturation (Novotny et al 2003; Barnhill, 2004, 2005b). In part, ASD is the behavioural expression of an individual adapting to the disruption of embryological and early infant development; OCD, OCSD, tic disorders and secondary forms of while OCD represent later developmental challenges. This hypothesis is consistent with the observation that insults occurring in utero impact the organization of the CNS rather than functional changes acquired once those systems are in place (Pauls et al, 2002). This observation raises another interesting question. Are infants who are already at risk for ASD more sensitive to post-natal distress that is influenced by aberrant processing facial/emotional stimuli, inability to use synchrony of interaction for self-regulation; difficulty linking pleasure with facial cues; deficits in emotional memory, and severe problems eliciting and responding to mutual or reciprocal social responses (Lerner et al, 2005; Baranek et al, 2007; Feldman et al, 2009)?

These aberrant responses also set up a situation in which neurophysiological differences create a feedback loop in which faulty signaling or aberrant patters of emotional responding fails to elicit appropriate parental responses. This derailment of early development in turn creates a situation in which disturbances in infant-caregiver interactions are analogous to disrupted emotional interchanges (Gunnar, 2007….) The de-synchronization of these critical early attachment behaviours may represent a second potential hit in the development of ASD. In part, this derailment of early mirroring (and activity of mirror neurons) may have an analogue in the adverse effects of maternal depression on infant brain organization and emerging social/emotional and stress/response pathways. The events amplify the adverse effects of infant's genetically at risk for mood disorders (Feldman etc, 2009). To date we have limited data regarding the impact of parents with the expanded phenotype for ASD have on the development of synchrony, reciprocity, joint attention and emerging theory of the mind (Andrews et al, 2003,). It is also unclear what effects parental OCD or Tourette's disorder might have on an infant at genetic risk for behavioral inhibition or the neurocognitive/neurobiological substrates for both disorders (Barnhill, 2005b; Althoff et al, 2010). At a molecular level, these epigenetic effects on key genes may play a key role in the development, penetrance resistence (resilience) to many neuro-psychiatric disorders emergence (Bird et la , 2008; Bucan et al, 2008, Ramocki et al, 2009; Balemans et al, 2010, Stahl, 2010).

IDD plays a major role in the clinical expression and severity of ASD (Novotny et al, 2003). There is also ample clinical evidence that ASD frequently co-occurs with ADHD, tic/obsessive compulsive disorders and mood/anxiety disorders (El-Fishaway et al, 2011). The overlap with ADHD and ASD involves problems with inhibitory controls, executive functions and deployment of attentional resources (Farone et al 2010). Tourette's disorder (TD) and tic-related forms of OCD share increased rates repetitive aberrant social behaviors and attention (inhibition of intrusive thoughts and urges); dysregulation of fronto-striatal-thalamic-frontal circuitry, regulation of dopamine, glutamate and GABA activity; hyper-excitability and changes in refractory periods in the pre-motor cortex (Leckman et al 2003). Mood and anxiety disorders share sensitivities to compromised adaptive skills; temperament associated with behavioral inhibition; several alleles that help regulate neurotransmitter availability; and intracellular regulation of cAMP, kinases/phosphorylases and lipase activity, Brain Derived Nerve Growth Factor (BDNF) and cytokine production; and corticotrophin releasing factors receptor availability and other aspects of neuro-endocrine activity (Post, 2007; Bucan et al, 2008; Avramopoulos, 2010); . These intracellular pathways play a key role in ASD (El-Fishaway, 2010) and OCD (Pauls et al, 2002) but are largely unexplored among persons with IDD and comorbid mental disorders (Barnhill, 2006a; Kiddle et al, 2011).

Many of these systems are also involved in regulating stress response systems. By extension they also affect a child's vulnerability to persistent effects from abuse, neglect and psychological trauma. For example, the "ss" "sl" alleles in the promoter region of the serotonin transporter protein receptor are associated with an increased vulnerability to trauma (Sugden et al, 2010). They may also play a role in amygdala enlargement, abnormalities in neuronal migration, neurogenesis, synaptic function and regulation of neuro-endocrine responses observed in ASD . The functional activity in Catecholamine- O- Methyltransferase (COMT) (Stein et al, 2006; Albaugh et al, 2010) and regulation of corticotrophin releasing factor production (CRF receptors) (Hiem et al, 2003) also contribute to early brain development play and stress response pathways that eventually be linked to anxiety, PTSD and mood disorders (Gorman 2010). Promoter genes regulating glutamic acid decarboxylase and interneuron development are also associated with a range of neuropsychiatric disorders, epilepsy, and vulnerability to trauma and mood disorders (Barnhill, 2004; Rueda et al, 2007). All influence the link between environmental stress and repetitive behaviors.

The impact of genetic errors on brain development can play out in several directions. One involves regional versus cell-line specific effects. The adverse effects on a cell population arises from defective neurogenesis, insensitivity to trophic factors during early brain development; malfunctioning gene activation/deactivation during neuronal differentiation and maturation; later availability and effectiveness of nerve growth factors and other peptides that maintain as well as protect the integrity and functional viability of neurotransmitter receptors and the intracellular pathways essential for their action. Since most neurons have extensive dendritic interconnections with diverse cell types, developmental errors in neurogenesis, neuron migration and maturation can ramify throughout the developing brain. They are also at the core of many syndromes associated with specific neuro- embryological abnormalities (Barnhill, 2006; Bird et al, 2008; Bagot et al, 2010). Ongoing epigenetic effects, myelination, dendritic neuroplasticity and pruning are triggered by gene activation/silencing. At a structural level these forces shape the neuroanatomical differences between IDD, ASD, tic disorders, OCSD and OCD (Vaccarino et al, 2003). But their greatest long term impact may on the functional integrity and integration of multiple circuits (coherence) (Bagot et al, 2010; Stahl, 2010). As noted earlier, the clinical phenotype of neurodevelopmental disorders is the ever-changing expression of multiple gene-environment transactions. These multi-directional forces are critical to social, emotional, social/emotional communication, and cognitive development(Volpe, 2000; Pomeroy, 2000; Franic et al, 2010). As we have seen, development is a transactional process that relies on neuroplasticity, interactive specialization and integration of multiple brain regions. The gene-environment interactions during early development set the stage and write the script; but epigenetic forces shape all developmental disorders serve as the director and stage manager during the performance and . This metaphor should remind us of the nature-via-nurture model proposed by Ridley (2002) and how this transaction shapes the probability rather than determines the outcome.

11. Conclusions

In this chapter we explored the boundaries of OCD in persons with IDD by comparing and contrasting it with other forms of repetitive behaviors associated with ASD and Tourette's disorder. In particular, this analysis addressed the relationship between OCD and stereotypies/repetitive behaviors in ASD and IDD, OC Spectrum and complex tic disorders. Our review of this relationship generated several questions:

1. How are can we differentiate the impact these developmental disorders from those associated with comorbid mood, OC spectrum disorders and subsyndromal OCD? For example, the co-occurrence of a mood disorders shapes the core anxieties associated with OCD. Hypomania is associated with mood elevation, increased reward seeking behaviors and impaired judgment (Rifkin et al, 2007; Barnhill, 2008b; Bucan et al, 2008). These changes can influence the neuro-behavioral foundation of OCD- change the negative valence of obsessions and/or a shift towards approach rather avoidance or escape functions of compulsions (Barnhill, 2008b).This shift is more consistent OC spectrum disorders. Unfortunately the answer to this question is still a work in progress.
2. Complex tics, OCD and OCSD present with a waxing waning course that can include irritability and worsening of impulse controls. How are these related to mood cycles associated with bipolar disorder? Clinicians can approach these as two distinct phenomena characterized by periodicity. We can distinguish them based on the synchronization of tics and mood-behavior changes (depression increases, hypomania may decrease tic frequency and severity); differentiate irritability associated with a mood disorder from trait-related problems found in many impulse control disorders (as in OCSD); and use genetic and neuroscience data to provide a biological basis for assessing them as independent phenomena (Barnhill, 2005b; Barnhill, 2007b).
3. Is OCD associated with Tourette's syndrome, other neuropsychiatric disorders, bipolar disorder and borderline personality the same condition that co-occurs with social anxiety disorder? In each combination, OCD fits existing diagnostic criteria but the validity of the exclusion criteria that include TD, ASD, or brain disorders is less certain in individuals with severe IDD (King et al, 2007). This blurring of boundaries suggests that both the overlap and specificity of cortico-striatal, limbic and ventral basal ganglia dysfunction may be further muddled by IDD.

As noted, the presence of IDD and ASD makes it decidedly more difficult to answer these questions. These difficulties are often the result of problems encountered in the diagnostic process, especially communication difficulties; impaired understanding of the psychiatric assessment and the capacity to self-report; and sensitivity to catastrophic reactions to disruptions in attachment needs (staff changes) as well as other social and environmental stresses (Fletcher et al 2007). In addition, decreased adaptability associated with IDD and ASD increases the probability that stress will increase the expression of stereotypies, ritual, tics, OC behaviors and ritualized behaviors.

Yet most affected individuals do not present to clinics complaining of depression or troublesome obsessions or compulsions. Most present with a more ambiguous picture of an increase in pre-existing repetitive behaviors- baseline exaggeration (Fletcher et al, 2007). Differentiating these generic behaviors from OCD requires a careful algorithmic approach that is analogous to that used in delineating endophenotypes in research protocols- using both clinical and research data to better differentiate OCD from other repetitive behaviors associated with ASD and severe-profound IDD (Barnhill, 2008). Under these circumstances, it may be more practical to begin the diagnostic paradigm by outlining an endophenotype of repetitive behaviors then progressing to the diagnosis of OCD. Yet to clinicians, this diagnostic paradigm approach might be most useful in the assessment and treatment planning for diagnostic puzzlers or treatment resistant cases.

For the reader, it probably seems practical to exclude these reducing clinical heterogeneity by expanding exclusion and inclusion criteria to include various endophenotypes of repetitive behaviours. The end result of this process is a "purer" form of OCD based on more specific neurophysiologic, neuroimaging, neuropharmacological and genetic subtyping. Although more time consuming, this approach fine tunes our current system of behavioural observation, rating scales and self-reporting of symptoms (Maitaix-Cols et al 2008). For example OCD could be classified as an anxiety-driven syndrome driven associated with behavioral inhibition, neurophysiological markers of anxiety; specific involvement of the fronto-striatal systems on functional neuroimaging and neuropsychological studies, and neurochemical findings consistent with disruptions in serotonin release and post synaptic action; and an exclusive reliance on compulsions as escape behaviors in the face of internalized conflicts or perceived threats (Zohar et al, 1991; Barnhill, 2008). Even though this endophenotypic approach would tighten the diagnostic rigor for OCD and enhance research studies, there still would be problems adapting such a model by clinicians working with patients who haveS/PIDD (King et al, 2007; Barnhill, 2008) or ASD (Anderson et al. 2004; Schaer et al, 2007; Pauls et al, 2003; Bird et al, 2008; Bucan et al 2008).

Although much work remains several there are several important accomplishments:

1. Laying the groundwork for reframing obsessive compulsive spectrum disorders (including OCD), stereotypies-mannerisms and tic-like behaviors in neurological conditions such as Tourette's disorder as potential endophenotypes of repetitive behaviors.
2. Developing an understanding of repetitive behaviors from a dimensional perspective. Taking this approach reinforces the concept that OCD and repetitive behaviors in persons with IDD/ASD are not easily explained by any single model.
3. Addressing the heterogeneity of OCD in terms of phenomenology and underlying psychobiology, reciprocal social interactions (ethology), interaction between genes and environment in shaping (epigenetics) risk and phenomenology, social-emotional development (infant and childhood development) and learning theory.
4. Synthesizing data from functional behavioral and neuro-psychiatric assessments into a model that integrates brain-behavior with learning models for OCD, OCSD and other repetitive behaviors.
5. Focusing on repetitive behaviors as a final common pathway with multiple etiologies and then addressing the impact of ASD and IDD on these pathways. This model is the centerpiece for defining OCD as an endophenotypes of repetitive behaviors.

In closing, we are back to the basic issues raised at the beginning of this chapter. The eventual solution lies in not only ongoing research but synthesizing current available data into an explanatory rather solely descriptive model. Hopefully we progress beyond the stage of describing, categorizes and quantifying data and focus instead on providing explanations of why this is so. This chapter is but one small step towards such a synthesis.

12. Acknowledgement

I would like to acknowledge the assistance of Susan Palmatier in the preparation of this manuscript

13. References

Albaugh MD Harder V, Althoof RR, Rettew DC, Ehli EA, Lengyl-Nelson T, Davies GE, Ayer L, Sulman J, Stanger C and Hudziak JJ. COMT Val158Met Genotype as a Risk

Factor for Problem Behaviors in Youth.. *J Amer Acad Child and Adol Psychiatry* 49(8), 2010, pp 841-49.

Alfano CA, Pina AA, Villalta IK, Beidel DC, Ammerma RT, Crosby LE. Mediators and Moderators of Outcome in the Behavioral Treatment of Social Phobia. *J Amer Acad Ch Adolesc Psychiatry,* 48(11), 2009, pp 945- 53.

Altamura AC, Dell'Osso B, D'Ursa N, Fumagalli S, Mundo E (2008). Duration of Untreated Illness as a Predictor of Treatment Response and Clinical Course of General Anxiety Disorder, *CNS Spectrums* 12 (5), 2007, pp 415-24.

Althoff RR, Verhulst FC, Rettew DC, Hudziak JJ, van der Ende J. Adult Outcomes of Childhood Dysregulation, *J Am Acad Ch and Adol Psychiatry* 49(11), 2010, pp 105-116

Anderson KE, Savage CR. Cognitive and Neurobiologic Findings in Obsessive-Compulsive Disorder. *Psychiatry Clin North Amer,* 27(1), 2004, pp 37-48.

Andrews G, Halford DS, Bunch KM, Bowden D, Jones T. Theory of Mind and Relation al Complexity, *Child Development* 74(5), 2003, pp 1476-1500

Asbahr FR, Garvey MA, Snider LA, Zanetta DM, Elkis H, Swedo S. Obsessive-Compulsive Symptoms among Patients with Sydenham's chorea , *Biol Psychiatry* 57, 2005, pp 1073-76.

Avramopoulos D. Genetics of Psychiatric Disorders. *Psychiatric Clin North Amer* 33(1), 2010, pp 1-14.

Bagot RC, Meaney MJ. Epigenetics and the Biological Basis of Gene X Environment Interactions. *J Amer Acad Child and Adol Psychiatry* 49(8), 2010, pp 752-71.

Baldwin DS, Brandish EK, Meron D). The Overlap of Obsessive-Compulsive Disorder and Social Phobia and Its Treatment *CNS Spectrums* 13(9) Suppl 4, 2008, pp 47-53.

Balemans MC, Huibers MM, Eikelenboom NW, van Summeren RC et al. Reduced Exploration, Increased Anxiety, and Altered Social Behavior: Autistic-like Features of Euchromatin Histrone Methyl transferase 1 Heterozygous Knockout Mice. *Behav Brain Res* 208(1, 2010, pp: 47-55

Baranek GT, Boyd BA, Poe M, et al. Hyperresponsive Sensory Patterns in Children with Autism, Developmental Delay and Typical Development. *Am J Intel Dev Disability,* 112(4), 2007, pp 233-45.

a. Barnhill J (2000), Anxiety Disorders in Developmental Disabilities. In *Assessment and Treatment of Anxiety Disorders in Persons with Mental Retardation,* Poindexter A (Ed), pp2-12, NADD Press, ISBN—1-57256-015-0, Kingston, NY .

b. Barnhill LJ (2000), Ethology, Anxiety Disorders and Developmental Disabilities. *Journal of Intellectual Disability Research,* Vol. 44, parts three and four, abstract no: 047, p. 200-201.

c. Barnhill LJ (2000), Epilepsy and Anxiety Disorders in Developmental Disorders. *Journal of Intellectual Disability Research,* Vol.44, parts three and four, abstract no: 046, p. 200.

Barnhill J. Neurobiology of Self-Injury: Is There a Relationship to Addictions *NADD Bull* 6(2), 2003a, pp 29-37.

Barnhill J. The Differential Diagnosis of Anxiety in Individuals With Epilepsy and Intellectual Disability. *Mental Health Aspects of Developmental Disabilities,* 7(4), 2004, pp 124-130.

a. Barnhill J. The Spectrum of Tourette's Disorder, Obsessive-compulsive Disorder, Pervasive Developmental Disorder: Two Cases. *NADD Bulletin* 8(3), 2005, pp 57-62.

b. Barnhill J. Body Dysmorphic Disorder: A Subset of Self-Injurious Behaviors with Intellectual Disability? *Mental Health Aspects of Developmental Disabilities*, 8(1), 2005, pp 5-12.

a. Barnhill J (2006), Developmental Neuropsychiatry: Embryology and Psychopathology. *NADD Bulletin*, 8(5), pp: 95-96.

b. Barnhill J. Stereotypic Movement Disorder. NADD Bulletin 9(2), 2006, pp 23-26.

a. Barnhill J, deKoning ND, Poindexter AR. Other Disorders of Infancy and Childhood In Fletcher R, Loschen E, Satavrakaki C, First M (eds). *Diagnostic Manual- Intellectual Disability: A Textbook of Diagnosis of Mental disorders in Persons with Intellectual Disability*, 2007, Kingston NY: NADD Press, pp183-202, ISBN-1-57256-125-4.

b. Barnhill LJ, Antonacci DJ, and Poindexter AR (2007), Tic Disorders. *In Diagnostic Manual- Intellectual Disability: A Textbook of Diagnosis of Mental Disorders in Persons with Intellectual Disability (DM-ID)*, Fletcher R, Loschen E., and Stavrakaki C, Micahel F., eds., NADD Press., pp 157-202, ISBN-1-57256-125-4, Kingston, NY.

c. Barnhill J, de Koning, Poindexter A, Other Disorders of Childhood and Adolescence. In Diagnostic Manual- Intellectual Disability: *A Textbook of Diagnosis of Mental Disorders in Persons with Intellectual Disability.* Fletcher R, Loeschen E, Stavrakaki C, First M (Eds), pp 183- 202,. NADD Press, ISBN-1-57256-125-4, Kingston NY .

Barnhill J. Body Dysmorphic Disorder in People with Intellectual Disability: A Biopsychosocial Approach . *Mental Health Aspects of Developmental Disabilities* 10(1), 2007, pp 1-12.

a. Barnhill J. Obsessive-Compulsive Disorder: Diagnosis and Treatment, *NADD Bulletin,* 11(4), 2008, pp: 70-74.

b. Barnhill J. What Exactly is OCD in Individuals with Intellectual and Developmental Disabilities. *Mental Health Aspects of Dev Disabil,* 11(3), 2008, pp 85-93.

Barnhill J. Is There a Relationship between Self-injurious Behaviors and Addictions: Redux, Part 1. *NADD Bull* 9 13(4), 2010, pp 61-66.

Beesdo K, Knappe S, Pine DS. Anxiety and Anxiety Disorders in Children and Adolescents: Developmental Issues and Implications for the DSM-V. *Psych Clin North Amer* 32(3), 2009, pp 483-522.

Betancur C (2010). Etiologic Heterogeneity in Autistic Spectrum Disorders: More Than 100 Genetic and Genomic Disorders and Still Counting. *Brain Res,* Nov 30, 2010, Epub.

Bird TD, Schellenberg G (2008), Genotype-Phenotype Correlations. In *The Molecular and Genetic Basis of Neurologic and Psychiatric Disease Fourth Edition,* Rosenberg RN, DiMauro S, Paulson HI, Ptacek L, Nestler EJ (Eds), pp 104113, Wolters Kluwer/Lippincott, Williams & Wilkins, ISBN- 13:978-0-7817-6956-3, Baltimore.

Black DW, Gaffney GR. Subclinical Obsessive-Compulsive Disorder in Children and Adolescents: Additional Results from a High Risk Study. *CNS Spectrums* 13(9) Suppl 4, 2008, pp 54- 61.

Britton JC, Lissek S, Grillon C, Norcross MA, Pine DS. Development of Anxiety: The Role of Threat Appraisal and Fear Learning. *Depress Anxiety* 28(1), 2010, pp 5-17.

Britton JC, Rauch S, Rosso IM, Kilgore WDS et al. Cognitive Inflexibility and Fronto-Cortical Activation in Pediatric Obsessive-Compulsive Disorder. *J Am Acad Ch Adol Psychiatry,* 49(9), 2010, pp 944-53.

Bucan M, Brodkin ES (2008), Psychiatric Diseases: Challenges in Psychiatric Genetics. In *The Molecular and Genetic Basis of Neurologic and Psychiatric Disease Fourth Edition,*

Rosenberg RN, DiMauro S, Paulson HI, Ptacek L, Nestler EJ (Eds), pp 749-59, Wolters Kluwer/Lippincott, Williams & Wilkins, ISBN- 13:978-0-7817-6956-3, Baltimore,

Chao HT, Chen H, Samaco RC, Xue M, ChahourM, Yoo J et al. Dysfunction in GABA Signaling Mediates Autism-like Stereotypies and Rett Syndrome Phenotypes. *Nature* 468(73210, 2010, pp 263-9.

Charney D, Drevets W (2002), The Neurobiological Basis of Anxiety Disorders In *Neuropsychopharmacology : The Fifth Generation of Progress.* Davis KL, Charney D, Coyle JT, Nemeroff C (Eds). pp 901-30,,Lippincott, Williams &Wilkins , ISBN- 0-7817- 2837-1, Baltimore.

Chavira DA, Stein MB. Childhood Social Anxiety Disorder, *Ch Adol Psychiatric Clin North America* 14(4), 2005, pp 797-818.

Cook EH. Genetics of Autism *Ment Retard Dev Dis Res* 1998, 4(2), pp 11-120.

Cooper N, Feder A, Southwick SM, Charney DS (2007), Resilience and Vulnerability to Trauma: Psychobiological Mechanisms. In *Adolescent Psychopathology and the Developing Brain,* Romer D and Walker EF (eds), pp 347-72, Oxford Univ Press:, ISBN 978-0-19-530625-5, New York.

Cooray S, Gabrielle S, Gaus V, Anxiety Disorders. *In Diagnostic Manual- Intellectual Disability: A Textbook of Diagnosis of Mental Disorders in Persons with Intellectual Disability,* Fletcher R, Loeschen E, Stavrakaki C, First M (Eds), pp 317-49, NADD Press:, , ISBN- 1-57256-125-4, Kingston NY..

Costello EJ, Egger Hl, Angold A. The Developmental epidemiology of Anxiety Disorders: Phenomenology, Prevalence and Comorbidity. *Ch Adol Psychiatric Clin North America* 14(4), 2005, pp 631-48.

Crews F, He J, Hodge C (2007). Adolescent Cortical Development: A Critical Period of Vulnerability in Adolescents. *Pharmacology, Biochemistry Behavior,* 2007. 86 (2), pp 189-99.

Davis M. Neurobiology of Fear Responses. *J Neuropsychiatry and Clin Neuroscience,* 9 (3), 1997, pp382-400.

Davis M (2002). Neural Circuitry of Anxiety and Stress Disorders In *Neuropsychopharmacology : The Fifth Generation of Progress.* Davis KL, Charney D, Coyle JT, Nemeroff C (Eds). pp 932-52, Lippincott, Williams &Wilkins, ISBN-0-7817-2837- 1, Baltimore.

Dawson G, Sterling L, Faja S (2009). Autism: Risk Factors, Risk Processes, and Outcome. In Handbook of Developmental Social Neuroscience, DE Haan M, Gunnar MR Eds), pp 435-58, Guilford Press, ISBN 978-1-60623-117-3., New York..

De Haan M, Matheson (2009). The Development of Social Information Processing Emotion in Faces and Voices. In Handbook of Developmental Social Neuroscience, DE Haan M, Gunnar MR Eds), pp 107-21, Guilford Press, ISBN 978-1-60623-117-3., New York.

De Mathis MA, Diniz JB, Rosario MC, Torres AR, Hoexter M, Hasler G, Miguel E. What Is the Optimal Way to Subdivide Obsessive-Compulsive Disorder, *CNS Spectrum* 11(10), 2006, pp 762-88.

De Schipper JC, Schuengel C . Attachment Behavior Towards Support Staff in Young People with Intellectual Disabilities: Associations with Challenging Behaviour. *J Int Disabil Res* 54(7), 2010, pp 584-96.

El-Fishaway P, Stite MW. Genetics of Autism: Key Issues, Recent Findings and Clinical Implications. *Psychiatric Clin North Amer* 33(1), 2011, pp 81-105.

Farone SV, Mick E. Molecular Genetics of Attention Deficit-Hyperactivity Disorder. *Psychiatr Clin North Amer* 33(1), 2010, pp 159- 80.

Feinstein C, Singh W (2007). Social Phenotype in Neurogenetic Syndromes., *Child Adol Psychiatric Clin North Amer,* 16(3), pp 631-48.

Feldman R, Granat A, Pariente C, Kanety H, Kuint J, Gilboa-Schechtman E (2009). Maternal Depression and Anxiety Across the Post-partum Year and Infant Social Engagement, Fear Regulation and stress Reactivity. *J Am Acad Adol Psychiatry* 48(9), 2009, pp 919-927.

Fineberg NA, Sharma P, Sivakumaran T, Sahakian B, Chamberlain S. Does Obsessive-Compulsive Personality Disorder Belong within the Obsessive-Compulsive Spectrum:. *CNS Spectrums,* 12 (6), pp 467-82.

Figer M, Mantione M, van den Munchkef P, Schuurmen R, Denys D. Targets for Deep Brain Stimulation in Obsessive-Compulsive Disorder. *Psychiatric Anns* 40(10), 2010, pp 492-8.

Flavell JE (ed) (1982) Self-injurious Behavior: Analysis and Intervention in Developmental Disabilities (Special Edition).

Fletcher R, Loeschen E, Stavrakaki C, First M (Eds) *Diagnostic Manual- Intellectual Disability: A Textbook of Diagnosis of Mental Disorders in Persons with Intellectual Disability,* 2007. NADD Press, ISBN-1—57256-125-4, Kingston NY,

Franic S, Middledorp CM, Dolan CV, Ligthart L, Boomsma DI (2010). Childhood and Adolescent Anxiety and Depression: Beyond Heritability. *J Amer Acad Child and Adol Psychiatry,* 49(8), 2010, pp820-29.

Fries ABW, Pollack SD(2007)., Emotion Processing and the Developing Brain. In *Human Behavior. Learning and the Developing Brain,* Coch D, Fischer KW, Dawson G (Eds), pp329-61 , Guilford Press, ISBN-13: 978-1-59385-136-1, New York.

Fudge JL, Emiliano AB. The Extended Amygdala and the Dopamine System. Another Piece of the Dopamine Puzzle *J Neuropsychiatry and Clin Neuroscience,* 15(3), 2003, pp 306- 15.

Gardner WI. Diagnostically-Based Treatments of Bio-Medical And Psychosocial Conditions that Influence Self-Injurious Behaviors: A Multimodal Contextual Case Formulation. *ADD Bull* 6(2), 2003, pp 23-28.

Ghidoni BBZ. Rett's Syndrome. *Child Adol Psychiatric Clin North Amer* 16(3), 2007, pp 723-44.

Gothelf D. Velocardiofacial Syndrome, *Child Adol Psychiatric Clinics North Amer* 13(3), 2007, pp 677-94.

Ginsberg GS, Kingery JN, Drake KL, Grados MA. Predictors of Treatment Response in Pediatric Obsessive-Compulsive Disorder, *J Am Acad Child Adol Psychiatry* 47(8). 2008, pp 868-78.

Gorman JM, Kent JM, Coplan JD (2002). Current and Emerging Therapeutics of Anxiety Disorders. In. *Neuropsychopharmacology : The Fifth Generation of Progress,* Davis KL, Charney D, Coyle JT, Nemeroff C (Eds), pp 967-80, Lippincott, Williams &Wilkins, ISBN- 0-.7817-2837-1, Baltimore.

Gorman JM, Docherty JP. A hypothesized Role for Dendritic Remodeling in the Etiology of Mood and Anxiety Disorders. *J Neuropsychiatry Clin Neurosci* 22(3), 2010, pp 256-64.

Grados MA. The Genetics of Obsessive-Compulsive Disorder and Tourette's Disorder: An Epidemiological and Pathway-Based Approach or Gene Discovery. *J Amer Acad Child and Adol Psychiatry* 49(8), 2010, pp 810-19.

Grafodatskaya D, Chung B, Szatmari P, Weksberg R. Autism Spectrum Disorder and Epigenetics. *J Amer Acad Child and Adol Psychiatry* 49(8), 2010, pp 794-809.

Grey I, Pollard J, McClean B, MacAuley N, Hastings R). Prevalence of Psychiatric Diagnoses and Challenging Behaviors in a Community-Based Population with Adults with Intellectual Disability. *J Ment Health Res in Dev Disabil*, 3(4), 2010, pp 202-209.

Griffiths DM, Gardner WI, Nugent JA (1998). Behavior Supports and Community Living. NC Dept of Human Resources.

Gunnar MR (2007)., Stress and the Developing Brain. In *Adolescent Psychopathology and the Developing Brain,* Romer D and Walker EF (eds), pp 127-47 Oxford Univ Press, ISBN 978-0-19-530625-5, New York, NY..

Haley DW, Stansbury K. Infant Stress and Parent Responsiveness: Regulation of Physiology and Behavior during Still-Face and Reunion. *Child Development* 74(5), 2003, pp 1534-1546.

Harmon-Jones E (2007), Asymmetrical Frontal Cortical Activity , Affective Valence, and Motivational Direction. . In *Social Neuroscience: Integrating Biological and Psychological Explanations of Social Behavior,* Harmon-Jones E, Winkielman P (Eds), pp 137-56, Guilford Press, ISBN 13: 978-1-59385-404-1, New York

Hall S and Oliver C. Differential Effects of Severe Self-injurious Behaviors on the Behavior of Others. *Behavioral Psychotherapy* 20 (3), 1992, pp 355-65

Hall S, Oliver C Murphy GH. Early Development of Severe Self-injurious Behavior: An Empirical Study.

Am J Mental Retardation, 106 (2), 2001, pp 189-99.

Harris JC. Ethology in Harris JC (1996). *Developmental Neuropsychiatry* I,. Oxford Press, 1995, pp169-91, ISBN-0-19-509849-3 (v 2), New York, NY.

Harris JC (2006), Intellectual Disability: Understanding Its Development, Causes, Classification, Evaluation and Treatment, Oxford University Press, ISBN-0-19-517885-8, New York.

Harris J, Gusci R, Nettelbeck T, Kirby N. Impact of Additional Disabilities on Adaptive Behavior and Support Profiles for People with Intellectual Disabilities. *J Amer Assoc Intellectual Dev Disabilities* 114(4), 2009, 237-53.

Hefner K, Whittle N, Juhasz J, Norcross M, Karlsson R-M, Sakisda LM, Bussey TJ, Singewald N, Holmes A. Impaired Fear Extinction Learning and Cortico-Amygdala Circuit Abnormalities in a Common Genetic Mouse Strain. *J Neuroscience* 28(32), 2008: 8047-85.

Heilman KM. The Neurobiology of Emotional Experience. *J Neuropsychiatry and Clin Neuroscience.* 9 (3), 1997, pp 439-448

Hiem AFT, Nemeroff CB (2003). Neurobiology of Early Life Stress and Its Disorders, In *Pediatric Psychopharmacology: Principles and Practice,* Martin A, Scahill L, Charney DS, Leckman JF (eds), 110-23, Oxford Univ Press, ISNB- 0-19-514173-3, New York.

Hoch TA, Long KA, McPeak MM, Rojahn R (2002), Self-Injurious Behavior in Mental Retardation. In *Behavior Modification for Persons with Developmental Disabilities Vol I*

,Matson JL, Laud RB, Matson ML (Eds), pp190-218, NADD, ISBN-0-306-41648-4, Kingston..

Hodes RL, Cook EW, Lang PJ. Individual Differences in Autonomic Response: Conditioned Association of Conditioned Fear. *Psychophysiology*, 22(5), 1985, pp 45-60.

Hofvander B, Delorme R, Chaste P, Nyden A, Wentz E et al (2009). Psychiatric and Psychosocial Problems in Adults with Normal-Intelligence Autistic Spectrum Disorders. *Psychiatry* 10 (9), 2009, pp35-44.

Hollander E, Stein D (eds), 1997. *Obsessive-Compulsive Disorder*. Marcel Dekker, 1997, ISBN-0-8247-9856-2, New York. .Houinie AG, Rosario-Campos MS, Diniz, JB, Shavitt RG et al. Obsessive Compulsive Disorder in Tourette Syndrome. *Advances in Neurology*, vol 99, 2006, pp 22-38.

Howenstein R. Systematic Desensitization of Phobias in Individuals with Developmental Disabilities. *NADD Bull* 9(3), 2006, pp 46-52.

Howlin P, Magiati I, Charman T. Systematic Review of Early Intensive Behavioral Interventions for Children with Autism. *Am J Intellect Dev Disability* 114(1), 2009, pp- 23-41.

Jacob S, Landeros- Weisenberger A, Leckman JF. Autism Spectrum and Obsessive-Compulsive Disorders- OC Behaviors, Phenotypes and Genetics. *Autism Res* 2,, 2009, pp 293-311.

Joosten AV, Bundy AC. Sensory Processing and Stereotypical and Repetitive Behaviour in Children with Autism and Intellectual Disability. *Aust Occup Ther J* 57(6):, 2010, pp 366-72.

Johnson CP, Myers SM, Council on Children with Disabilities . Identification and Evaluation of Children with Autism Spectrum Disorders, *Pediatrics* 120(5), 2007, pp 1183-1215.

Joy SP, Lord JS, Green L, Fein D (2003), Mental Retardation and Developmental Disabilities, In *Neuropsychiatry: Second Edition* Schiffer RB, Rao SM, Fogel BS (Eds), pp552-604, Lippincott, Williams & Wilkins, ISBN-0-7817-2655-7, Baltimore.

Kagan J, Snidman N (2007), Temperament and Biology. In *Human Behavior. Learning and the Developing Brain,* Coch D, Fischer KW, Dawson G (eds), pp219-46, Guilford Press, ISBN-13: 978-1-59385-136-1, New York.

Kana RK, Keller TA, Minshew NJ, Just MA. Inhibitory Control in High-functioning Autism: Decreased Activation and Underconnectivity in Inhibition Networks. *Biol Psychiatry* 62(3), 2007, pp 198-206.

King R. Complex Post-traumatic Stress Disorder: Implications for Individuals with Autism Spectrum Disorder. *NADD Bull* 13(5), 2010, pp 7-15.

Koh KB, Kang JL, Lee JD, Lee YL. Shared Neural Activity in Panic Disorder and Undifferentiated Somatoform Disorder Compared with Healthy Controls *J Clin Psychiatry* 71(12), 2010, pp 1576-81.

Kring SR, Greenberg JS, Setzer MM. Adolescents and Adults with Autism with and without Co-morbid Psychiatric Disorders: Disorders in Maternal Well Being. *J Mental Health Res in Intellect Dis* 1(2), 2008, pp 53-75.

Niedtfeld I, Schulze L, Kirsch P, Herpetz SC, Bohus M, Schmahl C. Affect Regulation and Pain in Borderline Personality Disorder: A Possible Link to the Understanding of Self-Injury *Biol Psychiatry* 68, 2010, pp 383-391.

Kiddle H, Dagnon D. Vulnerability to Depression in Adolescents with Intellectual Disabilities, *Advances in Mental Health and Intellectual Disab*ility 5(1), 2011, pp 3-8.

King BH, Bostic JQ. An Update on Pharmacological Treatments for Autism Spectrum Disorders. *Child Adol Psychiatr Clin North America* 15(1), 2006, pp 161-176.

King R, Stavrakaki C, Gedeye A (2007)., Obsessive-Compulsive Disorder In) *Diagnostic Manual- Intellectual Disability: A Textbook of Diagnosis of Mental Disorders in Persons with Intellectual Disability,* Fletcher R, Loeschen E, Stavrakaki C, First M (Eds). pp 349-364,NADD Press, ISBN—57256-125-4, Kingston NY.

Knapp P, Mastergeorge AM. Clinical Implications of Current Findings in Neurodevelopment. *Psychiatric Clin North Amer,* 32 (2), 2009, pp177-97.

Koda V, Charney DS, Pine D (2003). Neurobiology of Early-onset Anxiety Disorders, In *Pediatric Psychopharmacology: Principles and Practice,* Martin A, Scahill L, Charney DS, Leckman JF (eds), pp 138-49,. Oxford Univ Press, ISNB- 0-19-514173-3, New York.

Knutson B, Wimmer GE (2007), Reward: Neural Circuitry for Social Validation. In *Social Neuroscience: Integrating Biological and Psychological Explanations of Social Behavior.* Harmon-Jones E, Winkielman P (Eds), pp 157-75, Guilford Press, ISBN-13: 978-1-59385-404-1, New York.

Lang LR, Mahoney R, El Zein F, Delaune E, Amidon M. Evidence to Practice: Treatment of Anxiety in Individuals with Autism Spectrum Disorders. *Neuropsychitatr Dis Treat* 25(7), 2011, pp: 27-30.

Leckman JF, Yen C-B, Blier P (2003). Neurobiology of Tic Disorders including Tourette's Disorder. In *Pediatric Psychopharmacology: Principles and Practice,* Martin A, Scahill L, Charney DS, Leckman JF (eds) Oxford Univ Press, ISNB- 0-19-514173-3, New York, pp 164-74.

Lee JW. Catatonic Variance, Hyperthermic Exptrapyramidal Reactions and subtypes of Malignant Neuroleptic Syndrome. *Ann Clin Psychiatry* 19(1, 2007, pp: 9-16.

Lehman J, Heber SN. Neuro-circuitry Underlying Deep Brains Stimulation. *Psychiatric Ann* 40(10), 2010, pp 499-503

Leonard H Childhood Rituals and Superstitions: Developmental and Cultural Perspectives. In *Obsessive-Compulsive Disorder in Children and Adolescents.* Rapoport JL (Ed), 1989, pp 289-310, American Psychiatric Association Press, ISBN 0-88048-282-6, Washington DC.

Leonard H, Ale CM, Freeman JB, Garcia AM, Ng JS. Obsessive-Compulsive Disorder, *Ch Adol Psychiatric Clin North America* 14(4), 2005, pp 727-44.

Lerner JS, Gonzalez RM, Dahl RE, Hariri AR, Taylor SE. Facial Expressions of Emotion Reveal Neuro-endocrine and Cardiovascular Stress Responses, *Biol Psychiatry* 58, 2005, pp 743-50.

Levitas A, Dykens E, Finacune B, Kates M (2007), Behavioral Phenotypes in Genetic Disorders. Fletcher R, Loeschen E, Stavrakaki C, First M (Eds) In Diagnostic Manual- Intellectual Disability: A Textbook of Diagnosis of Mental Disorders in Persons with Intellectual Disability, p33-62,. NADD Press, pp33-62, ISBN-1-57259-125-4, Kingston NY..

Lombroso PJ, Ogren MP). Fragile X: Keys to Molecular Genetics and Synaptic Plasticity. *J Am Acad Ch Adol Psychiatry* 47(7), 2008, pp 736-39.

Lunsky Y, Bradley E, Gracey D et al. Gender Differences in Psychiatric Diagnosis among Individuals with and without Intellectual Disabilities. *Am J Intellectual and Dev Disorders* 114 (1), 2009, pp 52-60

Mataix-Cols D, Nakatani N, Heyman I. Structure of Obsessive-Compulsive Symptoms in Pediatric OCD, *J Am Acad Ch Adol Psychiatry,* 47(7), 2008, pp 773- 8.

Matthews SJ, Price RB, Charney DS. Recent Advances in the Neurobiology of Anxiety Disorders: Implications for Novel Therapeutics, *Am J Med Gen* 2008, pp 89-98.

Max JE, Keatly E, Wilde EA, Bigler ED, Levin HS et al. Anxiety Disorders in Children and Adolescents in the First Months after a Traumatic Brain Injury. *J Neuropsychiatry Clin Neurosci* 23(1), 2011, pp 29-39.

McClure, Pine DS, Stres (2007). Affect, and Neural Function in Adolescence. In *Adolescent Psychopathology and the Developing Brain,* Romer D and Walker EF (eds), Oxford Univ Press, ISBN 978-0-19-530625-5: New York, NY.

McNally L, Bhagwagor Z, Hannstead .). Inflammation, Glutamate and Glia in Depression: A Literature Review., *CNS Spectrum,* 13(4), 2008, pp 501-10.

Millham MP, Nugent AC, Drevets WC, Dickstein D, Leibenluft E, Ernst M, Charney D, Pine D. Selective Reduction in Amygdala Volume in Pediatric Anxiety Disorders. *Biol Psychiatry* 57, 2005, pp 961-66.

Menolascino FJ, Stark J (1985), Handbook of Mental Illness in the Mentally Retarded, Plenum Press, ISBN-0-306-41648-4, New York.

Merikangas KR). Vulnerability Factors for Anxiety Disorders in Children. *Ch Adol Psychiatric Clin North America* 14(4), 2005, pp 649-80.

Mitchell A, Clegg J (2005). Is Post-traumatic Stress Disorder a Helpful Concept for Adults with Intellectual Disability. *J Int Disability Research* 49(7), 2005, pp552-9.

Mobbs D, Eckert MA, Mills D, Korenberg J, et al. Fronto-striatal Dysfunction during Response Inhibition in Williams Syndrome. *Biol Psychiatry* 62(3), 2007, pp 256-61.

Mobbs D, Petrovic P, Marchant JL, Hanaabis D, Weiskopf N, Seymour B, Dolan RJ, Frith CD (2007). When Fear is Near: Imminence Elicits Prefrontal-peri-aqueductal Gray Shifts in Humans. *Science* 317, 2007, pp 1079-4.2007.

Mosconi MW, Kay M. DeCruz A-M, Gater S et al. Neurobehavioral Abnormalities in First-Degree Relatives of Individuals with Autism, *Arch Gen Psychiatry* 67(8), 2010, pp 830- 40.

Murphy TK, Voeller KKS, Blier P (2003). Neurobiology of Obsessive-Compulsive Disorder, *In Pediatric Psychopharmacology: Principles and Practice,* Martin A, Scahill L, Charney DS, Leckman JF (eds), pp 150-63. Oxford Univ Press, ISNB- 0-19-514173-3, New York.

Myers SM, Johnson CP. Management of Children with Autistic Spectrum Disorders, *Pediatrics* 120(5), 2007, pp 1162-1182.

Nestadt G, Grados M, Samuel JF. Genetics of Obsessive-Compulsive Disorder. *Psychiatr Clin North Amer,* 33(1), 2010, pp 141-158.

Niedtfeld I, Schulze L, Kirsch P, Herpetz SC, Bohus M, Schmahl C. Affect Regulation and Pain in Borderline Personality Disorder: A Possible Link to the Understanding of Self-Injury *Biol Psychiatry* 68, 2010, pp 383-391.

Neumeister A, Vythilinga M, Bonne O, Kaplan JS, Charney DS (2003). Anxiety, In *Neuropsychiatry, Second Edition* Schiffer RB, Rao SM, Fogel BS (Eds), pp760- 775, Lippincott, Williams & Wilkins, pp 750-775, ISBN- 0-7817-2655-7, Baltimore .

Noll LM, Barrett RP (2002). Stereotyped Acts, In *Behavior Modification for Persons with Developmental Disabilities* Vol I Matson JL, Laud RB, Matson ML (Eds), pp 219-78, NADD Press, ISBN- -0-306-41648-4, Kingston.

Northoff G. What Catatonia Can Tell Us About "Top-Down Regulation: A Neuropsychiatric Hypothesis. *Behav Brain Sci* 25(2, 2002, pp 578-604.

Novotny S, Evers M, Barboza K, Rawitt R, Hollander E (2003). Neurobiology of Affiliation: Implications for Autism Spectrum Disorders, In *Pediatric Psychopharmacology: Principles and Practice,* Martin A, Scahill L, Charney DS, Leckman JF (eds) Oxford Univ Press, ISNB- 0-19-514173-3, New York, pp 195-209.

Oliver C, Halls S, Murphy G. The Early Development of Self-injurious Behaviour: Evaluating the Role of Social Reinforcement. *J Intellectual Dis Res,* 49 (1), 2005, pp 59-99.

Pallanti S, Hollander E (2008). Obsessive-Compulsive Disorder Spectrum as a Scientific Metaphor. *CNS Spectrums* 13(9) Suppl 4, 2008, pp 6-15.

Parsons JA, May JG, Menolascino FJ (1985). The Nature and Incidence of Mental Illness in Mentally Retarded Individuals. In Melonascino FJ, Stark J (1985), *Handbook of Mental Illness in the Mentally Retarded,* pp 3-44, Plenum Press, ISBN-0-306-41648-4, New York.

Pauls DL, Mundo E, Kennedy JL (2002). The Pathophysiology and Genetics of Obsessive-Compulsive Disorder. In *Neuropsychopharmacology : The Fifth Generation of Progress,* Davis KL, Charney D, Coyle JT, Nemeroff C (Eds), pp 1609-1621, Lippincott, Williams &Wilkins, ISBN-0-7817-2837-1, Baltimore.

Perez-Edgar K. Fox NA. Temperament and Anxiety Disorders. *Ch, Adol Psychiatric Clin North America* 14(4), 2005, pp 681-706.

Perez-Edgar K, Henderson HA,Diaz V, Raggi VL, Fox NA. Stable Early Maternal Reports of Behavioral Inhibition Predicts Lifetime Social Anxiety. *J Amer Acad Ch Adolesc Psychiatry,* 48(9), 2009, pp. 928-35.

Petty J, Allen D, Oliver C Relationship among Challenging, Repetitive, and Communicative Behaviors in Children with Severe Intellectual Disabilities. *America J Intellectual Dev Disabilities,* 114 (5), 2009, pp 356-368.

Pierce K, Conant D, Hazin R, Stoner R, Desmond J (2011). Preference for Geometric Patterns Early in Life as a Risk Factor for Autism. *Arch Gen Psychiatry,* 68(1), 2011, pp 101-9.

Pomeory SL, Kim JYH. Biology and Pathobiology of Neuronal Development , *Mental Retard Dev Disabilities* Res Rev 6(1), 2000, pp 41-7 .

Portman ME, Starveric V, Beck AT. Challenges in the Assessment and Diagnosis Generalized Anxiety Disorder, *Psychiatric Ann* 41(2), 2011, pp 78-87.

Post RM, Weiss SS. Sensitization and Kindling Phenomena in Mood, Anxiety and Obsessive-Compulsive Disorders: The Role of Serotinergic Mechanisms in Illness Progression. *Biol Psychiatry* 44(3), 1998, pp 193-206.

Post RM. Kindling and Sensitization as Models for Affective Episode Recurrence, Cyclicity and Tolerance Phenomena, *Neurosci Biobehav Rev* 31(6), 2007, pp 858-73.

Prado HS, de Rosario MC, Lee J, Houine AG, Shavitt RG, Miguel E. Sensory Phenomena in Obsessive-Compulsive Disorder and Tic Disorders: A Review of the Literature, *CNS Spectrum* 14(5), 2008, pp 425-31.

Prosnin AR, Love TM, Koeppe RA, Zubieta JK, Silk KR. Dysregulation of Regional Endogenous Opioid Function in Borderline Personality Disorder. *Amer J Psychiatry,* 167(8), 2010, pp 925-33.

Qureshi SU, Long ME, Bradshaw MY, Pyne JM et al. Does PTSD Impair Cognition Beyond the Effects of Trauma, *J Neuropsychiatry Clin Neuroscience* 23(1), 2011, pp 16-28.

Ramocki MB, Peters SU, Tavyev YJ, Zhang F, Carvalho Et al. Autism and Other Neuropsychiatric Symptoms Are Prevalent in Individuals with MeCP2 duplication syndrome. *Ann Neurol* 66(6), 2009, pp: 771-83.

Rasmussen SA, Eisen JL (2002). The Course and Clinical Features of Obsessive-compulsive Disorder. In *Neuropsychopharmacology : The Fifth Generation of Progress,* Davis KL, Charney D, Coyle JT, Nemeroff C (Eds).pp 1593-1608, Lippincott, Williams &Wilkins, ISBN-0-7817-2837-1, Baltimore..

Reinblatt SP, Walkup JT. Pharmacological Treatment of Pediatric Anxiety Disorders. *Child Adol Psychiatr Clinics North Amer* 14(4),2006, pp 877-908.

Reiss S (2000). The Concept of Anxiety Sensitivity: Possible Implications of for Research on Dual Diagnosis, In *Assessment and Treatment of Anxiety Disorders in Persons with Mental Retardation,* Poindexter A (Ed),,pp65-67, NADD Press, ISBN 1-57256-015-0, Kingston NY .

Ruedrich S, Menolascino FJ (1985). Dual Diagnosis of Mental Retardation and Mental Illness : An Overview, In Menolascino FJ, Stark J (1985), *Handbook of Mental Illness in the Mentally Retarded,* pp 45-82, Plenum Press, ISBN-0-306-41648-4, New York.

Ridley M (2002). *Nature via Nurture: Genes, Experience and What Makes Us Human.* pp 125-200, Harper Collins Publishers,. ISBN-0-06-000678-1 New York.

Rifkin A and Barnhill LJ (2007), Impulse Control Disorders. *In Diagnostic Manual-Intellectual Disability: A Textbook of Diagnosis of Mental Disorders in Persons with Intellectual Disability (DM-ID),* Fletcher R, Loschen E., and Stavrakaki C, Micahel F (eds). pp 483-96, NADD Press. ISBN-1-27256-125-4, Kingston NY.

Robertson MM, Yakeley J (1996). Gilles de la Tourette's Syndrome and Obsessive – Compulsive Disorders. In *Neuropsychiatry,* Fogel BS, Schiffer RB, Rao S(eds), pp 827-70, Williams & Wilkins: Baltimore, 1996, pp 827-70, ISBN- 0-683-03305-0, Baltimore .

Roblek T, Piacentini J. Cognitive-Behavioral Therapy for Childhood Anxiety Disorders. *Child Adol Psychiatr Clinics North Amer* 14(4), 2005, pp 863-76.

Ronald A, Hoekstra RA. Autism Spectrum Disorders and Autistic Traits: A Decade of New Twin Studies. *Am J Med Genetics B Neuropsychiatry Genet,* 2011, Jan 13, E pub .

Rueda MR, Rothbart MK, Saccomanno L, Posner MI (2007), Modifying Brain Networks Underlying Self-Regulation. In *Adolescent Psychopathology and the Developing Brain,* Romer D and Walker EF (eds), pp401-19, Oxford Univ Press, ISBN 978-0-19-530625-5, New York, NY.

Saxena S. Neurobiology and Treatment of Compulsive Hoarding..*CNS Spectrums* 13(9) Suppl 4, 2008, pp 29-37.

Sayers SN, Oliver C, Ruddick L, Wallis B. Stereotyped Behavior in Children with Autism and Intellectual Disability: An Examination of the Executive Dysfunction Hypothesis. *J Intell Disabil Res, Jan E Pub,* 2011..

Schaer M, Eliezs (2007). From Genes to Brain: Understanding Brain Development in Neurogenetic Disorders Using Neuroimaging Techniques. *Child Adol Psychiatric Clinics of North Amer* 16(3), 2007, pp 557-80.

Schienle A, Hettema JM, Calceda R, Nemeroff CB (2011). Neurobiology and Genetics of Generalized Anxiety Disorder. *Psychiatric Annals* 41(2), 2011, pp 113- 121.

Simonoff E, Pickles A, Romero EG, Abram KM. Psychiatric Disorders in Children with Autistic Spectrum Disorders: Prevalence, Comorbidity and Associated Factors in Population-Derived Sample. *J Am Acad Child Adol Psychiatry* 47(8), 2008, pp 921-9.

Skuse D, Morris J, Lawrence K. The Amygdala and Development of the Social Brain. *Annals NY Academy Sciences* 1008, 2003, pp 91-101.

Smith KR, Matson. Psychopathology: Differences among Adults with Intellectual Disability, Comorbid Autism Spectrum Disorders and Epilepsy. *J Res Dev Disabil* 31(3), 2010, pp 743-9.

Stahl L, Pry R (2005). Attentional Flexibility and Perseveration: Developmental Aspects in Young Children 11(2): 175-89.

Stahl S, Wise DD (2008). The Potential Role of a Corticotrophin-Releasing Factor Antagonists in Psychiatric Disorders. *CNS Spectrums,* 13(6), 2008, pp 467-483.

Stahl SM. Methylated Spirits: Epigenetic Hypotheses of Psychiatric Disorders. *CNS Spectrum,* 15(4), 2010, pp 220-230.

Stein DJ. Psychobiology of Anxiety Disorders and Obsessive-Compulsive Spectrum Disorders. *CNS Spectrums* 13(9) Suppl 4, 2008, pp 23-29.

Stein DJ, Newman TK, Savitz J, Ramesar R (2006). Warriors versus Worriers: The Role of COMT Gene Variants, *CNS Spectrums* 11(10), 2006, pp 745- 748.

Stein DJ, Muller J. Cognitive-Affective Neuroscience of Somatization disorders and Functional Somatic Syndromes: Reconceptualizing the Triad of Depression-Anxiety-Somatic Symptoms, *CNS Spectrums* 13(5), 2008: 379- 84.

Stein MB, Lang AJ (2002), Anxiety and Stress Disorders: Course over the Lifetime. In *Neuropsychopharmacology : The Fifth Generation of Progress.* Davis KL, Charney D, Coyle JT, Nemeroff C (Eds), pp 859-66, Lippincott, Williams &Wilkins, ISBN-0-7817-2837-1, Baltimore.

Stewart E, Roasrio MC, Baer L, Carter A et al. Four-factor Structure of Obsessive-Compulsive Disorder: Symptoms in Children, adolescents and Adults. J *Am Acad Ch Adol Psychiatry* 47(7), 2008, 763- 72

Sturmey P, Berstein H (2002), Functional Analysis of Maladaptive Behavior. In *Behavior Modification for Persons with Developmental Disabilities* Vol I, Matson JL, Laud RB, Matson ML (Eds), pp 101-129. NADD Press, ISBN-0-306-41658-4, Kingston, NY.

Sukhodolsky DG, Landeras-Wineberger A, Schaill L, Leckman JF, Schultz RT. Neuropsychological Functioning in Children with Tourette's Syndrome with and without Attention deficit/Hyperactivity Disorder. *J Am Acad Ch Adol Psychiatry* 49(11), 2010, pp 1155-1164.

Suess L, Halpern MS. Obsessive-Compulsive Disorder: A Religious Perspective, 1989 , *In Obsessive-Compulsive Disorder in Children and Adolescents.* Rapoport JL (Ed), pp 311-261, American Psychiatric Association Press, ISBN 0-88048-282-6, Washington DC.

Sugden K, Arsenault L, Harrington H, Moffitt TE, Williams B, Avshalom C. Serotonin Transporter Genes Moderates the Development of Emotional Problems among Children Following Bullying Victimization. *J Amer Acad Child and Adol Psychiatry* 49(8), 2010, pp 830-40

Suveg C, Aschenbrand SG, Kendall PC. Separation Anxiety Disorder, Panic Disorder and School Refusal. *Ch Adol Psychiatric Clin North America* 14(4), 2005, pp 773-96.

Swedo S (1985), Rituals and Releasers: An Ethological Model of Obsessive-Compulsive Disorder, In *Obsessive-Compulsive Disorder in Children and Adolescents.* Rapoport JL

(Ed), pp269-88 1989, American Psychiatric Association Press, ISBN 0-88048-282-6, Washington DC.

Travis LL and Sigman M. Social Deficits and Interpersonal Relationships in Autism. *J Ment Retard and Dev Dis Res*, 4(2),1998, pp 73-80.

Turk CL, Mennin DS (2011). Phenomenology of Generalized Anxiety Disorder, *Psychiatric Ann* 41(2), 2011, pp 71-77.

Ursano A, Kartheiser P and Barnhill J (2007), Disorders of Infancy, Childhood and

Adolescence. In *Textbook of Psychiatry*, 5th edition, APA Press, pp 861-920, ISBN-978-58562-257-3, Washington DC..

Vaccarino FM, Leckman JF (2003). Overview of Brain Development, In *Pediatric Psychopharmacology: Principles and Practice,* Martin A, Scahill L, Charney DS, Leckman JF (eds), pp 3-19, Oxford Univ Press, ISNB- 0-19-514173-3, New York.

Vasa RA, Grados JP, Slomine B et al. Neuroimaging Correlates of Anxiety after Pediatric Traumatic Brain Injury, *Biol Psychiatry* 55 (2), 2004, pp 208-16.

Volpe JJ. Overview: Normal and Abnormal Human Brain Development. *Mental Retard Dev Disabilities Res Rev*, 6(1), 2000, pp 1-5.

Waslick B. Pharmacological Interventions for Pediatric Anxiety Disorders: a Research Update. *Child Adol Psychiatr Clinics North Amer* 14(4), 2006, pp 51-71.

Welchew DE, Ashwin C, Bekouk K, Salvador R, Suckling J, Baron-Cohen S and Bullmore E. Functional Disconnectivity of the Medial Temporal Lobe in Asperger's Syndrome, *Biol Psychiatry* 57, 2005, pp 991-8.

Witwer AN, Lecavalier L (2008). Psychopathology in Children with Intellectual Disability. *J Ment Health Res in Intellectual Disabilities* 1(1), 2008, pp 75-96.

Zohar J, Insel T, Rasmussen (eds) (1991). *The Psychobiology of Obsessive-Compulsive Disorders*. Springer, 1991, ISBN- 0-8261-7520-1, New York.

4

Reasoning in Anxiety, OCD and Related Disorders: Can Formal Reasoning Theories Inform Us About Psychopathology?

Kieron P. O'Connor[1,2] and Marie-Claude Pélissier[1]
[1]*Centre de recherche Fernand-Seguin, Montreal,*
[2]*University of Montreal, Montreal,*
Canada

1. Introduction

Early cognitive theories of psychopathology evoked the use of reasoning rules to the explanation of how people's behaviour was influenced by the way they think. In effect, Beck (1979) proposed that cognitive distortions were at the root of misguided thinking and that the faulty thinking could be corrected through cognitive therapy (cognitive restructuring). The therapist would point out how automatic rules had been formed through faulty thinking and help the client correct these rules and test out new ones.

Ellis (1962) also referred to irrational thinking as a source of psychopathology by suggesting how rules based on premises like 'If….then…' shaped action. Rational emotive, involves identifying these rules of causality with the client and then questioning the rules, as well as identifying which emotions are triggered when such faulty rules are acted upon. However, empirical data to support how the development of faulty reasoning progresses and is maintained are less clear. Although, the technique of cognitive restructuring has shown to be clinically relevant and helpful in cognitive therapy, the mechanisms by which restructuring operates, remain vague: how do people start changing their minds, that they start perceiving situations differently? Hence, it seems and mechanisms of change in cognitive therapy are not very well understood (Brewin, 1996).

The present review paper makes an attempt at connecting of general reasoning theories to pathological thinking, in particular in anxiety disorders. Its fundamental question is the following: As cognitive psychologists, can we benefit from theories of reasoning in order to understand psychopathology? This paper is based on the idea that reasoning, whether rational or irrational is what people do, all or most of the time and to understand psychopathology, we need to look at which reasoning strategies are used when people are 'seeing', 'saying' and 'doing' pathological things. Are these strategies the same or different inside and outside psychopathology?

2. Theories of human reasoning

Theories of how people reason can be described according to three leading currents. First, mental logic or inference-rule based theory dating back to early philosophers like Aristotle who portrayed human thinking as an operation requiring the use of principles of logic.

Second, is a theory of reasoning according to heuristics, developed by Tversky and Kanheman (1982), viewing human thinking as a biased process where incorrect probabilistic estimates filter judgement and decision making. Third, the theory of mental models developed by Johnson-Laird (1983) and Johnson-Laird and Byrne (1991), viewing reasoning as a coherent system that is not necessarily logical in a mathematical sense, but consistent within itself according to each person's construction of their own mental models.

2.1 Theory of inference rules

Reasoning research concerned with inference rules originates from philosophical tradition, where it was assumed a person used mental logic, that is, pursued the goal of thinking in a logical manner. Hence, those who fail to be logical could be trained to think more logically. As Rachman (1983) noted, in this view humans are not irrational, but simply fallible. Theories of inference rules are said to be normative, that is, they describe what is considered to be the ideal process of correct logical thinking.

2.2 Deductive reasoning

In deductive reasoning, conclusions are made on the basis of premises that are presumed to be true. In principle, deduction should yield valid conclusions, i.e. those in which the conclusion must be true if the premises are true (Johnson-Laird, 1999). The structure of the argument is what gives the conclusion its validity and not the content of the premises per se (Manktelow, 1999). The following form would represent this theoretical argument:

- Initial premise: All A are B
- Proposition A
- Conclusion: B

Supposing you added content to such an argument, you would find the following:

- All beaches are sandy.
- This is a beach.
- This beach is sandy.

Regardless of the fact that some beaches are NOT actually sandy, in its pure form, the argument is valid. This is so because, in deductive reasoning, all the information required in order to draw a conclusion is explicitly found in the premises. Hence a logical argument does not require any semantic knowledge to be solved. Other forms of deductive arguments concern conditional statements, like a proposition in the form of: 'if p then q'. This conditional framing is also called modus ponens. Here is an example of a modus ponens:

• If the mountain is high then the oxygen is rare. • The mountain is high.	(If p then q) (p)
• The oxygen is rare.	(q)

If you negate the antecedent (not p) you then draw a different conclusion. An example of denying the antecedent (DA) is the following:

• If the mountain is high then the oxygen is rare. • The mountain is not high.	(If p then q) (not p)
• The oxygen is not rare.	not q)

On the other hand, if you use affirmation of the consequent (AC), you would find the following:

• If the mountain is high then the oxygen is rare.	(If p then q)
• The oxygen is rare.	(q)
• The mountain is high.	(p)

And finally, the modus tollens which states 'if p then not-q' describes the instance when the consequent is denied, as shown in the following example:

• If the mountain is high then the oxygen is rare.	(If p then q)
• The oxygen is not rare.	(not q)
• The mountain is not high.	not p)

Such invalid deductive reasoning shows itself in several clinical variants.
Example of affirming the consequent:
People who are physically attractive are popular.
I'm not physically attractive.
Hence I'm not popular.
Example of denying the consequent:
Only cowards run away from challenges.
I avoid challenges.
So I'm a coward.
In mental logic, only two forms of deduction yield valid conclusions and they are the modus ponens and modus tollens. A valid deductive conclusion is one that is true if the premises are true. So if we assume that it is true that if the mountain is high then the oxygen is rare, the reverse (the mountain is not high, the oxygen is not rare) is not necessarily true (DA) and neither is the converse (if the oxygen is rare, then the mountain is high) (AC), so DA and AC do not necessarily lead to valid conclusions. To summarise, a conditional rule is one of *implication* where *p* implies *q* but the rule is not one of equivalence, that is *p* is not equivalent to *q*. That is precisely why DA and AC forms do not produce valid conclusions. For example, other conditions than 'high mountains' can produce rare oxygen (extreme high heat, a closed space, dehydration, etc.) but a high mountain implies that oxygen is rare, so oxygen MUST be rare if in a high mountain.

2.3 Conditional reasoning

Conditional reasoning is meant to illustrate logical forms of reasoning but if applied to a clinical example, it becomes apparent that the different conditional forms would not be judged by the same logical validity criteria in everyday reasoning:
Take for example a modus ponens using everyday thinking:

• If I am pleasant to everybody then everyone will like me.	(If p then q)
• I am pleasant to everybody.	(p)
• Everyone likes me.	(q)

The same example when denying the antecedent DA would yield the following:

• If I am pleasant to everybody then everyone will like me.	(If p then q)
• I am not pleasant with everybody.	not p)
• Nobody likes me.	(not q)

Or AC as in the following:

• If I am pleasant to everybody then everyone will like me.	(If p then q)
• Everyone likes me.	(q)
• I am pleasant to everybody.	(p)

And finally, the modus tollens as shows the following example:

• If I am pleasant to everybody than everyone will like me.	(If p then q)
• Nobody likes me.	(not q)
• I am not pleasant to everybody.	not p)

From a logical point of view, both modus ponens and modus tollens forms are correct however, from a clinical point of view, all four examples would be invalid and disputed by the cognitive therapist simply because the initial premise is debatable (being pleasant to everybody does not necessarily lead to everyone liking you!). In that sense, conditional reasoning paradigms concern verifying logical validity of an argument rather than observing the actual process of human thinking which means its use in terms of research into pathology may be limited. Moreover, people are not very successful when trying to solve conditional reasoning tasks, as illustrated in the case of one of the most documented experimental task of deductive reasoning called the Wason Selection Task (WST).

2.4 Wason selection task

The WST was created by Wason (1966) and has proved to be very informative about people's deductive reasoning abilities. In the WST, there are typically four cards with a letter or a number on each of them (for example A, M, 2 and 7). The following conditional rule: 'If there is a vowel on one side, then there is an even number on the other' is presented to a participant by the experimenter. The participant needs to indicate which card(s) MUST be turned over in order to find out if the conditional rule is true or false. It is expected that one uses the abstract rule of logic in both forms of modus ponens ('if p than q') in order to confirm the rule and in modus tollens, (if p than not-q), to seek evidence that would disconfirm the rule. Typically, people tend to use the modus ponens form, that is, they try and confirm the rule by turning over the 'A'. Fewer than 10% of people try to falsify the rule and this result has been consistent and replicated over the last two decades (Evans, 1982; 1989). Wason (1968) and Johnson-Laird and Wason (1970) supposed that the absence of falsification meant that people's reasoning was characterised by a *confirmation bias*, the tendency to look for confirming evidence without looking for disconfirmation. The confirmation bias proved useful to illustrate how people are simply not ruled by principles of logic. Hence here, what can be learned as cognitive psychologists, is that people are not inclined to look for falsifying evidence when it comes to abstract material. However, what it also seems to show is that abstract reasoning tasks do not describe thinking processes as they *are* per se, but more on how humans fail to be logical. In other words, by devising logical abstract tasks and testing people on the standard of their logical abilities, it becomes apparent that human's natural tendency is to think illogically. Wason (1969), attempted to prompt people to use contradicting evidence in order to falsify the rule and found that people still preferred confirming evidence and avoided using falsifying information.

The 'confirmation bias', underlined by the WST results prompted Evans (1972, as cited in Manktelow & Over, 1990) to look for another explanation than the inability to disconfirm a rule which he called a 'matching bias'. In effect, he thought it more plausible that participants had a tendency to make unjustified inferences where they would verify only the cards that showed information *named* in the rule (so for example, the vowel and the even number). Thus, Evans and Lynch (1973, as cited in Manktelow & Over, 1990) found evidence for the *matching bias* using a modified version of the WST, proving that participants can arrive at the correct conclusion (falsifying the rule) by pure accident, that is, selecting the falsifying card not for logical reasons but because something in the rule states it's falsifying condition. Evans (1989) later underlined that it is not because people don't want to falsify information but rather an inability to do so.

An effect such as the matching bias underlines how relevance and context can be involved in reasoning tasks. It also points out how abstract rules of reasoning are not necessarily used to solve a particular task because knowledge and context can yield a conclusion, whether valid or not. Nevertheless, reasoning biases do inform us about the particularities of human reasoning and the following section will further illustrate how these reasoning strategies influence the outcome of reasoning tasks in particular.

2.5 Reasoning biases

The majority of research focusing on reasoning biases stems from experiments in syllogistic and conditional reasoning. As was mentioned earlier, the matching bias was illustrated by modifying a conditional reasoning task (WST) and realising how people tend to be influenced by the manner in which the conditional rule is presented. In syllogistic problems, participants are also influenced by 'non logical' issues that is, aspects of the task which are not *meant* to interact with its resolution (Evans & Over, 1996). For example, the belief bias is the tendency for people to accept invalid arguments because they are faced with believable conclusions, not necessarily correct ones. Evans et al. (1983) empirically demonstrated that belief interacts with reasoning in a series of experiments showing how people had a strong tendency to uncritically accept believable conclusions, while being more careful in their assessment about unbelievable ones.

Two explanations were proposed by Evans (1989) for the belief bias. One is the possibility that people are misunderstanding the logical prerequisites of what constitutes a valid argument, what the author calls 'misinterpreted necessity'. In effect for most people, the fact that an argument may follow from a premise is good enough to conclude that it is valid, whereas in logic, a conclusion *must* follow from an argument to conclude that it is correct. A second explanation for the belief bias, the 'selective scrutiny' argument, is that before solving any reasoning problem, people possess a 'selective heuristic'. In other words in the case of an unbelievable conclusion, they may be more prone to use logical analysis because of how surprising the conclusion is, whereas in a believable conclusion, they may be less rigorous. Oakhill and Johnson-Laird (1985) also showed how that the belief bias was equally apparent when people generated their own conclusions and in fact, that the interpretation of premises was correct but that the reasoning process was still altered by beliefs.

Some researchers have tried to diminish the belief bias effect by adding information in the instructions to help the participants avoid using prior knowledge and understand that a logical valid conclusion must follow from the given premises and only IF they do, should they conclude it is valid, regardless of whether the conclusion is plausible. For example, experiments by Newstead et al. (1992, 1994, as cited in Evans & Over, 1996) showed that the belief bias could be greatly diminished with the use of these 'augmented instructions' but not completely eliminated. Another study replicated these results by further validating how the belief bias was apparent irrespective of participants' abstract reasoning abilities (Markovits & Nantel, 1989).

As was pointed out earlier, the results of the Wason Selection Task demonstrated the occurrence of a confirmation bias. A very important experiment which further empirically validated this idea was devised by Wason (1960). What is called the '2-4-6 Problem' is meant to test inductive reasoning. A series of three numbers (typically: 2 4 6) are presented to participants and they are told that they need to uncover a rule (known by the experimenter), to which the series of three numbers conforms. For the participant to find out the experimenter's rule, he or she needs to write down a series of three numbers that would illustrate it. For each group of proposed numbers, the experimenter will say whether the participants guess matches the rule but participants are instructed to disclose the rule only once they are sure it is the correct one. The participant writes down each of his hypotheses. The main and consistent effect of this task is that participants have a tendency to verify only positive instances of the hypothesised rule which shows again that falsification is not a primary reasoning strategy used by people in general.

2.6 Rationality and reasoning

In summary, people do not naturally resort to strategies that would help them solve logical reasoning tasks on the one hand and on the other hand, individuals seem to be influenced more by prior knowledge and context. This is of great concern to reasoning researchers and increases the difficulty to solve the debate as to *how* we reason and arrive at conclusions. An alternative solution proposed by Evans et al. (1993) and Evans and Over (1996) considers that these '*reasoning biases*' should not stand as proof of human irrationality but rather, as evidence that reasoning may include a dual process: rationality1, which describes reasoning in a way that is usually reliable and efficient for achieving one's goals (based on prior experiences and beliefs) and rationality2, meaning reasoning with principles of logic when one has reason to. The theory contends that both types of rationality are also bound by 'cognitive constraints', meaning people's ability to process information. Hence, it is proposed that individuals use one, or the other type of reasoning, according to what presents itself to be solved. That is, normal, everyday decision making situations would require practical reasoning (rationality1) where deciding on actual facts would require theoretical reasoning (rationality2). This proposal could account for why people fail to be logical when tested on formal reasoning tasks. Evans (1989) had even proposed that 'debiasing', a procedure meant to reduce or even eradicate the impact of reasoning biases could enhance people's ability to use rationality2, that is, solve logical reasoning tasks.

Evans and Over's rationality1 and 2 theory has not been accepted unanimously as some researchers have argued for a more unified competence whether it be based on the premise that people reason with practicability (only using rationality1) or that people reason with theoretical principles (using only rationality2). For Johnson-Laird (1999), the theory's strength is that it can indeed explain both reasoning competence and incompetence however, this would accommodate too much and thus become difficult to test and disprove.

2.7 Limits to reasoning studies

Some critics have contested the use of formal tests of reasoning and asked or not people reason with the mechanisms inferred by the experimenter. Cohen (1981) puts forth what he calls the 'normative system problem' whereby for example, people may be using a more personal system of probability (based on experience) while the experimenter expects and intends a more statistical probabilistic mechanism of reasoning to be used. A second drawback to a normative system of reasoning concerns the problem of the cognitive load such abstract tasks can put on a participant. Effectively, it's been proposed that qualifying someone as being irrational if that person cannot solve a task that is beyond the limits of their human cognitive processing abilities, is incorrect.

Oaksford and Chater (1993) have considered another argument concerning cognitive processing abilities, which refers to a problem of 'external validity'. That is, a normative system theory does not transpose well into real-life problems because previous knowledge and beliefs are taken into account in 'real-life reasoning'. Cohen (1981) also argues that, because laboratory experiments are artificial and not representative of normal thinking and reasoning, then external validity may be in danger.

Finally, a third argument of 'interpretation' may account for why participants may not be assessing reasoning problems in the way intended by the researcher. Henle (1962) argues that people's personal representation of the problems would yield to conclusions that were logical if one considers that person's specific representation of the premises. Hence in this view, mental logic is actually existent, only the formal tests are unfit to represent it adequately.

2.8 Reasoning with heuristics

Tversky and Kahneman (1973, 1982) developed a reasoning theory suggesting that reasoning is a decision making operation where premises are judged according to a restricted number of heuristics. Heuristics are general filters of reasoning which bypass calculating real probabilities. Yet, heuristics can lead to systematic errors because the assessment of premises is based on data of limited validity. Tversky and Kahneman (1982) claim that just as people's perceptions can distant reality, heuristics activate a bias on judgment of probability. So for example, the 'representativeness heuristic' leads a person to rely on the degree to which A resembles B, or how much A is a representative of B, e.g., social gatherings tend to be superficial so the people at my friend's party will be superficial. While this may be true, it is not always the case because base rates are not considered when the representativeness heuristic filters judgment. The 'availability heuristic' suggests that people estimate the frequency or probability of the occurrence of an event by bringing to mind the easiest example of a class of event, that is, instances of large classes of events are recalled quicker than infrequent ones. In other words, familiarity yields to erroneous decisions, according to the availability heuristic, e.g., I heard about a mugging lately on the news, so I could be mugged. The anchoring heuristic describes the fallacy of starting with an initial value biased to fit the final answer. In other words, the starting point seems to be suggested either by the formulation of the problem or by the result of a partial computation. Tversky and Kahneman (1982) report that several of the main heuristics described here are apparent even if participants are rewarded for correct answers and encouraged to be more accurate by the use of prompts. Heuristics research shows how common assumptions and the accessibility of information through personal experience can override logic.

2.9 Inductive reasoning

An inductive conclusion is drawn on the basis of selective evidence and tends to increase information. However in inductive reasoning, a conclusion is not necessarily true, since it is drawn from a person's own opinions, experiences and knowledge. Conclusions in inductive reasoning add information that is not necessarily in the premises which implies that contrary to deductive reasoning, here, the content of the argument cannot be separated from the form. Johnson-Laird (1993) proposes a comprehensive definition of inductive reasoning as 'any process of thought yielding a conclusion that increases the semantic information in its initial observations or premises'. Again, what this definition implies is that the content of the proposition has the implication of ruling out certain states of affairs. An important question that has preoccupied researchers is one concerning the 'correctness' of an inference, that is, how is induction justified? For Johnson-Laird (1994a), current research on induction is in a state of uncertainty and 'no adequate theory of the human inductive process exists' (p. 14). He argues that the mechanism of induction is almost inseparable from normal mental activity since it is part of how we make sense of the world and the way we do that is by having models based on the availability of pertinent knowledge to what we are reasoning about (see the 'availability heuristic' in Tversky & Kanheman, 1982). This leads us most of the time to use inductive reasoning in everyday life, which as we have seen, does not always lead to true conclusions. But it is the form that we use in everyday reasoning because valid deductions are not possible in the absence of all true or necessary information. Manktelow (1999) also reports on the dilemma that has prevailed for years on how one instance can yield a generalisation while at other times, many instances which should lead to a particular inference and yet, people do not generalise from them. A proposal from Johnson-Laird (1994a) concerns the strength of an argument and it suggests that such strength depends on the relation between the premises and the conclusion. That is, the strength of an inference will increase if the premises are considered consistent with the conclusion in at least one possible state of affairs. If there seems to be no counterexamples, the argument will stay strong, that is, the conclusion will be considered to follow reliably from the premises. To summarise, the strength of an inference is equivalent to the probability of the conclusion given the premises are true. This account is in relation to Johnson-Laird's theory of mental models, which will be exposed in the following section.

2.10 Mental models

Johnson-Laird (1983) initially developed his theory of mental models (MM) to explain verbal comprehension, inspired by the work of Kenneth Craik (1943, as cited in Johnson-Laird, 1994b) on how the mind creates 'small scale models' of reality. It is suggested that when people try to make sense of a proposition, they create a model in their mind of the situation that is discussed. The model itself can be a word or a visual image but most importantly, its structure corresponds with the way people organize their view of the world (Johnson-Laird, 1994a).

Johnson-Laird and Byrne (1991) broadened the MM theory, suggesting that there are three levels of thinking that people experience when they attempt to draw conclusions: First, people will try to understand the premises by using what they know in general. Then, they will construct models about what has been understood from these premises. The models can be images, words or instances of each premise. The next level involves combining the models in order to draw a description of the state of affairs they are trying to compose. This description must yield to a conclusion which includes new information, outside of the given premises. If the person doing the reasoning does not find such a conclusion, he or she will reason that anything follows from the premises. However, if one does find a conclusion, the last stage will involve searching for alternative models which would be coherent with the premises but where the hypothesized conclusion would be false. This last level then involves validating that no falsifying model compromises the conclusion, that is, that the conclusion is valid. If alternative models do falsify the conclusion then it is false and the person will search for a new conclusion that will not be proven wrong by an alternative model.

In summary, in this section, the main differences between deductive and inductive reasoning have been described and the main reasoning paradigms that have been used to test these inference processes were outlined. The key result from this research is that people in the general population have trouble resolving logical tasks. Effectively, they are prone to different reasoning biases which lead them to false conclusions. Moreover, certain forms of deduction are invalid and yet, people do not seem to be able to differentiate between those which are valid and those which are not. Theories like Johnson-Laird's mental models theory or Tversky and Kanheman's heuristics theory have helped to view reasoning as guided by factors other than formal logic, as it stands. For example, the mental models theory tells us that people have representations of 'how the world is' and they will draw inferences based on these models. If the model is incorrect, invalid conclusions may be drawn from it. Tversky and Kanheman (1982) have shown that heuristics seem to guide reasoning so that it is understood that people will look for the easiest way to judge a probability, not necessarily the most valid judgement. Hence, it appears that context is important to inference as well as people's individual cognitive structure. It thus becomes clear from this review that certain reasoning models can serve as theoretical paradigms to test pathological reasoning since 'thinking' is how people behave, whether pathological or not. Moreover, studies using reasoning paradigms explain thinking behaviour by observing thinking performance which offers a more parsimonious explanation than those of information processing theory and studies, which tend to hypothesise about remote abilities like 'selective attention' or 'memory' to explain thinking behaviour. The next section will elaborate on studies that have used reasoning paradigms to test pathological thinking and the comprehension that these study results yielded in terms of diverse mental disorders.

3. Reasoning paradigms with pathological thinking

Pathological expressions like repetitiveness, self contradiction and denial of facts have been observed and noted by authors like Wason and Johnson-Laird (1972) in their many reasoning studies. For example, the case of a participant persisting with a hypothesis in a task was presented by noting the participant's 'strong obsessional features', that is 'his fertile imagination, and intense preoccupation with original hypotheses, has narrowed his field of appreciation to the point where he has become blind to the obvious' (Wason & Johnson-Laird, 1972, p. 233). This trumping of the senses is typical of obsessional narratives which frequently lead to a conclusion in stark contradiction to the premise. Example: The car door is locked safely but maybe the sound wasn't quite right and the car is old and a friend of mine found the doors didn't lock properly and in any case anything can happen with these mechanical devices, so… the car door could well be unlocked (see O'Connor et al., 2005). The hint of a link between these observations and psychopathology which seems a valid invitation for exploring the field of reasoning and psychopathology. The following section reviews current state of research into reasoning and pathology looking at it from these two perspectives: 1) reasoning processes in psychopathology: how reasoning performance can inform us about the mechanisms of psychopathology and 2) the effect of content on reasoning competence: how manipulating content with characteristics of a psychopathology can influence reasoning competence.

3.1 Mechanisms of psychopathology

Researchers using reasoning paradigms as a means of understanding mechanisms of psychopathology consider that reasoning in itself, plays a determinant role in human behaviour. Observing variations in reasoning performance can inform us about the processes that guide behaviour. The advantages of working with reasoning paradigms are that the tasks used are well documented and have been tested in a variety of conditions in the general population. The results serve as an anchor for estimating differences. The following section describes a Bayesian probabilistic task, often used in clinical populations. This probabilistic task measures how people estimate the likelihood of an event and their decision making style.

3.2 A probabilistic reasoning paradigm

The task involves imagining 10 bags containing 100 poker chips each, while manipulating the ratio of red versus blue chips in each condition. Participants estimate how likely it was that a bag containing predominantly red or blue chips is chosen, on the basis of the experimenter's draws of chips from a (presumably) randomly chosen bag. In the original version developed by Phillips and Edwards (1966), the effects of probability estimates on different variables such as: prior probabilities, amount of data gathered before making a decision, diagnostic impact of data, payoffs and response modes were evaluated. The results from Phillips and Edwards (1966) showed that people in the general population had a tendency to request more information to come to a decision than logical probability calculus would predict.

Volans (1976), Huq et al. (1988) and Garety et al. (1991) used modified versions of the probabilistic task in a series of studies with people suffering from diverse psychological difficulties. For example, Huq et al. (1988) decided to test groups of deluded, psychiatric and normal controls. Clinical observations of people experiencing delusions led them to hypothesize that fixity of belief and intensity of conviction would lead the participants to be less conservative than the other two groups. Their hypotheses were that people with delusions would require less information before making a decision and be overconfident about these choices compared to normal controls or other psychiatric participants. The results confirmed both hypotheses since deluded participants showed a significantly higher level of conviction on their 'initial certainty' estimates, and requested less evidence before making a decision compared to the two other control groups. The authors concluded that people with delusions showed a 'jumping to conclusion' (JTC) style of reasoning. It remains to be understood how this translates into everyday decision making and if this reasoning 'bias' means that people with delusions jump to conclusion about any information that is presented to them. The fact that the task is neutral would indicate that this is the case but a more realistic context may yield different results.

The study from Huq et al. (1988) had included a group of people diagnosed with schizophrenia without distinction of deluded participants without hallucinations hence their findings needed to be replicated. Garety et al. (1991) thus extended the work using the probabilistic reasoning task with better defined diagnostic groups so in addition to a group diagnosed with schizophrenia, a 'pure delusional' group was included, that is, people diagnosed with DSM-III-R (American Psychiatric Association) criteria for delusional disorder (DD) (paranoia type). An anxious control group and a non-psychiatric control group served as comparisons. The hypothesis was that DD patients would show a greater bias in probabilistic reasoning than schizophrenic patients since their abnormal beliefs were more subtle, and they experienced no hallucinations. No significant differences were found between schizophrenic patients and paranoid delusional patients on their responses of the probabilistic task. Effectively, both these groups were overconfident and required less evidence before making a decision than the anxious and normal control group. Even if these results are consistent, more research is needed in order to differentiate between a possible task effect and a genuine different reasoning style. No other, studies have been conducted in order to test this idea, by using a different probabilistic task and exploring if this would lead to variations in style of reasoning. Further experiments using emotionally salient content confirmed these findings (see Dudley et al., 1997a, 1997b).

Dudley et al. (1997a) devised two separate experiments to examine whether people with delusions exhibited a general deficit in reasoning, when using different probabilistic material and by varying the ratio of beads from that of the standard probabilistic task. The first experiment verified performance on a 'biased coin task'. People with delusions, depressed controls and non-psychiatric controls needed to estimate the chance that a coin was biased to 'heads' when presented with a set of results from throwing the coin. The results on this task showed there were no differences in probabilistic estimates between the three groups. This finding is important because it indicates that people with delusions don't have any problems with estimating probabilities. However, the second experiment tested decision making with variations in the ratio of beads (an 85:15 condition and a 60:40 condition) the manipulation aimed to test whether a different base rate would yield a more cautious strategy from the delusional participants. Results showed that indeed, delusional patients took notice of the different base rate and were more cautious but still required less evidence than the two control groups for the same condition. Thus replication of the JTC bias was apparent. It seems that people with delusional disorder use the same reasoning process as normal controls but that they require less evidence to do so hence showing a different reasoning style. However, the question remains on how this translates into clinical reality, that is, how this applies to therapy. Colbert et al. (2010) suggest that jumping to conclusions may be a trait characteristic of those with a propensity to delusions and predictive of later symptomatology.

In their critical review of cognitive approaches to delusions, Garety and Freeman (1999) compare three main theories of development and maintenance of delusional disorder. Their own theory is the only one where reasoning is considered to play a part in delusions although they specify that this applies only to certain delusional types. Effectively, Garety (1991) and Garety and Hemsley (1994) propose a multifactorial model that includes past experience, affect, self-esteem and motivation as having a role in some delusions while biases in perception and judgment would be more crucial to other types. As described previously, the series of experiments using the probabilistic task have been consistent in demonstrating a JTC reasoning Style, later termed a 'data gathering deficit' (gathering less evidence to form a hypothesis) in people with delusions. The authors conclude that although erroneous conclusions are not always the result of this 'data-gathering deficit', it does predispose individuals to accept incorrect hypotheses. In a wider perspective, it also implies that people who suffer from delusions show this style of reasoning when faced with neutral material and that both diagnostic groups, delusional and schizophrenic, are prone to reason in this manner.

3.3 Reasoning processes and anxiety and obsessive compulsive disorders

Cognitive theories use terms like 'irrational thinking', 'cognitive errors' and 'irrational beliefs', etc., and yet, little information is available about the mechanisms involved in the development of such pathological irrationality. In fact, reasoning processes in anxiety disorders have been relatively less investigated than in thought disorders. One of the reasons may be that thought disorders are more easily associated with the hypothesis that 'faulty reasoning' plays an important role in bizarre idea formation. Behavioural models based on classical conditioning of the fear response associated to catastrophic thinking are the explanation mostly agreed on, concerning the development of anxiety. But how 'catastrophic thinking' develops in the first place is less clear. Reasoning performance on neutral tasks may inform us on of diverse reasoning strategies in different psycho-pathologies.

Whether psychopathology influences reasoning performance or whether it is the opposite, that is, reasoning strategies cause psychopathology remains an important question. A second query relates to the implications of reasoning results: how does reasoning performance inform us about a particular pathology? As Garety and Freeman (1999) suggested, longitudinal studies are required to respond to the question of causality between psychopathology and reasoning strategies. Second, translating reasoning findings into clinical applications remains an important challenge for clinical researchers. For example, pioneer authors like Milner et al. (1971) examined decision-making in obsessive-compulsive disorder (OCD). They compared performance of a group of people with OCD and a non-clinical control group on an auditory signal detection task. A faint tone embedded in white noise was presented and participants had to decide whether they needed additional trials before stating if the tone was present. The results suggested that before making a decision, OCD participants requested a higher number of trials than people in the control group. It was hypothesized that 'in obsessional disorder decisions may be deferred to an abnormal extent' (Milner et al., 1971, p. 88). This finding marked the beginning of a series of experiments yielding consistent results about people with OCD needing more information before being certain of their decision. Unfortunately, no explanations were offered on how these findings contributed to the development or maintenance of OCD. However, the request for less information before making a decision as reflected in the JTC bias seemed to form an element of reasoning defining poor insight. Whereas people with OCD tend to take longer making decisions, people with delusional disorder are significantly quicker. Body dysmorphic disorder (BDD) may be considered a group in between OCD and DD in terms of insight and overvalued ideation and BDD show only a modest JTC reasoning bias (Reese et al., 2010)

Volans (1976) investigated reasoning in OCD using the standard probabilistic task (described earlier) with one modification involving a YES-NO response mode (ex: as to which jar, A or B, was chosen). Again, draws to decision were significantly higher in the OCD group than for the normal control group and the phobic group. These significant results were replicated by Fear and Healy (1997) who tested probabilistic reasoning in both OCD and DD groups as well as a 'mixed' group (people with both delusional and obsessional beliefs) in comparison to anon-clinical control group. Results echoed those of Volans (1976), where the OCD group differed in their reasoning style from the DD and the mixed group by requesting more evidence before making a decision. So where people with DD seem to exhibit a 'data-gathering deficit' by requiring less evidence than normal control, they are still much closer to the norm than people with OCD. It would appear then, that people with OCD exhibit a 'data-gathering excess', because of their extreme deviation from the norm. Again, a clear explanation is lacking in terms of how this contributes to the conceptualization of OCD. In other words, which decisions in everyday life would be affected by this bias?

The 'data gathering excess' style of reasoning found in OCD was not present in another study using a probabilistic task. In effect, Rhéaume et al. (2000) used a modified version of the probabilistic task with people who showed pathological perfectionism. Here, the ratio of beads that was used was a proportion of 60:40, which renders the task more difficult and ambiguous because of the almost equal proportions of each colour of beads. Rhéaume et al. measured functional and dysfunctional perfectionism to form two separate groups. People with 'dysfunctional' perfectionism (which is hypothesized to be linked to OCD) required less draws before making a decision when compared to people with 'functional' perfectionism. Although the authors found a relationship between dysfunctional perfectionism and an obsessive-compulsive behaviour scale, current consensus does not yield perfectionism as a predictor of OCD (Frost et al., 2002) so it may be premature to draw any further conclusions.

The probabilistic reasoning paradigm was also used in a non clinical sample of people scoring high on the Intolerance of Uncertainty Questionnaire (IUQ) which distinguishes worriers meeting GAD criteria from those who do not. Ladouceur et al. (1997) used a modified version of the probabilistic task. Two levels of ambiguity, moderate and high, were created by varying the ratio of the coloured beads (moderate ambiguity = 85:15 and high ambiguity = 60:40). Results obtained from this sub-clinical population lead to contradicting conclusions. Indeed, the results suggested that under the moderate level of ambiguity condition, more people characterized with IU required a greater number of draws before making a decision. However, the effect disappeared in the high ambiguity condition and the authors explain the finding by postulating a lower threshold of perception of ambiguity by people with IU, which creates a need to precipitate a decision. The modification by the authors of the original probabilistic task meant that the order of appearance of the colour of the beads was undetermined. Therefore, the number of draws requested by the participants was determined by chance. Consequently, it is difficult to compare these results with previous probabilistic reasoning studies.

Probabilistic reasoning constitutes only one aspect of reasoning and other types of reasoning have been investigated in psychopathology like deductive and inductive reasoning processes. Effectively, Reed (1977, 1991) initiated such formal investigation with participants diagnosed with 'anankastic' personality disorder, the equivalent of the more modern diagnosis of obsessive-compulsive personality disorder (OCPD). In his study, he compared an OCPD group to psychiatric controls on a deductive reasoning arithmetic task and an inductive task requiring. Participants to infer a rule about a series of numbers. Results showed that the OCPD group performed better on the deductive task but that their results on the inductive task were inferior to that of the psychiatric control group. In the absence of a non-psychiatric control group and a better diagnostic definition, the results are not sufficiently representative. However, Reed's research emphasized the relevance of exploring inductive and deductive reasoning in people with obsessions and prompted further investigation of such mechanisms.

Hence, Pélissier and O'Connor (2002) examined formal deductive and inductive reasoning in OCD and to date, this study constitutes the only research to have extensively examined such processes in OCD. A group of twelve people with OCD was compared to ten people with GAD and a normal control group of ten other participants, on a series of six inductive and deductive tasks. The deductive tasks involved were: the Wason Selection Task, the 2-4-6 problem and a deductive exercise designed by the authors. Essentially, no significant differences were found between groups on either of these measures. The inductive tasks were three exercises designed by the authors based on reasoning literature: estimating plausibility of 40 different given inferences ('Finding the evidence'), linking two separate, unrelated premises ('Bridging') and estimating the validity of an arbitrary statement before and after supplying arguments to support it ('Supporting an arbitrary statement'). The results in the inductive tasks suggested group differences in two of the three exercises. Effectively, the OCD group took longer to initiate their inference process than the two control groups. Also, they seemed to doubt an arbitrary statement in a higher proportion than the two other groups, even after generating supporting evidence for this particular statement. Drawing from Johnson-Laird's mental model theory, the authors hypothesized that these findings were due to an excessive production of alternative mental models on the part of people with OCD.

In effect, Pélissier and O'Connor's (2002) proposed that producing too many alternative mental models led people with OCD to be less certain of their conclusion, whereas in reality supporting arguments created greater certainty. This interpretation of the results was challenged by the same authors in a more recent study where Pélissier et al. (2009) tested inductive reasoning using a modified version of Johnson-Laird's (1994a, 1994b) probabilistic inductive reasoning task. In effect, Pelissier et al. tested the mental models hypothesis by creating a task expressly designed to measure the impact of alternative possibilities on conviction level. This supposed that an important parameter influencing reasoning might be the source of the alternative possibilities more than the quantity of alternative models. Hence the task devised to test inductive reasoning and the impact of the source of arguments involved whether arguments were given by an external source or were self-generated by the participants. Results revealed that people with OCD are more influenced when the alternative conclusions are given by the experimenter, that is, their level of confidence decreases much more in this condition than in the self-generated condition. Such enhanced doubting of the initial inference was not apparent in the control group, that is, the non-OCD control group was not specifically sensitive to whether or not conclusions were inferred by themselves or given by the experimenter. So the results actually refute the interpretation of results from the previous Pélissier's study, that is, people with OCD do not produce too many models but rather, doubt seems to influence reasoning processes by according too much importance to mental models coming from outside sources. Simpson et al.. (2007) replicated the finding of differences in inductive reasoning in OCD and the higher level of doubt, and Keen et al. (2008), likewise, showed that participants with OCD were more influenced by simulation heuristics and able to simulate their OCD scenarios as if they were real.

3.4 Pathology in reasoning: effect of content on reasoning competence

There is a line of research in which diverse reasoning paradigms are modified by including themes that are relevant to diverse psychopathologies. These studies explore whether reasoning patterns remain the same or diverge when pathological content is included the reasoning paradigm. If the patterns of reasoning are the same or just more pronounced to those observed in the neutral condition, it is possible to hypothesize that this particular reasoning style plays a role in the maintenance of the pathological symptoms while not being a causal factor. However, if the reasoning style is different in the pathology related content condition compared to the neutral condition it would be hypothesised that a special case of reasoning is employed in that particular condition. The studies using modified reasoning paradigms also manipulate variables other than reasoning. For example, a conceptual variable like perfectionism may be tested using a reasoning paradigm, serving more as a template to test whether a pathological construct is relevant or not to a particular psychopathology.

3.5 Effects of content in affective and thought disorder

Young and Bentall (1997) developed an experiment to include content in a reasoning paradigm. The authors modified the Bayesian probabilistic task and replaced beads by descriptions of people (a person that was liked and a person that was disliked) to create a 'personality' condition. The condition was designed to test whether the salience of the material would influence the groups' probabilistic estimates and decision making style. Three groups were tested: deluded patients, depressed patients and non-clinical controls. Results demonstrated that overall, the three groups reached an initial level of certainty and revised these certainty levels more rapidly in the personality condition than in the neutral condition. However, this effect was more pronounced in the clinical groups compared to the normal control group. The authors concluded that emotionally salient themes may produce 'abnormalities' of probabilistic reasoning which would be expected in the development and maintenance of delusions.

The results of this study show that although the control group showed a quick decision making strategy, people in the clinical groups exhibit an even quicker bias towards concluding rapidly.

These results were replicated by subsequent research by Dudley et al. (1997b) who tested whether a 'jumping to conclusions' (JTC) (strategy of coming to a conclusion on the basis of less information) was observed when using realistic material versus abstract material in delusional patients. Three groups were tested: people with delusions, people who were depressed and normal controls. The participants were presented with two versions of the probabilistic task where both versions used realistic material but one of them had emotionally neutral content and the other used emotionally salient themes. Results of these two experiments show that people with delusions request less evidence before coming to a conclusion when presented with realistic content, so the JTC bias was generalized to realistic content. The second finding was that all groups requested less evidence when the material was more salient. Therefore, emotionally relevant material increases the JTC reasoning style for everyone, although the authors underline the tendency for people with delusions to require even less evidence than the two other groups but this was not statistically significant.

Drawing on the previous results, Dudley et al. (1998) set out to explore whether the JTC bias using salient material was present in other forms of reasoning in order to rule out a task effect. The authors modified the Wason Selection Task (WST) by manipulating the content going from neutral to being more realistic. Hence, conditional reasoning performance of people with delusional disorder was compared to a depressed and a non-clinical control group. Four versions of the WST were devised to vary in content of realism. Results showed that people with delusional disorder reasoned in the same manner as the two control groups on all but one of the four versions. In fact, the difference in reasoning was found in the most realistic version of the WST where people in the delusional group solved the task less efficiently than the normal control and depressed group. The results were unexpected since increased realism generally increases the WST performance. Thus Dudley et al. (1998) suggested that people with delusions may have a working memory deficit limiting them from manipulating all the necessary elements. The authors state that this remains to be determined in future studies but seemingly, a more realistic context leads clinical groups to a stronger bias. The results stress the importance of tailoring reasoning tasks to particular psychopathologies in order to resemble clinical reality. In an attempt to tease out distinctions in reasoning between anxiety, depression and paranoia, Bennett and Corcoran (2010) reported that elevated levels of depression were associated with the tendency to underestimate the likelihood of future positive and neutral events, whereas subclinical paranoia was associated with overestimation of the likelihood of future threatening events (Bennett & Corcoran, 2010). Further, there is also evidence that anxiety states may interact in paranoia to produce even greater jumping to conclusions (Lincoln et al., 2010).

3.6 Effects of content in anxiety disorders

Research using reasoning paradigms in anxious clinical populations uses salient material more than reasoning studies in thought disorders. Essentially, most paradigms Involve the modification of the WST by replacing the elements of the task (for example 'a vowel') with anxious content or simply using anxiety tailored scripts as the basis for requesting inferential performance. For instance, Arntz et al. (1995) investigated inductive reasoning processes biased toward danger and subjective anxiety in a population of anxious participants compared to non anxious controls. Their study involved four groups of anxious patients (52 spider phobics, 41 panic patients, 38 social phobics, and 31 other anxiety patients) compared to 24 normal control participants. All participants had to rate the perceived danger in anxiety-tailored scripts, where objective danger vs. objective safety as well as objective anxiety vs. objective non-anxiety information were varied. It was hypothesized that anxious patients would not only infer danger on the basis of objective danger cues but also infer danger on the basis of subjective anxiety information where non-clinical controls would not. The hypothesis was confirmed and the authors concluded that a process termed 'ex-consequentia reasoning' was responsible, where participants conclude that feeling anxious implies danger. One possible limit to the implications of these results is the fact that the task requires all participants to infer either 'danger' or 'not-danger'. This dichotomous choice may lead anxious participants to consistently infer danger, not necessarily because they have faulty reasoning strategies but precisely because they never experience having anxiety symptoms that yield conclusions of safety. The results then seem to underline the difference between being anxious and not being anxious. In other words, it is unclear if the inability to conclude 'if I feel anxious, then I am not in danger' (presumably the reasoning of normal controls), is based on faulty reasoning on the part of anxious participants or based on their symptoms. So although this would also need to be tested, it should not be ruled out that the inference of danger may simply be the absence of sufficient premises to permit a safety conclusion.

Spider fearful students were tested by de Jong et al. (1997) in two separate experiments: the first one tested phobic participants on a conditional reasoning task where they had to assess the validity of conditional statements in the context of general threats or phobic specific threats. Modified versions of the WST were used where danger rules (if p than danger) and safety rules (if p than safety) were proposed to two groups (high and low level of fear towards spider). In the second experiment, the same material was used but was administered to three groups: treated and untreated spider phobic women, and a group of non fearful control participants. The results of these two experiments showed that in the general threat condition, reasoning strategies were guided by utility judgment, that is, all participants in all groups relied on confirming evidence when faced with a danger rule (selecting the q card) and relied on disconfirming information when given a safety rule (selecting the not-q card). In the phobic threat condition, this pattern was even more pronounced especially in the non-treated spider phobic group. What these results seem to be saying is that the more salient the content for phobic participants, the more they use a reasoning strategy that the authors call 'fear-confirming reasoning' and which seems to be a natural progression on a continuum of these danger-safety reasoning strategies. However, presumably the control participants did not respond to the anxiety-salient condition because the content was irrelevant to them. This makes sense since they do not suffer from spider phobia. This 'fear-confirming pattern' was tested to validate it's consistency by verifying it's use in other anxiety disorders.

The 'fear-confirming reasoning' was tested by de Jong et al. (1998) in hypochondriacal patients on a series of modified versions of the WST. Echoing previous results with the spider phobics, hypochondriacal patients did use the fear confirming strategies but this was not significantly different from the control group. The authors conclude that the threat of health problems would be more prone to make even non-hypochondriacal people search for disconfirmation, because of it's universal nature where as spider information would be neutral to non-spider phobics. A group of hypochondriacal patients and controls using the same modified WST were tested by Smeets et al. (2000). However this time, the authors deleted a worry statement presumed to have influenced normal controls in the de Jong et al. (1998) study. The results of the revised study confirmed a fear-confirming reasoning style that was more pronounced in the health threat condition for hypochondriacal patients. So although it is not a specific trait of hypochondriasis to reason in a 'better safe than sorry' manner, this fear confirming reasoning pattern may serve to maintain the health fears in place. More recent work by Vroling and de Jong (2010) has attributed a threat confirming belief bias and its interference on logical reasoning to a better 'safe than sorry' heuristic. But the belief bias was not directly correlated with anxiety symptoms, which suggests the bias may be more likely a diathesis for the development of anxious psychopathology.

3.7 Ex-consequentia reasoning

Both judgements and interpretative biases are linked with anxiety and mood congruent effects. Emotion can exert complex effects on decision-making and reasoning, sometimes hindering adaptive thinking (Blanchette & Richards, 2010). One example is 'ex-consequentia reasoning' where feeling stages can dictate conclusions about the world, e.g., I feel bad, so there must be a reason. A further study devised by Engelhard et al. (2001) expanded on the concept of 'ex-consequentia-reasoning' (Arntz et al., 1995) by comparing 'emotion-based reasoning' (ER) with 'intrusion-based reasoning' (IR). Both concepts are described as the process of inferring danger respectively on the basis of emotion or on the basis of the occurrence of an intrusion (an upsetting thought about an anxiety-related stimulus). The study tested a population of Vietnam combat veterans suffering from posttraumatic stress disorder (PTSD) compared to a group not diagnosed with PTSD. The experimental task aimed to discovery if people inferred danger on the basis of anxiety responses in the case of ER and on the basis of intrusions in the case of IR when presented with objective danger information and objective safety information. The scenarios presented to all participants varied in content with objective danger/safety information and anxiety/no anxiety response for the ER condition and with objective danger/safety information and intrusions/ no intrusions for the IR condition. Inference of danger was measured by asking people to assess how dangerous each scenario was, by scoring a visual analogue scale for each of them. Results confirmed that all participants inferred more danger on the basis of objective danger information compared to objective safety information. Nevertheless, combat veterans with PTSD rated the scenarios as being significantly more dangerous on the basis of both anxiety responses and intrusions where non-PTSD participants did not show such a significant difference. Engelhard and colleagues (2001) suggested that ER and IR were linked to PTSD and may serve to maintain PTSD symptoms. That is, the maintenance of pathological symptoms may be characterized by the tendency for anxious people to infer danger on the basis of anxious symptoms and here, on the basis of anxious thoughts. However yet again, the question remains to be answered about whether this is due to a faulty reasoning strategy ('if I feel anxious and think about scary events, then there must be danger') or due to the induction process itself, which involves providing additional information to the premises, from which one infers conclusions. For instance, the additional information may be different for PTSD sufferers than for non-PTSD sufferers because by definition, people with PTSD must have experienced a richer array of anxiety symptoms and intrusions at the time of the experiment. In order to establish a causal link between ER/IR and the development of PTSD, a subsequent study was devised by the authors.

In this study, Engelhard et al. (2002) did not use the ER condition and simply tested the IR condition to establish whether IR predicted PTSD symptoms, following a train disaster. Twenty-nine participants who were directly exposed witnesses of a train crash were compared to fourteen non-witness people from a small Belgium town where this disaster occurred. The task used to assess the inference of danger was similar to Engelhard et al.'s (2001) previous study in that scenarios were designed to manipulate objective danger/safety information with intrusions/ no intrusions segments. Participants were required to assess how dangerous each scenario was, using the visual analogue scale. Results revealed to the people who were direct witnesses rated the scenarios with the intrusion segments as more dangerous than the scenarios without such intrusions and this was significantly different than the control group (non witnesses). Also, participants within the directly exposed group who showed higher ratings in IR reported higher levels of chronic PTSD symptoms at 3.5 months follow-up. The authors caution about their conclusion on how intrusions can predict PTSD symptoms by reminding us that completing a task involving intrusions may have prompted the witnesses to experience similar intrusions. Also, since the non-witnesses, by definition, were not exposed to the trauma, they may have found the intrusion segments unrelated to their own experience.

4. Discussion

The first section of this review article delineated the key differences between deductive and inductive reasoning and described the chief reasoning paradigms that have been used to test these reasoning processes. The main finding from this research is that people in the general population do not easily solve logical tasks. That is, people are prone to diverse reasoning biases which lead them to false conclusions. Thus theories like Johnson-Laird's mental models or Tversky and Kanheman's heuristics theory have helped to view reasoning as depending more on a person's own strategies than formal logical strategies. Hence, it seems context is important to inference as well as people's own cognitive structure. Studies using reasoning paradigms may explain thinking behaviour, be it normal or pathological, by observing thinking performance. The line of research going into reasoning seems to offer a simple, more direct way of studying cognitive aspects of psychopathology.

The second part of this article has outlined a novel line of research in clinical psychopathology. Effectively, research into reasoning and pathology is twofold: studies that manipulate content in order to understand reasoning processes in particular psychological disorders; and studies that inform us about psychopathology by using reasoning paradigms to show how reasoning performance can inform us about the mechanisms of pathology.

The question of how reasoning performance can inform us about psychopathology has been partly answered by replication of well devised studies on probabilistic reasoning. For instance, extensive work of Garety et al. (1991, 1994, 1999), Dudley et al. (1997a, 1997b, 1998) and Dudley and Over (2003) have yielded consistent results about delusional disorder and other thought disorders. Garety and Freeman (1999) do point out in their review of research in delusional disorders that most of the studies are not longitudinal and do not lead to any causal explanation of the disorders. However, the implication of their findings can be translated into clinical applications. For example, the 'data-gathering deficit' or 'jumping to conclusion' style of reasoning would prompt clinicians to develop techniques to help patients collect greater evidence before concluding or hypothesizing about events involving their delusional thoughts. In the case of anxiety disorders, consistent results of people with OCD exhibiting a 'data-gathering excess' may involve helping obsessionals accept less information before making a decision. In a way, exposure and response prevention encourages this strategy by asking patients to inhibit repetitive actions (excessive gathering of information) so they can process information without additional checking for example.

The second line of reasoning research concerning the effect of content on reasoning competence, yields less compelling answers for the understanding of psychopathology. Effectively, the results of most probabilistic studies show that emotionally salient themes increase the reasoning patterns already observed when using neutral content. So in essence, when it comes to personally relevant themes, people are increasingly biased in their reasoning pattern but how this applies to everyday life remains unclear. Research in anxiety and reasoning shows conclusively that anxious people infer danger on the basis of feeling anxious. But these results do present difficulties which have been underlined: inferring danger may not originate from faulty reasoning strategies but precisely because people who are anxious, by definition, have no credible experience that would help them to infer 'no danger' in the face of anxiogenous material, inhibiting them to conclude that 'if I feel anxious, then I am not in danger' (presumably the reasoning of normal controls). The induction process itself involves producing additional qualifiers to the premises and drawing conclusions. It may be that the additional qualifiers are different in people with anxiety than for non anxious people.

4.1 Future directions

Earlier, we cited the view of Rachman (1983) that cognitive research had taken two separate directions and that both could benefit our understanding much more if they were integrated: clinical cognitive theories versus cognitive reasoning research. In effect, Rachman suggests that clinical cognitive theories such as those developed by Beck could benefit from more empirical support with the use of reasoning theories, for example reasoning with heuristics, developed by Tversky and Kahnemann (1982). On the other hand, he proposed cognitive research should consider psychopathology when testing thinking.
Research including pathological content that is relevant to each psychological difficulty seems a potentially rewarding route to understand psychopathology. How people reason within the psychopathology should be observed but we are lacking in reliable empirical measures. Essentially, reasoning may not be simply about fragmented premises and the logical combination of such statements but a complex script which is hardly accessible through the formal standard reasoning paradigms. Hence, future studies should try to observe reasoning strategies in context, using tailored scripts or narratives taken from people suffering from psychological disorders and drawing conclusions from the reasoning processes involved in these narratives. This would mean tailoring exercises to reflect everyday reasoning process, as they occur and as close as possible to thinking as it presents itself in everyday reasoning.

5. References

Arntz, A., Rauner, M. & van den Hout, M. (1995). 'If I feel anxious, there must be danger': Ex-consequentia reasoning in inferring danger in anxiety disorders. *Behaviour Research and Therapy,* Vol. 33, No. 8, pp. 917-925.

Beck, A.T. (1979). *Cognitive therapy and the emotional disorders.* New York: International Universities Press.

Bennett, K. & Corcoran, R. (2010). Biases in everyday reasoning: Associations with subclinical anxiety, depression and paranoia. *Psychosis: Psychological, Social and Integrative Approaches*, Vol. 2, No. 3, pp. 227-237.

Blanchette, I. & Richards, A. (2010). The influence of affect on higher level cognition: A review of research on interpretation, judgement, decision making and reasoning. *Cognition and Emotion,* Vol. 24, No. 4, pp. 561-595.

Brewin, C.R. (1996). Theoretical Foundations of Cognitive-Behaviour Therapy for Anxiety and Depression. *Annual Review of Psychology,* Vol. 47, pp. 33-57.

Cohen, L. J. (1981). Can human irrationality be experimentally demonstrated? *Behavioural and Brain Sciences,* Vol. 4, pp. 317-370.

Colbert, S.M., Peters, El. & Garety, P. (2010). Jumping to conclusions and perceptions in early psychosis: Relationship with delusional beliefs. *Cognitive Neuropsychiatry*, Vol. 15, No. 4, pp. 422-440.

De Jong, P.J., Haenen, M-A., Schmidt, A. & Mayer, B. (1998). Hypochondriasis: the role of fear-confirming reasoning. *Behaviour Research and Therapy*, Vol. 36, pp. 65-74.

De Jong, P.J., Mayer, B & van den Hout, M. (1997). Conditional reasoning and phobic fear: evidence for a fear-confriming pattern. *Behaviour Research and Therapy*, Vol. 35, No. 6, pp. 507-516.

Dudley, R.E.J., John, C.H., Young, A.W. & Over, D.E. (1997a). Normal and abnormal reasoning in people with delusions. *British Journal of Clinical Psychology*, Vol. 36, pp. 243-258.

Dudley, R.E.J., John, C.H., Young, A.W. & Over, D.E. (1997b). The effect of self-referent material on the reasoning of people with delusions. *British Journal of Clinical Psychology*, Vol. 36, pp. 575-584.

Dudley, R.E.J. & Over, D.E. (2003). People with delusions jump to conclusions: A theoretical account of research findings on the reasoning of people with delusions. *Clinical Psychology and Psychotherapy*, Vol. 10, pp. 263-274.

Dudley, R.E.J., Young, A.W., John, C.H. & Over, D.E. (1998). Conditional reasoning in people with delusions: Performance on the Wason Selection Task. *Cognitive Neuropsychiatry*, Vol. 3, No. 4, pp. 241-258.

Ellis, A. (1962). Reason and emotion in psychotherapy: A comprehensive method of treating human disturbances. New York: Ellis Citadel Press.

Engelhard, I.M., Macklin, M.L., McNally, R.J., van den Hout, M.A. & Arntz, A. (2001). Emotion- and intrusion-based reasoning in Vietnam veterans with and without chronic posttraumatic stress disorder. *Behaviour Research and Therapy*, Vol. 39, pp. 1339-1348.

Engelhard, I.M., van den Hout, M.A., Arntz, A. & McNally, R.J. (2002). A longitudinal study of 'intrusion-based reasoning' and posttraumatic stress disorder after exposure to a train disaster. *Behaviour Research and Therapy*, Vol. 40, pp. 1415-1424.

Evans, J.St.B.T (1982). *The Psychology of Deductive Reasoning*. London: Routledge & Kegan Paul.

Evans, J.St.B.T (1989). *Bias in Human Reasoning: Causes and Consequences*. Hove, UK: Lawrence Erlbaum.

Evans, J.St.B.T., Barston, J.L. & Pollard, P. (1983). On the conflict between logic and belief in syllogistic reasoning. *Memory and Cognition*, Vol. 11, No. 3, pp. 295-306.

Evans, J.St.B.T & Over, D.E. (1996). *Rationality and Reasoning*. Hove, UK: Psychology Press.

Evans, J.St.B.T., Over, D.E. & Manktelow, K.I. (1993). Reasoning, decision making and rationality. *Cognition*, Vol. 49, No. 1-2, pp. 165-87.

Fear, C.F. & Healy, D. (1997). Probabilistic reasoning in obsessive-compulsive and delusional disorders. *Psychological Medicine*, Vol. 27, No. 1, pp. 199-208.

Frost, R.O., Novara, C. & Rhéaume, J. (2002). Perfectionism in Obsessive-Compulsive Disorder. In R.O. Frost and G. Steketee (Eds). *Cognitive Approaches to Obsessions and Compulsions: Theory, Assessment and Treatment*. (pp. 91-105). Oxford, UK: Elsevier

Garety, P.A. (1991). Reasoning and delusions. *British Journal of Psychiatry*, Vol. 159, No. Supp. 14, pp. 14-18.

Garety, P.A. & Freeman, D. (1999). Cognitive approaches to delusions: A critical review of theories and evidence. *British Journal of Clinical Psychology*, Vol. 38, pp. 113-154.

Garety, P.A. & Hemsley, D.R. (1994). *Delusions: Investigations into the psychology of delusional reasoning*. Hove, UK: Psychology Press.

Garety, P.A., Hemsley, D.R., & Wessely, S. (1991). Reasoning in deluded schizophrenia and paranoid patients. Biases in performance on a probabilistic task. *The Journal of Nervous and Mental Disease*, Vol. 179, No. 4, pp. 194-201.

Henle, M. (1962). On the Relation between Logic and Thinking. Psychological Review, Vol. 69, No. 4, pp. 366-378.

Huq, S.F., Garety, P.A. & Hemsley, D.R. (1988). Probabilistic judgements in deluded and non-deluded subjects. *The Quaterly Journal of Experimental Psychology*, Vol. 40A, No. 4, pp. 801-812.

Johnson-Laird, P.N. (1983). *Mental Models: Towards a Cognitive Science of Language, Inference and Consciousness.* Cambridge, MA: Cambridge University Press.

Johnson-Laird, P.N. (1993). *Human and machine thinking*. Hove, UK: Lawrence Erlbaum.

Johnson-Laird, P.N. (1994a). Mental Models and Probabilistic Thinking. *Cognition*, Vol. 50, pp. 189-209.

Johnson-Laird, P.N. (1994b). A model theory of induction. *International Studies in the Philosophy of Science*, Vol. 8, No. 1, pp. 5-29.

Johnson-Laird, P.N. (1999). Deductive Reasoning. *Annual Reviews Psychology*, Vol. 50, pp. 109-135.

Johnson-Laird, P.N. & Byrne, R.M.J. (1991). *Deduction.* Hillsdale, NJ: Erlbaum.

Johnson-Laird, P.N. & Wason, P.C. (1970). A theoretical analysis of insight into a reasoning task. *Cognitive Psychology*, Vol. 1, pp. 134-148.

Keen, N., Brown, G.P. & Wheatley, J. (2008). Obsessive compulsive symptoms and the simulation of future negative events. *British Journal of Clinical Psychology,* Vol. 47, No. 3, pp. 265-279.

Ladouceur, R., Talbot, F. & Dugas, M.J. (1997). Behavioural Expressions of Intolerance of Uncertainty in Worry. *Behaviour Modification*, Vol. 21, No. 3, pp. 355-371.

Lincoln, T.M., Lange, J., Burau, J., Exner, C. & Moritz, S. (2010). The effect of state anxiety on paranoid ideation and jumping to conclusions. An experimental investigation. *Schizophrenia Bulletin,* Vol. 36, No. 6, pp. 1140-1148.

Manktelow, K,I. (1999). *Reasoning and Thinking.* Hove, UK: Psychology Press.

Manktelow, K,I. & Over, D.E. (1990). *Inference and Understanding. A philosophical and Psychological Perspective.* New York: Routledge.

Markovits, H. & Nantel, G. (1989). The belief-bias effect in the production and evaluation of logical conclusions. *Memory and Cognition*, Vol. 17, No. 1, pp. 11-7.

Milner, A.D., Beech, H.R. & Walker, V.J. (1971). Decision processes and obsessional behaviour. *British Journal of Social and Clinical Psychology*, Vol. 10, pp. 88-89.

O'Connor, K.P., Aardema, F. & Pélissier, M.-C. (1985). *Beyond reasonable doubt: Reasoning process in obsessive compulsive disorder*. John Wiley & Sons.

Oakhill, J.V. & Johnson-Laird, P.N. (1985). Rationality, memory and the search for counterexamples. *Cognition*, Vol. 20, No. 1, pp. 79-94.

Oaksford, M.R. & Chater, N. (1993). Reasoning theories and bounded rationality. In K.I. Manktelow & D.E.Over (Eds.). *Rationality.* London: Routledge.

Pélissier, M.C. & O'Connor, K.P. (2002). Deductive and Inductive Reasoning in Obsessive-Compulsive Disorder. *British Journal of Clinical Psychology*, Vol. 41, pp. 15-27.

Pélissier, M.-C., O'Connor, K.P. & Dupuis, G. (2009). When doubting begins: Exploring inductive reasoning in obsessive-compulsive disorder. *Journal of Behavior Therapy and Experimental Psychiatry*, Vol. 40, No. 1, pp. 39-49.

Phillips, L. & Edwards, W. (1966). Conservatism in a simple probability inference task. *Journal of Experimental Psychology*, Vol. 72, No. 3, pp. 346-354.

Rachman, S. (1983). Irrational Thinking, with Special Reference to Cognitive Therapy. *Journal of Advancement in Behaviour Research and Therapy*, Vol. 5, pp. 63-88.

Reed, G. (1977). Obsessional cognition: performance on two numerical tasks. *British Journal of Psychiatry*, Vol. 130, pp. 184-185.

Reed, G. (1991). The cognitive characteristics of obsessional disorder. In P.A. Magaro (Ed), *Cognitive Bases of Mental Disorders* (pp. 77-99). London: Sage Publication.

Reese, H.E., McNally, R.J. & Wilhelm, S. (2010). Probabilistic reasoning in patients with body dysmorphic disorder. *Journal of Behavior Therapy and Experimental Psychiatry*, Vol. 43, No. 3, pp. 270-276.

Rhéaume, J., Freeston, M.H., Ladouceur, R., Bouchard, C., Gallant, L., Talbot, F. et al., (2000). Functional and dysfunctional perfectionists: are they different on compulsive-like behaviours? *Behaviour Research and Therapy*, Vol. 38, pp. 119-128.

Simpson, J., Cove, J., Fineberg, N., Msetfi, R.M. & Ball, L. (2007). Reasoning in people with obsessive-compulsive disorder. *British Journal of Clinical Psychology*, Vol. 46, No. 4, pp. 397-411.

Smeets, G, de Jong, PJ. & Mayer, B. (2000). If you suffer from a headache, then you have a brain tumour: domain-specific reasoning 'bias' and hypochondriasis. *Behaviour Research and therapy*, Vol. 38, pp. 763-776.

Tversky, A. & Kahneman, D. (1973). Availability: a heuristic for judging frequency and probability. *Cognitive Psychology*, Vol. 5, pp. 207-232.

Tversky, A. & Kahneman, D. (1982). *Judgement Under Uncertainty: Heuristics and Biases.* In D. Kahneman, P. Slovic and A. Tversky (Eds.) Cambridge: Cambridge University Press.

Volans, P.J. (1976). Styles of decision-making and probability appraisal in selected obsessional and phobic patients. *British Journal of Social and Clinical Psychology*, Vol. 15, pp. 305-317.

Vroling, M.S. & de Jong, P.J. (2009). Threat-confirming belief bias and symptoms of anxiety disorders. *Journal of Behavior Therapy and Experimental Psychiatry,*, Vol. 41, No. 2, pp. 110-116.

Wason, P.C. (1960). On the failure to eliminate hypotheses in a conceptual task. *Quarterly Journal of Experimental Psychology*, Vol. 12, pp. 129-140.

Wason, P.C. (1966). Reasoning. In B. Foss (Ed), *New horizons in psychology* (pp. 135-151). Harmondsworth, UK: Penguin Books.

Wason, P.C. (1968). Reasoning about a rule. *Quaterly Journal of Experimental Psychology*, Vol. 20, pp. 273-281.

Wason, P.C. (1969). Regression in Reasoning? *British Journal of Psychology*, Vol. 60, No. 4, pp. 471-480.

Wason, P.C. & Johnson-Laird, P.N. (1972). *Psychology of reasoning: structure and content.* Cambridge, MA: Harvard University.

Young, H.F. & Bentall, R.P. (1997). Probabilistic reasoning in deluded, depressed and normal subjects: effects of task difficulty and meaningful versus non-meaningful material. *Psychological Medicine*, Vol. 27, pp. 455-465.

Part 2

Neuroscience

5

Animal Models of Anxiety Vulnerability - The Wistar Kyoto Rat

X. Jiao[1], K.D. Beck[1,2,3], K.C.H. Pang[1,2,3] and R.J. Servatius[1,2,3]
[1]Stress and Motivated Behavior Institute
[2]GSBS, NJMS-UMDNJ, Newark, NJ;
[3]Neurobehavioral Research Laboratory (129), VANJHCS, East Orange, NJ, U.S.A.

1. Introduction

1.1 Anxiety

Anxiety disorders are the most common psychiatric disorders with a worldwide lifetime prevalence of 16-29% (Kessler *et al.*, 2005; Somers *et al.*, 2006). People with anxiety disorders are likely to suffer from depression and drug (or alcohol) abuse in an effort to gain relief from their symptoms, therefore, eliciting secondary disorders (Kessler *et al.*, 2005). Although each subtype (i.e. generalized anxiety disorder, obsessive-compulsive disorder (OCD), panic disorder, post traumatic stress disorder (PTSD) and social phobia) has unique features, the core symptom of all anxiety disorders is excessive avoidance. The etiology of anxiety disorders remains elusive (the presumed role of trauma in PTSD notwithstanding). What is abundantly clear is anxiety disorders arise as a complex interaction of genetic, epigenetic, sociocultural factors with life experiences; that is, anxiety disorders are best explained with diathesis models (Kendler *et al.*, 2002; Mineka and Zinbarg, 2006; Zinbarg and Barlow, 1996).

Among a variety of neurobiological and neurobehavioral factors representing a source of risk for anxiety disorders, inhibited temperament is consistently linked to anxiety disorders (Biederman *et al.*, 1993; Fox *et al.*, 2005a; Hirshfeld *et al.*, 1992; Hirshfeld-Becker *et al.*, 2007; Kagan *et al.*, 1987; Rosenbaum *et al.*, 1993; Smoller *et al.*, 2003). Behavioral inhibition is characterized as extreme withdrawal in the face of social and nonsocial challenges (Fox *et al.*, 2005b; Kagan *et al.*, 1989; Rosenbaum *et al.*, 1991). Those with inhibited temperament exhibit excessive physiological reactivity to environmental challenges (Kalin *et al.*, 2000; Kalin and Shelton, 2003; Keltikangas-Jarvinen *et al.*, 1999; Perez-Edgar *et al.*, 2007; Schwartz *et al.*, 2003; Smoller *et al.*, 2005; Tyrka *et al.*, 2006; Tyrka *et al.*, 2008).

Although there is support for temperament as a risk factor, the translation of risk to actualized disorder is unclear. Acquisition, expression and retention of avoidance may be the final common pathway to anxiety disorders. The particularly debilitating feature of avoidance is that, left untreated, avoidance increases over time and leads to a worsening of symptoms. Avoidance acquisition is more apparent in PTSD; the growth of avoidance traces the full expression of PTSD (Karamustafalioglu *et al.*, 2006; Kashdan *et al.*, 2006; North *et al.*, 2004; O'donnell *et al.*, 2006a). Given this prominent position, avoidance learning may represent an endophenotype for anxiety disorders (Gould and Gottesman, 2006).

Here, we present the case for inbred WKY rats to serve as a model for risk of anxiety disorders. Evidence is presented for the concordance of neurobehavioral, neuroendocrine, and neurochemical features to that observed in humans at risk for expressing an anxiety disorder. Particular emphasis is placed on enhanced avoidance acquisition and resistance to extinction as an endophenotype for vulnerability to anxiety disorders. Implications for treatment and efficacy are discussed.

2. Putative animal model for vulnerability to anxiety disorders - The WKY rat

The Wistar Kyoto (WKY) rat strain was first developed as a normotensive control strain for the spontaneously hypertensive rat (SHR) strain derived from the Wistar (WIS) rat (Okamoto and Aoki, 1963). Unlike its parent strain WIS rat, the WKY rat exhibits many unique behavioral characteristics differing from an out-bred rat strain. The most significant features are behavioral withdrawal, propensity to avoid, hyper-responsiveness to stress and hypervigilance (Drolet *et al.*, 2002; Lemos *et al.*, 2011; McAuley *et al.*, 2009; Pare, 1992a; Pare, 1989b; Pare, 1992b; Pare, 1993; Solberg *et al.*, 2001).

2.1 Temperament: Behavioral inhibition

The WKY rat displays features of inhibited temperament in a variety of situations (Braw *et al.*, 2008; Ferguson and Cada, 2004; Malkesman *et al.*, 2005; Pare, 1992b; Pare, 1994; Pare, 1996; Pare *et al.*, 2001; Servatius *et al.*, 1998; Tejani-Butt *et al.*, 2003). For example, Figure 1 depicts activity in the open field test comparing WKY rats to outbred SD rats. Upon placement into the center of the open field (which is brightly lit), the WKY rat remains immobile for a period of time; the latency to leave the center segment is often 2-3 times as long as exhibited by outbred strains (Drolet *et al.*, 2002; Ferguson and Cada, 2003; Nosek *et al.*, 2008). This reluctance to leave the center segment is followed by slow deliberate exploration. However, activity will generally increase over several minutes. Hypolocomotion is not

Open field activity in male and female WKY and SD rats

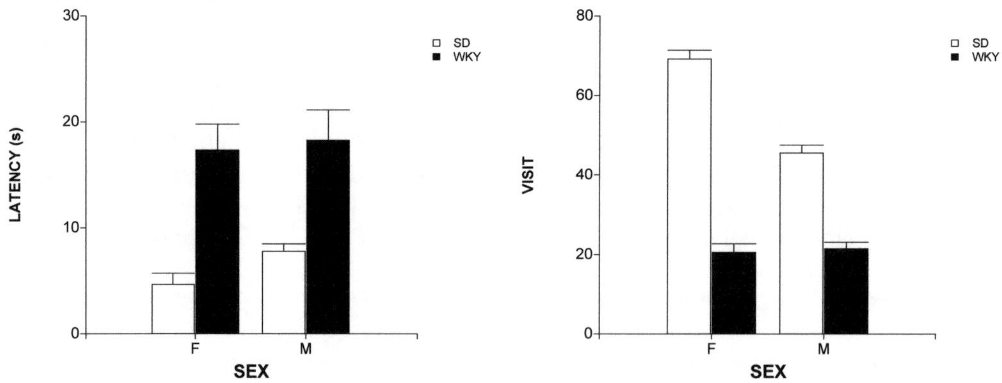

Fig. 1. Both female and male WKY rats display longer latencies to leave the center segment and overall lower numbers of segments crossed in a 2-min open field test. These data represent several studies (male: N = 60/strain; female: N=25/strain) and are obtained as the initial assessment of phenotype two weeks after delivery from breeders.

secondary to a motoric disturbance, in that WKY rats exhibit normal motor activity in a running wheel (Ferguson and Cada, 2003), a rotarod (Ferguson *et al.*, 2003b) and a turning wheel avoidance task (Pare, 1992a). Together, these data suggest that the lack of movement is not physical, but psychological. Moreover, inhibited temperament is displayed by both female and male WKY rats compared to their outbred counterparts.

Inhibited temperament extends to more explicit nonsocial and social threats. In terms of social interactions, WKY rats generally exhibit normal play behaviors with conspecifics (Braw *et al.*, 2006; Malkesman *et al.*, 2006b), but reductions in play and more subordinate-type behaviors when faced with outbred rats (Ferguson and Cada, 2004). In response to an electrified probe, normal rats bury the probe; WKY rats simply freeze (Ahmadiyeh *et al.*, 2005; Carr and Lucki, 2010; Gutiérrez-Mariscal *et al.*, 2008; Pare, 1994). Thus, WKY rats represent an animal model of behavioral withdrawal in the face of social and non-social challenges.

2.2 Anxiety signs and symptoms

As stated earlier, the core feature of anxiety disorders is avoidance. There are a variety of expressions of avoidance; however, all will have a common process of acquisition and resistance to extinction. In addition to avoidance as a learned response, common features of anxiety disorders are altered arousal, social interaction, communication, attention, learning and memory. Still, each anxiety disorder has distinct features. Thus, endophenotypes may relate to the core features of avoidance learning, common characteristics (e.g., heighten arousal), or disorder-specific features (e.g., compulsions). Accordingly, behavioral assessments may be sensitive to a particular aspect or a general process concordant with anxiety.

2.2.1 Arousal

Arousal has two general aspects, the basal or undisturbed state and the relative magnitude of response to challenges. Moreover, arousal may be indexed through neuroendocrine or neurobehavioral measures. For each, the WKY has documented abnormalities.

Neuroendocrine and neurochemical. Within the hypothalamic-pituitary-adrenal axis (HPAA), levels of corticosterone (CORT) and adrenocorticotropic hormone (ACTH) are measured to evaluate arousal levels as affected by circadian rhythms and stress (Ottenweller *et al.*, 1994). WKY rats has been proposed as a model of stress vulnerability, exhibiting exaggerated HPAA responses to stress regimens compared to common rat strains (Pare *et al.*, 1999b; Pare and Kluczynski, 1997; Pare and Redei, 1993b; Redei *et al.*, 1994). Basal peripheral ACTH and CORT levels are generally higher in WKY rats and remained significantly higher after the diurnal peak as compared to WIS rats (Solberg *et al.*, 2001). Moreover, WKY rats exhibit a sustained CORT response to acute stress and an enhanced plasma ACTH response to various stressors (De La Garza II and Mahoney III, 2004; Malkesman *et al.*, 2006a; Pare and Redei, 1993a; Rittenhouse *et al.*, 2002). Others reported that CRH content and mRNA binding are not different in WKY rats relative to other strains suggesting that a defective negative feedback system may contribute to hyperresponsive HPAA in WKY rats (Gomez *et al.*, 1996; Redei *et al.*, 1994). Together, neuroendocrine evidence suggests that WKY rats are inherently hyperresponsive to stress. Exaggerated HPAA activity is reminiscent of inhibited temperament (Smoller *et al.*, 2003; Smoller *et al.*, 2005).

In general the neurochemical profile of the WKY rat is aberrant compared to outbred rats. WKY rats have inherently low butyrylcholinesterase level (Figure 2) and activity (Servatius *et al.*, 1998), leading to greater sensitivity to cholinomimetics (Beck *et al.*, 2001). Among the neurotransmitters, WKY rats have altered levels of monoamines, namely norepinephrine (NE), dopamine (DA) and serotonin (5-HT), and their metabolites as compared to out-bred strains with a high degree of specificity in various regions (De La Garza II and Mahoney III, 2004; Ferguson *et al.*, 2003a; Pardon *et al.*, 2003; Scholl *et al.*, 2010). Moreover, these monoamine systems show greater responsiveness in the face of acute stress (Pardon *et al.*, 2002; Pardon *et al.*, 2000) and chronic stress (Pardon *et al.*, 2003). We will discuss this point in a later section (section 5).

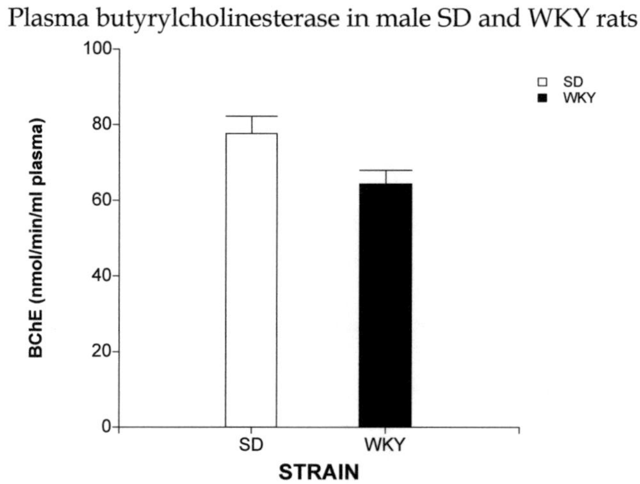

Fig. 2. WKY rats exhibit significant lower level of butyrylcholinesterase compared to SD rats. (n=19-20/strain, $p<.05$)

Neurobehavioral. The acoustic startle response (ASR) is a simple reflex used to index arousal and vigilance in mammals (Ardekani *et al.*, 1989). The ASR can be used to reveal differences in sensitivity (threshold to elicit a reflex response), responsivity (the magnitude of response), latency, as well as nonassociative processes of habituation, dishabituation and sensitization.

We and others demonstrated that WKY rats made larger startle responses to a white noise within a wide range (92dB to 120dB) as compared to other inbred and outbred rat strains (Glowa and Hansen, 1994; McAuley *et al.*, 2009; Servatius *et al.*, 1998). Of 45 inbred and outbred rat strains including SD rats, male WKY rats exhibited the highest ASR magnitude when exposed to 8 trials of 110dB white noise (Glowa and Hansen, 1994). We found that WKY rats exhibited significantly higher startle responsivity at 92 and 102dB white noise after correction for each subject's body weight (Figure 3a). In addition to greater startle responsivity, male WKY showed higher sensitivity compared to male SD rats, measured by a multi-intensity startle test (3-ASR) (Figure 3b). Although both male and female WKY exhibit substantially higher ASRs compared to SD rats, only male rats demonstrate habituation when single intensity startle test (1-ASR) was used (Figure 4). Yet others reported that WKY show similar or lower ASR magnitude compared to SD rats (Buuse,

2004; Palmer *et al.*, 2000). We reasoned the inconsistency may be due to variant procedures used and whether subjects' body weight was factored into the startle response.

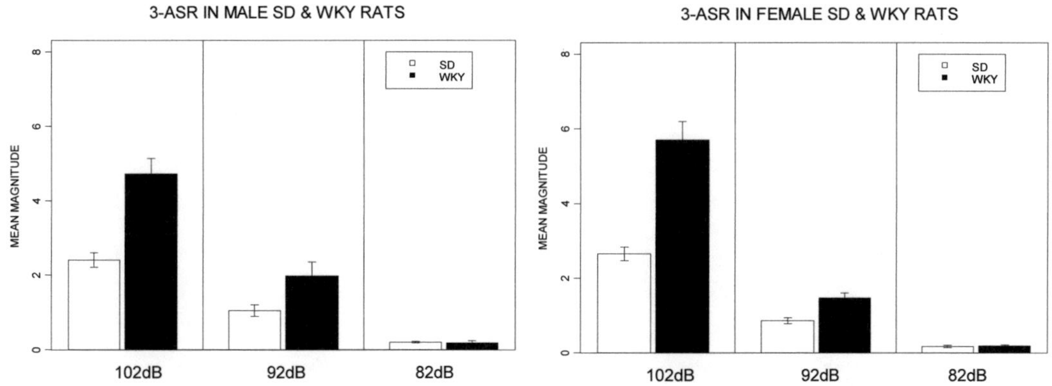

(3a) Startle responsivity in male and female SD and WKY rats.

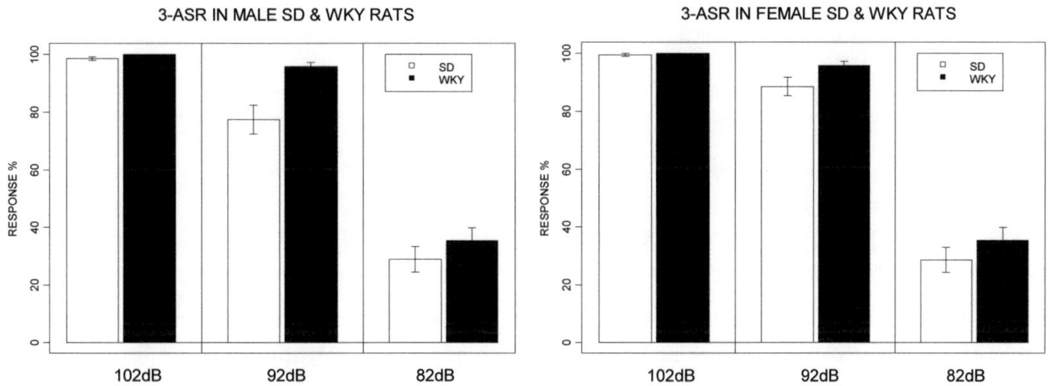

(3b) Startle sensitivity in male and female SD and WKY rats

Fig. 3. WKY rats display higher startle magnitude compared to the same sex outbred SD rats regardless of sex (n=12-17/strain/sex) (a). WKY rats of both sexes also exhibited greater sensitivity to respond, responding more to acoustic stimuli of moderate intensity (b).

WKY rats exhibited exaggerated stress response and elevated arousal following stress stimulation. Stress has been described as one of the key risk factors of anxiety disorders (Chantarujikapong *et al.*, 2001; Grillon *et al.*, 2007b; Mineka and Zinbarg, 1996). As described in previous literatures, WKY rats are behaviorally hyperresponsive to stress with the stress-induced exaggerated HPAA response (Redei *et al.*, 1994; Solberg *et al.*, 2001). Inasmuch as the basal behavioral state of WKY is abnormal, assessing the impact of stress on behavioral reactivity has been problematic. For example, assessing freezing to context or to cues is difficult given the propensity to freeze in novel situations. However, prior acute stress have been noted to increase freezing behavior and reduce activity in the OFT and elevated plus maze in WKYs (Nosek *et al.*, 2008). When challenged in the forced swim test (FST), the WKY rat predominantly exhibits floating behavior and fewer struggling responses compared to other strains. The lack of struggling has been interpreted as 'behavioral despair', a sign of depression-like behavior in rodents (Malkesman and Weller, 2009; Pare, 1992a; Pare and

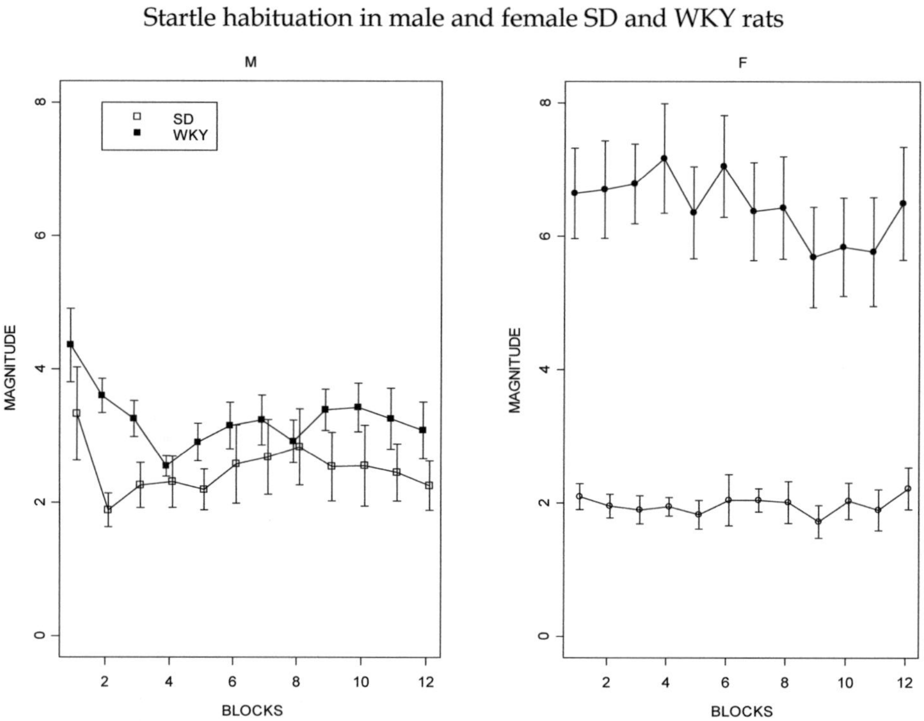

Fig. 4. Habituation of acoustic startle responses in WKY and SD rats: nonassociative processes. Although WKY rats generally display larger ASRs than SD rats, habituation appears normal (n=8/strain/sex).

Redei, 1993a). The heightened stress reactivity is most clearly evident in the enhanced susceptibility to develop stress-induced ulcers in WKY rats compared to outbred strains (Pare, 1989a; Pare, 1989c; Pare and Schimmel, 1986). Pretreatment with drugs that elevate central monoamines reduce the severity of ulceration (Pare *et al.*, 1999a; Tejani-Butt *et al.*, 2003). Evidence from elevated arousal or exaggerated stress response in WKY rats may provide insight to the alterations in the CNS neurochemistry that may be responsible for anxiety. The effects of stress are discussed in the following sections in more detail.

2.2.2 Sleep disturbances

Sleeping disruption is one of the major symptoms of anxiety disorder and a hallmark of PTSD (Ross et al., 1989). WKY rats exhibit altered sleep-wake cycle and longer rapid eye movement sleep (REMS) episodes compared to other strains (Dugovic et al., 2000). REMS fragmentation was significantly altered following stress in WKY rats compared to control strain (DaSilva *et al.*, 2011; Dugovic *et al.*, 2000; Laitman *et al.*). Altered sleep patterns may also preexist as a vulnerability to anxiety, that are further disturbed after exposure to psychological distress.

2.2.3 Avoidance

As the core symptom of all anxiety disorders, avoidance behavior differs between patients with anxiety disorder and normal population (Foa *et al.*, 2006; O'Donnell *et al.*, 2006b). In humans avoidance is characterized in the form of emotions, ideations, and behaviors. In animal models, avoidance is characterized as passive (withholding a likely response to avoid aversive stimulation) and active (performing a target response to prevent aversive stimulation). Early work showed WKY rats exhibit superior acquisition in passive avoidance tasks compared to SD or WIS rats (Pare 1993; Pare 1996). Given that being immobile/freezing is the dominant coping strategy for WKY rats, superior acquisition of passive avoidance is not a surprise. However, when tested with a wheel-turning avoidance task, WKY performed equally well compared to WIS rat (Pare, 1992a). In contrast, Berger and Starzec found that WKY rats performed poorly in lever-press avoidance task compared to SHR rats (Berger and Starzec, 1988). As an arbitrary target response, a leverpress is not among the species specific defense reactions (Bolles, 1970). We reasoned that the inconsistency between studies and laboratories may due to the procedure applied, the nature of the test and the reference strain to which WKYs were compared.

In our institute, we utilized a signalled lever-press avoidance paradigm to study anxiety and its vulnerability in rats. It is known that anxiety is a disorder that develops over a period of time, so is the avoidance. Thus, a lever-press avoidance learning model allows the acquisition of avoidance to develop over an extended period of time, mimicking the developmental process of anxiety in humans. Our data indicated that the learning of WKY rats is superior in the lever-press avoidance task compared to a noninhibited reference strain, the SD rat (Beck et al., 2010; Jiao et al., 2011; Servatius et al., 2008). The superior active avoidance performance of WKY rats is in stark contrast to other rat strains with features of trait behavioral inhibition such as the Maudsley High Reactive (Blizard and Adams, 2002), which are generally poor in active avoidance. Moreover, rats bred for superior active avoidance are typically the least behaviorally inhibited (Syracuse high avoiders, Roman high avoiders and Australian high avoiders) (Aguilar *et al.*, 2004; Brush, 2003; Driscoll, 1986; Overstreet *et al.*, 1990; Overstreet *et al.*, 1992).

Over the past several years we have amassed a substantial database concerning the avoidance performance of WKY rats. For one, the avoidance performance of WKY rats reaches asymptotic levels that approach unity; that is, once acquired WKY rats typically exhibit near perfect avoidance (Figure 5.). That perfect avoidance begins with the first trial of a session. Outbred rats display a typical pattern of avoidance performance in which each session begins with escape responses, although avoidance was expressed at the end of the previous session (i.e., warm up) (Hineline, 1978a; Hineline, 1978b). WKY rats generally do not exhibit warm up as acquisition progresses. This near perfect expression of avoidance resembles human avoidance. Facilitated avoidance acquisition is apparent in both female and male rats compared to their respective outbred counterparts. The near perfect avoidance behavior also insulates the rat from experiencing changes in shock contingencies. Accordingly, WKYs display perseveration of avoidance responding in the absence of shock, but continued presence of the explicit safety signal (Servatius *et al.*, 2008). Perseveration/resistance to extinction has been implicated in neuropathology of anxiety (Barad, 2005; Myers and Davis, 2002).

WKY rats also display another interesting and potentially clinically-relevant feature. Each training session begins with a 60-s stimulus free period prior to the first warning signal. As WKY rats acquire avoidance they emit bar presses, which are not reinforced, during this period (Figure 6.). This pattern of response is only exhibited prior to the first trial; nonreinforced responses are rarely displayed on subsequent trials. These nonreinforced responses may be akin to worry (Mineka, 2004), accompanying avoidance acquisition only in those at risk.

Acquisition and extinction in a lever-press avoidance task

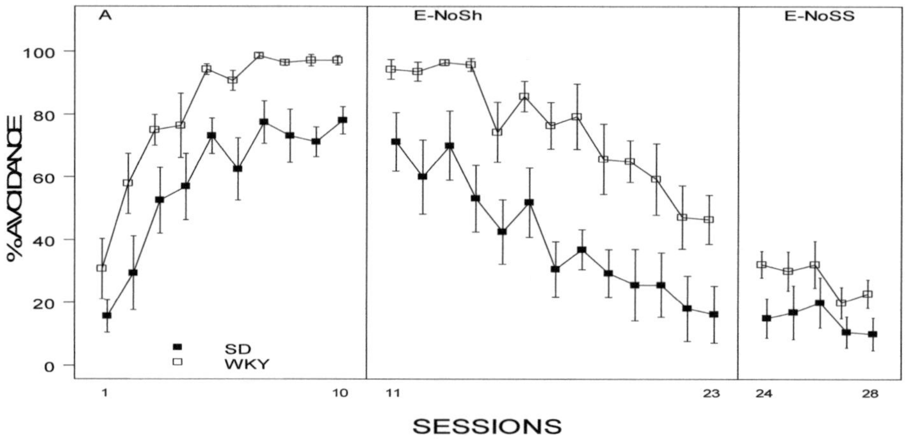

Fig. 5. Avoidance responses made during acquisition and extinction in WKY and SD rats. WKY rats acquired lever-press avoidance faster and to a higher degree (sessions 1-10). However, WKY rats extinguished slower during early extinction phase while the transition between acquisition and extinction was more significant in SD rats (sessions 11-23, shock-off, safety signal on; sessions 24-28, shock-off, safety signal off). (N=8/strain)

Lever-press during the 1st min of each session in male and female SD and WKY rats

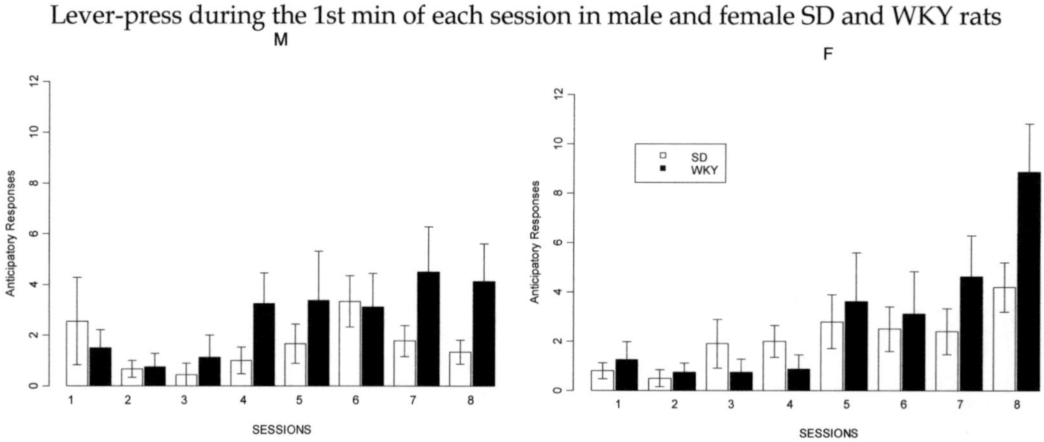

Fig. 6. WKY rats emitted more anticipatory lever-presses during the initial minute of each session during acquisition. (N=8-10/strain/sex)

On the other hand, stress intensity is often cited as a contributing factor in the development of anxiety disorders (Braunstein-Bercovitz *et al.*, 2001; Foa *et al.*, 2006; Grillon *et al.*, 2007b; Grillon *et al.*, 2007a; Mineka and Zinbarg, 1996; Silver *et al.*, 2002). Given the relationship between anxiety disorders and avoidance, one expects stress to accelerate avoidance acquisition, raise the asymptotic levels, or affect extinction. The results from a recent study suggest that stressor intensity only affects extinction. Training with a greater shock intensity than our standard, did not affect the acquisition curves of either SD or WKY rats (Figure 7.) (Jiao *et al.*, 2011). Of course, there is little room to enhance asymptotic performance of WKY rats, but the rate to reach this level could differ. However, WKY rats trained with higher intensity shock exhibited perseveration of avoidance response during extinction compared to WKY rats trained with the lower intensity shock; extinction curves of SD rats resembled WKY rats trained with a lower intensity.

A long standing discrepancy between the basic science literature and clinical descriptions concerns the relationship between avoidance acquisition and arousal. In rats, arousal decreases as avoidance is acquired (Coover *et al.*, 1973). However, arousal is sustained in humans with anxiety disorders and who are employing avoidance. Therefore, we assessed ASRs prior to avoidance acquisition and toward the end of acquisition training. Whereas the ASRs of SD rats are virtually unchanged between the measures, the ASRs of WKY rats *increase* (Figure 8.). The increase is evident at a period of training in which WKY rarely, if at all, experience shock. This increase is beyond the basal exaggerations normally noted between strains. There is emerging data that exaggerated ASRs in PTSD may be increases beyond preexisting ASR differences; that is, exaggerated ASRs are an amplification of a preexisting condition (Guthrie and Bryant, 2005). These data suggest that exaggerated ASRs are an interaction of subject vulnerabilities and avoidance acquisition.

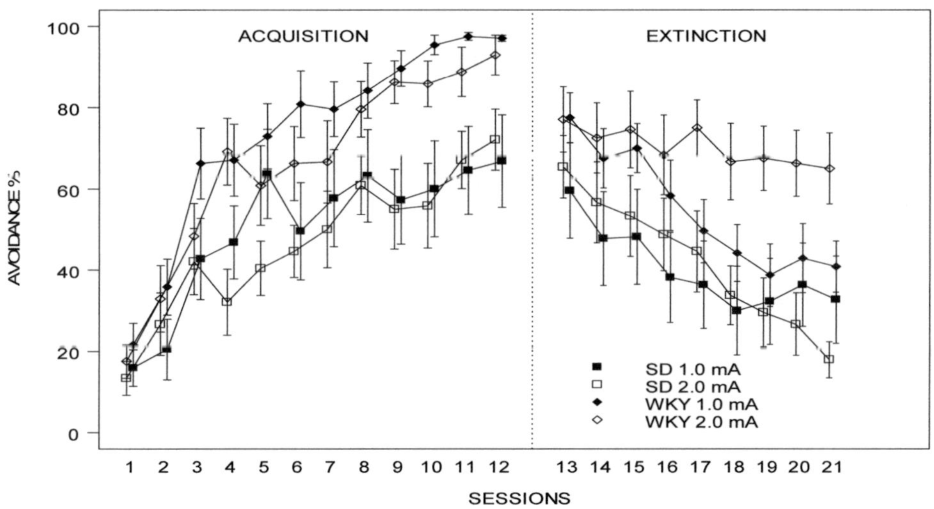

Fig. 7. WKY rats acquired lever-press avoidance faster and to a higher degree regardless of shock intensity. However, WKY rats trained with 2.0-mA foot-shock resisted extinction while the transition between acquisition and extinction was more significant in all SD rats and WKY rats trained with 1.0-mA foot-shock (Jiao *et al.*, 2011).

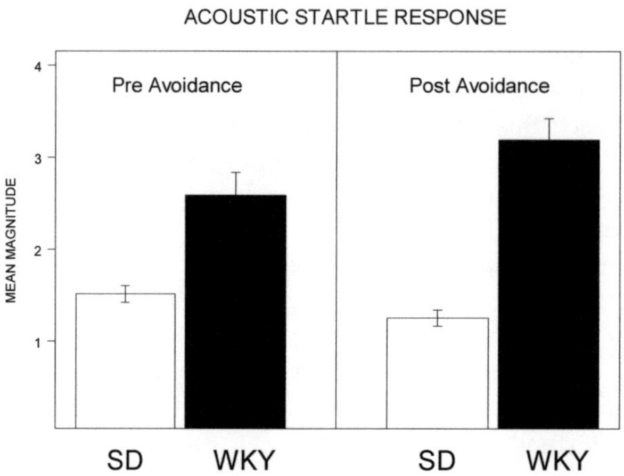

Fig. 8. WKY and SD rats were tested for 1-ASR before and after 10 sessions of avoidance acquisition. In both tests, WKY startled with a higher magnitude than SD rats. WKY rats exhibited elevated startle response following acquisition training while SD showed similar startle magnitude in both tests. (N=24/strain; strain difference, $p<.05$; test difference, $p<.05$)

3. Genetic components

Genetic components (trait vulnerability) play an important role in various psychiatric disorders, including anxiety disorders. Quantitative trait loci (QTL) analysis indicated that common loci, which influence certain behavioral characteristics tested by OFT and defensive bury test in rats, may represent genetic factors contributing to anxiety and depression (Ahmadiyeh *et al.*, 2005; Boyle and Gill, 2001; Cloninger *et al.*, 1998; Henderson *et al.*, 2000; Solberg *et al.*, 2004). Several QTL (*Imm 1* D2Rat188, *Imm3* D5Rat40, *Imm6* D16Arb5, *Climb2* D1Rat147, *FST1* D16Rat75) were identified for climbing, immobility and swimming in WKY rats, sharing common target regions with susceptibility loci mapped by genome scan analyses for emotionality QTL in rodents and human genetic linkage to emotional disorder (Solberg *et al.*, 2004). Significance of microarray analysis (SAM) revealed that expression of 66 genes was increased in the locus coeruleus (LC) of WKY compared to SD rats (Pearson *et al.*, 2006), including genes that encoded for enzymes involved in NE turnover. Moreover, the mRNA of catechol-O-methyltransferase *(COMT)*, a key enzyme in the catabolism of catecholamines, was found at levels four- to sevenfold higher in the cerebral cortex in WKYs than SDs (Walker *et al.*, 2004). Thus, this rat strain may be genetically predisposed to psychiatric disorders that are linked to altered monoaminergic system.

4. Brain anatomy and neuronal activity

Converging data from structural and functional magnetic resonance imaging (MRI) studies suggest that differential patterns of anatomical brain abnormalities appear to be involved in mood and anxiety disorders (Brambilla *et al.*, 2002; Lind *et al.*, 2006; Milad *et al.*; Ohara *et al.*, 2004). Abnormalities were found in orbital frontal lobe, basal ganglia, temporal lobe and hippocampus in patients with various subtypes of anxiety (Brambilla *et al.*, 2002; Bystritsky *et al.*, 2001; McEwen, 2005). Moreover, imaging data from humans suggest that medial prefrontal cortex, amygdala, thalamus and periaquaductal gray are involved in avoidance acquisition (Mobbs *et al.*, 2007; Samanez-Larkin *et al.*, 2008; Simmons *et al.*, 2006; Straube *et al.*, 2009; Suslow *et al.*, 2009). However, the neurocircuitry underlying avoidance extinction and its perseveration in anxiety states is largely a matter of speculation. Mainly supported by fear extinction studies, mPFC plays a key role in both humans and experimental animals (rodents). Anxiety patients exhibit reduced activity of the anterior cingulate cortex and thalamus during episodes of re-experiencing (Hopper *et al.*, 2007; Lanius *et al.*, 2003), leading to a suggestion that reduced cortical influence on structures such as the amygdala may explain the resistance to extinction. Reduced cortical influence on the amygdala is also presumed to underlie the persistent expression of heightened arousal (e.g., increased acoustic startle) observed in PTSD patients (Nutt and Malizia, 2004).

The knowledge of anatomical difference between WKY and other rats is quite limited. A recent volumetric study evaluated hippocampus in female rats in which the hippocampal volume of WKY rats is 20% less than that of WIS rats (Lemos *et al.*, 2011). On the other hand, alterations in neuronal activation are demonstrated in the expression of c-Fos or brain derived neurotrophic factor (BDNF) in various brain regions in WKY rats compared to out-bred rat strains (Ma and Morilak, 2004; O'Mahony *et al.*, 2011). We recently reported that the c-Fos immunoreactivity is lower in the medial prefrontal cortex in the WKY rat than the SD rat at the end of extinction of a lever-press avoidance task, whereas a reduced GABAergic activation was found in basal amygdala in the WKY rat trained with higher shock intensity (Jiao *et al.*, 2011).

However, the structures that are critical for acquisition and extinction of lever press avoidance are relatively unknown. In our initial work, we assessed c-Fos immunoreactivity in various regions in the SD rat at multiple time points within the phases of acquisition and extinction. Our results indicated that there is a trend of increased c-Fos expression in the prefrontal regions as extinction starts and proceeds. Interestingly, a similar pattern was observed in the lateral and basolateral amygdala where a reduced activity was expected during extinction. A further analysis targeting GABAergic neuron revealed that GABAergic activation arises during the extinction phase. An elevated GABAergic activation (detected by the double staining for c-Fos and parvalbumin (PV, a calcium binding protein that is expressed in 50-60% amygdalar GABAergic neurons (Kemppainen and Pitkanen, 2000)) in the basolateral and lateral amygdala would reduce the excitatory output from the amygdala as GABA neurons in the basolateral amygdala are mainly interneurons that make synaptic contact on projection neurons (Rosenkranz and Grace, 2001). Thus an elevated GABAergic activity may be responsible for the increased neuronal activation during extinction phase in the basolateral amygdala. However, this assumption needs further investigation since parvalbumin positive neurons represent 50-60% of GABAergic neurons in the basolateral amygdala (Kemppainen and Pitkanen, 2000). We do not as yet know whether these neuronal alterations are present or different in WKY rats.

From a different perspective, enhanced avoidance learning may be secondary to deficits in neurotrophins. Converging data supports the role of neurotrophins in mood disorders; one of the latest theories of the neuropathology of anxiety and depression disorders (Chen *et al.*, 2006; Martinowich *et al.*, 2007). For example, low levels of the brain derived neurotrophic factor (BDNF) are found in stress-related disorders in humans (Duman and Monteggia, 2006). In general, lower BDNF is related to anxiety and depression disorders that are not responsive to serotonergic antidepressant treatment (Duman, 2004; Kalueff *et al.*, 2006). Consistent with this perspective, a recent study illustrated that BDNF levels are significantly lower in the CA3 of hippocampus in WKY rats compared to SD rats (Malkesman *et al.*, 2009).

5. Potential mechanisms in psychopharmacology

Alterations in neurochemistry in the CNS are implicated in various psychiatric disorders (i.e. depression, addiction and anxiety). Recent investigations targeting central neurochemical pathways have enhanced our understanding of anxiety disorders.

5.1 Serotonin (5-HT)

Evidence for the association of altered serotonergic activity in anxiety, that decreasing serotonergic function is anxiogenic and increasing it anxiolytic, is mostly supported by the use of selective serotonin reuptake inhibitors (SSRIs) in various sub-types of anxiety disorders (Bremner, 2006; Vaswani *et al.*, 2003). WKY rats showed significant lower basal 5-HT tissue level in limbic regions and cell body area compared to WIS or SD rats (De La Garza II and Mahoney III, 2004; Scholl *et al.*, 2010). Acute stress elicits an increased tissue level of 5-HT in the amygdala in WIS but not in WKY rats, it increased 5-HT turnover rate in the mPFC only in WKY rats (De La Garza II and Mahoney III, 2004). When exposed to chronic stress, WKY rats failed to show stress-induced reduction of 5-HT tissue level as SD rats did, whereas the turnover rate was increased in both WKY and SD rats (O'Mahony *et al.*, 2011). Previous studies showed increased binding of 5-HT_{1a} receptors in hippocampus and hypothalamus, but decreased binding of 5-HT transporters in the cell body area in WKY rats following chronic stress, compared to SD rats (Pare and Tejani-Butt, 1996). However WKY rats are insensitive to serotonergic drugs (e.g. SSRIs and receptor agonists) in terms of activity in the EPM and OFT, immobility in the FST, or severity of gastric ulceration after stress (Chaouloff *et al.*, 1998; Griebel *et al.*, 1999; Lahmame and Armario, 1996; Lopez-Rubalcava and Lucki, 2000; Pare *et al.*, 2001; Tejani-Butt *et al.*, 2003), suggesting serotonergic manipulation may not affect the temperamental behaviors of these rats.

5.2 Dopamine (DA)

Converging literatures demonstrate that an aberrant DA circuitry is associated with anxiety disorders (Gendreau *et al.*, 1998; Hamner and Diamond, 1996; Mathew *et al.*, 1981; Taylor *et al.*, 1982).WKY rats exhibit altered dopaminergic function in various brain regions. DA levels in WKY rats do not differ between WIS or SD rats in most brain areas; DA turnover is higher in the nucleus accumbens shell in the WKY rat compared to the WIS rat (De La Garza II and Mahoney III, 2004; Ferguson *et al.*, 2003a; Scholl *et al.*, 2010). Receptor and transporter binding studies show that WKY rats have altered dopaminergic pathways compared to control strains. The results from those studies reveal a significant strain difference, with WKY rats exhibiting lower levels of D1 receptor binding in the caudate putamen and nucleus accumbens core, but higher binding levels in the substantia nigra pars reticulata compared to WIS rats (Novick *et al.*, 2008). D1 receptors in the substantia nigra are involved in mediating the startle response (Meloni and Davis, 1999), thus a higher D1 receptor level in this region may lead to heightened ASR magnitude in WKY rats. Results from a recent study demonstrated that WKY rats exhibited higher D2 receptor binding levels in the nucleus accumbens shell and ventral tegmental area, but lower D2 receptor binding in the caudate putamen, nucleus accumbens core and hypothalamus compared to WIS rats (Yaroslavsky *et al.*, 2006). It is known that the D1 and D2 receptors represent critical sites where DA acts to modify behavior related to anxiety and reward; the altered expression of this receptor in the WKY rat may be reflective of the anxiety susceptibility noted in this rat strain. Moreover, DA transporter binding levels were lower in the nucleus accumbens core, amygdala and cell body regions (ventral tegmental area and substantia nigra), but higher in the hippocampus and hypothalamus compared to SD and WIS rats (Jiao *et al.*, 2003). The observed differences in the density and distribution of DAT sites in WKY rats may lead to altered modulation of synaptic DA levels in the cell body and mesolimbic regions, thereby contributing to the noted anxiety- and depression-like behaviors reported in this rat strain. This speculation was supported by a further study in which some of the alterations in DAT binding was reversed by chronic nomifensine (i.e. a dopamine transporter blocker) treatment (Jiao *et al.*, 2006). Moreover, after 8-12 days of nomifensine administration, WKY rats showed significantly increased head poke responses in the emergence test, reduced latency to leave the center in an open field and increased activity in the FST (Tejani-Butt *et al.*, 2003). Therefore, the WKY rat may represent a good model for a sub-type of anxiety disorder exhibiting imbalanced DA distribution in the CNS.

5.3 Norepinephrine (NE)

Defective noradrenergic function is one of the major mechanisms in the neuropathology of anxiety in human (Bremner *et al.*, 1996; Charney and Redmond, Jr., 1983; Hamner and Diamond, 1996; Neumeister *et al.*, 2005; Sullivan *et al.*, 1999). The WKY appears to have normal tissue levels of NE (De La Garza II and Mahoney III, 2004; O'Mahony *et al.*, 2011; Scholl *et al.*, 2010) and tyrosine hydroxylase (TH, the rate-limiting enzyme in NE synthesis) (Mann and Bell, 1991; Vachette *et al.*, 1993). In response to acute stress, noradrenergic reactivity appears to be blunted. For example, acute stress-induced increases of NE tissue levels in the lateral bed nucleus of the stria terminalis (BSTL) were significantly lower in WKY compared to SD rats (Pardon *et al.*, 2002; Pardon *et al.*, 2003). Moreover, the acute stress-induced increases in neuronal activity (cFos expression) in medial amygdala and locus ceruleus (LC) was lower in WKY rats compared to SD rats (Ma and Morilak, 2004). Alternatively, NE reactivity may be delayed. Acute stress-induced increases of TH mRNA level in WKY rats were apparent, but delayed by 2-hr in WKY rats compared to control strains (Pardon *et al.*, 2002; Sands *et al.*, 2000). Although reactivity to acute stress is blunted, chronic stress appears to sensitize NE in WKY rats. After chronic exposure to cold stress, increased BSTL NE release was induced by acute stress challenge only in WKY rats, but not in SD rats (Pardon *et al.*, 2003). Chronic stress decreases NE transporter binding in the cell body area and decreases $\alpha 2$ and β receptor binding in terminal regions, suggesting aberrant NE modulatory responses towards stress in WKY rats (Tejani-Butt *et al.*, 1994; Zafar *et al.*, 1997). Although the NE response to acute stress is blunted, , WKY rats may exhibit less habituation to stress appearing as larger levels of reactivity as the reactivity of SD rats declines. A sustained NE response may underlie hypervigilance and elevated arousal in response to specific or generalized stress (Cameron *et al.*, 2004; Lahdesmaki *et al.*, 2002; Maes *et al.*, 2002; Schramm *et al.*, 2001). The efficacy of NE-targeted drugs in altering behaviors relevant to anxiety is limited. Much of the past research has focused on altering behaviors in the FST. Drugs which act by blocking NE transporters reduced immobility in FST and increase activity in the OFT in WKY rats (Lahmame and Armario, 1996; Lucki and Nobler, 1985; Pare, 1992b; Pare *et al.*, 2001; Will *et al.*, 2003). Thus, increasing NE availability affects inhibited temperament of WKY rats.

5.4 Others

There is a dearth of knowledge about strain difference between the WKY rat and comparison strains in the glutamatergic and the GABAergic pathways. A recent autoradiographic study demonstrated that WKY rats exhibited lower N-methyl-d-aspartate (NMDA) receptor binding in anterior cingulate cortex, caudate putamen, nucleus accumbens, CA1 of hippocampus and substantia nigra compared to WIS rats (Lei *et al.*, 2009). Interestingly, chronic stress increased NMDA receptor binding in the prefrontal cortex, caudate putamen and nucleus accumbens only in the WKY rat (Lei and Tejani-Butt, 2010). Thus the authors speculated that NMDA receptors in these regions may be more sensitive to stress in WKY rats. Consistent with the previous report (Jiao *et al.*, 2011), our recent preliminary data suggest that naïve WKY rats exhibited altered density of PV immunoreactive cells in the amygdala and prefrontal cortex compared to SD rats (Table 1.). Although basal tissue level of GABA does not differ between WKY and WIS rats, stress increased it only in WKY rats (O'Mahony *et al.*, 2011). Moreover, the levels of GABA-A receptor binding are higher in amygdala, caudate putamen, CA2 and CA3 of hippocampus, periaqueductal gray and substantia nigra in WKY compared to WIS rats (Lei *et al.*, 2009). Given the role of GABA and GABA-A receptor in the pathophysiology of stress and anxiety, future investigation should emphasize GABAergic system in order to understand the unique behavioral aspects in WKY rats, a field that has not been studied sufficiently in this strain. So far only one report demonstrated the effect of diazepam on WKY rats measured by emergence test (Pare *et al.*, 2001). Single dose of diazepam reduced WKY rats' activity in an OFT. Thus the effects of pharmacological manipulation on GABAergic system need further investigation in WKY rats.

REGIONS	STRAIN	MEAN PV (ir) CELL DENSITY ± S.E.M. (CELL COUNTS/mm3)
Anterior Cingulate	SD	2208.08 ± 716.27
	WKY	3503.53 ± 111.97
Prelimbic Cortex	SD	2364.65 ± 281.96
	WKY	3181.51 ± 241.74
Infralimbic Cortex	SD	2891.72 ± 408.16
	WKY	2989.72 ± 442.44
Basal Amygdala	SD	2939.07 ± 211.16
	WKY	1786.03 ± 445.31
Lateral Amygdala	SD	2294.93 ± 251.59
	WKY	1427.58 ± 265.70

Table 1. PV (ir) positive cell densities in the prefrontal cortex and amygdala in WKY and SD rats. (N=4/strain)

5.5 Summary

The WKY rat exhibits a neurochemical profile reminiscent of anxiety disorders. The profile is also reminiscent of behavioral inhibition in nonhuman primates (Kalin, 2004; Kalin and Shelton, 2003; Kalin *et al.*, 2007). Past research has focused on the WKY as animal model of depression owing to the stress reactivity, susceptibility to ulcers, and reduced FST. Faster avoidance acquisition, avoidance perseveration and sustained arousal induced by avoidance learning are strong signs of anxiety vulnerability. Thus, investigation of psychotropic drugs in their ability to affect avoidance may have relevance for treatment of human anxiety. Recent findings of GABAergic activity selective to avoidance acquisition and extinction in WKY rats suggest a novel target for this class of anxiolytics.

6. Overall summary

Anxiety disorders develop as an interaction of trait vulnerabilities (e.g., behavioral inhibition), early life experiences and environmental exposures. The interplay of these influences determines success or failures to effectively cope, especially under stress. WKY rats model trait inhibited temperament, a risk factor for anxiety disorders. Accordingly, WKY rats have neurobehavioral, neuroanatomical, neurochemical and neuropharmacological features consistent with inhibited temperament. In particular, WKY rats acquire active avoidance faster; avoidance that is resistant to extinction. Moreover, WKY rats display two behavioral features which are hallmarks of anxiety as avoidance develops: worry and increased arousal. In the respect of neurochemistry and neuroendocrine, WKY rats demonstrated over stimulated NE circuitry and exaggerated HPAA activity in response to stress stimulation, and innate 5-HT deficit together with altered receptors function in monoamine systems and GABAergic system, which all contribute to hyper-reactivity towards stress and the phenotypes that related to anxiety behavior in this rat strain. Together, these significant findings suggest that the WKY rats should be studied as an animal model of vulnerability to develop anxiety disorders.

7. Acknowledgement

This research was supported by NIH grants and a Department of Veterans Affairs Merit Review research program and the Stress & Motivated Behavior Institute of the New Jersey Medical School. The described experimentations were conducted with approval by the VANJHCS Institutional Animal Care and Use and Research and Development Committees. The authors would like to thank the technical expertise of Toni Marie Dispenziere, Tracey Longo and Amanda Agley in the behavioral testing of the animals in these experiments.

8. References

Aguilar, R., Gil, L., Fernandez-Teruel, A., and Tobena, A. (2004) Genetically-based behavioral traits influence the effects of Shuttle Box avoidance overtraining and extinction upon intertrial responding: a study with the Roman rat strains. *Behav. Processes* 66, 63-72.

Ahmadiyeh, N., Churchill, G. A., Solberg, L. C., Baum, A. E., Shimomura, K., Takahashi, J. S., and Redei, E. E. (2005) Lineage is an epigenetic modifier of QTL influencing behavioral coping with stress. *Behav. Genet.* 35, 189-198.

Ardekani, A. M., Walker, S. J., Donohue, S. J., Stitzel, R. E., Connors, J. M., and Vrana, K. E. (1989) Adrenocorticotropin and corticosterone levels in pre-weanling spontaneously hypertensive rats. *Life Sciences* 44, 919-925.

Barad, M. (2005) Fear extinction in rodents: basic insight to clinical promise. *Current Opinion in Neurobiology* 15, 710-715.

Beck, K. D., Zhu, G., Beldowicz, D., Brennan, F. X., Ottenweller, J. E., Moldow, R. L., and Servatius, R. J. (2001) Central nervous system effects from a peripherally acting cholinesterase inhibiting agent: interaction with stress or genetics. *Ann. N. Y. Acad. Sci.* 933, 310-314.

Berger, D. F. and Starzec, J. J. (1988) Contrasting Lever-Press Avoidance Behaviors of Spontaneously Hypertensive and Normotensive Rats (Rattus norvegicus). *Journal of Comparative Psychology* 102, 279-286.

Biederman, J., Rosenbaum, J. F., Bolduc-Murphy, E. A., Faraone, S. V., Chaloff, J., Hirshfeld, D. R., and Kagan, J. (1993) A 3-year follow-up of children with and without behavioral inhibition. *J. Am. Acad. Child Adolesc. Psychiatry.* 32, 814-821.

Blizard, D. A. and Adams, N. (2002) The Maudsley Reactive and Nonreactive strains: a new perspective. *Behav. Genet.* 32, 277-299.

Bolles, R. C. (1970) Species-specific defense reactions and avoidance learning. *Psychological Review* 77, 32-48.

Boyle, A. E. and Gill, K. (2001) Sensitivity of AXB/BXA recombinant inbred lines of mice to the locomotor activating effects of cocaine: a quantitative trait loci analysis. *Pharmacogenetics* 11, 255-264.

Brambilla, P., Barale, F., Caverzasi, E., and Soares, J. C. (2002) Anatomical MRI findings in mood and anxiety disorders. *Epidemiol. Psichiatr. Soc.* 11, 88-99.

Braunstein-Bercovitz, H., mentman-Ashkenazi, I., and Lubow, R. E. (2001) Stress affects the selection of relevant from irrelevant stimuli. *Emotion.* 1, 182-192.

Braw, Y., Malkesman, O., Dagan, M., Bercovich, A., Lavi-Avnon, Y., Schroeder, M., Overstreet, D. H., and Weller, A. (2006) Anxiety-like behaviors in pre-pubertal rats of the Flinders Sensitive Line (FSL) and Wistar-Kyoto (WKY) animal models of depression. *Behavioural Brain Research* 167, 261-269.

Braw, Y., Malkesman, O., Merenlender, A., Bercovich, A., Dagan, M., Overstreet, D. H., and Weller, A. (2008) Withdrawal emotional-regulation in infant rats from genetic animal models of depression. *Behavioural Brain Research* 193, 94-100.

Bremner, J. D. (2006) The relationship between cognitive and brain changes in posttraumatic stress disorder. *Ann. N. Y. Acad. Sci.* 1071, 80-86.

Bremner, J. D., Krystal, J. H., Southwick, S. M., and Charney, D. S. (1996) Noradrenergic mechanisms in stress and anxiety: II. Clinical studies. *Synapse* 23, 39-51.

Brush, F. R. (2003) The Syracuse strains, selectively bred for differences in active avoidance learning, may be models of genetic differences in trait and state anxiety. *Stress.* 6, 77-85.

Buuse, M. v. d. (2004) Prepulse inhibition of acoustic startle in spontaneously hypertensive rats. *Behavioural Brain Research* 154, 331-337.

Bystritsky, A., Pontillo, D., Powers, M., Sabb, F. W., Craske, M. G., and Bookheimer, S. Y. (2001) Functional MRI changes during panic anticipation and imagery exposure. *Neuroreport* 12, 3953-3957.

Cameron, O. G., Abelson, J. L., and Young, E. A. (2004) Anxious and depressive disorders and their comorbidity: Effect on central nervous system noradrenergic function. *Biological Psychiatry* 56, 875-883.

Carr, G. V. and Lucki, I. (2010) Comparison of the kappa-opioid receptor antagonist DIPPA in tests of anxiety-like behavior between Wistar Kyoto and Sprague Dawley rats. *Psychopharmacology (Berl)* 210, 295-302.

Chantarujikapong, S. I., Scherrer, J. F., Xian, H., Eisen, S. A., Lyons, M. J., Goldberg, J., Tsuang, M., and True, W. R. (2001) A twin study of generalized anxiety disorder symptoms, panic disorder symptoms and post-traumatic stress disorder in men. *Psychiatry Res.* 103, 133-145.

Chaouloff, F., Aguerre, S., and Mormede, P. (1998) GR 127935 and (+)-WAY 100135 do not affect TFMPP-induced inhibition of 5-HT synthesis in the midbrain and hippocampus of Wistar-Kyoto rats. *Neuropharmacology* 37, 1159-1167.

Charney, D. S. and Redmond, D. E., Jr. (1983) Neurobiological mechanisms in human anxiety. Evidence supporting central noradrenergic hyperactivity. *Neuropharmacology* 22, 1531-1536.

Chen, Z. Y., Jing, D., Bath, K. G., Ieraci, A., Khan, T., Siao, C. J., Herrera, D. G., Toth, M., Yang, C., McEwen, B. S., Hempstead, B. L., and Lee, F. S. (2006) Genetic variant BDNF (Val66Met) polymorphism alters anxiety-related behavior. *Science* 314, 140-143.

Cloninger, C. R., Van, E. P., Goate, A., Edenberg, H. J., Blangero, J., Hesselbrock, V., Reich, T., Nurnberger, J., Jr., Schuckit, M., Porjesz, B., Crowe, R., Rice, J. P., Foroud, T., Przybeck, T. R., Almasy, L., Bucholz, K., Wu, W., Shears, S., Carr, K., Crose, C., Willig, C., Zhao, J., Tischfield, J. A., Li, T. K., Conneally, P. M., and . (1998) Anxiety proneness linked to epistatic loci in genome scan of human personality traits. *Am. J. Med. Genet.* 81, 313-317.

Coover, G. D., Ursin, H., and Levine, S. (1973) Plasma-corticosterone levels during active-avoidance learning in rats. *J. Comp Physiol Psychol.* 82, 170-174.

DaSilva, J. K., Lei, Y., Madan, V., Mann, G. L., Ross, R. J., Tejani-Butt, S., and Morrison, A. R. (2011) Fear conditioning fragments REM sleep in stress-sensitive Wistar-Kyoto, but not Wistar, rats. *Progress in Neuro-Psychopharmacology and Biological Psychiatry* 35, 67-73.

De La Garza II, R. and Mahoney III, J. J. (2004) A distinct neurochemical profile in WKY rats at baseline and in response to acute stress: implications for animal models of anxiety and depression. *Brain Research* 1021, 209-218.

Driscoll, P. (1986) Roman high- and low-avoidance rats: present status of the Swiss sublines, RHA/Verh and RLA/Verh, and effects of amphetamine on shuttle-box performance. *Behav. Genet.* 16, 355-364.

Drolet, G., Proulx, K., Pearson, D., Rochford, J., and Deschepper, C. F. (2002) Comparisons of behavioral and neurochemical characteristics between WKY, WKHA, and Wistar rat strains. *Neuropsychopharmacology* 27, 400-409.

Dugovic, C., Solberg, L. C., Redei, E., Van, R. O., and Turek, F. W. (2000) Sleep in the Wistar-Kyoto rat, a putative genetic animal model for depression. *Neuroreport* 11, 627-631.

Duman, R. S. (2004) Role of neurotrophic factors in the etiology and treatment of mood disorders. *Neuromolecular. Med.* 5, 11-25.

Duman, R. S. and Monteggia, L. M. (2006) A neurotrophic model for stress-related mood disorders. *Biol. Psychiatry* 59, 1116-1127.

Ferguson, S. A. and Cada, A. M. (2003) A longitudinal study of short- and long-term activity levels in male and female spontaneously hypertensive, Wistar-Kyoto, and Sprague-Dawley rats. *Behav. Neurosci.* 117, 271-282.

Ferguson, S. A., Gough, B. J., and Cada, A. M. (2003a) In vivo basal and amphetamine-induced striatal dopamine and metabolite levels are similar in the spontaneously hypertensive, Wistar-Kyoto and Sprague-Dawley male rats. *Physiol Behav.* 80, 109-114.

Ferguson, S. A., Gray, E. P., and Cada, A. M. (2003b) Early behavioral development in the spontaneously hypertensive rat: a comparison with the Wistar-Kyoto and Sprague-Dawley strains. *Behav. Neurosci.* 117, 263-270.

Ferguson, S. A. and Cada, A. M. (2004) Spatial learning/memory and social and nonsocial behaviors in the Spontaneously Hypertensive, Wistar-Kyoto and Sprague-Dawley rat strains. *Pharmacology Biochemistry and Behavior* 77, 583-594.

Foa, E. B., Stein, D. J., and McFarlane, A. C. (2006) Symptomatology and psychopathology of mental health problems after disaster. *J. Clin. Psychiatry* 67 Suppl 2, 15-25.

Fox, N. A., Henderson, H. A., Marshall, P. J., Nichols, K. E., and Ghera, M. M. (2005a) Behavioral inhibition: linking biology and behavior within a developmental framework. *Annu. Rev. Psychol.* 56, 235-262.

Fox, N. A., Henderson, H. A., Marshall, P. J., Nichols, K. E., and Ghera, M. M. (2005b) Behavioral inhibition: linking biology and behavior within a developmental framework. *Annu. Rev. Psychol.* 56, 235-262.

Gendreau, P. L., Petitto, J. M., Gariepy, J. L., and Lewis, M. H. (1998) D2-like dopamine receptor mediation of social-emotional reactivity in a mouse model of anxiety: Strain and experience effects. *Neuropsychopharmacology* 18, 210-221.

Glowa, J. and Hansen, C. (1994) Differences in response to an acoustic startle stimulus among forty-six rat strains. *Behavior Genetics* 24, 79-84.

Gomez, F., Lahmame, A., de Kloet, E. R., and Armario, A. (1996) Hypothalamic-pituitary-adrenal response to chronic stress in five inbred rat strains: differential responses are mainly located at the adrenocortical level. *Neuroendocrinology* 63, 327-337.

Gould, T. D. and Gottesman, I. I. (2006) Psychiatric endophenotypes and the development of valid animal models. *Genes Brain Behav.* 5, 113-119.

Griebel, G., Cohen, C., Perrault, G., and Sanger, D. J. (1999) Behavioral Effects of Acute and Chronic Fluoxetine in Wistar-Kyoto Rats. *Physiology & Behavior* 67, 315-320.

Grillon, C., Avenevoli, S., Daurignac, E., and Merikangas, K. R. (2007a) Fear-Potentiated Startle to Threat, and Prepulse Inhibition Among Young Adult Nonsmokers, Abstinent Smokers, and Nonabstinent Smokers. *Biol. Psychiatry.*

Grillon, C., Duncko, R., Covington, M. F., Kopperman, L., and Kling, M. A. (2007b) Acute Stress Potentiates Anxiety in Humans. *Biol. Psychiatry.*

Guthrie, R. M. and Bryant, R. A. (2005) Auditory startle response in firefighters before and after trauma exposure. *Am. J. Psychiatry* 162, 283-290.

Gutiérrez-Mariscal, M., de Gortari, P., López-Rubalcava, C., Martínez, A., and Joseph-Bravo, P. (2008) Analysis of the anxiolytic-like effect of TRH and the response of amygdalar TRHergic neurons in anxiety. *Psychoneuroendocrinology* 33, 198-213.

Hamner, M. B. and Diamond, B. I. (1996) Plasma dopamine and norepinephrine correlations with psychomotor retardation, anxiety, and depression in non-psychotic depressed patients: a pilot study. *Psychiatry Research* 64, 209-211.

Henderson, A. S., Korten, A. E., Jorm, A. F., Jacomb, P. A., Christensen, H., Rodgers, B., Tan, X., and Easteal, S. (2000) COMT and DRD3 polymorphisms, environmental exposures, and personality traits related to common mental disorders. *Am. J. Med. Genet.* 96, 102-107.

Hineline, P. N. (1978a) Warmup in avoidance as a function of time since prior training. *J. Exp. Anal. Behav.* 29, 87-103.

Hineline, P. N. (1978b) Warmup in free-operant avoidance as a function of the response-shock = shock-shock interval. *J. Exp. Anal. Behav.* 30, 281-291.

Hirshfeld, D. R., Rosenbaum, J. F., Biederman, J., Bolduc, E. A., Faraone, S. V., Snidman, N., Reznick, J. S., and Kagan, J. (1992) Stable behavioral inhibition and its association with anxiety disorder. *J. Am. Acad. Child Adolesc. Psychiatry.* 31, 103-111.

Hirshfeld-Becker, D. R., Biederman, J., Henin, A., Faraone, S. V., Davis, S., Harrington, K., and Rosenbaum, J. F. (2007) Behavioral inhibition in preschool children at risk is a specific predictor of middle childhood social anxiety: a five-year follow-up. *J. Dev. Behav. Pediatr.* 28, 225-233.

Hopper, J. W., Frewen, P. A., van der Kolk, B. A., and Lanius, R. A. (2007) Neural correlates of reexperiencing, avoidance, and dissociation in PTSD: symptom dimensions and emotion dysregulation in responses to script-driven trauma imagery. *J. Trauma Stress.* 20, 713-725.

Jiao, X., Pang, K. C., Beck, K. D., Minor, T. R., and Servatius, R. J. (2011) Avoidance perseveration during extinction training in Wistar-Kyoto rats: An interaction of innate vulnerability and stressor intensity. *Behav. Brain Res.* 221, 98-107.

Jiao, X., Pare, W. P., and Tejani-Butt, S. (2003) Strain differences in the distribution of dopamine transporter sites in rat brain. *Progress in Neuro-Psychopharmacology and Biological Psychiatry* 27, 913-919.

Jiao, X., Pare, W. P., and Tejani-Butt, S. M. (2006) Antidepressant drug induced alterations in binding to central dopamine transporter sites in the Wistar Kyoto rat strain. *Progress in Neuro-Psychopharmacology and Biological Psychiatry* 30, 30-41.

Kagan, J., Reznick, J. S., and Gibbons, J. (1989) Inhibited and uninhibited types of children. *Child Dev.* 60, 838-845.

Kagan, J., Reznick, J. S., and Snidman, N. (1987) The physiology and psychology of behavioral inhibition in children. *Child Dev.* 58, 1459-1473.

Kalin, N. H. (2004) Studying non-human primates: a gateway to understanding anxiety disorders. *Psychopharmacol. Bull.* 38 Suppl 1, 8-13.

Kalin, N. H. and Shelton, S. E. (2003) Nonhuman primate models to study anxiety, emotion regulation, and psychopathology. *Ann. N. Y. Acad. Sci.* 1008, 189-200.

Kalin, N. H., Shelton, S. E., and Davidson, R. J. (2000) Cerebrospinal fluid corticotropin-releasing hormone levels are elevated in monkeys with patterns of brain activity associated with fearful temperament. *Biol. Psychiatry* 47, 579-585.

Kalin, N. H., Shelton, S. E., and Davidson, R. J. (2007) Role of the Primate Orbitofrontal Cortex in Mediating Anxious Temperament. *Biological Psychiatry* 62, 1134-1139.

Kalueff, A. V., Avgustinovich, D. F., Kudryavtseva, N. N., and Murphy, D. L. (2006) BDNF in anxiety and depression. *Science* 312, 1598-1599.

Karamustafalioglu, O. K., Zohar, J., Guveli, M., Gal, G., Bakim, B., Fostick, L., Karamustafalioglu, N., and Sasson, Y. (2006) Natural Course of Posttraumatic Stress Disorder: A 20-Month Prospective Study of Turkish Earthquake Survivors. *J. Clin. Psychiatry* 67, 882-889.

Kashdan, T. B., Elhai, J. D., and Frueh, B. C. (2006) Anhedonia and emotional numbing in combat veterans with PTSD. *Behaviour Research and Therapy* 44, 457-467.

Keltikangas-Jarvinen, L., Kettunen, J., Ravaja, N., and Naatanen, P. (1999) Inhibited and disinhibited temperament and autonomic stress reactivity. *Int. J. Psychophysiol.* 33, 185-196.

Kemppainen, S. and Pitkanen, A. (2000) Distribution of parvalbumin, calretinin, and calbindin-D(28k) immunoreactivity in the rat amygdaloid complex and colocalization with gamma-aminobutyric acid. *J. Comp Neurol.* 426, 441-467.

Kendler, K. S., Myers, J., and Prescott, C. A. (2002) The etiology of phobias: an evaluation of the stress-diathesis model. *Arch. Gen. Psychiatry* 59, 242-248.

Kessler, R. C., Chiu, W. T., Demler, O., Merikangas, K. R., and Walters, E. E. (2005) Prevalence, severity, and comorbidity of 12-month DSM-IV disorders in the National Comorbidity Survey Replication. *Arch. Gen. Psychiatry* 62, 617-627.

Lahdesmaki, J., Sallinen, J., MacDonald, E., Kobilka, B. K., Fagerholm, V., and Scheinin, M. (2002) Behavioral and neurochemical characterization of alpha(2A)-adrenergic receptor knockout mice. *Neuroscience* 113, 289-299.

Lahmame, A. and Armario, A. (1996) Differential responsiveness of inbred strains of rats to antidepressants in the forced swimming test: are Wistar Kyoto rats an animal model of subsensitivity to antidepressants? *Psychopharmacology (Berl)* 123, 191-198.

Laitman, B. M., DaSilva, J. K., Ross, R. J., Tejani-Butt, S., and Morrison, A. R. Reduced Gamma Range Activity at REM Sleep Onset and Termination in Fear-Conditioned Wistar-Kyoto Rats. *Neuroscience Letters* In Press, Accepted Manuscript.

Lanius, R. A., Williamson, P. C., Hopper, J., Densmore, M., Boksman, K., Gupta, M. A., Neufeld, R. W., Gati, J. S., and Menon, R. S. (2003) Recall of emotional states in posttraumatic stress disorder: an fMRI investigation. *Biol. Psychiatry* 53, 204-210.

Lei, Y. and Tejani-Butt, S. M. (2010) N-methyl-d-aspartic acid receptors are altered by stress and alcohol in Wistar-Kyoto rat brain. *Neuroscience* 169, 125-131.

Lei, Y., Yaroslavsky, I., and Tejani-Butt, S. M. (2009) Strain differences in the distribution of N-methyl-d-aspartate and gamma ([gamma])-aminobutyric acid-A receptors in rat brain. *Life Sciences* 85, 794-799.

Lemos, J. C., Zhang, G., Walsh, T., Kirby, L. G., Akanwa, A., Brooks-Kayal, A., and Beck, S. G. (2011) Stress-Hyperresponsive WKY Rats Demonstrate Depressed Dorsal Raphe Neuronal Excitability and Dysregulated CRF-Mediated Responses. *Neuropsychopharmacology* 36, 721-734.

Lind, K., Jonsson, M., Karlsson, I., Sjogren, M., Wallin, A., and Edman, A. (2006) Depressive symptoms and white matter changes in patients with dementia. *Int. J. Geriatr. Psychiatry* 21, 119-125.

Lopez-Rubalcava, C. and Lucki, I. (2000) Strain differences in the behavioral effects of antidepressant drugs in the rat forced swimming test. *Neuropsychopharmacology* 22, 191-199.

Lucki, I. and Nobler, M. S. (1985) The acute effects of antidepressant drugs on the performance of conditioned avoidance behavior in rats. *Pharmacology Biochemistry and Behavior* 22, 261-264.

Ma, S. and Morilak, D. A. (2004) Induction of FOS expression by acute immobilization stress is reduced in locus coeruleus and medial amygdala of Wistar-Kyoto rats compared to Sprague-Dawley rats. *Neuroscience* 124, 963-972.

Maes, M., Van, G. A., Delmeire, L., Kenis, G., Bosmans, E., and Song, C. (2002) Platelet alpha2-adrenoceptor density in humans: relationships to stress-induced anxiety, psychasthenic constitution, gender and stress-induced changes in the inflammatory response system. *Psychol. Med.* 32, 919-928.

Malkesman, O., Asaf, T., Shbiro, L., Goldstein, A., Maayan, R., Weizman, A., Kinor, N., Okun, E., Sredni, B., Yadid, G., and Weller, A. (2009) Monoamines, BDNF, Dehydroepiandrosterone, DHEA-Sulfate, and Childhood Depression-An Animal Model Study. *Adv. Pharmacol. Sci.* 2009, 405107.

Malkesman, O., Braw, Y., Zagoory-Sharon, O., Golan, O., Lavi-Avnon, Y., Schroeder, M., Overstreet, D. H., Yadid, G., and Weller, A. (2005) Reward and anxiety in genetic animal models of childhood depression. *Behavioural Brain Research* 164, 1-10.

Malkesman, O., Maayan, R., Weizman, A., and Weller, A. (2006a) Aggressive behavior and HPA axis hormones after social isolation in adult rats of two different genetic animal models for depression. *Behav. Brain Res.* 175, 408-414.

Malkesman, O. and Weller, A. (2009) Two different putative genetic animal models of childhood depression--A review. *Progress in Neurobiology* 88, 153-169.

Malkesman, O., Braw, Y., Maayan, R., Weizman, A., Overstreet, D. H., Shabat-Simon, M., Kesner, Y., Touati-Werner, D., Yadid, G., and Weller, A. (2006b) Two Different Putative Genetic Animal Models of Childhood Depression. *Biological Psychiatry* 59, 17-23.

Mann, R. and Bell, C. (1991) Neuronal metabolism and DOPA decarboxylase immunoreactivity in terminal noradrenergic sympathetic axons of rat. *J. Histochem. Cytochem.* 39, 663-668.

Martinowich, K., Manji, H., and Lu, B. (2007) New insights into BDNF function in depression and anxiety. *Nat Neurosci* 10, 1089-1093.

Mathew, R. J., Ho, B. T., Taylor, D. L., and Semchuk, K. M. (1981) Catecholamine and dopamine-[beta]-hydroxylase in anxiety. *Journal of Psychosomatic Research* 25, 499-504.

McAuley, J. D., Stewart, A. L., Webber, E. S., Cromwell, H. C., Servatius, R. J., and Pang, K. C. (2009) Wistar-Kyoto rats as an animal model of anxiety vulnerability: Support for a hypervigilance hypothesis. *Behav. Brain Res.*

McEwen, B. S. (2005) Glucocorticoids, depression, and mood disorders: structural remodeling in the brain. *Metabolism* 54, 20-23.

Meloni, E. G. and Davis, M. (1999) Enhancement of the acoustic startle response in rats by the dopamine D1 receptor agonist SKF 82958. *Psychopharmacology (Berl)* 144, 373-380.

Milad, M. R., Quirk, G. J., Pitman, R. K., Orr, S. P., Fischl, B., and Rauch, S. L. A Role for the Human Dorsal Anterior Cingulate Cortex in Fear Expression. *Biological Psychiatry* In Press, Corrected Proof, -454.

Mineka, S. and Zinbarg, R. (1996) Conditioning and ethological models of anxiety disorders: stress-in-dynamic-context anxiety models. *Nebr. Symp. Motiv.* 43:135-210., 135-210.

Mineka, S. and Zinbarg, R. (2006) A contemporary learning theory perspective on the etiology of anxiety disorders: it's not what you thought it was. *Am. Psychol.* 61, 10-26.

Mineka, S. (2004) The positive and negative consequences of worry in the aetiology of generalized anxiety disorder: A learning theory perspective. [References]. pp. 24-48.

Mobbs, D., Petrovic, P., Marchant, J. L., Hassabis, D., Weiskopf, N., Seymour, B., Dolan, R. J., and Frith, C. D. (2007) When fear is near: threat imminence elicits prefrontal-periaqueductal gray shifts in humans. *Science* 317, 1079-1083.

Myers, K. M. and Davis, M. (2002) Behavioral and neural analysis of extinction. *Neuron* 36, 567-584.

Neumeister, A., Daher, R. J., and Charney, D. S. (2005) Anxiety disorders: noradrenergic neurotransmission. *Handb. Exp. Pharmacol.* 205-223.

North, C. S., Pfefferbaum, B., Tivis, L., Kawasaki, A., Reddy, C., and Spitznagel, E. L. (2004) The course of posttraumatic stress disorder in a follow-up study of survivors of the Oklahoma City bombing. *Ann. Clin. Psychiatry* 16, 209-215.

Nosek, K., Dennis, K., Andrus, B. M., Ahmadiyeh, N., Baum, A. E., Solberg Woods, L. C., and Redei, E. E. (2008) Context and strain-dependent behavioral response to stress. *Behav. Brain Funct.* 4, 23.

Novick, A., Yaroslavsky, I., and Tejani-Butt, S. (2008) Strain differences in the expression of dopamine D1 receptors in Wistar-Kyoto (WKY) and Wistar rats. *Life Sciences* 83, 74-78.

Nutt, D. J. and Malizia, A. L. (2004) Structural and functional brain changes in posttraumatic stress disorder. *J. Clin. Psychiatry* 65 Suppl 1, 11-17.

O'donnell, M. L., Elliott, P., Lau, W., and Creamer, M. (2006b) PTSD symptom trajectories: From early to chronic response. *Behav. Res. Ther.*

O'donnell, M. L., Elliott, P., Lau, W., and Creamer, M. (2006a) PTSD symptom trajectories: From early to chronic response. *Behav. Res. Ther.*

O'Mahony, C. M., Clarke, G., Gibney, S., Dinan, T. G., and Cryan, J. F. (2011) Strain differences in the neurochemical response to chronic restraint stress in the rat: relevance to depression. *Pharmacol. Biochem. Behav.* 97, 690-699.

Ohara, K., Nishii, R., Nakajima, T., Kokai, M., and Morita, Y. (2004) [Alterations of symptoms with borderline personality disorder after fronto-temporal traumatic brain injury. A case study]. *Seishin Shinkeigaku Zasshi* 106, 458-466.

Okamoto, K. and Aoki, K. (1963) Development of a strain of spontaneously hypertensive rats. *Jpn. Circ. J.* 27, 282-293.

Ottenweller, J. E., Servatius, R. J., and Natelson, B. H. (1994) Repeated stress persistently elevates morning, but not evening, plasma corticosterone levels in male rats. *Physiology & Behavior* 55, 337-340.

Overstreet, D. H., Rezvani, A. H., and Janowsky, D. S. (1990) Impaired active avoidance responding in rats selectively bred for increased cholinergic function. *Physiology & Behavior* 47, 787-788.

Overstreet, D. H., Rezvani, A. H., and Janowsky, D. S. (1992) Genetic animal models of depression and ethanol preference provide support for cholinergic and serotonergic involvement in depression and alcoholism. *Biological Psychiatry* 31, 919-936.

Palmer, A. A., Dulawa, S. C., Mottiwala, A. A., Conti, L. H., Geyer, M. A., and Printz, M. P. (2000) Prepulse Startle Deficit in the Brown Norway Rat: A Potential Genetic Model. *Behavioral Neuroscience* 114, 374-388.

Pardon, M.-C., Gould, G. G., Garcia, A., Phillips, L., Cook, M. C., Miller, S. A., Mason, P. A., and Morilak, D. A. (2002) Stress reactivity of the brain noradrenergic system in three rat strains differing in their neuroendocrine and behavioral responses to stress: implications for susceptibility to stress-related neuropsychiatric disorders. *Neuroscience* 115, 229-242.

Pardon, M. C., Joubert, C., Perez-Diaz, F., Christen, Y., Launay, J. M., and Cohen-Salmon, C. (2000) In vivo regulation of cerebral monoamine oxidase activity in senescent controls and chronically stressed mice by long-term treatment with Ginkgo biloba extrac3t (EGb 761). *Mechanisms of Ageing and Development* 113, 157-168.

Pardon, M. C., Ma, S., and Morilak, D. A. (2003) Chronic cold stress sensitizes brain noradrenergic reactivity and noradrenergic facilitation of the HPA stress response in Wistar Kyoto rats. *Brain Research* 971, 55-65.

Pare, A. M. T., Pare, W. P., and Kluczynski, J. (1999a) Negative Affect and Voluntary Alcohol Consumption in Wistar-Kyoto (WKY) and Sprague-Dawley Rats. *Physiology & Behavior* 67, 219-225.

Pare, W. P. (1992a) Learning behavior, escape behavior, and depression in an ulcer susceptible rat strain. *Integr. Physiol Behav. Sci.* 27, 130-141.

Pare, W. P., Blair, G. R., Kluczynski, J., and Tejani-Butt, S. (1999b) Gender differences in acute and chronic stress in Wistar Kyoto (WKY) rats. *Integr. Physiol Behav. Sci.* 34, 227-241.

Pare, W. P. and Kluczynski, J. (1997) Differences in the stress response of Wistar-Kyoto (WKY) rats from different vendors. *Physiol Behav.* 62, 643-648.

Pare, W. P. and Redei, E. (1993a) Depressive behavior and stress ulcer in Wistar Kyoto rats. *Journal of Physiology-Paris* 87, 229-238.

Pare, W. P. and Redei, E. (1993b) Sex differences and stress response of WKY rats. *Physiol Behav.* 54, 1179-1185.

Pare, W. P. and Tejani-Butt, S. M. (1996) Effect of stress on the behavior and 5-HT system in Sprague-Dawley and Wistar Kyoto rat strains. *Integr. Physiol Behav. Sci.* 31, 112-121.

Pare, W. P. (1989a) "Behavioral despair" test predicts stress ulcer in WKY rats. *Physiology & Behavior* 46, 483-487.

Pare, W. P. (1989b) "Behavioral despair" test predicts stress ulcer in WKY rats. *Physiology & Behavior* 46, 483-487.

Pare, W. P. (1989c) Stress ulcer susceptibility and depression in Wistar Kyoto (WKY) rats. *Physiology & Behavior* 46, 993-998.

Pare, W. P. (1992b) The performance of WKY rats on three tests of emotional behavior. *Physiology & Behavior* 51, 1051-1056.

Pare, W. P. (1993) Passive-avoidance behavior in Wistar-Kyoto (WKY), Wistar, and Fischer-344 rats. *Physiology & Behavior* 54, 845-852.

Pare, W. P. (1994) Open field, learned helplessness, conditioned defensive burying, and forced-swim tests in WKY rats. *Physiology & Behavior* 55, 433-439.

Pare, W. P. (1996) Enhanced retrieval of unpleasant memories influenced by shock controllability, shock sequence, and rat strain. *Biological Psychiatry* 39, 808-813.

Pare, W. P. and Schimmel, G. T. (1986) Stress ulcer in normotensive and spontaneously hypertensive rats. *Physiology & Behavior* 36, 699-705.

Pare, W. P., Tejani-Butt, S., and Kluczynski, J. (2001) The emergence test: effects of psychotropic drugs on neophobic disposition in Wistar Kyoto (WKY) and Sprague Dawley Rats. *Progress in Neuro-Psychopharmacology and Biological Psychiatry* 25, 1615-1628.

Pearson, K. A., Stephen, A., Beck, S. G., and Valentino, R. J. (2006) Identifying genes in monoamine nuclei that may determine stress vulnerability and depressive behavior in Wistar-Kyoto rats. *Neuropsychopharmacology* 31, 2449-2461.

Perez-Edgar, K., Roberson-Nay, R., Hardin, M. G., Poeth, K., Guyer, A. E., Nelson, E. E., McClure, E. B., Henderson, H. A., Fox, N. A., Pine, D. S., and Ernst, M. (2007) Attention alters neural responses to evocative faces in behaviorally inhibited adolescents. *Neuroimage.* 35, 1538-1546.

Redei, E., Pare, W. P., Aird, F., and Kluczynski, J. (1994) Strain differences in hypothalamic-pituitary-adrenal activity and stress ulcer. *Am. J. Physiol* 266, R353-R360.

Rittenhouse, P. A., Lopez-Rubalcava, C., Stanwood, G. D., and Lucki, I. (2002) Amplified behavioral and endocrine responses to forced swim stress in the Wistar-Kyoto rat. *Psychoneuroendocrinology* 27, 303-318.

Rosenbaum, J. F., Biederman, J., Bolduc-Murphy, E. A., Faraone, S. V., Chaloff, J., Hirshfeld, D. R., and Kagan, J. (1993) Behavioral inhibition in childhood: a risk factor for anxiety disorders. *Harv. Rev. Psychiatry.* 1, 2-16.

Rosenbaum, J. F., Biederman, J., Hirshfeld, D. R., Bolduc, E. A., Faraone, S. V., Kagan, J., Snidman, N., and Reznick, J. S. (1991) Further evidence of an association between behavioral inhibition and anxiety disorders: results from a family study of children from a non-clinical sample. *J. Psychiatr. Res.* 25, 49-65.

Rosenkranz, J. A. and Grace, A. A. (2001) Dopamine attenuates prefrontal cortical suppression of sensory inputs to the basolateral amygdala of rats. *J. Neurosci.* 21, 4090-4103.

Samanez-Larkin, G. R., Hollon, N. G., Carstensen, L. L., and Knutson, B. (2008) Individual differences in insular sensitivity during loss anticipation predict avoidance learning. *Psychol. Sci.* 19, 320-323.

Sands, S. A., Strong, R., Corbitt, J., and Morilak, D. A. (2000) Effects of acute restraint stress on tyrosine hydroxylase mRNA expression in locus coeruleus of Wistar and Wistar-Kyoto rats. *Molecular Brain Research* 75, 1-7.

Scholl, J. L., Renner, K. J., Forster, G. L., and Tejani-Butt, S. (2010) Central monoamine levels differ between rat strains used in studies of depressive behavior. *Brain Research* 1355, 41-51.

Schramm, N. L., McDonald, M. P., and Limbird, L. E. (2001) The {alpha}2A-Adrenergic Receptor Plays a Protective Role in Mouse Behavioral Models of Depression and Anxiety. *J. Neurosci.* 21, 4875-4882.

Schwartz, C. E., Wright, C. I., Shin, L. M., Kagan, J., and Rauch, S. L. (2003) Inhibited and uninhibited infants "grown up": adult amygdalar response to novelty. *Science* 300, 1952-1953.

Servatius, R. J., Jiao, X., Beck, K. D., Pang, K. C. H., and Minor, T. R. (2008) Rapid avoidance acquisition in Wistar-Kyoto rats. *Behavioural Brain Research* 192, 191-197.

Servatius, R. J., Ottenweller, J. E., Beldowicz, D., Guo, W., Zhu, G., and Natelson, B. H. (1998) Persistently exaggerated startle responses in rats treated with pyridostigmine bromide. *J. Pharmacol. Exp. Ther.* 287, 1020-1028.

Silver, R. C., Holman, E. A., McIntosh, D. N., Poulin, M., and Gil-Rivas, V. (2002) Nationwide longitudinal study of psychological responses to September 11. *JAMA* 288, 1235-1244.

Simmons, A., Strigo, I., Matthews, S. C., Paulus, M. P., and Stein, M. B. (2006) Anticipation of aversive visual stimuli is associated with increased insula activation in anxiety-prone subjects. *Biol. Psychiatry* 60, 402-409.

Smoller, J. W., Rosenbaum, J. F., Biederman, J., Kennedy, J., Dai, D., Racette, S. R., Laird, N. M., Kagan, J., Snidman, N., Hirshfeld-Becker, D., Tsuang, M. T., Sklar, P. B., and Slaugenhaupt, S. A. (2003) Association of a genetic marker at the corticotropin-releasing hormone locus with behavioral inhibition. *Biol. Psychiatry.* 54, 1376-1381.

Smoller, J. W., Yamaki, L. H., Fagerness, J. A., Biederman, J., Racette, S., Laird, N. M., Kagan, J., Snidman, N., Faraone, S. V., Hirshfeld-Becker, D., Tsuang, M. T., Slaugenhaupt, S. A., Rosenbaum, J. F., and Sklar, P. B. (2005) The corticotropin-releasing hormone gene and behavioral inhibition in children at risk for panic disorder. *Biol. Psychiatry.* 57, 1485-1492.

Solberg, L. C., Baum, A. E., Ahmadiyeh, N., Shimomura, K., Li, R., Turek, F. W., Churchill, G. A., Takahashi, J. S., and Redei, E. E. (2004) Sex- and lineage-specific inheritance of depression-like behavior in the rat. *Mamm. Genome* 15, 648-662.

Solberg, L. C., Olson, S. L., Turek, F. W., and Redei, E. (2001) Altered hormone levels and circadian rhythm of activity in the WKY rat, a putative animal model of depression. *Am. J. Physiol Regul. Integr. Comp Physiol* 281, R786-R794.

Somers, J. M., Goldner, E. M., Waraich, P., and Hsu, L. (2006) Prevalence and incidence studies of anxiety disorders: a systematic review of the literature. *Can. J. Psychiatry* 51, 100-113.

Straube, T., Schmidt, S., Weiss, T., Mentzel, H. J., and Miltner, W. H. (2009) Dynamic activation of the anterior cingulate cortex during anticipatory anxiety. *Neuroimage.* 44, 975-981.

Sullivan, G. M., Coplan, J. D., Kent, J. M., and Gorman, J. M. (1999) The noradrenergic system in pathological anxiety: a focus on panic with relevance to generalized anxiety and phobias. *Biol. Psychiatry* 46, 1205-1218.

Suslow, T., Kugel, H., Rauch, A. V., Dannlowski, U., Bauer, J., Konrad, C., Arolt, V., Heindel, W., and Ohrmann, P. (2009) Attachment avoidance modulates neural response to masked facial emotion. *Hum. Brain Mapp.*

Taylor, D. P., Riblet, L. A., Stanton, H. C., Eison, A. S., Eison, M. S., and Temple, D. L. (1982) Dopamine and antianxiety activity. *Pharmacology Biochemistry and Behavior* 17, 25-35.

Tejani-Butt, S. M., Pare, W. P., and Yang, J. (1994) Effect of repeated novel stressors on depressive behavior and brain norepinephrine receptor system in Sprague-Dawley and Wistar Kyoto (WKY) rats. *Brain Res.* 649, 27-35.

Tejani-Butt, S., Kluczynski, J., and Pare, W. P. (2003) Strain-dependent modification of behavior following antidepressant treatment. *Progress in Neuro-Psychopharmacology and Biological Psychiatry* 27, 7-14.

Tyrka, A. R., Mello, A. F., Mello, M. F., Gagne, G. G., Grover, K. E., Anderson, G. M., Price, L. H., and Carpenter, L. L. (2006) Temperament and hypothalamic-pituitary-adrenal axis function in healthy adults. *Psychoneuroendocrinology* 31, 1036-1045.

Tyrka, A. R., Wier, L. M., Price, L. H., Rikhye, K., Ross, N. S., Anderson, G. M., Wilkinson, C. W., and Carpenter, L. L. (2008) Cortisol and ACTH responses to the Dex/CRH test: influence of temperament. *Horm. Behav.* 53, 518-525.

Vachette, C., Bourde, O., Gillon, J. Y., Pujol, J. F., and Renaud, B. (1993) Decrease in the reactivity of locus coeruleus neurons to hypotension after an increase in their tyrosine hydroxylase content: a subregional in vivo voltammetry study in the rat. *Eur. J. Neurosci.* 5, 261-268.

Vaswani, M., Linda, F. K., and Ramesh, S. (2003) Role of selective serotonin reuptake inhibitors in psychiatric disorders: a comprehensive review. *Progress in Neuro-Psychopharmacology and Biological Psychiatry* 27, 85-102.

Walker, J. R., Su, A. I., Self, D. W., Hogenesch, J. B., Lapp, H., Maier, R., Hoyer, D., and Bilbe, G. (2004) Applications of a rat multiple tissue gene expression data set. *Genome Res.* 14, 742-749.

Will, C. C., Aird, F., and Redei, E. E. (2003) Selectively bred Wistar-Kyoto rats: an animal model of depression and hyper-responsiveness to antidepressants. *Mol. Psychiatry* 8, 925-932.

Yaroslavsky, I., Colletti, M., Jiao, X., and Tejani-Butt, S. (2006) Strain differences in the distribution of dopamine (DA-2 and DA-3) receptor sites in rat brain. *Life Sciences* 79, 772-776.

Zafar, H. M., Pare, W. P., and Tejani-Butt, S. M. (1997) Effect of acute or repeated stress on behavior and brain norepinephrine system in Wistar-Kyoto (WKY) rats. *Brain Res. Bull.* 44, 289-295.

Zinbarg, R. E. and Barlow, D. H. (1996) Structure of anxiety and the anxiety disorders: a hierarchical model. *J. Abnorm. Psychol.* 105, 181-193.

6

Influence of Trait-Anxiety on Inhibition Function: Evidence from ERP Studies

Yue-jia Luo, Ruolei Gu and Yu-xia Huang
State Key Laboratory of Cognitive Neuroscience and Learning,
Beijing Normal University
China

1. Introduction

1.1 Influence of anxiety on Inhibition function: Emotional processing

Many researchers have reported that anxiety patients are more sensitive to emotional stimuli, particularly negative stimuli. This phenomenon is suggested to be linked with high-anxiety people's inhibition dysfunction when facing emotional stimuli (Barkley, 1997; Enright & Beech, 1993). Supporting this idea, there has been an increasing amount of literature addressing the inhibition mechanisms in high-anxiety individuals. For instance, many previous studies indicated that high-anxiety people may find it harder than low-anxiety people to inhibit the processing of emotional stimuli, especially the threatening contents (Derakshan, Ansari, Hansard, Shoker, & Eysenck, 2009; Mogg & Bradley, 1998; Mogg, Bradley, Williams, & Mathews, 1993). Yee & Vaughan (1996) suggest that anxiety disorders may associate with inhibition failure, and the inhibition processes in the executive function affects individuals as early as during childhood (see also Livesley, Jang, & Vernon, 1998).

In this study, we attempted to compare the difference in inhibition function between high and low trait-anxiety individuals during emotional processing. With reference to previous studies, we adopted the oddball paradigm involving novel stimuli (i.e., inserting an additional stimulus as the interference when subjects were performing the discrimination task) (Fichtenholtz et al., 2004). In order to complete cognition tasks, subjects should inhibit the emotional distracting stimuli. This paradigm is suitable to investigate inhibition mechanisms of emotional interferences and has been widely used in studies on attention and emotion (Yamasaki, LaBar, & McCarthy, 2002).

A total of 210 undergraduate students completed the Chinese version of Spielberger's trait anxiety (Shek, 1993) which has good validity and reliability evidenced by a large sample survey (Spielberger, Gorsuch, Lushene, Vagg, & Jacobs, 1983; Zheng et al., 1993). The average trait-anxiety score from participants investigated in the current study was 40.1 ± 10.1. Participants whose trait-anxiety scores were over 45 were grouped as high-trait anxiety (HTA) individuals, whereas the low-trait anxiety (LTA) group comprised subjects whose scores were equal or less than 35.

It is indicated that the response bias may influence the reliability of psychological assessment and measurement, especially in the self-report measurement. In order to decrease the bias from the socially desirable responding, we asked the participants to complete the Marlowe-Crowne Social Desirability Scale (MCSD) (Crowne & Marlowe, 1960;

Wang, Wang, & Ma, 1999). The mean MCSD score from the sample of university students was 15.5 ± 4.4 (Wang et al., 1999). In the current study the average MCSD score was 15.6 ± 4.4. Participants whose scores were over 20 were excluded from the EEG data acquisition.

Finally, the study comprised 28 right-handed subjects without neurological or mental illness, ranging in age from 18 to 25 years (mean age: 22 years). In this sample, 14 participants were assigned to the HTA group (6 men and 8 women) and 14 participants to the LTA group (4 men and 10 women). The trait-anxiety score of the HTA group was significantly higher than that of the LTA group (51.6 vs. 27.9, $p < 0.001$). The difference in MCSD scores between the two groups was not salient (13.9 versus 12.1, $p > 0.05$). Participants signed the informed consent before the experiment, and received remuneration on completion of the study.

The formal task contained three types of stimuli: standard ones, target ones, and novel ones. Standard stimuli and target stimuli were geometric figures (round, square, or triangle). Target stimuli were larger than standard figures by 5%. There were 1440 standard stimuli and 180 target stimuli. Novel stimuli were 180 color pictures selected from the Chinese Affective Picture System (CAPS) (Bai, Ma, Huang, & Luo, 2005), including 60 positive pictures (e.g., delicious food), 60 neutral pictures (e.g., household appliances), and 60 negative pictures (e.g., scene of a car accident). The emotional valence in positive and negative pictures was significantly different from that in the case of neutral pictures (7.42 versus 5.11, $p < 0.01$; 2.40 versus 5.11, $p < 0.01$); also, positive and negative pictures caused significantly higher arousal of emotion than neutral pictures (5.89 vs. 3.43, $p < 0.01$; 5.84 versus 3.43, $p < 0.01$). The valence extremity and the arousal level were matched across positive and negative pictures. The rating scores of pictures were from a body of Chinese university students who had similar backgrounds with participants of the current study. Subjects' eyes were 1 m away from the screen. The height of the pictures was 8.0 cm and length was 10.6 cm. The visual angle of the pictures was 6.07° × 4.58°.

Prior to the experiment, subjects were asked to complete the STAI again. The trait-anxiety scores of the HTA and LTA groups were 53.4 and 29.4, respectively. There was no significant difference in trait-anxiety level between the two tests. The experimental paradigm was the oddball task with three types of stimuli, of which, 75% were standard stimuli; 12.5%, target stimuli; and 12.5% novel stimuli. The entire experiment consisted of 6 blocks including 240 standard stimuli, 30 target stimuli, and 30 novel stimuli (10 pieces of positive, neutral, and negative pictures each) in each block. The trials were presented in a random order within each block. Among them, the target stimuli and standard stimuli were geometric figures with subtle differences in size, and each novel stimulus was only presented once during the entire experiment. Standard stimuli were presented for 500 ms, the target and the novel stimuli were presented for 750 ms at the center of the screen. The interval between them randomly ranged from 900 to 1000 ms. Subjects were required to focus on the subtle size difference between the standard and target stimuli and press the space bar immediately after seeing the target stimuli. The response hands and the order of blocks were counterbalanced between subjects. There was a short break between each block. We instructed the subjects to concentrate on the discrimination task and try their best to inhibit the influence of novel stimuli.

The electroencephalogram (EEG) was recorded during the task. Each participant's data were aggregated based on the type of novel stimuli (positive, neutral, or negative). Thus, three kinds of averages were generated from each participant. We measured the baseline-peak amplitudes and the peak latencies of N1 (time window: 90–150 ms), P2 (time window: 150–200 ms), N2 (time window: 200–280 ms), and P3 component (time window: 280–430 ms). A repeated-measure ANOVA was used with anxiety level (high/low), emotion property (positive/neutral/negative), laterality (left/right/midline), and anteriority (frontal/fronto-central/central/centro-parietal) as statistical factors. The Greenhouse—Geisser epsilon correction was applied to adjust the degrees of freedom of the F-ratios when necessary.

The analysis on the reaction time was conducted on the trials with correct responses. The reaction time of the HTA group and the LTA group was 527.37 ± 39.13 ms and 534.55 ± 42.89 ms, respectively. The difference between the groups was not significant (t = 7.17, $p > 0.05$). The mean response accuracies of both groups were about 70%. We compared the ERP data induced by negative and positive pictures, with the neutral condition as the control group. Three types of emotional pictures all evoked N1, P2, N2, and P3 components in the scalp.

The only significant effect of the N1 amplitude was found on the anteriority factor ($F (3, 78) = 58.48$, $p < 0.01$). N1 amplitudes were relatively higher in the anterior scalp. ANOVA conducted on P2 amplitudes revealed significant main effects of the emotion property factor ($F (2, 52) = 16.44$, $p < 0.01$).

P2 amplitudes evoked by negative pictures were relatively lower than those evoked by other types of stimuli. P2 latencies also showed main effects for emotion property ($F (2, 52) = 7.83$, $p < 0.01$). Negative stimuli elicited relatively shorter P2 latencies. With respect to N2 amplitudes, the main effect for emotion property was significant ($F (2, 52) = 23.72$, $p < 0.01$). N2 amplitudes were highest when induced by negative pictures, and those induced by neutral pictures were the lowest. N2 amplitudes were also found to peak over the midline of the scalp, and the amplitudes over the right hemisphere were greater than those over the left hemisphere ($F (2, 52) = 14.39$, $p < 0.01$). The anxiety level significantly affected N2 latencies ($F (1, 26) = 5.07$, $p < 0.05$), which was shorter in HTA individuals. There was a main effect of N2 latencies for emotion property as well ($F (2, 52) = 5.59$, $p < 0.01$). N2 latencies were the shortest under the negative condition and longest under the neutral condition.

A significant main effect of P3 amplitudes was observed on emotion property ($F (2, 52) = 20.08$, $p < 0.01$). P3 amplitudes were the largest under the neutral condition and smallest under the negative condition. Laterality of P3 amplitudes was similar to the results of the N2 component, which revealed that P3 amplitudes were largest over the midline of the scalp, and the right hemispheric amplitudes were larger than the left hemispheric amplitudes ($F (2, 52) = 11.80$, $p < 0.01$). There were significant interactions between the anxiety level and the emotion property ($F (2, 52) = 10.31$, $p < 0.01$). Further, simple effect analysis showed that there was a difference in P3 amplitudes between the HTA group and the LTA group. P3 amplitudes induced by positive stimuli in the HTA group were significantly smaller than those in the LTA group. Another interaction effect of P3 amplitude was between the laterality and the anteriority factor ($F (6, 156) = 26.70$, $p < 0.01$). P3 amplitudes peaked at CPz site. In conclusion, the arrangement rules of the P3 component elicited by the three types of pictures were different between the HTA and LTA groups. The difference between the groups largely embodied the differentiation of P3 amplitudes evoked by positive stimuli.

In this study, we found that in both groups, the P3 amplitude induced by negative pictures was smaller than that induced by neutral pictures. This result implies that subjects inhibited the influence of negative stimuli. In the LTA group, the P3 amplitude showed no significant difference between the positive and the neutral conditions, while the P3 amplitude induced by positive pictures in the HTA group was smaller than that induced by neutral pictures.

These results indicate that high-anxiety individuals use the same inhibition strategy towards positive and negative pictures. In other words, they show a tendency of excessive inhibition regardless of the emotional valences of the stimuli.

Some researchers emphasize the importance of endogenous components, such as N2-P3-P4, in the studies on inhibition function (Ilan & Polich, 1999). The P3 component is considered to be the index of inhibition to task-irrelevant information. Falkenstein, Hoormann, & Hohnsbein (1999) proposed that P3 marks the completion of the entire inhibition process. Moser et al. (2006) found that the LPP amplitude was significantly decreased when subjects were required to actively inhibit the influence of negative pictures. Fallgatter, Bartsch, & Herrmann (2002) also suggested that P3 may associate with high-load inhibition.

This study used an improved oddball paradigm, in which subjects would more likely pay attention to novel stimuli that interfered with the discrimination of standard and target stimuli. Subjects have to actively inhibit the interference in order to successfully complete the discrimination tasks. This anti-interference effort was manifested by significantly decreased P3 amplitudes in both high-anxiety and low-anxiety individuals under the negative condition compared to those under the neutral condition. The major difference between those two groups was that they showed different degrees of inhibition to positive information. Compared to the neutral condition, P3 amplitudes elicited by positive pictures were decreased in high-anxiety individuals, while there was no significant difference among the low-anxiety individuals. The results indicate that low-anxiety individuals selectively inhibit negative stimuli but do not make much effort to inhibit the positive stimuli since they are not so intrusive. In contrast, high-anxiety individuals feel that positive stimuli are very disturbing also, so they treat the two types of stimuli in the same way and show an over-inhibited tendency. Behavior inhibition model postulated by McNaughton & Gray (2000) suggests that BAS would be activated when one perceives some reward or beneficial information, while BIS would be activated when people meet conflicting stimuli (including non-reward stimuli, punishment stimuli, and novel stimuli which are irrelevant to the ongoing task). The activation of BIS would increase the level of response inhibition as well as enhance the attentional vigilance. This study provides evidences of the abnormal activation of BIS in high-anxiety individuals.

Many previous studies (Derakshan et al., 2009; Mogg & Bradley, 1998; Mogg et al., 1993) indicate that high-anxiety individuals may find it harder than low-anxiety individuals to inhibit the processing of emotional stimuli, especially threatening contents. However, high-anxiety participants in this study did not show differences in P3 amplitudes, unlike low-anxiety participants, when they were shown the negative pictures. One possible reason is that the high-anxiety people might try it harder to resist the interference from emotional stimuli because of their inhibition tendency. That may compensate their deficiency in inhibition function to some extent. The reaction time didn't show any significant difference between the high and low-anxiety groups, which could result from the same compensation effect. We suspect that when the task is not too difficult, high-anxiety people, to some degree, can balance the stimulus driven attentional system and the top-down, goal-driven attentional system (Critchley, Mathias, & Dolan, 2001; Eysenck, Derakshan, Santos, & Calvo, 2007). These efforts may help them resist the disruption of task-irrelevant negative stimuli. Meanwhile, the inhibition tendency might result in excessive inhibition of positive stimuli, which is evidenced in this study. This suggestion is speculative and should await future investigations.

In this study, the inhibition function localized by source analysis reveal that most of the P3 variations were attributed to the activation of the right centro-posterior cingulate cortex (PCC). As proposed by McNaughton (1997, 2006), anxiety might result from hyper-activity of the septohippocampal system which includes hippocampus, entorhinal cortex and PCC. The PCC contributes to a dynamic re-mapping of the physical state of the organism in response to current behavioral and environmental contexts (Critchley et al., 2001). In Li et al.'s study (2005), abstinent cocaine users showed an inverse correlation between the craving rating and the activity in the right PCC when they were presented stressful images. The results indicate that the PCC might exert a regulatory role in inhibiting craving responses. The PCC may be the brain region where the behavioral inhibition system executes the conflict supervision and response inhibition function.

2. Influence of anxiety on inhibition function: Decision making

In economic models, risk is defined as a cost that a decision-maker compares with the expected value so as to make a choice (Rushworth & Behrens, 2008). In the experimental psychological branch of decision-making research, the participants are often provided two options for them to choose. Between them, the option that is linked with higher level of risk is called a risky choice, while the other is called a risk-avoidant choice, or 'safe' choice (i.e. Goyer, Woldorff, & Huettel, 2008). Risk-avoidance tendency, therefore, refers to the preference of consistently picking the risk-avoidant option. Higher levels of trait anxiety are positively correlated with risk-avoidance in decision-making studies. That is, high-anxiety people are more prone to avoid risky choices when finishing decision-making tasks, compared to low-anxiety people (Eisenberg, Baron, & Seligman, 1998; Maner et al., 2007; Maner & Schmidt, 2006; Miu, Heilman, & Houser, 2008; Shepperd, Grace, Cole, & Klein, 2005; Wray & Stone, 2005). The reason for this phenomenon is still under debate.

The abnormality of inhibition function is suggested to be linked with higher levels of anxiety. Nigg (2000, 2001) distinguishes between two kinds of inhibition function: behavioral inhibition and motivational inhibition. The first type is related to response inhibition, while the second type is related to personality traits such as anxiety levels. High-anxiety subjects find it harder to inhibit the recall of threatening memory, compared to non-threatening information (Reidy & Richards, 1997). In addition, high-anxiety people are more likely to overreact to negative stimuli, indicating the dysfunction of inhibition control (Etkin, Klemenhagen, & Dudmen, 2004; Li, Wang, Poltakoff, & Luo, 2007). Bar-Haim, Lamy, & Glickman (2005) point out that the attentional bias (paying more attention to negative valence emotional stimuli) in high-anxiety participants reflects difficulty in disengaging attention from the stimuli once it has been attended, rather than speeded engagement of attention. Some researchers highlight the inability to inhibit fear-generating processing as the reason of attentional bias (Mayer & Merckelbach, 1999). Consistent with this idea, the level of trait anxiety is correlated with activation level of lateral prefrontal cortex (Bishop, 2009; Bishop, Duncan, & Lawrence, 2004), which is also linked with inhibition control (Dias, Robbins, & Roberts, 1997).

The inhibition function is suggested to play an important role in the process of decision making, since deliberate decision (the decisions marked by consideration of available behavioral choices as well as their consequences) need people to inhibit inappropriate behaviors (Sakagami, Pan, & Uttl, 2006). In agreement with this viewpoint, recent studies reveal that ADHD children's dysfunction in inhibition control might have something to do with their decision-making deficit (see Geurts, van der Oord, & Crone, 2006). Similar results have been founded in individuals with alcoholism (Noel, Bechara, Dan, Hanak, & Verbanck, 2007). Patients with lesions in the ventral lateral prefrontal cortex (VLPFC), a region that is linked with uncertain or risky decision making (Goel & Dolan, 2000; McClure, Laibson, Loewenstein, & Cohen, 2004), also show difficulties on behavioral inhibition measures (Aron, Fletcher, Bullmore, Sahakian, & Robbins, 2003), implying the potential relationship between the inhibition function and the ability of making decisions (see also Sakagami et al., 2006). In our opinion, the impact of anxiety on inhibition control might account for high-anxiety people's risk-avoidance tendency.

Below we would introduce a study that focuses on the potential influence of inhibition function on high-anxiety people's decision-making strategies. A version of Gehring & Willoughby (2002) monetary gambling task was applied while the subjects were under electroencephalogram (EEG) recording. The ERP component P3 was chosen for analysis, for its significance to ERP research on decision making (Christie & Tata, 2009; P. Li et al., 2010; Polezzi, Sartori, Rumiati, Vidotto, & Daum, 2010; Wu & Zhou, 2009). The P3 component is a centro-parietal positivity approximately 300–600 ms post-stimulus. In the area of decision-making research, enhanced P3 has been linked to motivationally salient and rewarding outcomes (Bellebaum & Daum, 2008; Hajcak, Moser, Holroyd, & Simons, 2007; Martin & Potts, 2004a). The relationship between P3 amplitude and decision-making behavior has been implicated in clinical studies, such as research on alcoholics (Maurage et al., 2007) and impulsive individuals (Martin & Potts, 2004b).

In this study, 253 undergraduate students (all Chinese) participated in a mass screening with the Chinese version of Spielberger's trait anxiety (STAI-T) inventory. This scale has demonstrated good internal consistency, as well as convergent and discriminant validity (Shek, 1993; Spielberger et al., 1983). Subsequently, students who scored high in trait anxiety (in the upper 25% of the distribution) were considered as high-trait anxiety people, while the students who scored low (in the lower 25% of the distribution) were considered as low-trait anxiety (LTA) people. From those who fit these criteria, we randomly chose 41 students and invited them to participate in the experiment. 20 of them were assigned to the high-trait anxiety (HTA) group (8 females), while 21 were assigned to the low-trait anxiety (LTA) group (10 females). An independent-samples t-test revealed that the two groups differed significantly in trait anxiety score, but not in age.

During each trial of the formal task, the subjects were asked to select one of the two alternative options. One of the option was presented as number '9' and the other was '99', indicating the amount of score that was potentially linked with the subjects' choice. After the decision was made, the result of the subject's choice was presented on the screen. There were four kinds of outcome valence: positive ('+'), negative ('-'), neutral ('0'), and ambiguous ('*'). The positive outcome indicated that the subject won as many points as he/she chose in this trial, while the negative outcome indicated the reverse. The neutral outcome meant the subject neither won nor lost. The ambiguous outcome was uninformative, of which the valence could be positive, negative or neutral. Unbeknownst to the subject, the outcomes were provided according to a pre-determined pseudorandom sequence, and all subjects received exactly 160 of each kind of outcome. At the end of the task, the subject was informed of the total score that he/she had earned. Then they were paid 60-80 Chinese Yuan for their participation (the exact number was depended on task performance).

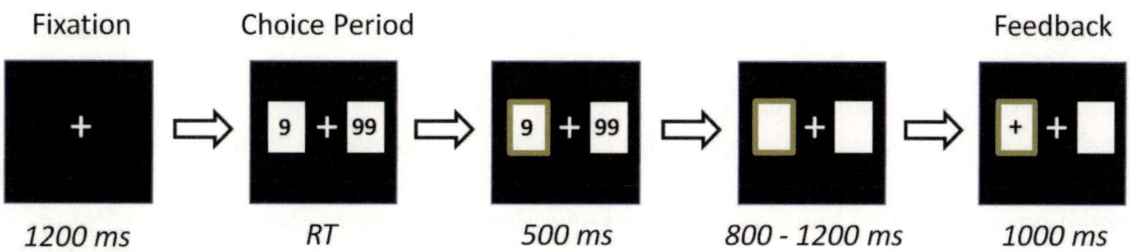

Fig. 1. The sequence of events within a single trial of the monetary gambling task, applied in the experiment.

We defined the choice of '9' to be the risk-avoidant choice (low-risk & low return) in our experiment, predicting that subjects would make this choice to avoid the possibility of a large loss ('-99'). However, by making this choice, they also gave up the opportunity to receive the larger reward ('+99'). In contrast, the choice of '99' was defined as the risky choice (high-risk & high-return). Correspondingly, the outcomes following risk-avoidant choices were defined as 'small outcomes', while the outcomes following risky choices were defined as 'large outcomes'.

For the purpose of investigating the potential influence of different kinds of outcome on ongoing decision-making, we calculated the ratio of risk-avoidant choice associated with each kind of outcome. To accomplish this, we divided the number of risk-avoidant choices following each kind of outcome by the total number of choices following the corresponding outcome. The results are described below as 'risk-avoidant ratio'. Please note that it is not necessary to calculate the 'risky ratio', since 'risky ratio' would be equal to 1 minus 'risk-avoidant ratio'.

The P3 amplitude was measured base-to-peak as the most positive value within a 300–600 ms window. The data were derived from all electrodes. However, only the electrodes at which the component reached its maximum were entered into analysis. According to the observation on scalp topography, the amplitude of P3 was maximal at centro-parietal areas of the scalp, at electrode position CPz. Accordingly, the P3 peak amplitude of electrode CPz, as well as 8 adjacent electrodes (C1, Cz, C2, CP1, CP2, P1, Pz, P2), were chosen to enter into analysis.

A repeated-measure ANOVA was used with anxiety level (high/low), outcome valence (positive/negative/neutral/ambiguous), outcome magnitude (9/99, or small/large), and electrode (9 sites) as statistical factors. The Greenhouse—Geisser epsilon correction was applied to adjust the degrees of freedom of the F-ratios when necessary. A two-tailed Pearson correlation was calculated between risk-avoidant ratios following each kind of outcome, and the P3 amplitude following the corresponding outcome. Interestingly, we found some part of the correlation results of the P3 amplitude were significant (see Table 1). When the outcome magnitude was small, the correlations between risk-avoidant ratio and P3 amplitude reached significance only when the outcome valence was neutral. In comparison, following a large outcome, the correlations between risk-avoidant ratio and P3 amplitude were significant, regardless of the outcome valence. These correlations were positive, indicating the relationship between P3 amplitude and individual difference in decision-making strategy was that the subjects, who showed larger P3 in response to larger outcomes, were more likely to be risk-avoidant (after receiving these kinds of outcomes) compared to those who showed smaller P3 responses.

In order to examine the potential effect of anxiety, the two-tailed Pearson correlation between risk-avoidant ratio and P3 amplitude was calculated in HTA group and LTA group independently. The results were also presented in Table 1. We suggest these results implied that the correlation between risk-avoidant ratio and P3 response was stronger in HTA group than in LTA group. In HTA group, when participants received a large outcome, the correlations between P3 amplitude and risk-avoidant ratio were significant regardless of the outcome valence. However in LTA group, the correlation was significant only when the outcome valence was 'ambiguous'.

	outcomes following risky choice (large outcome)			
	positive(+)	negative(-)	neutral(0)	ambiguous(*)
Total	$r = 0.460$ ($p = 0.004$)	$r = 0.447$ ($p = 0.005$)	$r = 0.482$ ($p = 0.002$)	$r = 0.568$ ($p < 0.001$)
HTA	$r = 0.695$ ($p = 0.001$)	$r = 0.516$ ($p = 0.028$)	$r = 0.628$ ($p = 0.005$)	$r = 0.709$ ($p = 0.001$)
LTA	$r = 0.271$ ($p = 0.248$)	$r = 0.419$ ($p = 0.066$)	$r = 0.383$ ($p = 0.096$)	$r = 0.462$ ($p = 0.040$)

Table 1. The two-tailed Pearson correlations between risk-avoidant ratio and the amplitude of P3 associated with different kind of outcomes, in the entire sample (first line), in HTA group (second line), and in LTA group (third line). The amplitude of P3 used to calculate correlation was the mean of the records at 9 sites (C1, Cz, C2, CP1, CPz, CP2, P1, Pz and P2). The p values are given below the corresponding correlation values. The significant results are highlighted in red.

In this study, the 'risk-avoidant ratio' and the P3 amplitude following large outcomes were positively correlated. These results indicated that the subjects, who showed larger P3 after receiving large outcomes, were more likely to make risk-avoidant choice following such outcomes. In other words, the amplitude of P3 in response to large outcomes served as an indicator of individual decision-making strategy. Presumably, the motivational significance of small outcomes is not strong enough to produce individual difference in outcome evaluation (for the relationship between the P3 amplitude and motivational significance, see Nieuwenhuis, Aston-Jones, & Cohen, 2005). Thus, most of the correlations between risk-avoidant ratio and P3 following small outcomes did not reach significance.

Our results suggest that the correlations between P3 amplitude and decision-making strategy might be mediated by individual difference in personalities. In particular, these correlations are likely to be influenced by levels of anxiety. Among the high-anxiety people, the correlation between P3 amplitude and risk-avoidant ratio was stronger. This phenomenon is linked with the opinion that there is a relationship between anxiety and risk-avoidant inclination (Eisenberg et al., 1998; Raghunathan & Pham, 1999). However, our results suggest that this relationship might be indirect, since the main effect of anxiety on behavior data or the P3 amplitude did not reach significance. Accordingly, we suggest the risk-avoidant tendency might be determined by the interaction between anxiety and other kinds of personalities (e.g., sensitivity for punishment and reward. See Franken & Muris, 2005).

Aside from anxiety, previous studies have reported that the impulsive individuals, who manifest pathological gambling behavior, show smaller P3 than control subjects (Martin & Potts, 2004a), which is consistent with the pattern of our results. Future research measuring individual differences in personality traits related to risky behavior (e.g. impulsivity and reward-seeking) will elucidate the problem (see Hsee & Hastie, 2006).

According to some researchers, the P3 amplitude is a reflection of inhibitory activity level (Sanz, Molina, Martin-Loeches, Calcedo, & Rubia, 2001). The frontal lobe is directly related to this inhibitory process, while many authors have emphasized the participation of the frontal lobe in P3 generation (Alexander, DeLong, & Strick, 1986; Savage et al., 1994). In our opinion, the relationship between the P3 component and risk-avoidant tendency in this study might imply the impact of inhibition function on decision making. That is, the P3 amplitude reflects the subject's effort to inhibit his/her desire to search for high-return benefit. It is not surprising that this relationship is more prominent in the HTA group, since high-anxiety people are more willing to avoid potential risk. Therefore, they are more likely to successfully inhibit the impulse to make a risk-seeking decision, indicated by the higher correlation between P3 amplitude and risk-avoidant ratio.

We suggest that our results provide new insight into the relationship between anxiety level, inhibition function, and decision making. High-anxiety people are more prone to make risk-avoidant choices, because the activity of inhibition control impacts their decision-making behavior more strongly, compared to low-anxiety people. To take a step further, we argue that our discovery is not limited in the area of economic decision making. Anxiety urges us to make conservative decision in the same way that it protects us from potential threats (see Maner et al., 2007).

Interestingly, the overall risk-avoidant ratio was not sensitive to the level of anxiety in this study, which might be inconsistent with the results of previous research (Eisenberg et al., 1998; Miu et al., 2008; Raghunathan & Pham, 1999; Shepperd et al., 2005). It might be worth pointing out that in previous studies, the subjects' decision-making tendencies were investigated with questionnaires, and no feedback would be expected in this kind of experiment (i.e. Eisenberg et al., 1998). In contrast, participants would immediately receive the outcome associated with their choice after a decision had been made in our task. We suggest that throughout our task, the participants always adjusted their decision-making strategies according to the outcomes they got. That is to say, the task is actually a process of probability learning for the participants. Therefore, it is not surprising that the influence of anxiety on overall behavioral performance was not significant. According to this theory, when the outcome is not available in each trial, the impact of anxiety on decision-making tendency should be stronger. This hypothesis is supported by one of our recent studies, in which the 'framing effect' paradigm was applied and no outcome was provided after the participants made their decision. In that study, we confirm that high-anxiety people chose the risk-avoidant option more often than low-anxiety people.

To sum up, in the current study, high-anxiety and low-anxiety participants did not significantly differ in their decision-making tendency. Nevertheless, anxiety impacted decision-making behavior in an indirect way. The P3 amplitude elicited by the outcome was significantly correlated with the risk-avoidant ratio, while this phenomenon was more prominent in the high-anxiety group than the low-anxiety group. In our opinion, the relationship between P3 amplitude and risk-avoidant ratio reflects the role of inhibition function in decision making. This relationship is stronger among high-anxiety people, because they are more likely to inhibit their desire to choose high-risk/high-return option. The results of this study extend our understanding about the impact of high-anxiety people's inhibition function on their behavior.

3. Conclusion

This chapter provides a review of two of our recent studies, which are interested in the relationship between anxiety and inhibition function. Although they focus on different aspects of human behavior (emotional processing and economic decision making, respectively), both of them indicate the importance of inhibition function to high-anxiety people's behavior. According to the ERP results, in the emotional processing study, low-anxiety subjects selectively inhibited the processing of negative stimuli, while high-anxiety subjects treated positive and negative stimuli equally. In the decision making study, there existed a relationship between risk-avoidant tendency and the subjects' effort to inhibit their impulse to choose high-risk/high-return option. Both findings imply that high-anxiety people might exhibit some degree of excessive inhibition (Huang et al., 2009), which is inconsistent with some previous research (i.e. Derakshan et al., 2009; Mayer & Merckelbach, 1999; Sanz et al., 2001). Further investigation would be necessary to verify whether high-anxiety people's inhibition function is hypoactive or hyperactive, compared to low-anxiety people. In our opinion, both of the hypotheses might be true. Strong anxious feeling interferes with the activity of the brain regions that are associated with the inhibition function, such as prefrontal cortex (Bishop, 2007; Bishop et al., 2004). Therefore, the high-anxiety peoples' inhibition function might act abnormally in the way that either a hypoactive or a hyperactive state would appear, depending on the circumstance. Future research on this issue will prove beneficial to both clinical and non-clinical studies.

In both of our studies, the impact of the inhibition function is indexed by the amplitude of ERP P3 component. Inspired by some previous research (i.e. Falkenstein et al., 1999; Righi, Mecacci, & Viggiano, 2009; Sanz et al., 2001), we associate P3 amplitude and the inhibition function in our research. In other studies, the P3 (including so-call 'P3a' and 'P3b') is also suggested to be linked with different types of cognitive abilities, such as working memory updating (Donchin & Coles, 1988), allocation of processing resources (Imai & Tsuji, 2004; Utku, Erzengin, Cakmak, & Karakas, 2002), perceptual awareness (Hon, Epstein, Owen, & Duncan, 2006), sensory discrimination (Molnar, 1999), revision of the mental representation (Pontifex, Hillman, & Polich, 2009), or cognitive self-evaluation (Righi et al., 2009). It would be worthwhile to see if the P3 actually reflects the activity of a fundamental cognitive component of these abilities. In addition, P3 amplitude reduction has long been associated with various kinds of problem behaviors, e.g., alcoholism (Maurage et al., 2007), drug abuse (Iacono & Mcgue, 2006), obsessive-compulsive disorder (Sanz et al., 2001), and pathological gambling (Stojanov et al., 2003). In the near future, we might see the P3 be regarded as a supplemental diagnostic indicator in the area of clinical psychology, like the case of P50 in schizophrenia (de Wilde, Bour, Dingemans, Koelman, & Linszen, 2007; Kurayama et al., 2009; Sanchez-Morla et al., 2008).

4. Acknowledgement

This work was supported by Ministry of Sci & Tech (973 Program, 2011CB711000), the National Natural Science Foundation of China (30930031, 30800298), National Key Technologies R&D Program (2009BAI77B01), Global Research Initiative Program, and United States National Institute of Health grants (1R01TW007897, P50DA05312). The authors thank the writing center in the University of Kentucky for help with language editing.

5. Reference

Alexander, G. E., DeLong, M. R., & Strick, P. L. (1986). Parallel organization of functionally segregated circuits linking basal ganglia and cortex. *Annu Rev Neurosci, 9*, 357-381.

Aron, A. R., Fletcher, P. C., Bullmore, E. T., Sahakian, B. J., & Robbins, T. W. (2003). Stop-signal inhibition disrupted by damage to right inferior frontal gyrus in humans. *Nature Neuroscience, 6*(2), 115-116.

Bai, L., Ma, H., Huang, Y. X., & Luo, Y. J. (2005). The development of native chinese affective picture system - a pretest in 46 college students. *Chinese Journal of Mental Health, 19*, 719–722.

Bar-Haim, Y., Lamy, D., & Glickman, S. (2005). Attentional bias in anxiety: A behavioral and ERP study. *Brain and Cognition, 59*(1), 11-22.

Barkley, R. A. (1997). Behavioral inhibition, sustained attention, and executive functions: Constructing a unifying theory of ADHD. *Psychological Bulletin, 121*(1), 65-94.

Bellebaum, C., & Daum, I. (2008). Learning-related changes in reward expectancy are reflected in the feedback-related negativity. *European Journal of Neuroscience, 27*(7), 1823-1835.

Bishop, S. J. (2007). Neurocognitive mechanisms of anxiety: an integrative account. *Trends in Cognitive Sciences, 11*(7), 307-316.

Bishop, S. J. (2009). Trait anxiety and impoverished prefrontal control of attention. *Nature Neuroscience, 12*(1), 92-98.

Bishop, S. J., Duncan, J., & Lawrence, A. D. (2004). Prefrontal cortical function and anxiety: controlling attention to threat-related stimuli. *Nature Neuroscience, 7*(2), 184-188.

Christie, G. J., & Tata, M. S. (2009). Right frontal cortex generates reward-related theta-band oscillatory activity. *Neuroimage, 48*(2), 415-422.

Critchley, H. D., Mathias, C. T., & Dolan, R. J. (2001). Neuroanatomical basis for first- and second-order representations of bodily states. *Nature Neuroscience, 4*(2), 207-212.

Crowne, D. P., & Marlowe, D. (1960). A new scale of social desirability independent of psychopathology. *J Consult Psychol, 24*, 349-354.

De Martino, B., Kumaran, D., Seymour, B., & Dolan, R. J. (2006). Frames, biases, and rational decision-making in the human brain. *Science, 313*(5787), 684-687.

de Wilde, O. M., Bour, L. J., Dingemans, P. M., Koelman, J. H., & Linszen, D. H. (2007). A meta-analysis of P50 studies in patients with schizophrenia and relatives: differences in methodology between research groups. *Schizophr Res, 97*(1-3), 137-151.

Derakshan, N., Ansari, T. L., Hansard, M., Shoker, L., & Eysenck, M. W. (2009). Anxiety, Inhibition, Efficiency, and Effectiveness An Investigation Using the Antisaccade Task. *Experimental Psychology, 56*(1), 48-55.

Dias, R., Robbins, T. W., & Roberts, A. C. (1997). Dissociable forms of inhibitory control within prefrontal cortex with an analog of the Wisconsin Card Sort Test: Restriction to novel situations and independence from "on-line" processing. *Journal of Neuroscience, 17*(23), 9285-9297.

Donchin, E., & Coles, M. G. H. (1988). Is the P300 component a manifestation of context updating? . *Behavioral and Bran Sciences, 11*(3), 355-372.

Eisenberg, A. E., Baron, J., & Seligman, M. E. P. (1998). Individual difference in risk aversion and anxiety. *Psychological Bulletin, 87*, 245-251.

Enright, S. J., & Beech, A. R. (1993). Reduced cognitive inhibition in obsessive-compulsive disorder. *Br J Clin Psychol, 32 (Pt 1)*, 67-74.

Etkin, A., Klemenhagen, K., & Dudmen, J. T. (2004). Individual difference in trait anxiety predict the response of the basolateral amygdala to unconsciously processed fearful faces. *Neuron, 44*, 1043-1055.

Eysenck, M. W., Derakshan, N., Santos, R., & Calvo, M. G. (2007). Anxiety and cognitive performance: attentional control theory. *Emotion, 7*(2), 336-353.

Falkenstein, M., Hoormann, J., & Hohnsbein, J. (1999). ERP components in Go Nogo tasks and their relation to inhibition. *Acta Psychologica, 101*(2-3), 267-291.

Fallgatter, A. J., Bartsch, A. J., & Herrmann, M. J. (2002). Electrophysiological measurements of anterior cingulate function. *Journal of Neural Transmission, 109*(5-6), 977-988.

Fichtenholtz, H. M., Dean, H. L., Dillon, D. G., Yamasaki, H., McCarthy, G., & LaBar, K. S. (2004). Emotion-attention network interactions during a visual oddball task. *Cognitive Brain Research, 20*(1), 67-80.

Franken, I. H. A., & Muris, P. (2005). Individual differences in reward sensitivity are related to food craving and relative body weight in healthy women. *Appetite, 45*(2), 198-201.

Funahashi, S. (2001). Neuronal mechanisms of executive control by the prefrontal cortex. *Neurosci Res, 39*(2), 147-165.

Gehring, W. J., & Willoughby, A. R. (2002). The medial frontal cortex and the rapid processing of monetary gains and losses. *Science, 295*(5563), 2279-2282.

Geurts, H. M., van der Oord, S., & Crone, E. A. (2006). Hot and cool aspects of cognitive control in children with ADHD: decision-making and inhibition. *J Abnorm Child Psychol, 34*(6), 813-824.

Goel, V., & Dolan, R. J. (2000). Anatomical segregation of component processes in an inductive inference task. *Journal of Cognitive Neuroscience, 12*(1), 110-119.

Goyer, J. P., Woldorff, M. G., & Huettel, S. A. (2008). Rapid Electrophysiological Brain Responses are Influenced by Both Valence and Magnitude of Monetary Rewards. *Journal of Cognitive Neuroscience, 20*(11), 2058-2069.

Hajcak, G., Moser, J. S., Holroyd, C. B., & Simons, R. F. (2007). It's worse than you thought: The feedback negativity and violations of reward prediction in gambling tasks. *Psychophysiology, 44*(6), 905-912.

Hon, N., Epstein, R. A., Owen, A. M., & Duncan, J. (2006). Frontoparietal activity with minimal decision and control. *Journal of Neuroscience, 26*(38), 9805-9809.

Hsee, C. K., & Hastie, R. (2006). Decision and experience: why don't we choose what makes us happy? *Trends in Cognitive Sciences, 10*(1), 31-37.

Huang, Y. X., Bai, L., Ai, H., Li, W., Yua, C., Liu, J., et al. (2009). Influence of trait-anxiety on inhibition function: Evidence from ERPs study. *Neuroscience Letters, 456*(1), 1-5.

Iacono, W. G., & Mcgue, M. (2006). Association between P3 event-related brain potential amplitude and adolescent problem behavior. *Psychophysiology, 43*(5), 465-469.

Ilan, A. B., & Polich, J. (1999). P300 and response time from a manual Stroop task. *Clinical Neurophysiology, 110*(2), 367-373.

Imai, A., & Tsuji, K. (2004). Event-related potential correlates of judgment categories and detection sensitivity in a visual detection task. *Vision Research, 44*(8), 763-773.

Kurayama, T., Nakazawa, K., Matsuzawa, D., Yoshida, S., Nanbu, M., Suto, C., et al. (2009). Alterations of Auditory P50 Suppression in Human Fear Conditioning and Extinction. *Biological Psychiatry, 65*(6), 495-502.

Li, C. S. R., Kosten, T. R., & Sinha, R. (2005). Sex differences in brain activation during stress imagery in abstinent cocaine users: A functional magnetic resonance imaging study. *Biological Psychiatry, 57*(5), 487-494.

Li, P., Jia, S. W., Feng, T. Y., Liu, Q. A., Suo, T., & Li, H. (2010). The influence of the diffusion of responsibility effect on outcome evaluations: Electrophysiological evidence from an ERP study. *Neuroimage, 52*(4), 1727-1733.

Li, X. Y., Wang, M., Poltakoff, E., & Luo, Y. J. (2007). Attention to threat in high and low trait-anxious individuals: A study using extremely threatening pictorial cues. *Perceptual and Motor Skills, 104*(3), 1097-1106.

Livesley, W. J., Jang, K. L., & Vernon, P. A. (1998). Phenotypic and genetic structure of traits delineating personality disorder. *Archives of General Psychiatry, 55*(10), 941-948.

Lust, S. A., & Bartholow, B. D. (2009). Self-reported and P3 event-related potential evaluations of condoms: Does what we say match how we feel? *Psychophysiology, 46*(2), 420-424.

Maner, J. K., Richey, J. A., Cromer, K., Mallott, M., Lejuez, C. W., Joiner, T. E., et al. (2007). Dispositional anxiety and risk-avoidant decision-making. *Personality and Individual Differences, 42*(4), 665-675.

Maner, J. K., & Schmidt, N. B. (2006). The role of risk avoidance in anxiety. *Behavior Therapy, 37*(2), 181-189.

Martin, L. E., & Potts, G. F. (2004a). Impulsivity and decision-making: An event related potential investigation. *Psychophysiology, 41*, S66-S66.

Martin, L. E., & Potts, G. F. (2004b). Reward sensitivity in impulsivity. *Neuroreport, 15*(9), 1519-1522.

Maurage, P., Philippot, P., Verbanck, P., Noel, X., Kornreich, C., Hanak, C., et al. (2007). Is the P300 deficit in alcoholism associated with early visual impairments (P100, N170)? An oddball paradigm. *Clinical Neurophysiology, 118*(3), 633-644.

Mayer, B., & Merckelbach, H. (1999). Unconscious processes, subliminal stimulation, and anxiety. *Clin Psychol Rev, 19*(5), 571-590.

McClure, S. M., Laibson, D. I., Loewenstein, G., & Cohen, J. D. (2004). Separate neural systems value immediate and delayed monetary rewards. *Science, 306*(5695), 503-507.

McNaughton, N. (1997). Cognitive dysfunction resulting from hippocampal hyperactivity--a possible cause of anxiety disorder? *Pharmacol Biochem Behav, 56*(4), 603-611.

McNaughton, N. (2006). The role of the subiculum within the behavioural inhibition system. *Behav Brain Res, 174*(2), 232-250.

McNaughton, N., & Gray, J. A. (2000). Anxiolytic action on the behavioural inhibition system implies multiple types of arousal contribute to anxiety. *Journal of Affective Disorders, 61*(3), 161-176.

Miu, A. C., Heilman, R. M., & Houser, D. (2008). Anxiety impairs decision-making: Psychophysiological evidence from an Iowa Gambling Task. *Biological Psychology, 77*(3), 353-358.

Mogg, K., & Bradley, B. P. (1998). A cognitive-motivational analysis of anxiety. *Behav Res Ther, 36*(9), 809-848.

Mogg, K., Bradley, B. P., Williams, R., & Mathews, A. (1993). Subliminal processing of emotional information in anxiety and depression. *J Abnorm Psychol, 102*(2), 304-311.

Molnar, M. (1999). The dimensional complexity of the P3 event-related potential: area-specific and task-dependent features. *Clinical Neurophysiology, 110*(1), 31-38.

Moser, J. S., Hajcak, G., Bukay, E., & Simons, R. F. (2006). Intentional modulation of emotional responding to unpleasant pictures: An ERP study. *Psychophysiology, 43*(3), 292-296.

Nieuwenhuis, S., Aston-Jones, G., & Cohen, J. D. (2005). Decision making, the p3, and the locus coeruleus-norepinephrine system. *Psychological Bulletin, 131*(4), 510-532.

Nigg, J. T. (2000). On inhibition/disinhibition in developmental psychopathology: views from cognitive and personality psychology and a working inhibition taxonomy. *Psychol Bull, 126*(2), 220-246.

Nigg, J. T. (2001). Is ADHD a disinhibitory disorder? *Psychological Bulletin, 127*(5), 571-598.

Noel, X., Bechara, A., Dan, B., Hanak, C., & Verbanck, P. (2007). Response inhibition deficit is involved in poor decision making under risk in nonamnesic individuals with alcoholism. *Neuropsychology, 21*(6), 778-786.

Polezzi, D., Sartori, G., Rumiati, R., Vidotto, G., & Daum, I. (2010). Brain correlates of risky decision-making. *Neuroimage, 49*(2), 1886-1894.

Pontifex, M. B., Hillman, C. H., & Polich, J. (2009). Age, physical fitness, and attention: P3a and P3b. *Psychophysiology, 46*(2), 379-387.

Raghunathan, R., & Pham, M. T. (1999). All Negative Moods Are Not Equal: Motivational Influences of Anxiety and Sadness on Decision Making. *Organizational Behavior and Human Decision Processes, 79*(1), 56-77.

Reidy, J., & Richards, A. (1997). Anxiety and memory: a recall bias for threatening words in high anxiety. *Behav Res Ther, 35*(6), 531-542.

Righi, S., Mecacci, L., & Viggiano, M. P. (2009). Anxiety, cognitive self-evaluation and performance: ERP correlates. *Journal of Anxiety Disorders, 23*(8), 1132-1138.

Roiser, J. P., de Martino, B., Tan, G. C. Y., Kumaran, D., Seymour, B., Wood, N. W., et al. (2009). A Genetically Mediated Bias in Decision Making Driven by Failure of Amygdala Control. *Journal of Neuroscience, 29*(18), 5985-5991.

Rushworth, M. F. S., & Behrens, T. E. J. (2008). Choice, uncertainty and value in prefrontal and cingulate cortex. *Nature Neuroscience, 11*(4), 389-397.

Sakagami, M., Pan, X. C., & Uttl, B. (2006). Behavioral inhibition and prefrontal cortex in decision-making. *Neural Networks, 19*(8), 1255-1265.

Sanchez-Morla, E. M., Garcia-Jimenez, M. A., Barabash, A., Martinez-Vizcaino, V., Mena, J., Cabranes-Diaz, J. A., et al. (2008). P50 sensory gating deficit is a common marker of vulnerability to bipolar disorder and schizophrenia. *Acta Psychiatr Scand, 117*(4), 313-318.

Sanz, M., Molina, V., Martin-Loeches, M., Calcedo, A., & Rubia, F. J. (2001). Auditory P300 event related potential acid serotonin reuptake inhibitor treatment in obsessive-compulsive disorder patients. *Psychiatry Research, 101*(1), 75-81.

Savage, C. R., Weilburg, J. B., Duffy, F. H., Baer, L., Shera, D. M., & Jenike, M. A. (1994). Low-level sensory processing in obsessive-compulsive disorder: an evoked potential study. *Biol Psychiatry, 35*(4), 247-252.

Shek, D. T. (1993). The Chinese version of the State-Trait Anxiety Inventory: its relationship to different measures of psychological well-being. *J Clin Psychol, 49*(3), 349-358.

Shepperd, J. A., Grace, J., Cole, L. J., & Klein, C. (2005). Anxiety and outcome predictions. *Personality and Social Psychology Bulletin, 31*(2), 267-275.

Spielberger, C. D., Gorsuch, R. L., Lushene, R., Vagg, P. R., & Jacobs, G. A. (1983). Manual for the state-trait anxiety inventory. *Palo Alto, CA: Consulting Psychologist Press.*

Stojanov, W., Karayanidis, F., Johnston, P., Bailey, A., Carr, V., & Schall, U. (2003). Disrupted sensory gating in pathological gambling. *Biological Psychiatry, 54*(4), 474-484.

Utku, H., Erzengin, O. U., Cakmak, E. D., & Karakas, S. (2002). Discrimination of brain's neuroelectric responses by a decision-making function. *J Neurosci Methods, 114*(1), 25-31.

Wang, X. D., Wang, X. L., & Ma, H. (1999). *Rating Scales for Mental Health.* Beijing: Chinese Mental HealthPress.

Wray, L. D., & Stone, E. R. (2005). The role of self-esteem and anxiety in decision making for self versus others in relationships. *Journal of Behavioral Decision Making, 18*(2), 125-144.

Wu, Y., & Zhou, X. L. (2009). The P300 and reward valence, magnitude, and expectancy in outcome evaluation. *Brain Research, 1286*, 114-122.

Yamasaki, H., LaBar, K. S., & McCarthy, G. (2002). Dissociable prefrontal brain systems for attention and emotion. *Proc Natl Acad Sci U S A, 99*(17), 11447-11451.

Yee, P. L., & Vaughan, J. (1996). Intergrating cognitive, personality, and social approaches to cognitive interference and distractibility. In G. R. Pierce, B. R. Sarason & I. G. Sarason (Eds.), *Cognitive Interference: Theories, Methods, and Findings* (pp. 77-98). Mahwah, NJ: Lawrence Erlbaum Associates.

Zheng, X. H., Shu, L., Zhang, A. L., Huang, G. L., Zhao, J. F., Sun, M., et al. (1993). Test of State-Trait Anxiety Inventory in Changchun. *Chinese Journal of Mental Health, 7*(2), 60-62.

7

Zebrafish, a Potential Novel Research Tool for the Analysis and Modeling of Anxiety

Robert Gerlai
University of Toronto Mississauga
Canada

1. Introduction

Although numerous medications have been developed for anxiety disorders and related neuropsychiatric conditions including phobias, these diseases still represent a large unmet medical need. This may be because despite the concerted research and drug development efforts by pharmaceutical research companies and academic laboratories alike, the mechanisms of these disorders still remain to be fully elucidated. Animal models have been proposed to accelerate research in this area. The current chapter focuses on a somewhat novel and underutilized laboratory organism, the zebrafish, which may have great utility in anxiety research.

Zebrafish have been successfully utilized in developmental biology, a discipline that often employs molecular biology and genetic methods. As a result of the past three decades of intensive investigation with zebrafish, this species has become one of the favourite model organisms of geneticists. The accumulated genetic knowledge about, and the genetic methods specifically developed for the zebrafish now make this species particularly attractive for several research fields other than developmental biology. One of these fields is behavioural neuroscience. Indeed, the number of zebrafish publications in the latter field has started to exponentially increase. This may be because zebrafish strikes an optimal compromise between system complexity and practical simplicity. On the one hand it is a complex organism with brain anatomy, neurophysiology, and molecular characteristics (e.g. nucleotide sequence of its genes) highly similar to those of other vertebrates including mammals. On the other hand, it is small, easy and cheap to maintain in the laboratory and has been highly amenable to high-throughput screening (e.g. forward genetic or drug screens). The latter is particularly noteworthy for the purposes of unravelling of the genetic (and in general the biological) mechanisms of complex brain functions and the disorders of these functions. High-throughput screens may have the ability to identify a good proportion of the potentially large number of molecular players involved in these functions.

The chapter discusses how the zebrafish may be utilized in the modeling of human anxiety disorders and in the analysis of the mechanisms of these disorders. Admittedly, the zebrafish is rather novel in this research and does not have a proven track record. The chapter is focussed on behavioural test paradigms that may have the capacity to induce anxiety related behavioural responses. The chapter argues that the foundation of research into the mechanisms of anxiety disorders is such behavioural paradigms as they will allow the quantification of functional changes in the brain induced by mutations or drugs and thus will facilitate the discovery of underlying mechanisms and drug targets. The chapter also argues that the most successful behavioural test paradigms will be those that represent ethological validity, i.e. consider the species-specific characteristics and the ecology and evolutionary history of the zebrafish. The chapter reviews several such recently developed test paradigms and presents data, for example, on the behavioural effects of the natural and synthetic alarm substances, a chemical that is released from the skin of injured fish, as well as on other test methods that utilize visual stimuli, including computer animated (moving) images of sympatric predators of zebrafish. The chapter also provides a detailed description of the behavioural responses these stimuli induce and makes recommendations for further development of these methods and how they may be employed in forward genetic screening for mutations involved in anxiety related phenotypes. The chapter concludes that, although the zebrafish is rather novel in anxiety research, the increasing number of publications with this species suggests a successful future.

2. Human anxiety remains a major unmet medical need despite decades of preclinical and clinical research

First let us define some basic terms. I use "fear" to describe the behaviour or internal state of the subject (human or non-human animal) that is elicited by aversive stimuli that can potentially harm the subject and/or signal such harm or forms of danger. For the sake of simplicity, I define anxiety as an abnormally prolonged, exaggerated, or misdirected form of fear. Please note that these definitions do not assume the presence or the absence of consciousness, awareness, or understanding of fear or of the stimuli that induce it and thus are employed equally to human and non-human animals.

Human anxiety is one of the most prevalent neuropsychiatric conditions. Approximately 5% of people living in westernized countries will suffer from general anxiety disorder during their life time and, for example, just in the United States as many as 10 million patients suffer from this disease at any given time point (Weisberg, 2009). The numbers are likely larger for other parts of the world and certainly even more staggering if one considers other types of anxiety disorders such as panic disorders, post-traumatic stress disorders (PTSD), phobias, or less severe forms of anxiety (Garakani et al., 2006; Choy et al., 2007; Klein, 1996). Despite decades of research, the quality of life of individuals suffering from anxiety related disorders is still significantly reduced even in patients with mild forms of the disease (for a review see Mendlowicz & Stein, 2000) because the treatment options, including pharmacological approaches, have been limited, variable or ineffective.

Most agree that the key to the development of appropriate treatment methods is the understanding of the mechanisms of the disease. Unfortunately, the mechanisms of anxiety related disorders have not been fully understood (Matthew et al., 2008). This is not to say that we do not know anything. Clearly a lot of knowledge has been accumulated already. For example, neuroanatomical and neuroimaging studies have confirmed that the amygdala and its reciprocal connections with the prefrontal cortex play a central role (for review see Matthew et al., 2008) but other brain regions, e.g. the periaqueductal gray (Misslin, 2003; Takahashi et al., 2008), have also been implicated in fear responses and anxiety related abnormalities. Progress has been made at levels of investigation other than neuroanatomy too. Numerous neurotransmitter systems, neurochemicals and hormones have been shown to be significantly altered in anxiety disorders (for review see Matthew et al., 2008). For example, the concentration of Corticotropin-Releasing Factor (CRF) has been shown to be elevated in some anxiety disorders, pharmacological blockade of glucocorticoids and noradrenaline has been proposed for trauma-related anxiety, and the glutamatergic system has been implicated in other forms of anxiety (for review see Matthew et al., 2008). The role the serotoninergic system may play in anxiety disorders has also been extensively studied (e.g. Leonardo & Hen, 2006). The involvement of neuropeptides substance P, neuropeptide Y, oxytocin, orexin, and galanin have also been demonstrated in anxiety (e.g. Matthew et al., 2008). While many of the above mechanisms represent potentially good pharmacological targets allowing the eventual development of drug therapies, the complexity of these disorders and the limited understanding of the mechanisms behind them warrants further detailed inquiries into the neurobiology of the disease.

3. Laboratory animals: Efficient tools of discovery

Numerous human neuropsychiatric disorder have been successfully modelled or some of the mechanisms underlying these diseases investigated using laboratory animals (Flint & Shifman, 2008). Anxiety disorders are no exception to this (see e.g. Hohoff, 2009). This is not surprising given that at every level of biological organization, i.e. from behavioural traits to the nucleotide sequence of genes, evolutionary conservation of features has been repeatedly demonstrated. This is of course not to say that there are no species specific characteristics. But if one is interested in the fundamentally important questions, evolutionary conservation allows the experimenter to efficiently utilize model organisms especially if the laboratory species is closely related to human. Most anxiety related studies have been conducted with rats, a mammalian species that shows high DNA nucleotide sequence homologies to human. The interest in this species therefore is not surprising. For example, a medline (PubMed) literature search with keywords "anxiety" and "rat" returns close to 8 thousand publications. Another model organism, the house mouse, which is perhaps even more frequently used in biomedical research, is also well utilized in anxiety research. A medline search with this species also reveals close to 5 thousand published studies. In addition to the rodents utilized in the laboratory, other model organisms, including the dog (almost 5 hundred publications) or non-human primates (62 publications) have also been employed in the analysis of anxiety. Even such evolutionarily distant species to us as the fruit fly (Drosophila melanogaster) has been proposed as a research tool for the understanding of the mechanisms of human anxiety (Iliadi, 2009). The rich literature on anxiety research clearly demonstrates the major effort to utilize model organisms for the analysis and/or modeling of human anxiety.

There are two principal reasons why one would like to use model organisms for the analysis of human disorders. First, is a practical consideration: laboratory organisms represent a compromise. These species can be kept and analyzed more cheaply than humans and they face fewer ethical roadblocks. Second, as argued above the evolutionary relatedness of laboratory organisms to us means that there may be numerous functional, e.g., neurobiological, physiological, biochemical and genetic homologies that the researcher can utilize in her/his quest for the understanding of the mechanisms of human anxiety (for examples see review by Denver (2009).

4. Naturalistic (ethological) approaches should be employed when the question concerns the biological mechanisms of behaviour

Many successful lines of investigation into the mechanisms of a broad range of behaviours have (e.g. Gerlai et al., 1999; Lu et al., 1997; Grant et al., 1992; Silva et al., 1992) utilized behavioural, electrophysiological, neuroanatomical and molecular genetics methods to investigate the mechanisms of brain function and how such mechanisms lead to the behavioral output. But when it comes to the method or approach of behavioural experimentation some controversies may need to be cleared. There may be many ways one can study animal and human behaviour. In the past and especially in North America classical psychologists argued that one has to be nature blind and ignore the unique species specific features of different organisms. This is the only way, went the argument, one could study the common, and thus most important, features of the phenomenon under investigation. This tenet led to an important controversy as to how to measure behaviour (Gerlai, 2001). It has been pointed out that, while not necessarily mutually exclusive, two fundamentally distinct approaches emerged, classical psychology and ethology. The classical psychology approach has emphasized the analysis of species invariant features that cut across multiple species, i.e. allow generalization of findings. The argument was that analysis of species independent features is expected to lead to easier translation from animal to human. On the other hand, the ethological approach has put more weight on naturalistic studies sensitive to species-specific features and the evolutionary and ecological relevance of the methods employed. Many, including I too, have argued that the ethological approach is more appropriate especially when one is interested in the question of biological mechanisms of behaviour (Crusio & Abeelen, 1986; Csányi & Gerlai, 1988; Gerlai & Clayton, 1999; Blanchard et al., 2003). There are two main reasons why this argument is made. One, alleles of genes that influence any trait under investigation have been selected by natural selection and the influence they exert on the phenotype is the result of evolution, the phylogenetic argument (Crusio, 1995). Two, analysis of the mechanisms underlying the phenotypical characteristics can only be conducted appropriately if the characteristics are not artificial constructs but are defined in a biologically meaningful manner. Although the question of what is biologically meaningful is not always easy to answer, in case of behaviour, the above argument translates to choosing methods that allow the quantification of natural, species-specific, responses that are the product of the studied organism and not of the experimenter's subjective bias, the phenogenetic argument (Crusio, 1995). Briefly, one needs to design his/her experiments according to the natural behaviour of the studied species. Notably, results of nature-blind experiments may not be easier to generalize to the human clinic. As I put it previously, "offering a sizeable financial reward to a rat and giving tasty rat chow to humans might not represent 'rigorous laboratory control' of motivation: ignoring species-specific characteristics can lead to less obvious, but similar, mistakes in behavioural research" (Gerlai & Clayton, 1999b).

5. Antipredatory behaviour: An ethologically relevant method to study anxiety

Naturalistic approaches thus may have an important place in research whose ultimate goal is to understand the biological mechanisms of abnormal fear responses in vertebrates including our own species (for discussion specific to fear/anxiety see Lister, 1990; Blanchard et al., 2003; Rosen et al., 2008; Gerlai et al., 2009). But behavioral analysis is often deceptively simple (Gerlai, 2001) and this is especially true for anxiety paradigms (Bouwknecht & Paylor, 2008). It is therefore important to consider what approach, behavioral method, has the highest possibility for success. Classical laboratory rodents including the rat and the mouse have been successfully employed in anxiety research using antipredatory paradigms (e.g. Hendrie et al., 1996). In these tests the subject is exposed to stimuli specific to its natural predator, and the species-typical antipredatory responses of the subject (e.g. freezing) are quantified. Rosen et al. (2008), for example, use trimethylthiazoline, a chemical that is present in the fox's urine and is known to be effective for rodents. Barros et al. (2008), who studied the marmoset, used a cat (a taxidermied wild oncilla cat, the natural predator of the marmoset) as a predator stimulus. Apfelbach et al. (2005) review a large variety of predator odors and their fear inducing effects in different prey species, including cat odor induced antipredatory responses in the rat. Others have utilized eye spots or eye like structures placed on objects mimicking the appearance of predators, an approach that has been effective in a variety of species including rodents, birds and fish (e.g. Gerlai et al., 2000; Miklosi et al., 1997 and references therein). The argument for using ethologically relevant stimuli and measuring species-specific responses in laboratory model organisms is principally based upon the notion that human anxiety disorders are likely to develop as a result of abnormal functioning of neurobiological mechanisms (brain areas, circuits and/or molecular mechanisms) that have evolved to subserve avoidance of predators or other harmful or dangerous agents in nature during our evolutionary past. Given that our species shares its evolutionary past with those of others this approach may have translational relevance. For example, Denver (2009) reviews the structural and functional evolution of vertebrate neuroendocrine stress systems and explains that "Recent findings suggest that the proteins, gene structures, and signaling pathways of the HPA [hypothalamus-pituitary-adrenal] axis were present in the earliest vertebrates and have been maintained by natural selection owing to their critical adaptive roles". This author also concludes that numerous neurotransmitters and neuromodulators influencing stress-related behaviors, such as anxiety and fear, are evolutionarily conserved. Others also argue that the basic neuronal mechanisms are shared across mammalian species, and, for example, the same set of genes may regulate critical aspects of anxiety in humans and in lower species (e.g. Hovatta and Barlow, 2008). Briefly, the translational relevance of fear/anxiety paradigms is expected to be high as long as the mechanisms that evolved in the brain to subserve these behaviors are properly engaged by the experimental set up.

6. Zebrafish in the analysis of fear and anxiety

As outlined above there have been a large number of studies devoted to the analysis of the biological mechanisms of anxiety and a considerable amount of effort has been invested in the development of pharmacological treatments of anxiety related disorders For preclinical research most of these studies used rodents. As we have accumulated a large amount of data on these rodent species, it may be logical to think that building upon this excellent foundation may be the only way to proceed. In the subsequent pages, however, I will try to persuade the reader that although abandonment of rodent research is certainly not to be recommended, utilization of another vertebrate, the zebrafish may be a good idea.

6.1 Practical simplicity meets system complexity: zebrafish as an optimal compromise for research

A commonplace in research known to many scientists is shown by the following equation: C = E x T, where E is a measure of the ease of use of a research species in the laboratory, T is the translational relevance of this species, and C is a constant. In other words, the more translationally relevant a species is for human, the less easy it is to use in the lab, and vica versa. Importantly, however, C, as defined above, may not be a universal constant: for some species C may be higher than for others. I argue that zebrafish represents an optimal compromise between practical simplicity and system complexity, i.e. its C is large. It is a small (4 cm long) freshwater fish which is easy to maintain and breed in the laboratory. Due to its highly social nature (shoaling) and its small size, a large number of zebrafish can be housed in small fish tanks. A single female may lay 2-300 eggs at every spawning and may spawn 2-3 times a week. Briefly, a large number of experimental subjects can be obtained quickly and utilized for research in a cost effective manner. These features make the zebrafish particularly appropriate for high-throughput screening applications including forward genetic mutagenesis screens or large scale drug (pharmacological compound) screens. But there are other important features of zebrafish one needs to consider for translational research.

Notably, zebrafish possess high nucleotide sequence homology (60-80%) with that of human genes. Importantly, this sequence homology is functionally relevant as the amino acid sequence of zebrafish proteins (60-90% sequence homology) especially at the functionally relevant catalytic or ligand binding domains of the proteins (approaching 100% sequence homology), has been found highly similar between zebrafish and human (Renier et al., 2007; Reimers et al., 2004), which demonstrates evolutionary conservation of function and allows one to use this relatively distantly related species for translational research. It is notable that evolutionary conservation, i.e. functional and structural homologies, do not end at the nucleotide or amino acid sequence levels, but have been demonstrated at numerous other levels of the biological organization of zebrafish, including, for example, its neurotransmitter systems (Mueller et al., 2004; Panula et al., 2006; also see Chatterjee & Gerlai, 2009; Gerlai et al., 2009) and its neuroendocrine responses to stress (Alsop & Vijayan, 2008). Conservation of function (at the gene expression level) has been found in zebrafish even in such responses as neuro-adaptation to drugs of abuse (Kily et al., 2008). Therefore I and others (Shin & Fishman, 2002) have argued that the zebrafish is an appropriate model organism for the analysis of a range of human diseases.

6.2 Genetics: the strength of zebrafish

A strength of zebrafish as a research tool is that by now an arsenal of genetic tools have been developed for this species and the amount of information on the zebrafish genome has also become substantial. For example, a large number of genetic markers crucial for the localization and identification of randomly induced mutations have been established. These include rapid amplification of polymorphic DNA (RAPD) and amplified fragment length polymorphisms (AFLP) (Donovan et al., 2000; Guo et al., 2000; Zhang et al., 1998), polymorphic microsatellite markers and radiation hybrid maps with microsatellite markers and expressed sequence tags (ESTs) (Geisler et al., 1999) as well as single nucleotide polymorphisms (SNPs) (Stickney et al., 2002). The latter study also utilized oligonucleotide microarrays, the gene chip technology that is rapidly spreading in zebrafish research (Sipe & Saha, 2007). A viral infection-based mutagenesis technique has been established for the generation of insertional mutations that could be rapidly cloned due to the presence of the viral tag in the genome (Amsterdam et al., 1999). An entire company was formed to use this methodology and by now a large library of mutants has been generated (see e.g.

http://www.znomics.com/; also see Wang et al., 2007). A gene-breaking transposon-based method to generate mutations has also been developed for zebrafish (Sivasubbu et al., 2006). In addition to forward genetic approaches, reverse genetic methods have been implemented. Morpholino antisense knockdown allows the inactivation of known genes in embryos (Nasevicius & Ekker, 2000; also see Bill et al. 2009 for more recent review). Targeted-induced local lesions in genomes (TILLING) has been successfully adapted to zebrafish (Wienholds et al., 2002). Targeted gene disruption has also been achieved with the use of zinc-finger nucleases (Doyon et al., 2008). More recently, a Gal4/Upstream Activating Sequence approach has been employed for the flexible deployment of transgenes in the analysis of expression patterns of target genes (Scott, 2009), and a transposon-based genetic approach has been proposed for zebrafish (Ni et al., 2009). Importantly, all these tools and pieces of information are in the public domain (e.g., GenBank, Sanger Center website, and ZFIN, see Sprague et al., 2001). Briefly, the zebrafish has become one of the most preferred laboratory animal species of geneticists.

6.3 Behaviour: The weakness of zebrafish

An important drawback one has to face when using zebrafish is that the behaviour of this species is not well characterized. This is not to say that there are no behavioural studies on zebrafish or that these behavioural studies are unimportant or inappropriate. On the contrary, there is an increasing number of behavioural neuroscience studies published on zebrafish. Nevertheless, compared to classical laboratory study species such as the rat, mouse, or even the fruit fly zebrafish behavioural research is in its infancy, the number of studies, and with it the amount of information on the behaviour of this species is orders of magnitude less than what is available for classical laboratory model organisms (Sison et al., 2006). Without proper behavioural tests, and without thorough understanding of the behavioural features of zebrafish, it is not possible to utilize behavioural phenotyping of mutation or drug effects, and how these manipulations may influence brain function becomes difficult to investigate (Gerlai 2002). Briefly, behavioural analysis is s a major bottleneck in zebrafish research. A simple literature search in Medline with the keyword "behavior" and "rat" reveals over 100 thousand papers, and another with keywords "behavior" and "mouse" returns about 50 thousand papers. But even for the fruit fly one finds about 5 thousand publications in this area of investigation while for zebrafish this number is less than 100. Although this number is indeed orders of magnitude less than the above, it is notable that the majority of these zebrafish publications were published only recently demonstrating a clear upsurge of interest in this species. It appears that, behavioural brain research and behaviour genetics have discovered the utility of zebrafish. Perhaps one of the best studied of the behaviour of zebrafish is their fear responses. Below I briefly discuss what we know about zebrafish fear and its quantification with an emphasis on how screening applications may be developed and utilized.

6.4 Induction of fear in zebrafish using ecologically relevant stimuli: The effect of the natural alarm substance

Predator-prey encounters have not been documented for zebrafish in nature but numerous piscivores have been found to inhabit the slowly moving creeks and small lakes of India and Nepal where zebrafish have been found (Engeszer et al., 2007). The zebrafish belongs to the

Osterophisan superorder of fishes, and numerous species of this superorder have been demonstrated to respond to alarm substances, natural "pheromones" first described by von Frisch (1938; 1941). These substances are released from epidermal club cells of the fish upon infury of the skin (e.g. Pfeiffer, 1972). The zebrafish was known to respond to its natural alarm substance (Schutz, 1956; Pfeiffer, 1963) and later a number of other fish species were also found to exhibit such a response (for a review see Pfeiffer, 1977). The range of behavioural reactions exhibited by fish in response to the alarm substance was also described in a detailed manner (Pfeiffer, 1977) and it was concluded that these responses may significantly differ from species to species but may include "A) fish swimming excitedly with their heads against the bottom and with their bodies at an angle of about 60° to the floor; B) becoming motionless and showing no movement for several minutes; C) sinking to the bottom and spitting gas for a considerable time; D) fleeing to the surface when they are alarmed, crowding together there and swimming hastily, frequently jumping out of the water; or E) fleeing towards the depth where they form a dense school". Waldman (1982) analyzed the effect of alarm substance on shoaling as well as the position of zebrafish in the vertical column of the water and found that it induces fish staying closer to each other and closer to the bottom tank he used. Waldman also described his personal observation regarding a potential developmental trajectory of the alarm substance induced behavioural reactions and theorized that zebrafish may only start exhibiting the alarm reaction after their age of 50 days post-hatching. Pfeiffer and Waldman had no access to technologically advanced video-recording and analysis methods such as tracking systems, thus many of their observations may only be regarded as working hypotheses. By now the technology allows us to precisely track the location as well as movement pattern of fish (see e.g. Blaser & Gerlai, 2006; Miller & Gerlai, 2007; 2008), which has enabled us to confirm many of the intuitions of the above authors. Furthermore, these behaviour quantification methods now allow automated measuring of behaviour, a prerequisite for high-throughput screening.

Another important factor one has to discuss is the origin of the fish used in the behavioural studies. In the early studies with the alarm substance, the zebrafish studied were purchased from local pet-stores and thus numerous factors potentially influencing the behaviour of the experimental fish could not be controlled. For example, the age, potential exposure to other fish species, housing density, type and amount of food prior to experimentation, temperature and water chemistry were all among the environmental conditioned that remained uncontrolled prior to arrival of the fish to the laboratory. The first paper in which the effect of alarm substabce was analyzed with all these factors rigorously monitored and experimentally controlled was conducted by Speedie & Gerlai (2008). This study confirmed that zebrafish not previously exposed to any predatory, harmful, or aversive stimuli would still show a robust alarm reaction to the natural alarm substance, i.e. the alarm response to the substance is innate and represents a genetic predisposition. Speedie & Gerlai (2008) found a significant increase of shoal cohesion, i.e. a decrease of distance between members of the zebrafish group being tested in response to administration of the alarm substance. These authors also found the duration and the number of episodes of erratic movement (zig-zagging) to increase. Freezing (complete immobility) and bottom dwell time also appeared to increase as a result of exposure to the substance. Notably, the alarm substance induced behavioural changes were observed independently of whether the experimental zebrafish were or were not exposed to a live predator during the experiment. In other words, the alarm substance alone could elicit the full repertoire of alarm reactions (Speedie & Gerlai, 2008).

In summary, the induction of fear responses in zebrafish was found possible under controlled laboratory conditions. This is an important step foreward but the difficulty with the studies employing the natural alarm substance has been that the exact concentration of the substance cannot be determined. The dose response analysis in the above cited zebrafish studies was based upon relative doses only, i.e. the experimenters utilized a dilution sequence but could not really ascertain what and how much was in the starting solution. This may not be an important issue as long as the relative doses are compared WITHIN a study. The absolute amount of alarm substance to be extracted from the skin of zebrafish almost certainly varied from study to study no matter how precisely the extraction protocol was followed and thus comparison of effects BETWEEN experiments was impossible to make. Without establishing the exact chemical identity of the alarm substance and without precisely measuring its concentration it was impossible to establish identical doses across different studies. This is a major issue for large scale behavioural screens.

6.5 H3NO, the synthetic alarm substance

The above problem was successfully addressed recently (Parra et al., 2009): a synthetic alarm substance was found just as effective in inducing fear in zebrafish as the natural alarm substance. Alarm substances of the Osteriophysan superorder of fishes were identified from numerous species in the past (Pfeiffer, 1977; Pfeiffer et al., 1985). A common chemical structure shared across these multiple species was found (Kelly et al., 2006; Brown et al., 2000; 2003). Based upon this discovery, a compound mimicking this common chemical element was synthesized. The compound is called hypoxanthine 3-N-oxide, or H3NO, a purine derivative oxidized at the 3-position. Hypoxanthine 3-N-oxide has now been shown to induce alarm responses in numerous fish species including the ones that belong to the Osteriophysan superorder (Pfeiffer, 1977; Pfeiffer et al., 1985; Brown et al., 2003; 2002; 2001; 2000). Zebrafish also belong to this superorder and thus it was hoped that this species too would respond to the synthetic alarm substance with species specific alarm reactions. This is what Parra et al. (2009) have now demonstrated. Their findings are not surprising from an evolutionary stand point. If a prey species is too selective about the taxonomic origin of the odour cue that signals danger, members of such a species would be in a disadvantage as they would not be able to recognize imminent danger, the presence of a hunting predator. It should really not matter what prey species the predator catches, and thus being selective about the alarm cue would be an evolutionary failure. Indeed as Parra et al. (2009) found, the synthetic alarm substance did induce a full fledged alarm reaction in zebrafish. These reactions included erratic movements and jumps, typically observed in response to the natural alarm substance. Thus, now we have a compound whose concentration can be precisely determined and thus its alarm inducing effects are no longer dependent upon the method of alarm substance extraction. Briefly, now we can expect high replicability across laboratories or across different independent experiments or across a large number of experimental subjects, prerequisites for high throughput screening.

6.6 Visual cues as fear inducing stimuli: The sight of the sympatric predator

It is important to realize that although the use of alarm substance in anxiety research is highly promising, the utility of olfactory cues such as this may be limited, or at least complicated from a practical standpoint. For example, although such an olfactory cue is clearly ethologically relevant and induces robust and species specific fear responses, odour cues are not easy to control in terms of the timing of their delivery, their removal, and their spatial localization. Briefly, its hard to precisely control when and where they are perceived. For example, although one may think the precise delivery time is easy to establish, it must be noted that it may take time for the substance to diffuse well enough to reach the target subject. It is also notable that removal of such an odour cue is also complicated. For example, residual odour cues left behind from a prior session may influence the behaviour of subsequent subjects. Cleaning the test tanks is labour intensive, and one may not be entirely certain whether the cleaning indeed removed all cues. Ascertaining that the substance used remains active also requires some attention. For example, in our hand even when stored in dry powder format at -20 ^{o}C, H3NO did deteriorate over a period of several months. Also, as explained above, the on-set and offset of the administration of the odour cue is not precise and for example, multiple on and off time periods are next to impossible to accomplish. Therefore it is likely that cues of other modalities, particularly visual cues, may hold better practical utility (Bass & Gerlai, 2008).

Sympatric predators may induce alarm responses as prey species that coinhabit and thus co-evolved with them may have developed genetic predisposition to innately "recognize" such predators. This was, for example, shown with another fish species, paradise fish (*Macropodus opercularis*), which was found to respond both to the sight and the smell of the snakehead fish (*Chana*) without any prior exposure to this predatory fish (Gerlai, 1993). Paradise fish were also found to exhibit some flexibility and learn to associate otherwise harmless visual stimuli with aversive stimuli (pain or predators), a response that was dependent upon genetic factors (Miklosi et al., 1997 and references therein). These results suggest that innate predator recognition and plastic learning-based antipredatory responses are not mutually exclusive features. Zebrafish have also been found to exhibit learning based alarm reactions (Hall & Suboski, 1995) and more recently they were also shown to respond to their sympatric predator without prior learning (Bass & Gerlai, 2008). The latter authors found zebrafish to exhibit elevated number of jumps in response to the sight of the Indian leaf fish (*Nandus nandus*), a sympatric predator that lives in the same geographical region where zebrafish are found. Importantly, the antipredatory response was elicited by the Indian leaf fish the very first time the experimental subjects were presented with it, demonstrating the lack of need to learn. Also importantly, when zebrafish were exposed to an allopatric predator or to non-predatory fish species, they did not exhibit the antipredatory reactions, which demonstrates that the Indian leaf fish induced responses were indeed specific to this sympatric predator. It is also notable that the Indian leaf fish was not presented in the same water where the experimental zebrafish were swimming, that is the predatory fish was physically isolated from the zebrafish subjects (Bass & Gerlai, 2008). Thus, the only modality the experimental zebrafish could utilize was visual. Admittedly predator-prey interaction between the Indian leaf fish and zebrafish has not been observed in nature (Engeszer et al., 2007). Nevertheless, the above results imply that the zebrafish may have a genetic predisposition to be sensitive to the visual cues that characterize its sympatric predators. From a practical perspective this is great news for the experimenter. Visual cues are easy to control and thus perhaps high throughput behavioural screening may be more feasible using such cues. In the above studies, however, live stimulus fish were presented. This poses a problem. The live predatory fish may change its behaviour from trial to trial. That is, consistent stimulus presentation across multiple experimental zebrafish subjects is difficult to ascertain. This may be a crucial issue for high throughput screening where thousands of zebrafish may need top be tested in a consistent and highly controlled manner before a behavioural outlier, presumably a mutant, may be identified. One way to address the issue of experimental control and consistent stimulus delivery is to walk away from the presentation of live stimulus fish and use instead computerized images. Could the image of a sympatric predator induce alarm reactions?

6.7 The computerized predator: Animated image to induce fear

To answer the above question, Gerlai et al. (2009) experimented with using computerized image presentation to induce fear responses in zebrafish. The authors presented animated (moving) images of the Indian leaf fish to zebrafish and demonstrated that this stimulus elicited erratic movement and jumping from zebrafish, behaviours that were found to be also induced by the alarm substance or by the live Indian leaf fish. At this point it is not known what feature(s) of the computerized image induced the fear responses. In other words, we do not know what makes a good predator for zebrafish. Possible visual properties of the predator zebrafish may respond to include color and pattern (brown patches and markings on a silver background), size (about 10-12 cm long), body proportions (relatively large head and mouth), and/or movement pattern (slow or stationary ambush predator) or any combination of these features. It is possible that when certain key features of a sympatric predator are exaggerated one could induce a further elevated fear response in zebrafish. And clearly, many parameters of the fear paradigm may need to be optimized. Since the publication of the Gerlai et al. (2009) paper, we have already completed another study in which all we did was to lengthen the test tank. The slight change in the dimension of the test apparatus resulted in a robust behavioural change in the zebrafish. In this apparatus, the image of the Indian leaf fish now induced a robust avoidance reaction (increased distance from the image) as well as an increased bottom dwell time. This is noteworthy for two reasons. One concerns the different strategies prey may engage in under specific circumstances. When the prey is within striking distance from the appearing predator swimming away may not be an optimal antipredatory response. Thus in a small test tank other behaviours may be seen, which in our case included erratic movement and jumping. However, if a larger (longer) tank is used, the natural behavioural response of zebrafish to the approaching predator is escape, i.e. increase of the distance between the predator and the prey presumably because this larger tank placed the zebrafish subject outside of the striking distance of the (image of the) predator. The second point concerns the practical aspect of this finding. Measuring distance is much easier and can be better automated than measuring a complex motor pattern like erratic movement. Thus, the longer tank offers the ability to automate the behavioural test. But other modifications beyond changing the dimensions of the tank may also enhance its ability to induce and record fear responses. For example, freezing may be more robustly induced if the tank provides hiding places (e.g. artificial plants). Again, quantification of immobility is achievable using video-tracking systems and thus this behaviour, similarly to measuring distance, can be precisely quantified using automated methods. In summary, the computerized presentation of visual cues have already been shown to induce robust fear and the induced fear responses have been shown to be quantifiable using also computerized video-tracking methods. Thus, the fear paradigm presented above is fully automatable and is ready for high throughput screening of mutations or compounds that alter such fear responses.

6.8 Automation is the key for high throughput screening

As explained above, automated stimulus delivery and automated quantification of behaviour are the two important components of high throughput behavioural tests because such automation allows one to run the tests in parallel, i.e. scale up. In this section I explore further the question of automation. Undoubtedly, so far the most sophisticated pattern detection device has been the human brain: the experimenter can identify complex motor and posture patterns as he/she observes the behaving fish (e.g. Gerlai & Csányi, 1990). This is what classical ethologists have been advocating for decades: observe your subject and measure the elements of the ethogram, i.e. how much time the animal spends doing certain things and how often these things (behaviours) occur. A notable drawback of this method, however, is that it is painstakingly slow and extremely labour intensive. The experimenter has to watch video-recordings and key in his/her observations. This is definitely not high throughput! Observation-based behaviour analysis thus have no place in large scale screens. But this method does have merits and certainly makes sense at the earliest phases of characterization of behavioural responses. This is because it allows one to obtain highly detailed information about animal behaviour and perhaps unexpected changes in the behaviour. But once this preliminary idea-generating pilot work is complete and once the experimenter established how the animal responds in the given behavioural task the next step must be to develop automated behaviour quantification techniques. As we have seen, automated induction and quantification of fear responses is already a reality for zebrafish research.

Numerous commercially produced video-tracking systems are available for the researcher and the utility of video-tracking as compared to other behavioural quantification methods has already been systematically analyzed specifically for zebrafish (e.g. Blaser & Gerlai, 2006). But other automated behaviour measuring methods including the force transducer method may also be considered (e.g. Fitch et al. (2002) that allow automated quantification of behaviour. Some commercially available force transducer based methods are claimed to be able to detect particular "force-prints" that correspond to specific motor and posture patterns. If indeed these force prints correspond to motor patterns, the force transducer method could in principle replace the labour intensive observation-based method of ethologists. For aquatic organisms, however, force transducer-based detection is inappropriate because in the water environment the test subject will not generate acceleration forces detectable by the system. Video-image or video-tracking analysis systems have not been successfully employed in motor pattern quantification, although the claim has been made that they are capable of doing so at least for the house mouse (for a review see e.g. Gerlai, 2002). Despite the infrequent use of zebrafish in behavioural studies, we already have evidence showing that videotracking-based automated quantification of fear responses of zebrafish can reveal significant changes in complex motor patterns (Gerlai et al., 2009). For example, reduced swimming speed, increased within individual temporal variability of swimming speed, increased turn angle and increased within individual temporal variability of turn angle upon presentation of the predator image correlated well with certain complex motor patterns, such as erratic movement and jumping, one would expect to be able to quantify only using observation based methods. The close correlation between the above video-tracking and observation based parameters is not surprising: erratic movement is associated with rapid changes in the direction and speed of swimming, i.e. increased variability of swim speed and increased turn angle and increased variability of turn angle. Similarly, jumping is a rapid and transient increase of swim speed which is expected to translate to increased swim speed variability. In summary, quantification of fear responses has already been automated using videotracking so has the induction of fear responses thus, as we already argued above, a high-throughput fear paradigm is now available for zebrafish (Gerlai et al., 2009).

6.9 Light vs. dark, novel vs. familiar places: Other methods to measure fear responses

There may be several ways one can induce and study the effect of fear. Novelty has long been known to induce fear responses in a variety of species including humans. For example, the open field task has been extensively used with rodents (e.g. Prut & Belzung, 2003; Crusio & Abeelen, 1984) or other animals including fish (Egan et al., 2009; Csányi & Gerlai, 1988). In this task, the subject is exposed to an unfamiliar environment. The response to this novel environment is believed to arise as a result of a compromise between opposing forces or tendencies: exploration, which is believed to be associated with active responses, and fear, which is often associated with passive responses. Exploratory activity is considered adaptive as it may lead to finding food, mates and escape routes, for example, while passive fear induced responses (immobility) is argued to reduce predation risk (Crusio & Abeelen, 1986). The adaptive aspect of these responses may seem speculative but quantitative genetic analyses did confirm ambidirectional selection force underlying open field behaviour. That is, in the evolutionary past of the house mouse individuals that performed at intermediate levels (not too active but not too passive either) had been favoured (Crusio & Abeelen, 1986), a finding that extends to other vertebrates including fish (Gerlai et al., 1990). It is likely that the evolutionary past of zebrafish is similar and this species too has been under ambidirectional selection as far as novelty induced behavioural responses are concerned. Therefore, exposing this fish to a novel environment is expected to induce moderate levels of fear reactions. Importantly, behavioural experimentation always includes at least some level of handling of animals by humans, which is also expected to induce fear.

Novelty induced fear responses have been analyzed in zebrafish by Levin et al. (2007) who showed an initially low level of exploratory activity of zebrafish that gradually increased with time. These authors also described a "diving" response, i.e. increased amount of time spent on the bottom of the test tank, a response that slowly habituated as the fish got accustomed to their novel environment. Egan et al. (2009) also reported similar findings. Levin et al. (2007) showed nicotine had anxiolytic properties as this drug reduced novelty induced fear responses. In addition to novelty, different levels of illumination have also been explored to induce and test fear responses.

The light-dark preference paradigm has been often utilized especially with rodents (e.g. Hascöett et al., 2001; Belzung & Griebel, 2001), but more recently with zebrafish too (see below). The assumption underlying this paradigm is that the nocturnal rodent is expected to prefer, i.e. hide in dark places and avoid well illuminated areas. The evolutionary, i.e. adaptive significance of this behaviour is believed to be associated with predator avoidance. A well illuminated rodent can be easily picked up by an aerial or terrestrial predator. Whether zebrafish prefer well illuminated or dark places, has been somewhat controversial in the literature. The starting assumption was that as a result of the zebrafish being diurnal, active during the day and sleeping during the dark phase of the photoperiod, this species should prefer well illuminated areas where it can visually detect approaching predators more easily. And indeed, this was exactly what was found in a light dark preference task: zebrafish avoided the dark compartment and preferred a well illuminated compartment of a two compartment shuttle box (Gerlai et al., 2000). However, Serra et al. (1999) showed that zebrafish prefer areas of the test environment with a dark background. The difference in the results of these two studies is not easy to explain but may be due to numerous methodological differences. For example, Serra et al (1999) used a dark background but the compartment was well illuminated. Whereas Gerlai et al. (2000) used a dark compartment that was truly dark as it was covered on all sides and the top. One may argue that a dark background, however well illuminated it may be, allows zebrafish to camouflage well (zebrafish has a dark olive-brown back), but a dark cave may harbour predators that remain undetectable for the diurnal zebrafish that uses vision as one of its primary senses.

6.10 Pharmacological analysis of fear responses of zebrafish: The first pioneering studies

Many pharmaceutical research companies have been searching for anxiolytic compounds. This is despite that there are numerous prescription medications already available for anxiety and related disorders. The reason for the continued search for better drugs is that we do not really have a complete understanding of how anxiety develops and what biological mechanisms may underlie this disease cluster. The other reason is that the currently available, however numerous, drugs are often not efficacious or do not work for all patients. Briefly, there is still a large unmet medical need for anxiety related disorders. One way zebrafish may be beneficial for such research is to speed up discovery of the biological mechanisms. This may be achieved using, for example forward genetic screens that identify mutations leading to the isolation of underlying genes. Another completely different approach has been to search for compounds, small molecules as they are called in pharmaceutical research jargon, which may alter fear responses. It is thus important to consider what is known about the psychopharmacological properties of zebrafish in the context of fear and anxiety. For example, could one detect the efficacy of known anxiolytic drugs using zebrafish. That is does the zebrafish model have predictive validity. Predictive validity is an important question for the use of novel model organisms. The main point with regard to the translational relevance of laboratory model organisms concerns the notion "evolutionary of homology", i.e. conservation of biological function across previously utilized species (e.g. rodents), the novel laboratory species (e.g. zebrafish), and humans. Admittedly, zebrafish have been used very infrequently in psychopharmacological analyses. Nevertheless, the few studies that have been completed suggest a possibly bright future for drug development with the use of zebrafish.

Alcohol (ethanol, ethyl alcohol or EtOH) is one of the best studied drugs in zebrafish research. For example, the effect of developmental alcohol exposure was shown to be strain dependent (Loucks & Carvan, 2004), early embryonic alcohol exposure were found to exert significant behavioural effects in the adult (Fernandes & Gerlai, 2009), adaptation (tolerance) after chronic alcohol exposure as well as alcohol withdrawal induced behavioural responses were all demonstrated (Gerlai et al., 2009; 2006), and numerous changes induced by acute alcohol administration have also been revealed (Gerlai et al., 2000). Importantly, alcohol has both anxiolytic (for the effects of lower doses of alcohol in zebrafish see Gerlai et al., 2000, also see Egan et al., 2009) as well as anxiogenic properties (for the effects of prolonged exposure to alcohol and during withdrawal in zebrafish see Gerlai et al., 2009, also see Egan et al., 2009) depending on concentration and mode or regime of its administration. Other drugs of abuse have also been shown to exert significant behavioural effects in zebrafish. For example, the rewarding properties of cocaine have been shown and mutants with altered cocaine reinforced place preference have already been identified in forward genetic screens (Darland & Dowling, 2001). The reinforcing properties of drugs of abuse have also been analyzed (Ninkovic & Bally-Cuif, 2006). Drugs of abuse, similarly to alcohol, often have anxiety altering properties again depending on concentration and dosing regimen employed. For example, a cocaine withdrawal induces anxiety responses in zebarfish (Lopez-Patino et al., 2008). Some classical anti-anxiety drugs have also been tested using zebrafish, e.g. α-fluromethylhistidine exhibited an anxiolytic profile (Peitsaro et al., 2003), diazepam reversed cocaine withdrawal induced anxiety, and the benzodiazepine inverse agonist FG-7142 induced anxiety in zebrafish (Lopez-Patino et al., 2008). Also, acute administration of caffeine, known to induce anxiety in humans (e.g. Childs et al., 2008) and rodents (e.g. El Yacoubi et al., 2000), also led to increased anxiety responses, e.g. reduced frequency of visits to the upper water layer and increased erratic movements in zebrafish (Egan et al., 2009).

Levels of stress hormones have also been analyzed in zebrafish (Alsop & Vijayan, 2008a) and numerous similarities between zebrafish and human stress responses have been revealed, which strengthen the translational relevance of zebrafish in fear and anxiety research. For example, the sight of a predator elevates cortisol levels in zebrafish (Barcellos et al., 2007). It is important to note that cortisol, as in zebrafish, is also the primary stress hormone of the HPA axis in human but not in rodents. In the latter corticosterone plays a more important role instead. Last, treatment with the widely prescribed antidepressant Prozac, i.e. fluoxetine (a selective serotonin reuptake inhibitor) zebrafish reduced their fear responses and spent more time in the top portion of a novel tank and also performed fewer erratic movements. Interestingly, these behavioural changes were accompanied by reduced whole-body cortisol levels (Egan et al., 2009), responses that parallel those seen in rodents (Dulawa et al., 2004).

7. Outlook to the future

It is difficult to forecast how useful zebrafish may become in the modeling and analysis of the biological mechanisms of human fear and anxiety. At this point, however, it seems that the main components necessary for such a research to be successful in the future already exist. While only distantly related to human, the zebrafish has already proven its translational relevance. But perhaps the most important advantage of this species as a laboratory tool may be best described with one word: numbers. Complex biological phenomena are associated with large number of mechanisms. These may be discovered using broad screens, genetic or pharmacological. Zebrafish have been proven to be ideal for large scale screens due to several of its features, but mainly to the fact that a large number of these little fish can be produced fast and can be maintained and now tested efficiently in the laboratory. Given the complexity of the mechanisms of fear and anxiety, one may expect the need to identify a large number of molecular players, i.e. genes and their protein products and the biochemical interactions between the proteins. I argue that this complexity may be best tackled, at least initially, using large scale screens for mutations and drugs. These screens are the key to the identification of potential targets and leads that may subsequently be followed up on by more targeted hypothesis driven analyses. These big "fishing" experiments may be best conducted using the easy to keep and highly prolific zebrafish. It is important to note that I am not advocating the screening approach as the only possible or only potentially fruitful one. Obviously as our knowledge accumulates, increasingly directed and hypothesis driven in depth analyses become possible. But what I am arguing is that the notion of hypotheses having to drive our research somewhat clouded our judgement and we perhaps started the in depth analyses too soon. There expected to be a large number of unknown mechanisms waiting to be discovered and their discovery may be significantly facilitated by "blind", i.e. unbiased, screening applications. And this is exactly where zebrafish has a major advantage over other laboratory organisms.

8. Acknowledgements

Supported by NIH/NIAAA 1R01AA015325-01A2.

9. References

Ahmed O, Seguin D, Gerlai R (2011). An automated predator avoidance task in zebrafish. *Behav. Brain Res.* 216:166-171.

Alsop D, Vijayan M. (2008a) The zebrafish stress axis: Molecular fallout from the teleost specific genome duplication event. *Gen Comp Endocrinol* ; 161:62-66.

Alsop D, Vijayan MM. (2008b) Development of the corticosteroid stress axis and receptor expression in zebrafish. Am J Physiol Regul Integr Comp Physiol; 294: R711–719.

Amsterdam A, Burgess S, Golling G, Chen W, Sun Z, Townsend K, Farrington S, Haldi M, Hopkins N. (1999) A large-scale insertional mutagenesis screen in zebrafi sh. *Genes Dev*; 13:2713–2724.

Apfelbach R, Blanchard CD, Blanchard RJ, Hayes RA, McGregor IS. (2005) The effects of predator odors in mammalian prey species: a review of field and laboratory studies. *Neurosci Biobehav Rev*; 29: 1123-1144.

Barcellos LJG, Ritter F, Kreutz LC, Quevedo RM, Bolognesi da Silva L, Bedin AC, et al. (2007) Whole-body cortisol increases after direct and visual contact with a predator in zebrafish Danio rerio. *Aquaculture*; 272: 774–778.

Barros M, Maior RS, Huston JP, Tomaz C (2008) Predatory stress as an experimental strategy to measure fear and anxiety-related behaviors in non-human primates. *Rev Neurosci.*; 19: 157-169.

Bass SLS, Gerlai R. (2008) Zebrafish (*Danio rerio*) responds differentially to stimulus fish: The effects of sympatric and allopatric predators and harmless fish. *Behavioural Brain Research*; 186: 107–117.

Belzung, C. & Griebel, R. (2001) Measuring normal and pathological anxiety-like behaviour in mice: A review. *Behavioural Brain Research*; 138: 200-209.

Bill BR, Petzold AM, Clark KJ, Schimmenti LA, Ekker SC. (2009) A primer for morpholino use in zebrafish. *Zebrafish*; 6:69-77.

Blanchard DC, Griebel G, Blanchard RJ. (2003) Conditioning and residual emotionality effects of predator stimuli: some reflections on stress and emotion. *Prog Neuropsychopharmacol Biol Psychiatry*; 27: 1177–1185.

Blaser R, Gerlai R. (2006) Behavioral phenotyping in Zebrafish: Comparison of three behavioral quantification methods. *Behav Res Methods*; 38: 456-469.

Bouwknecht JA, Paylor R. (2008) Pitfalls in the interpretation of genetic and pharmacological effects on anxiety-like behaviour in rodents. *Behav Pharmacol.*; 19: 385-402.

Brown GE, Adrian JC Jr, Nabil TN, Mark CH, Jocelyn MK. (2003) Nitrogen-oxides elicit antipredator responses in juvenile channel catfish, but not convict cichlids or rainbow trout: conservation of the Ostariophysan alarm pheromone. *J Chem Ecol*; 29: 1781-1796.

Brown G. E., Adrian J. C. Jr., Lewis M. G., Tower J. M. (2002) The Effects of Reduced pH on Chemical Alarm Signaling in Ostariophysan fishes. *Canadian Journal of Fisheries and Aquatic Sciences*; 59: 1331-1338.

Brown G. E., Adrian J. C., Jr., Shih M. L. (2001) Behavioural Responses of Fathead Minnows (*Pimephales promelas*) to Hypoxanthine-3-N-oxide at Varying Concentrations. *Journal of Fish Biology*; 58: 1465-1470.

Brown G. E, Adrian JC Jr, Smyth E, Leet H, Brennan S. (2000) Ostariophysan alarm substances: Laboratory and field tests of the functional significance of nitrogen oxides. *J Chem Ecol*; 26: 139-154.

Chatterjee D, Gerlai R. (2009) High Precision Liquid Chromatography Analysis of Dopaminergic and Serotoninergic Responses to Acute Alcohol Exposure in Zebrafish. *Behavioural Brain Research*; 200: 208–213.

Childs E, Hohoff C, Deckert J, Xu K, Badner J, de Wit H. (2008) Association between ADORA2A and DRD2 polymorphisms and caffeine-induced anxiety. *Neuropsychopharmacology*; 33: 2791–2800.

Choy Y, Fyer AJ, Goodwin RD. (2007) Specific phobia and comorbid depression: a closer look at the National Comorbidity Survey data. *Comprarative Psychiatry*; 48: 132–136.

Crusio. W.E. (1995) Natural selection on hippocampal circuitry underlying exploratory behaviour in mice: Quantitative-genetic analysis. In: E. Alleva, A. Fasolo, H.-P. Lipp, L. Nadel, and L. Ricceri (Eds.), *Behavioural Brain Research in Naturalistic and Seminaturalistic Settings*, Kluwer Academic Press, Dordrecht, The Netherlands, pp. 323-342,.

Crusio WE, Abeelen JHF van (1984) The genetic architechture of behavioural responses to novelty in mice, *Heredity*; 56: 55-63.

Csányi, V. & Gerlai, R. (1988) Open-field behavior and the behavior-genetic analysis of the paradise fish (*Macropodus opercularis*). *J Comp Psychol.*; 102: 326-336.

Darland T, Dowling JE. (2001) Behavioral screening for cocaine sensitivity in mutagenized zebrafish. *Proc Natl Acad Sci USA*;98:11691–6.

Donovan A, Brownlie A, Zhou Y, Shepard J, Prat SJ, Moynihan J, Paw BH, Drejer A, Barut B, Zapata A. (2000) Positional cloning of zebrafish ferroportin 1 identifies a conserved vertebrate iron exporter. *Nature*; 403: 776–781.

Denver RJ. (2009) Structural and functional evolution of vertebrate neuroendocrine stress systems.*Ann N Y Acad Sci.*; 1163: 1-16.

Doyon Y, McCammon JM, Miller JC, Faraji F, Ngo C, Katibah GE, Amora R, Hocking TD, Zhang L, Rebar EJ, Gregory PD, Urnov FD, Amacher SL. (2008) Heritable targeted gene disruption in zebrafish using designed zinc-finger nucleases. *Nat Biotechnol*; 26: 702-708.

Dulawa SC, Holick KA, Gundersen B, Hen R. (2004) Effects of chronic fluoxetine in animal models of anxiety and depression. *Neuropsychopharmacology*; 29: 1321–1330.

Egan RJ, Bergner CL, Hart PC, Cachat JM, Canavello PR, Elegante MF, Elkhayat SI, Bartels BK, Tien AK, Tien DH, Mohnot S, Beeson E, Glasgow E, Amri H, Zukowska Z, Kalueff AV. (2009) Understanding behavioral and physiological phenotypes of stress and anxiety in zebrafish. *Behav Brain Res.* 205: 38-44

El Yacoubi M, Ledent C, Parmentier M, Costentin J, Vaugeois JM. (2000) The anxiogeniclike effect of caffeine in two experimental procedures measuring anxiety in the mouse is not shared by selective A(2A) adenosine receptor antagonists. *Psychopharmacology* (Berl); 148: 153–163.

Engeszer RE, Patterson LB, Rao AA, Parichy DM. (2007) Zebrafish in the wild: a review of natural history and new notes from the field. *Zebrafish.*; 4 :21-40.

Fernandes Y, Gerlai R. (2009) Long-term behavioral changes in response to early developmental exposure to ethanol in zebrafish. *Alcoholism: Clinical and Experimental Research*; 33: 601-609.

Fitch, T., Adams, B, Chaney, S., Gerlai, R. (2002) Force transducer based movement detection in fear conditioning in mice: A comparative analysis. *Hippocampus*; 12: 4-17.

Flint J, Shifman S. (2008) Animal models of psychiatric disease. *Curr Opin Genet Dev.*; 18: 235-240.

Frisch, K. von. (1938). Zur Psychologie des Fisch- Schwarmes. *Naturwissenschaften* 26:601-606.

Frisch, K. von (1941). Uber einen Schreckstо'f der Fisch- haut und seine biologische Bedeutung. *Z. vergl. Physiol.* 29:46-145.

Garakani A, Mathew SJ, Charney DS. (2006) Neurobiology of anxiety disorders and implications for treatment. *Mt Sinai J Med.*; 73: 941-949.

Geisler R, Rauch GJ, Baier H, Van Bebber F, Brobeta L, Dekens MP, Finger K, Fricke C. (1999) A radiation hybrid map of the zebrafish genome. *Nat Genet*; 23:86–89.

Gerlai, R. (2002) Phenomics: Fiction or the Future? *Trends Neurosci.*; 25: 506-509.

Gerlai, R. (2001) Behavioral tests of hippocampal function: Simple paradigms, complex problems. *Behav. Brain Res.*; 125: 269 – 277.

Gerlai, R. (1993) Can paradise fish (*Macropodus opercularis*) recognize its natural predator? An ethological analysis. *Ethology*; 94, 127-136.

Gerlai, R., Clayton, N. S. (1999a) Analysing hippocampal function in transgenic mice: An ethological perspective. *Trends Neurosci.*; 22: 47-51.

Gerlai R, Clayton NS. (1999b) Tapping artificially into natural talents - Reply. *Trends Neurosci,*; 22: 301-302.

Gerlai, R. & Csányi V. (1990) Genotype environment interaction and the correlation structure of behavioral elements in paradise fish (*Macropodus opercularis*). *Physiol Behav.*; 47, 343 356.

Gerlai R, Chatterjee D, Pereira T, Sawashima T, Krishnannair R. (2009) Acute and Chronic alcohol dose: Population differences in behavior and neurochemistry of zebrafish. *Genes, Brain and Behavior*; 8: 586–599.

Gerlai R, Lee V, Blaser R. (2006) Effects of acute and chronic ethanol exposure on the behavior of adult zebrafish (*Danio rerio*). *Pharmacol Biochem Behav*; 85: 752-761.

Gerlai, R., Lahav, M., Guo, S., Rosenthal, A. (2000) Drinks like a fish: Zebra fish (Danio rerio) as a behavior genetic model to study alcohol effects. *Pharmacol. Biochem. Behav.*; 67:773-782.

Gerlai, R., Shinsky, N. , Shih, A. , Williams, P., Winer, J., Armanini, M., Cairns, B., Winslow, J., Gao, W-Q., Phillips, H. S. (1999) Regulation of learning by EphA receptors: A protein targeting study. *J. Neurosci*; 19: 9538-9549.

Gerlai, R., Crusio, W. E., Csányi, V. (1990) Inheritance of species-specific behaviors in the paradise fish (Macropodus opercularis): A diallel study. *Behav Genet*,; 20, 487-498.

Grant SG, O'Dell TJ, Karl KA, Stein PL, Soriano P, Kandel ER. (1992) Impaired long-term potentiation, spatial learning, and hippocampal development in fyn mutant mice. *Science*.; 258: 1903-1910.

Guo S, Yamaguchi Y, Schilbach S, Wada T, Lee J, Goddard A, French D, Handa H, Rosenthal A. (2000) A regulator of transcriptional elongation controls vertebrate neuronal development. *Nature*; 408:366–369.

Hall D, Suboski MD. (1995) Visual and olfactory stimuli in learned release of alarm reactions by zebra danio fish (*Brachydanio rerio*). *Neurobiol Learn Mem*; 63:229–240.

Hascöett, M., Bourin, M. & Dhonnchadha, B. A. N. (2001) The mouse light-dark paradigm: A review. *Progress in Neuro-Psychopharmacology and Biological Psychiatry*; 25: 141-166.

Hendrie CA, Weiss SM, Eilam D. (1996) Exploration and predation models of anxiety: evidence from laboratory and wild species. *Pharmacol Biochem Behav*.; 54:13-20.

Hohoff C. (2009) Anxiety in mice and men: a comparison. *J Neural Transm*.; 116: 679-687.

Hovatta I, Barlow C. (2008) Molecular genetics of anxiety in mice and men. *Ann Med*.; 40: 92-109.

Iliadi KG. (2009) The genetic basis of emotional behavior: has the time come for a Drosophila model? *J Neurogenet*.; 23:136-146.

Kelly JM, Adrian JC Jr, Brown GE. (2006) Can the ratio of aromatic skeletons explain cross-species responses within evolutionary conserved Ostariophysan alarm cues?: testing the purine-ratio hypothesis. *Chemoecology*; 16: 93-96.

Kily LJ, Cowe YC, Hussain O, Patel S, McElwaine S, Cotter FE, et al. (2008) Gene expression changes in a zebrafish model of drug dependency suggest conservation of neuro-adaptation pathways. *J Exp Biol*; 211:1623–1634.

Klein DF. (1996) Panic disorder and agoraphobia: hypothesis hothouse. *J Clin Psychiatry*; 57 Suppl 6: 21–27.

Leonardo ED, Hen R. (2006) Genetics of affective and anxiety disorders. *Annu Rev Psychol*.; 57: 117-137.

Levin ED, Bencan Z, Cerutti DT. (2007) Anxiolytic effects of nicotine in zebrafish. *Physiology and Behavior*; 90: 54-58.

Lister RG. (1990) Ethologically-based animal models of anxiety disorders. *Pharmacol Ther*.; 46:321-340.

Lopez-Patino MA, Yu L, Cabral H, Zhdanova IV. (2008) Anxiogenic effects of cocaine withdrawal in zebrafish. *Physiol Behav*; 93: 160–171.

Loucks E, Carvan III MJ. (2004) Strain-dependent effects of developmental ethanol exposure in zebrafish. *Neurotoxicol Teratol;* 26: 745–55.
Lu, Y-M., Jia, Z., Janus, C., Henderson, J. T., Gerlai, R., Wojtowicz, J. M., Roder, J. C. (1997) Mice lacking metabotropic glutamate receptor 5 show impaired learning and reduced CA1 LTP, but normal CA3-LTP. *J Neurosci;* 17: 5196-5205.
Mathew SJ, Price RB, Charney DS. (2008) Recent advances in the neurobiology of anxiety disorders: implications for novel therapeutics. *Am J Med Genet C Semin Med Genet.*;148C: 89-98
Mendlowicz MV, Stein MB. (2000) Quality of life in individuals with anxiety disorders. Am *J Psychiatry.*;157: 669-682.
Miklósi, Á., Csányi, V., Gerlai, R. (1997) Behavior genetic analysis of predator avoidance and inspection behavior in paradise fish: The effect of parental care (Macropodus opercularis). *Behavior Genetics* ; 27:191-200.
Miller N, Gerlai R. (2008) Oscillations in Shoal Cohesion in Zebrafish (*Danio rerio*) *Behav. Brain Res;* 193: 148-151.
Miller N, Gerlai R. (2007) Quantification of Shoaling Behaviour in Zebrafish (*Danio rerio*). *Behav. Brain Res.;* 184:157-166.
Misslin R. (2003) The defense system of fear: behavior and neurocircuitry. *Neurophysiol Clin.;* 33: 55-66.
Mueller T, Vernier P, Wullimann MF. (2004) The adult central nervous cholinergic system of a neurogenetic model animal, the zebrafish (*Danio rerio*). *Brain Res;* 1011:156–169.
Nasevicius A, Ekker SC. (2000) Effective targeted gene "knockdown" in zebrafish. *Nat Genet;* 26:216–220.
Ni J, Clark KJ, Fahrenkrug SC, Ekker SC. (2008) Transposon tools hopping in vertebrates. *Brief Funct Genomic Proteomic.*;7:444-453.
Ninkovic J, Bally-Cuif L. (2006) The zebrafish as amodel system for assessing the reinforcing properties of drugs of abuse. *Methods;* 39:262–274.
Panula P, Sallinen V, Sundvik M, Kolehmainen J, Torkko V, Tiittula A, et al. (2006) Modulatory neurotransmitter systems and behavior: towards zebrafish models of neurodegenerative diseases. *Zebrafish;* 3: 235–247.
Parra KV, Adrian JC Jr, Gerlai R. (2009) The synthetic substance hypoxanthine 3-N-oxide elicits alarm reactions in zebrafish (*Danio rerio*). *Behav Brain Res.* 205: 336-341.
Pfeiffer W. (1963) Alarm substances. *Experientia* (Basel); 19:113-123.
Pfeiffer W. (1977) The distribution of fright reaction and alarm substance cells in fishes. *Copeia;* 4: 653–665.
Pfeiffer W, Riegelbauer G, Meier G, Scheibler B. (1985) Effect of hypoxanthine 3-N-oxide and hypoxanthine 1-N-oxide on central nervous excitation of the black tetra, *Gymnocorymbus ternetzi* (*Characaidae, Ostariophysi, Pisces*) indicated by dorsal light response. *J Chem Ecol;* 11: 507-523.
Peitsaro N, Kaslin J, Anichtchik OV, Panula P. (2003) Modulation of the histaminergic system and behaviour by alpha-fluoromethylhistidine in zebrafish. *J Neurochem;* 86: 432–441.
Prut, L. & Belzung, C. (2003) The open field as a paradigm to measure the effects of drugs on anxiety-like behaviors: A review. *European Journal of Pharmacology;* 463: 3-33

Reimers MJ, Hahn ME, Tanguay RL. (2004) Two zebrafi sh alcohol dehydrogenases share common ancestry with mammalian class I, II, IV, and V alcohol dehydrogenase genes but have distinct functional characteristics. *J Biol Chem*;279:38303–38312.

Renier, C; Faraco, JH; Bourgin, P; Motley, T; Bonaventure, P; Rosa, F; Mignot, E. (2007) Genomic and functional conservation of sedative-hypnotic targets in the zebrafish. *Pharmacogenetics and Genomics*; 17: 237-253.

Rosen JB, Pagani JH, Rolla KL, Davis C. (2008) Analysis of behavioral constraints and the neuroanatomy of fear to the predator odor trimethylthiazoline: a model for animal phobias. *Neurosci Biobehav Rev.*; 32: 1267-1276.

Schutz, F. Vergleichende (1956) Untersuchungen iiber die Schreckreaktion bei Fischen und deren Verbreitung *Z. vergl. Physiol.*; 38:84-135.

Scott EK. (2009) The Gal4/UAS toolbox in zebrafish: new approaches for defining behavioral circuits. *J Neurochem.*; 110: 441-456.

Serra, E. L., Medalha, C. C. & Mattioli, R. (1999) Natural preference of zebrafish (*Danio rerio)* for a dark environment. *Brazilian Journal of Medical and Biological Research*; 32: 1551-1553.

Shin JT, Fishman MC. (2002) FromZebrafish to human: modular medical models. *Annu Rev Genomics Hum Genet*; 3:311–340.

Silva AJ, Paylor R, Wehner JM, Tonegawa S. (1992) Impaired spatial learning in alpha-calcium-calmodulin kinase II mutant mice. *Science.*; 257: 206-211.

Sivasubbu S, Balciunas D, Davidson AE, Pickart MA, Hermanson SB, Wangensteen KJ, Wolbrink DC, Ekker SC. (2006) Gene-breaking transposon mutagenesis reveals an essential role for histone H2afza in zebrafish larval development. *Mech Dev*; 123: 513-529.

Speedie N, Gerlai R. (2008) Alarm substance induced behavioral responses in zebrafish (*Danio rerio*) *Behav. Brain Res.*; 188: 168-177.

Sprague J, Doerry E, Douglas S, Westerfield M. (2001) The zebrafi sh information network (ZFIN): A resource for genetic, genomic and developmental research. *Nucleic Acids Res*; 29:87–90.

Stickney HL, Schmutz J, Woods IG, Holtzer CC, Dickson MC, Kelly PD, Myers RM, Talbot WS. (2002) Rapid mapping of zebrafish mutations with SNPs and oligonucleotide microarrays. *Genome Res*; 12: 1929–1934.

Sipe CW, Saha MS. (2007) The use of microarray technology in nonmammalian vertebrate systems. *Methods Mol Biol.*; 382:1-16.

Takahashi LK, Chan MM, Pilar ML. (2008) Predator odor fear conditioning: current perspectives and new directions. *Neurosci Biobehav Rev.*; 32: 1218-1227.

Zhang J, Talbot WS, Schier AF. (1998) Positional cloning identifies zebrafish one-eyed pinhead as a permissive EGF-related ligand required during gastrulation. *Cell*; 92:241–251.

Waldman B. (1982) Quantitative and developmental analysis of the alarm reaction in the zebra Danio *Brachydanio rerio*. *Copeia*; 1: 1–9.

Wang D, Jao LE, Zheng N, Dolan K, Ivey J, Zonies S, Wu X, Wu K, Yang H, Meng Q, Zhu Z, Zhang B, Lin S, Burgess SM. (2007) Efficient genome-wide mutagenesis of zebrafish genes by retroviral insertions. *Proc Natl Acad Sci U S.*; A 104: 12428-12433.

Weisberg RB. (2009) Overview of generalized anxiety disorder: epidemiology, presentation, and course. *J Clin Psychiatry.*; Suppl 2: 4-9.

Wienholds E, Schulte-Merker S, Walderich B, Plasterk RHA. (2002) Target selected inactivation of the zebrafish rag1 gene. *Science*; 297: 99–102.

8

Acute Stress in Patients with Panic Disorder Produces Effects on Salivary Amylase and Cortisol

Jotaro Akiyoshi et al.*
Department of Neuropsychiatry,
Oita University Faculty of Medicine, Oita,
Japan

1. Introduction

Salivary alpha-amylase (sAA) has been suggested to reflect stress-related body changes. Psychosocial stress increases the release of salivary alpha-amylase, which reflects the activity of the sympathetic-adrenal-medullary (SAM) system. Therefore, it is presumed that sAA measurement is a useful tool for evaluating the SAM system. In addition, previous studies examining the response of sAA levels to SAM system activity showed that increased sAA levels were correlated with increased plasma catecholamine, indicating sympathetic nervous system activation. So far, numerous studies have shown that changes in sAA levels are dependent on stress stimuli. It is difficult to objectively evaluate the emotional and physical state. sAA measurement can be performed easily and quickly, and therefore, could be used to aid the evaluation of the psychosocial and/or physical stress levels. It is very important to be able to evaluate and understand the level of psychosocial and/or physical stress (distress) experienced by patients. The measurement of sAA is expected to be useful tool as a patient distress.

In panic disorder, stressful events are frequently comprised of both neutral and emotionally arousing information, yet the impact of stress on emotional and neutral events is still not fully understood. The hippocampus contains dense concentrations of receptors for stress hormones (such as cortisol), and elevated stress hormone levels can impair performance on hippocampal-dependent memory tasks. Yet, cortisol can also facilitate memory for emotional information, and this involves interactions between the hippocampus and amygdala. Physiological and psychological stresses have the short-term effects on salivary amylase (sAA) and salivary cortisol levels during both emotional and neutral episodes. The stress manipulation results sAA and salivary cortisol responsiveness. The stress manipulation also increases salivary cortisol levels, catecholamine function as indicated by

* Yoshihiro Tanaka, Koichi Isogawa, Yoshinobu Ishitobi, JusenTsuru, Tomoko Ando, Aimi Kawano, Shizuko Okamoto, Masayuki Kanehisa, Yoshihiro Maruyama, Haruka Higuma, Taiga Ninomiya, Hiroaki Hanada and Kensuke Kodama
Department of Neuropsychiatry, Oita University Faculty of Medicine, Oita, Japan

the presence of alpha-amylase, heart rate, and subjectively reported stress levels. Stressed patients with panic disorder reported more anxiety compared to non-stressed control subjects, and these anxiety levels are positively correlated with salivary amylase and cortisol levels, providing evidence for a relationship between stress and hormonal responses. Stress produces physiological responsiveness under neutral versus emotional episodes in panic disorder.

2. Relationship between the hippocampus, amygdala, cortisol and amylase

The hippocampus is a bilateral, subcortical brain structure with an elongated shape and complex microcircuitry. This structure functions in both declarative memory (episodic memory and semantic memory) and spatial memory (Squire, 1992). Along with the amygdala, the hippocampus is one of the most frequently studied brain regions in terms of neuronal plasticity. Neuronal plasticity is thought to represent the cellular mechanism associated with both learning and the storage of memories (Cooke and Bliss, 2006). The hippocampus is also a region susceptible to damage via both hypoxic encephalopathy and Alzheimer's disease. The amygdala is an almond-shaped, bilateral structure located inside the temporal lobes. Previously, the amygdala was considered a functionally vague area of the brain, and did not generate much scientific interest. However, today it is one of the most frequently studied brain regions as an essential location of fear and anxiety mechanisms. In addition to animal experiments using fear conditioning methods, fMRI studies in humans have become increasingly important for these investigations. The lateral nucleus of the amygdala is considered an important region for the formation and storage of emotional memory. During the formation of emotional memories, associations between stimuli and emotional responses are thought to be encoded by neural plasticity in the lateral amygdala. The lateral amygdala also communicates this information with other brain regions involved in fear memory storage and functional output. For example, the central nucleus of amygdala is a critical region of emotional output (Phelps EA, LeDoux JE 2005). Cortisol is a steroid hormone secreted from the adrenal cortex. Cortisol levels are increased by stress (Simon and Gorman, 2004) and, as a result, blood pressure and blood sugar levels are also increased, while immune function and fertility are compromised. The digestive enzyme amylase is contained in pancreatic fluids and saliva and breaks down starch and glycogen. Salivary amylase is also secreted by stress via activation of the sympathetic nervous system and the action of β-adrenergic receptors (van Stegeren et al. 2006). Chronic stress over long periods leads to cortisol secretion in large quantities, and such excessive cortisol levels can result in hippocampal atrophy. Patients with depression (Campbell and Macqueen 2004) or post-traumatic stress disorder (PTSD) (Woon et al. 2010) are likely to be susceptible to this mechanism. Excessive cortisol administration in rats also causes increased corticotropin-releasing factor (CRF) levels in the amygdala, along with increased amygdala excitability. In turn, activation of the amygdala further potentiates cortisol release. Thus, in contrast to the traditional negative feedback systems limiting cortisol activity via the hypothalamus, cortisol produces a positive feedback signal regulating its levels via the amygdala (Makino et al 1994).

Recently Inagaki et al., (2011) reported that saliva samples were taken at three points, and sAA activity was measured using a hand-held monitor before the test, immediately after the test, and 10 min after the test. In the study, a marked increase in sAA activity due to physiological stress and a rapid return to the baseline level were observed. This physiological stress method might be useful for evaluating stress. Engert et al., (2011) reported that there was the cross-correlation of salivary cortisol and sAA responses to psychological stress. The participants were exposed to a psychological laboratory stressor with high frequency saliva sampling in two independent studies. Synchronized time series of sAA and cortisol measures before, during and after stress induction were obtained. Cross-correlation analysis was applied to test for the association of sAA and cortisol levels at various stages relative to the onset of the stressor. Positive and negative cross-correlations between lagged pairs of sAA and cortisol measures were found in both studies. The strongest correlation was found for sAA preceding cortisol release. With a smaller effect size cortisol also significantly preceded sAA. sAA and cortisol stress responses are reliably associated at various time lags throughout a stressful situation. As a possible connection site between HPA axis and SNS that may underlie sAA-cortisol associations.

3. Panic disorder and salivary amylase

Panic disorder (PD), one of the most severe anxiety syndromes, is characterized by recurrent and unprovoked panic attacks. During these attacks, a variety of physical symptoms may occur accompanied by a sense of doom and a strong desire to escape present situations (Weissman et al., 1990). Extensive research has attempted to associate panic disorder with an abnormal functioning of the hypothalamic-pituitary-adrenal (HPA) system. Various reports have suggested increased basal cortisol production, yet blunted ACTH and cortisol responsiveness to CRF infusion, along with other subtle differences in feedback sensitivity of the HPA axis (Roy-Byrne et al., 1986; Holsboer et al., 1987; Gurguis et al., 1991; Schreiber et al., 1996; Abelson et al., 2007). Such seemingly inconsistent findings have persisted throughout the literature for decades. Interestingly, reports of naturally occurring panic attacks found that these attacks occur without an obvious secretion of cortisol in most instances (Cameron et al., 1987; Bandelow et al., 2000). The prominent lack of cortisol response to a situation often subjectively perceived by patients as life threatening is confusing, since HPA activity is well known to rapidly increase in times of threat or when encountering a harmful situation (Mason, 1968). However, most patients studied for acute endocrine responses to panic attacks (either naturally or in the lab) have most likely experienced many previous instances of panic attacks. Thus, it is tempting to speculate that the blunted cortisol response to acute panic attack simply reflects successful habituation to repeated stimulation by complex emotional events. In healthy volunteers, a rapid habituation of cortisol responsiveness can be observed when subjects are repeatedly exposed to stressful stimuli in the same environmental context (Kirschbaum et al., 1995; Schommer et al., 2003). As an extension of these studies, we have focused on salivary cortisol levels in patients with panic disorder following electrical stimulation stress. The SAM system is associated with both arousal and anxiety (Aston-Jones et al. 1994; Aston-Jones et al. 1998; Southwick et al. 1999; Berridge and Waterhouse 2003). As a part of this system, stress can trigger locus coeruleus (LC) firing and subsequent widespread norepinephrine neurotransmission in the brainstem, amygdala and prefrontal cortex (Liddell et al. 2005). Activity in these regions leads to behavioral responses such as orienting to threat, fear, arousal and inhibition of general activity (Gray 1982; Redmond 1987; Coull et al. 2001; Liddell et al. 2005). sAA is secreted by the parotid gland in response to adrenergic activity and is suppressed by β-adrenoreceptor blockade. Alpha-amylase has emerged as a new biomarker for responses to psychosocial stress within the sympathetic nervous system (Ehlert et al., 2006; Granger et al., 2007), and it has been suggested that alpha-amylase levels could be used as an index of SAM activity. Acute investigational stressors induce alpha-amylase secretion, although chronic stress may be associated with reduced alpha-amylase output. Amylase secretion is independent of salivary flow rate and has an endogenous diurnal rhythm (Nater et al., 2007). However, some reports suggest that parasympathetic activation can also induce alpha-amylase release (Nater et al., 2006). Alpha-amylase is not a reliable marker of catecholamine levels. Therefore, alpha-amylase activity may best be described as an autonomic biomarker, complementing but not replacing the measurement of catecholamines and cardiac activity.

There is a strong relationship between anxiety and the degree of attention allocated towards threat-related cues. In a meta-analysis of 172 studies, Bar-Haim et al. (2007) found that anxious, but not healthy, subjects exhibit a selective attentional bias towards threatening cues. The direction of threat prejudice can be modulated by state and contextual factors. For example, situation anxiety increases attentional bias to threats (e.g., MacLeod and Mathews, 1988), but this bias diminishes if attention is directed towards an internal focus, e.g., self-awareness of physiological symptoms (Mansell et al. 2003) or external threats other than the threat stimuli presented during the attention task (Mathews and Sebastian 1993; Williams et al. 1996). In a previous study, patients with panic disorder who displayed panic attacks (46%) had markedly greater anticipatory anxiety before the delivery of 5% carbon dioxide, and this alteration was accompanied by increased β-adrenergic cardiac tone (Roth et al., 1992).

Some reports indicated a possible change in cortisol responsiveness to stress/novel situations in panic disorder subjects (Stones et al., 1999). This was considered to be consistent with previous suggestions of HPA axis dysregulation in panic disorder patients, although some research indicated under-responsiveness rather than a hyper-responsiveness to stress/novel situations in this group. Recently, Petrowski et al. (2010) reported a blunted cortisol response to moderate or intense psychosocial stress in a group of patients with panic disorder. Other studies also reported a hypo- or non-responsiveness to stress in patients with panic disorder (Leyton et al., 1996; Hoehn et al., 1997; Garcia-Leal et al., 2005).

sAA and salivary cortisol levels might differ according to the length of time a study participant had been in the hospital (Balodis et al., 2010). Further studies are needed to try to incorporate drug-free patients and make comparisons between treated and non-treated populations. sAA levels might be a predictive biological marker for antidepressant-responsiveness in patients with panic disorder. Additional studies incorporating more frequent measurements and additional combinations of stress markers will be needed in order to establish a predictive model for successful treatment of patients with panic disorder.

4. Conclusion

Hippocampus and amygdala are important brain regions for learning and storage of memory. Hippocampus involves declarative memory and spatial memory, amygdala involves emotional memory. Excessive cortisol level can result in hippocampal atrophy. Cortisol decreases CRF secretion in hypothalamus, but increase CRF level in amygdala.sAA is parallel movement to stress and cortisol in blood vessel; it is a convenient method for stress.

sAA could be used as an index of SAM activity. The SAM system is associated with both arousal and anxiety. Acute investigational stressors induce alpha-amylase secretion, although chronic stress may be associated with reduced alpha-amylase output. SAA levels might be a predictive biological marker for antidepressant- responsiveness in patients with panic disorder.

5. References

Abelson JL, Khan S, Liberzon I, Young EA. 2007. HPA axis activity in patients with panic disorder: review and synthesis of four studies. Depress Anxiety 24: 66-76.

Aston-Jones G, Rajkowski J, Kubiak P, Alexinsky T. 1994. Locus coeruleus neurons in monkey are selectively activated by attended cues in a vigilance task. J Neurosci 14: 4467-4480.

Aston-Jones G, Rajkowski J, Ivanova S, Usher M, Cohen J. 1998. Neuromodulation and cognitive performance: recent studies of noradrenergic locus ceruleus neurons in behaving monkeys. Adv Pharmacol 42: 755-759.

Balodis IM, Wynne-Edwards KE, Olmstead MC. 2010. The other side of the curve: examining the relationship between pre-stressor physiological responses and stress reactivity. Psychoneuroendocrinology 35: 1363-1373.

Bandelow B,Wedekind D, Pauls J, Broocks A, Hajak G, Ru¨ther E. 2000. Salivary cortisol in panic attacks. Am. J. Psychiatry 157: 454-456.

Bar-Haim Y, Lamy D, Pergamin L, Bakermans-Kranenburg MJ, van IJzendoorn MH. 2007. Threat-related attentional bias in anxious and nonanxious individuals: a meta-analytic study. Psychol Bull 133: 1-24.

Berridge CW, Waterhouse BD. 2003. The locus coeruleus-noradrenergic system: modulation of behavioral state and state-dependent cognitive processes. Brain Res Brain Res Rev 42: 33-84.

Cameron OG, Lee MA, Curtis GC, McCann DS. 1987. Endocrine and physiological changes during "spontaneous" panic attacks. Psychoneuroendocrinology 12: 321-331.

Campbell S, Macqueen G. 2004. The role of the hippocampus in the pathophysiology of major depression. J Psychiatry Neurosci 29: 417-426.

Cooke SF, Bliss TV. 2006. Plasticity in the human central nervous system. Brain 129:1659-73.

Coull JT. 2001. Modulation of attention by noradrenergic alpha2-agents varies according to arousal level. Drug News Perspect 14: 5-11.

Ehlert U, Erni K, Hebisch G, Nater U. 2006. Salivary alphaamylase levels after yohimbine challenge in healthy men. J Clin Endocrinol Metab 91: 5130-5133.

Engert V, Vogel S, Efanov SI, Duchesne A, Corbo V, Ali N, Pruessner JC. 2011. Investigation into the cross-correlation of salivary cortisol and alpha-amylase responses to psychological stress. Psychoneuroendocrinology. (Epub ahead of print)

Garcia-Leal C, Parente AC, Del-Ben CM, Guimara˜es FS, Moreira AC, Elias LL, Graeff FG. 2005. Anxiety and salivary cortisol in symptomatic and nonsymptomatic panic patients and healthy volunteers performing simulated public speaking. Psychiatry Res 133: 239-252.

Granger DA, Kivlighan KT, el-Sheikh M, Gordis EB, Stroud LR. 2007. Salivary alpha-amylase in biobehavioral research: recent developments and applications. Ann N Y Acad Sci 1098: 122-144.

Gray P, Cooney J. 1982. Stress-induced responses and open-field behavior in estrous and nonestrous mice. Physiol Behav 29: 287-292.

Gurguis GN, Mefford IN, Uhde TW. 1991. Hypothalamic-pituitary- adrenocortical activity in panic disorder: Relationship to plasma catecholamine metabolites. Biol Psychiatry 30: 502-506.

Hoehn T, Braune S, Scheibe G, Albus M. 1997. Physiological, biochemical and subjective parameters in anxiety patients with panic disorder during stress exposure as compared with healthy controls. Eur Arch Psychiatry Clin Neurosci 247: 264-274.

Holsboer F, von Bardeleben U, Buller R, Heuser I, Steiger A. 1987. Stimulation response to corticotropin-releasing hormone (CRH) in patients with depression, alcoholism and panic disorder. Horm Metab Res Suppl 16: 80-88.

Inagaki T, Ieda M, Yamashita S, Miyaoka T, Horiguchi J. 2011. Salivary alpha-amylase reactivity under psycho-physiological stress. A nonverbal communication measurement tool? J Behav Brain Sci 1: 12-15.

Kirschbaum C, Pruessner JC, Stone AA, Federenko I, Gaab J, Lintz D, Schommer N, Hellhammer DH. 1995. Persistent high cortisol responses to repeated psychological stress in a subpopulation of healthy men. Psychosom Med 57: 468-474.

Leyton M, Be´langer C, Martial J, Beaulieu S. 1996. Cardiovascular, neuroendocrine, and Monoaminergic responses to psychological stressors: Possible differences between remitted panic disorder patients and healthy controls. Biol Psychiatry 5: 353-360.

Liddell BJ, Brown KJ, Kemp AH, Barton MJ, Das P, Peduto A, Gordon E, Williams LM. 2005. A direct brainstem-amygdala-cortical 'alarm' system for subliminal signals of fear. Neuroimage 24: 235-243.

MacLeod C, Mathews A. 1988. Anxiety and the allocation of attention to threat. Q J Exp Psychol A 40: 653-670.

Makino S, Gold PW, Schulkin J. 1994. Corticosterone effects on corticotropin-releasing hormone mRNA in the central nucleus of the amygdala and the parvocellular region of the paraventricular nucleus of the hypothalamus. Brain Res 640: 105-112.

Mansell W, Clark DM, Ehlers A. 2003. Internal versus external attention in social anxiety: an investigation using a novel paradigm. Behav Res Ther 41: 555-572.

Mason JW. 1968. A review of psychoendocrine research on the pituitary-adrenal cortical system. Psychosom Med 30: 576-607.

Mathews A, Sebastian S. 1993. Suppression of emotional Stroop effects by fear-arousal. Cognition and Emotion 7: 517-530.

Nater UM, Rohleder N, Schlotz W, Ehlert U, Kirschbaum C. 2007. Determinants of the diurnal course of salivary alpha-α-amylase. Psychoneuroendocrinology 32: 392-401.

Nater UM, La Marca R, Florin L, Moses A, Langhans W, Koller MM, Ehlert U. 2006. Stress-induced changes in human salivary alpha-α-amylase activity—associations with adrenergic activity. Psychoneuroendocrinology 31: 49-58.

Petrowski K, Herold U, Joraschky P, Wittchen HU, Kirschbaum C. 2010. A striking pattern of cortisol non-responsiveness to psychosocial stress in patients with panic disorder with concurrent normal cortisol awakening responses. Psychoneuroendocrinology 35: 414-421.

Phelps EA, LeDoux JE. 2005. Contributions of the amygdala to emotion processing: from animal models to human behavior. Neuron 48: 175-87.

Redmond DE Jr. 1986. The possible role of locus coeruleus noradrenergic activity in anxiety-panic. Clin Neuropharmacol 9: 40-42.

Roth WT, Margraf J, Ehlers A, Taylor CB, Maddock RJ, Davies S, Agras WS. 1992. Stress test reactivity in panic disorder. Arch Gen Psychiatry 49: 301-310.

Roy-Byrne PP, Uhde TW, Post RM, Gallucci W, Chrousos GP, Gold PW. 1986. The corticotropin- releasing hormone stimulation test in patients with panic disorder. Am J Psychiatry 143: 896-899.

Schommer NC, Hellhammer DH, Kirschbaum C. 2003. Dissociation between reactivity of the hypothalamus-pituitary-adrenal axis and the sympathetic-adrenal-medullary system to repeated psychosocial stress. Psychosom Med 65: 450-460.

Schreiber W, Lauer CJ, Krumrey K, Holsboer F, Krieg JC. 1996. Dysregulation of the hypothalamic-pituitary-adrenocortical system in panic disorder. Neuropsychopharmacology 15: 7-15.

Simon A, Gorman J. 2004. Psychopharmacological possibilities in the acute disaster setting . Psychiatr Clin North Am 27: 425–458.

Southwick SM, Paige S, Morgan CA3rd, Bremner JD, Krystal JH, Charney DS. 1999. Neurotransmitter alterations in PTSD: catecholamines and serotonin. Semin Clin Neuropsychiatry 4: 242-248.

Squire, Larry R. Memory and the hippocampus. 1992. A synthesis from findings with rats, monkeys, and humans. Current issue feed Psychological Review, 99: 195-231.

Stones A, Groome D, Perry D, Hucklebridge F, Evans P. 1999. The effect of stress on salivary cortisol in panic disorder patients. J Affect Disord 52: 197-201.

van Stegeren A, Rohleder N, Everaerd W, Wolf OT. 2006. Salivary alpha amylase as marker for adrenergic activity during stress: effect of betablockade. Psychoneuroendocrinology 31: 137-141.

Weissman MM, Markowitz JS, Ouellette R, Greenwald S, Kahn JP. 1990. Panic disorder and cardiovascular/cerebrovascular problems: results from a community survey. Am J Psychiatry 147: 1504-1508.

Williams JMG, Mathews A and MacLeod C. 1996. The emotional Stroop task and psychopathology. Psychological Bulletin 120: 3-24.

Woon FL, Sood S, Hedges DW. 2010. Hippocampal volume deficits associated with exposure to psychological trauma and posttraumatic stress disorder in adults: a meta-analysis. Prog Neuropsychopharmacol Biol Psychiatry 34: 1181-1188.

Part 3

Assessment

9

Measuring States of Anxiety with Clinician-Rated and Patient-Rated Scales

Per Bech
Psychiatric Research Unit, Frederiksborg General Hospital, University of Copenhagen Denmark

1. Introduction

Most of the scales we use in clinical psychiatry when measuring mood and anxiety were developed more that three decades ago. Thus the Hamilton Anxiety Scale (HAM-A) (Hamilton 1969) is still the internationally most used clinician-rated scale within states of clinical anxiety, whereas Spielberger's State Anxiety Scale (Spielberger, Gorsuch & Lushene 1970) or the Symptom Checklist (SCL-90) (Derogatis et al. 1974) are among the most frequently used patient-rated questionnaires.

In her comprehensive content analysis of the items included in 27 different rating scales or questionnaires for clinical anxiety, de Bonis (1974) concluded that the HAM-A seems to cover the clinically most representative items for states of generalized anxiety. This can be considered in itself as one way of demonstrating the clinical validity of the HAM-A.

As concerns questionnaires, the Spielberger State Anxiety Scale covers the psychic anxiety symptoms whereas the anxiety subscale of the SCL-90 contains more somatic anxiety symptoms than psychic anxiety symptoms (Derogatis et al. 1974).

Although the SCL 90 includes some specific anxiety subscales, e.g., a phobia and an obsessive-compulsive (OCD) subscale, these anxiety subscales are also not sufficiently valid. The measurement of panic attacks is probably most validly measured in terms of minor versus major attacks, i.e. global assessments. The measurement of states of OCD is probably most validly measured by the duration of this state of anxiety, e.g. less or more than two hours daily. The Anxiety-Symptom-Scale (ASS) is shown in the Appendix as an example of a very short screening questionnaire covering the many subtypes of states of anxiety. In the following, it is the general state of anxiety as measured archetypically by the HAM-A, and by the corresponding self-rating scales that will be treated.

The psychometric validation of these general anxiety scales became important with reference to the classes of drugs most frequently investigated in trials of anti-anxiety medication, namely tricyclic antidepressants (e.g., imipramine) versus benzodiazepines (e.g., diazepam). Early on, Derogatis et al (1974) demonstrated that whereas imipramine was superior to diazepam when using the SCL-90 subscale of depression, no differences were obtained when using the SCL-90 anxiety subscale. The landmark study in this respect was the study by Rickels et al (1993) which demonstrated that when treating patients with generalized anxiety disorder with imipramine versus diazepam in a placebo-controlled, randomised trial, imipramine was superior to benzodiazepine on the psychic factor in the HAM-A but not on the somatic factor in the HAM-A.

These results led to a change in the algorithm of generalized anxiety from DSM-III to DSM-IV so that the number of somatic anxiety symptoms was reduced. However in the ICD-10 diagnostic manual (World Health Organization 1993) the number of somatic anxiety symptoms outranged the number of psychic anxiety symptoms in the algorithm of generalized anxiety disorder.
The following will treat the specific psychometrically valid methods (principal components analysis, factor analysis and item response theory analysis) in order to indicate how to use HAM-A and SCL-90 in trials of anti-anxiety drugs.

2. Methods

In clinical psychometrics we often describe principal components analysis (PCA) or factor analysis (FA) as the classical methods of validation while item response theory analysis (IRT) is seen as the modern method (Bech et al. 2011).
Historically, PCA was published at a later date than Spearman's two factor models of intelligence (Spearman 1904, Spearman 1927), namely by Hotelling (1933). When modifying a factor analysis with our sophisticated electronic programs, e.g. SPSS or SAS, we start today with PCA and then, if necessary, go for various forms of rotations in the so-called exploratory FA (Child 2006).
IRT analysis is used to evaluate to what extent the total score of a scale is sufficient when measuring the clinical effect of anti-anxiety drugs. We have both a parametric IRT model (Rasch 1960) and a non-parametric model (Mokken 1971). In the following, only Mokken analysis will be referred to.

3. Results

3.1 The Hamilton anxiety scale (HAM-A)

The first version of the HAM-A (Hamilton 1959) consisted of 13 items, whereas the revised version (Hamilton 1969) included 14 items (see Appendix). Hamilton released his HAM-A_{14} with reference to principal components analysis (PCA) on 115 patients (including patients with both primary anxiety states (N = 42) and patients with anxiety secondary to somatic disorders (N = 53)). Table 1 shows the results. The first principal component is clearly a general factor in which all the 14 items have positive loadings. The second principal component is a bi-directional, or dual factor with positive loadings on the psychic symptoms of anxiety and negative loadings on the somatic anxiety symptoms. Table 1 also shows the results from the study by Pichot et al (1981) on 411 patients from the family doctor setting with a mixture of primary and secondary states of anxiety. Pichot et al (1981) employed both a PCA approach and an exploratory factor analysis (FA) with varimax rotation. Essentially, Pichot et al (1981) found no extra information in the FA with rotation. As shown in Table 1, the PCA results of Pichot et al (1981) are very similar to those obtained by Hamilton (1969). The first principal component is obviously a general factor while the second principal component is a bi-directional factor. In the original publication by Pichot et al (1981) the sign of the second principal component loadings is actually the opposite of the signs published by Hamilton (1969), but this type of loading (negative and positive) is just a technical or topographical issue (Child 2006). The second principal component identified by Pichot et al (1981) contrasts psychic versus somatic symptoms of anxiety corresponding to Hamilton (1969).

Items	General factor		Dual factor	
	Hamilton (1969)	Pichot et al (1981)	Hamilton (1969)	Pichot et al (1981)
Anxious mood	0.66	0.50	0.50	0.39
Tension	0.83	0.62	0.32	0.35
Fears	0.49	0.45	0.29	0.35
Insomnia	0.52	0.65	0.05	0.26
Concentration	0.69	0.62	0.37	0.27
Depressed mood	0.69	0.66	0.33	0.38
Somatic (muscular)	0.52	0.54	-0.53	-0.25
Somatic (sensory)	0.73	0.58	-0.30	- 0.40
Cardiovascular	0.68	0.53	-0.41	- 0.48
Respiratory	0.56	0.52	-0.40	-0.43
Gastro-intestinal	0.66	0.29	-0.16	-0.39
Genito-urinary	0.45	0.33	-0.25	-0.31
Other autonomic	0.67	0.52	-0.14	-0.30
Behaviour at interview	0.60	0.70	0.10	- 0.09

Table 1. Principal Component Analysis of the Hamilton Anxiety Scale by Hamilton (1969) [N = 115] and Pichot et al (1981) [N = 411]

The usefulness of this two factor model of the HAM-A_{14} was demonstrated by Rickels et al (1993) in a double-blind, placebo-controlled trial comparing diazepam with imipramine in patients with a DSM-III diagnosis of generalized anxiety disorder. Imipramine was found superior to diazepam on the psychic anxiety symptoms (Table 1) on HAM-A, while both imipramine and diazepam were superior to placebo on the somatic anxiety symptoms (Table 1). However, among the psychic anxiety symptoms in HAM-A (Table 1) are such items as depressed mood and sleep.

Clinical validity was examined in a trial focussing on a 6-item HAM-A subscale (HAM-A_6) comprising five psychic anxiety symptoms (anxious mood, psychic tension, fears, intellectual difficulties, and anxious behaviour) and one somatic anxiety symptom (muscular tension) (Bech 2007). This group of HAM-A symptoms covering the core symptoms of generalized anxiety disorder is in accordance with the study by Snaith et al (1982).

The analyses performed by Meoni et al (2001) revealed that the HAM-A_6 items were among the symptoms in patients with DSM-IV generalized anxiety disorder with the most significant discrimination between venlafaxine and placebo.
The HAM-A_6 was compared to the HAM-A_{14} in order to evaluate the two scales' psychometric validity, using Mokken's non-parametric IRT model (Bech 2007). In this study the four placebo-controlled trials with fixed doses of pregabalin in patients with generalized anxiety disorder were combined, and Mokken analysis identified a coefficient of homogeneity of 0.35 for HAM-A_{14} while HAM-A_6 reached 0.46 (Bech 2007). A coefficient of homogeneity of 0.40 or higher is, in accordance with Mokken (1971), required to able to state that the total score of a scale is a sufficient statistic.
The pregabalin dose-response relationship study was performed on six of the available placebo-controlled trials (Bech 2007). One US trial was excluded from the analysis because more than 30% of the patients dropped out during the planned trial period of 4 weeks. The quality of a trial is, among other things, evaluated by the percentage of patients completing the planned short-term study, and 70% is used in this context (Angst et al. 1989). Another trial (Montgomery et al. 2006) was excluded because the HAM-A_{14} baseline mean score was higher than the mean score of the other trials (27.4 versus 24.5 ($P \leq 0.01$)) and because the age of the patients was high (44.0 (12) versus 37.2 (10) ($P \leq 0.01$)) (Bech 2007).
Effect size was used as response criterion in this pooled analysis of the four trials with sufficient homogeneity. An effect size of 0.40 or higher was considered to be evidence of a clinically significant effect of pregabalin compared to placebo (Bech 2007). A dose of 150 mg pregabalin over four weeks proved to obtain an effect size between 0.17 and 0.22 on HAM-A_6; and between 0.24 and 0.38 on HAM-A_{14}, i.e. not clinically significant. In a dose range between 200 mg and 450 mg daily, the pregabalin effect size was between 0.44 and 0.55 on the HAM-A_6 and 0.37 and 0.68 on the HAM-A_{14}. A dose of 600 mg pregabalin daily did not increase the effect size, as the range on the HAM-A_6 was between 0.36 and 0.50 (Bech 2007).
The trial excluded from this pooled analysis due to a significantly higher baseline HAM-A_{14} and patient age is the study by Montgomery et al (Montgomery et al. 2006). Table 2 shows the results after 4 weeks of therapy in the Montgomery et al study (2006), using effect size as response criterion. The HAM-A_6 effect size of both 400 and 600 mg pregabalin was between 0.28 and 0.30, while the effect size of 75 mg venlafaxine daily over four weeks reached a level of 0.40 (Bech 2007). In Table 2 the effect size for the HAM-A item of sleep is included, here the results show that the effect size was clearly above 0.40 for both doses of pregabalin whereas the venlafaxine effect size was below 0.40; indicating that venlafaxine is a non-sedating drug.

Treatment	Effect size		
	HAM-A_6	HAM-A_{14}	Sleep
Pregabalin 400 mg daily (N = 97)	0.30	0.38	0.65
Pregabalin 600 mg daily (N = 110)	0.28	0.31	0.54
Venlafaxine 75 mg daily (N = 113)	0.40	0.31	0.33

Table 2. The placebo-controlled trial by Montgomery et al (2006) with two fixed pregabalin doses and the active comparator venlafaxine. In the placebo arm N = 101. The results with effect size according to Bech (2007)

Lydiard et al (2010) have made an analysis of all six placebo-controlled pregabalin trials in generalized anxiety disorder, showing the change from baseline to endpoint on the individual HAM-A items. This analysis confirmed that no difference was seen between 450 mg and 600 mg pregabalin daily compared to placebo for the HAM-A_6 items. For the HAM-A_{14} item of depressed mood, however, 600 mg pregabalin was statistically more effective than 450 mg when compared to placebo ($P \leq 0.01$ versus $P \leq 0.05$), (Lydiard et al. 2010).
There are still very few instances in which HAM-A_6 and HAM-A_{14} have been used in trials with new generation antidepressants in patients with generalized anxiety disorder. An effect size of 0.38 was obtained on HAM-A_{14} in a placebo-controlled trial with sertraline (Allgulander et al. 2004). For venlafaxine Mitte et al (2005) obtained an effect size of 0.30 on HAM-A_{14} when pooling five placebo-controlled trials in patients with generalized anxiety disorder.
For duloxetine we only have one fixed dose trial in a placebo-controlled design in the treatment of generalized anxiety disorder over a 9 week period (Koponen et al. 2007). Based on the published results it was not possible to calculate effect size correctly (Koponen et al. 2007). However, the estimation of sample size in the Koponen et al study (2007) was based on the assumption that the pooled standard deviation of the change score on HAM-A_{14} from baseline to endpoint was 6.0, and that the difference in mean change score was 2.0 for duloxetine minus placebo. In this case, the effect size of 2/6, or 0.33, was accepted, i.e. at the level of venlafaxine (Table 2) for the HAM-A.

3.2 Symptom checklist (SCL-90)

The most comprehensive anxiety self-rating scale is the Symptom Checklist (SCL-90). Hamilton never developed a self-rating scale corresponding to his HAM-A_{14}. The original form of the SCL was developed by Parloff et al (1954). Historically, the final version was developed by Derogatis et al (1974), while the different subscales were most precisely defined by Bech (1993) . In a review Cyr et al (1985) discussed the factor structure of the SCL-90, concluding that principal component analysis (PCA) seems to identify the first principal component as a general factor, because all the 90 items are more or less positively correlated. However, exploratory factor analysis with varimax rotation as performed by Lipman et al (1977), obtaining a nine factor solution, has been used in several studies with the SCL-90. The anxiety subscale from this solution has never been accepted as a sufficient scale in trials of anti-anxiety drugs.
When using an unselected sample of patients treated in our Day Hospital at the Psychiatric Centre of North Zealand in Denmark (N = 555) we demonstrated with the SCL-90 that PCA identified as the first principal component a general factor reflecting that all the 90 items are more or less positively correlated (Bech et al. 2010). The second principal component was a bi-directional factor with depression items at one pole and anxiety items at the opposite.
We had previously identified a SCL depression subscale (SCL-D_6) with six items corresponding to the HAM-D_6. Now we selected from the second principal component the anxiety items with the highest loadings. When these items had been subjected to another PCA, we could demonstrate the contrast between psychic anxiety items and somatic anxiety items. This SCL-A_{20} anxiety subscale is very similar to the HAM-A_{14}. The SCL-D_6 and the SCL- A_{20} are shown in the Appendix.
Table 3 shows the results from a data set obtained by Danish psychiatrists in private practice (chaired by Drs. Bodil Andersen, Bettina N. Holm and Niels-Anton Rasmussen) who now use the SCL-90 in their daily routine. In Table 3 the four most frequent ICD-10 depression

diagnoses are shown at the top. The mean score on the depression scale (SCL-D_6) for dysthymia is approximately 10; this is the cut-off score for clinical depression. The mean scores on SCL-D_6 do increase from the category of mild depression to that of severe depression (Table 3). With regard to the anxiety subscale (SCL-A_{20}), the cut-off score for clinical anxiety is 30. The category of dysthymia obtained a mean score on the SCL-A_{20} just below 30 whereas the mean score for the depression categories increased with increasing degree of depression.

Diagnosis Code	**Category**	**Number of observations**	**SCL-D_6**	**SCL-A_{20}**
F 34.1	Dysthymia	(N = 43)	10.38	29.40
F 32.0	Depression, mild	(N = 192)	11.70	33.00
F 32.1	Depression, moderate	(N = 171)	12.12	34.00
F 32.2	Depression, severe	(N = 52)	13.20	37.00
F 34.1	Dysthymia	(N = 43)	10.38	29.40
F 43.0	Acute stress reaction	(N = 58)	9.36	27.00
F 41.2	Mixed anxiety/depression	(N = 28)	9.90	29.00
F 41.1	Generalized anxiety disorder	(N = 68)	11.28	36.40
F 43.1	Posttraumatic stress disorder	(N = 40)	13.50	43.20

Table 3. Standardization: SCL-D_6: A total score of 10 or more equals clinical depression
SCL-A20: A total score of 10 or more equals clinical anxiety

Table 3 also shows the four most frequent ICD-10 categories for anxiety, namely acute stress reaction, mixed anxiety-depression, generalized anxiety disorder, and PTSD (post-traumatic stress disorder). On the SCL-D_6, the cut-off score of 10 is obtained for GAD and PTSD, but not for mixed anxiety-depression which is in accordance with the ICD-10 criteria for this category. On the SCL-A_{20} the cut-off score for clinical depression is obtained for GAD and PTSD but not for mixed anxiety-depression, which is in concordance with the ICD-10 criteria for this category.

4. Discussion

Compared to the Hamilton Depression Scale (HAM-D) the Hamilton Anxiety Scale (HAM-A) has obtained a status as the international standard for anxiety measurement with a major impact on the item profiles of generalized anxiety disorder from DSM-IV to DSM-IV. We do not yet have the final version of DSM-V. As regards the ICD-10, research with HAM-A_{14} has shown that the category of generalized anxiety disorder according to ICD-10 is too biased in favour of the somatic anxiety symptoms. A revision of ICD-10, ICD-11, will be released around 2015. In the mean time the HAM-A_{14} is the most appropriate measure for generalized anxiety research. The HAM-A_{14} version shown in the Appendix was developed with the acceptance of Max Hamilton himself (Bech, Kastrup & Rafaelsen 1986). The correct use of the HAM-A is to focus on the $HAM\text{-}A_6$ in which the total score should be considered as a sufficient statistic.

Max Hamilton never constructed a self-rating version of his $HAM\text{-}A_{14}$. The $SCL\text{-}A_{20}$ included in the Appendix can be considered as a form of self-reported state of anxiety corresponding to $HAM\text{-}A_{14}$. As indicated in the Appendix, nine of the symptoms measure psychic anxiety and 11 items measure the somatic anxiety syndrome.

5. Conclusion

The measurement of states of anxiety by use of symptom rating scales such as the $HAM\text{-}A_{14}$ is psychometrically most valid in generalized anxiety. Within such states of anxiety the factors of psychic anxiety versus somatic anxiety are important. The $HAM\text{-}A_6$ covers the core items of the DSM-IV syndromes of generalized anxiety with most emphasis on the psychic anxiety symptoms. The $SCL\text{-}A_{20}$ is the SCL-90 subscale to most validly cover the $HAM\text{-}A_{14}$ symptoms.

The Anxiety Symptom Scale (ASS) is useful as a screening instrument to cover the whole field of anxiety states, including phobia, panic, or OCD.

6. Appendix

All the scales shown below are in the public domain.

1. Anxiety Symptom Scale (ASS)
2. The Hamilton Anxiety Scale ($HAM\text{-}A_{14}$)
   a. Scoring Sheet
   b. Manual
3. $SCL\text{-}D_6$
4. $SCL\text{-}A_{20}$

6.1 Anxiety symptom scale (ASS)

The following questions ask about how you have been feeling over the past two weeks. Please put a tick in the box that is closest to how you have been feeling.

	How much of the time during the past two weeks have you been bothered by	All the time	Most of the time	Slightly more than half the time	Slightly less than half the time	Some of the time	At no time
1	nervousness, tension or inner unrest?	5	4	3	2	1	0
2	worrying too much about even the most insignificant things in your daily life?	5	4	3	2	1	0
3	having to avoid certain things, places or activities as anxiety-provoking?	5	4	3	2	1	0
4	incipient anxiety attacks (panic)?	5	4	3	2	1	0
5	Actual anxiety attacks	5	4	3	2	1	0

6	**recurrent, unpleasant compulsive thoughts that won't stop?**	5	4	3	2	1	0
7	**having to check everything you do, again and again?**	5	4	3	2	1	0
8	**having to repeat the same actions, e.g. washing or counting**	5	4	3	2	1	0
9	**feeling very shy in company, for example when eating or drinking in front of other people?**	5	4	3	2	1	0
10	**difficulty in performing your daily activities because of these symptoms?**	5	4	3	2	1	0

When interpreting the ASS, first determine whether Item 10 (symptom impact on daily functioning) has a score of 3 or more. If this is the case, then determine which of the nine anxiety symptoms has the highest score, and thereafter whether there is a score on the top three symptoms; these are the true anxiety symptoms.
When measuring treatment effect it is of course possible to use the total score.

6.2 Hamilton anxiety scale
6.2.1 HAM-A$_{14}$ Scoring sheet

No.	Symptom	Score	
1	Anxious mood	0-4	
2	Tension	0-4	
3	Fears	0-4	
4	Insomnia	0-4	
5	Difficulties in concentration and memory	0-4	
6	Depressed mood	0-4	
7	General somatic symptoms (Muscular symptoms)	0-4	
8	General somatic symptoms (Sensory)	0-4	
9	Cardiovascular symptoms	0-4	
10	Respiratory symptoms	0-4	
11	Gastrointestinal symptoms	0-4	
12	Genito-urinary symptoms	0-4	
13	Other autonomic symptoms	0-4	
14	Behaviour during interview	0-4	
	Total score	0-56	

Symptoms scored from 0 to 4	Sum
0 = not present	6 to 14 = mild anxiety
1 = mild degree	15 to 28 = moderate anxiety
2 = moderate degree	29 to 52 = severe anxiety
3 = marked degree	
4 = maximum degree	

6.2.2 HAM-A14 Manual

1. Anxiety

This item covers the emotional condition of uncertainty about the future, ranging from worry, insecurity, irritability, apprehension to overpowering dread. The patient's report of worrying, insecurity, uncertainty, fear and panic, i.e, the psychic, or mental ("central") anxiety experience is to be found significant.
0: The patient is neither more nor less insecure or irritable than usual.
1: The patient reports more tension, irritability or feeling more insecure than usual.
2: The patient expresses more clearly to be in a state of anxiety, apprehension or irritability, which he may find difficult to control. It is thus without influence on the patient's daily life, because the worrying still is about minor matters
3: The anxiety or insecurity is at times more difficult to control because the worrying is about major injuries or harms which might occur in the future. E.g.: The anxiety may be experienced as panic, i.e. overpowering dread. Has occasionally interfered with the patient's daily life.
4: The feeling of dread is present so often that it markedly interferes with the patient's daily life.

2. Tension

This item includes inability to relax, nervousness, bodily tensions, trembling and restless fatigue.
0: The patient is neither more nor less tense than usual.
1: The patient indicates to be somewhat more nervous and tense than usual.
2: The patient expresses clearly to be unable to relax, full of inner unrest which he finds difficult to control, but still without influence on the patient's daily life.
3: The inner unrest and nervousness is so intense or so frequent that it occasionally has interfered with the patient's daily work.
4: Tensions and unrest interfere with the patient's life and work at all times.

3. Fears

A type of anxiety that arises when the patient finds himself in special situations. Such situations may be open or closed rooms, to queue, to ride a bus or a train. The patient shall experience relief by avoiding such situations. It is important to notice at this evaluation, whether there has been more phobic anxiety during the present episode than usual.
0: Not present.
1: Doubtful if present.
2: The patient has experienced phobic anxiety, but was able to fight it.
3: It has been difficult for the patient to fight or overcome his phobic anxiety which has thus to a certain extent interfered with the patient's daily life and work.
4: The phobic anxiety has clearly interfered with the patient's daily life and work.

4. Insomnia

This item covers only the patient's subjective experience of sleep length (hours of sleep per 24-hour-period) and sleep depth (superficial and interrupted sleep versus deep and steady sleep). The rating is based on the three preceding nights. Note: Administration of hypnotics or sedatives shall be disregarded.

0: Usual sleep length and sleep depth.
1: Sleep length is doubtfully or slightly reduced (e.g.due to difficulties failing asleep), but no change in sleep depth.
2: Sleep depth is now also reduced, sleep being more superficial. Sleep as a whole somewhat disturbed.
3: Sleep duration as well as sleep depth is markedly changed. The broken sleep periods total only a few hours per 24-hour-period.
4: It is here difficult to ascertain sleep duration as sleep depth is so shallow that the patient speaks of short periods of slumber or dosing, but no real sleep.

5. Difficulties in concentration and memory

This item covers difficulties in concentration, making decisions about everyday matters, and memory.
0: The patient has neither more nor less difficulties in concentration and/or memory than usual.
1: It is doubtful whether the patient has difficulties in concentration and/or memory.
2: Even with a major effort it is difficult for the patient to concentrate on his daily routine work.
3: More pronounced difficulties with concentration, memory, or descision making. E.g. has difficulties to read an article in a newspaper or watch a television programme right through. Scores 3 as long as the loss of concentration or poor memory has not clearly influenced the interview.
4: When the patient during the interview has shown difficulty in concentration and/or memory, and/or when decisions are reached with considerable delay.

6. Depressed mood

This item covers both the verbal and the non-verbal communication of sadness, depression, despondency, helplessness and hopelessness.
0: Natural mood.
1: When it is doubtful whether the patient is more despondent or sad than usual. E.g. the patient indicates vaguely to be more depressed than usual.
2: When the patient more clearly is concerned with unpleasant experiences, although he still is without helplessness or hopelessness.
3: The patient shows clear non-verbal signs of depression and/or hopelessness.
4: The patient's remarks on despondency and helplessness or the non-verbal ones dominate the interview in which the patient cannot be distracted.

7. General somatic symptoms (muscular symptoms)

This item includes weakness, stiffness, soreness merging into real pain, which is more or less diffusely localised in the muscles. E.g. jaw ache or neck ache.
0: The patient is neither more nor less sore or stiff in his muscles than usual.
1: The patient indicates to be somewhat more sore or stiff in his muscles than usual.
2: The symptoms have gained the character of pain.
3: The muscle pains interfere to some extent which the patient's daily life and work.
4: The muscle pains are present most of the time and interfere clearly with the patient's daily life and work.

8. General somatic symptoms (sensory symptoms)

This item includes increased fatigability and weakness merging into real functional disturbances of the senses. Including: Tinnitus, blurring of vision, hot and cold flushes and prickling sensations.
0: Not present
1: It is doubtful whether the patient's indications of pressing or prickling sensations (e.g.,in ears, eyes or skin) are more pronounced than usual.
2: The pressing sensations in the ear reach the character of buzzing in the ears, in the eye as visual disturbances, and in the skin as prickling or itching sensations (paraesthesias).
3: The generalized sensory symptoms interfere to some extent with the patient's daily life and work.
4: The generalized sensory symptoms are present most of the time and interfere clearly with the patient's daily life and work.

9. Cardiovascular symptoms

This item includes tachycardia, palpitations, oppression, chest pain, throbbing in the blood vessels, and feelings of fainting.
0: Not present.
1: Doubtful if present.
2: Cardiovascular symptoms are present, but the patient can still control the symptoms.
3: The patient has now and again difficulties in controlling the cardiovascular symptoms which thus to some extent interfere with the patient's daily life and work.
4: The cardiovascular symptoms are present most of the time and interfere clearly with the patient's daily life and work.

10. Respiratory symptoms

This item includes feelings of constriction or contraction in throat or chest, dyspnoea merging into choking sensations and sighing respiration.
0: Not present.
1: Doubtful if present.
2: Respiratory symptoms are present, but the patient can still control the symptoms.
3: The patient has now and again difficulties in controlling the respiratory symptoms which thus to some extent interfere with the patient's daily life and work.
4: The respiratory symptoms are present most of the time and interfere clearly with the patient's daily life and work.

11. Gastro-intestinal symptoms

The item includes difficulties in swallowing, "sinking" sensation of the stomach, dyspepsia (heartburn or burning sensations in the stomach, abdominal pains related to meals, fullness, nausea and vomiting), abdominal rumbling and diarrhoea.
0: Not present.
1: Doubtful if present (or doubtful if different from the patient's ordinary gastrointestinal sensations).
2: One or more of the above-mentioned gastro-intestinal symptoms are present, but the patient can still control the symptoms.

3: The patient has now and again difficulties in controlling the gastrointestinal symptoms which thus to some extent interfere with the patient's daily life and work. E.g. tendency of losing control over the bowels.
4: The gastrointestinal symptoms are present most of the time and interfere clearly with the patient's daily life and work. E.g. losing control over the bowels.

12. Genito-urinary symptoms

This item includes non-organic or psychic symptoms such as frequent or more pressing passing of urine, menstrual irregularities, anorgasmia, dyspareunia, premature ejaculation, loss of erection.
0: Not present.
1: Doubtful if present (or doubtful if different from the ordinary genito-urinary sensations).
2: One or more of the above-mentioned genito-urinary symptoms are present, but they do not interfere with the patient's daily life and work.
3: The patient has now and again one or more of the above mentioned genito-urinary symptoms to such a degree that they to some extent interfere with the patient's daily life and work. E.g. tendency to lose control over micturition.
4: The genito-urinary symptoms are present most of the time and interfere clearly with the patient's daily life and work. E.g. losing control over micturition.

13. Autonomic symptoms

This item includes dryness of mouth, blushing or pallor, sweating and dizziness. 0: Not present.
1: Doubtful if present.
2: One or more of the above-mentioned autonomic symptoms are present, but they do not interfere with the patient's daily life and work.
3: The patient has now and again one or more of the above-mentioned autonomic symptoms to such a degree that they to some extent interfere with the patient's daily life and work.
4: The autonomic symptoms are present most of the time and interfere clearly with the patient's daily life and work.

14. Behaviour at interview

This item is based on patient behaviour during the interview. Did the patient appear tense, nervous, agitated, restless, fidgeting, tremulous, pale, hyperventilating, or sweating?
On the basis of such observations a global estimate is made:
0: The patient does not appear anxious.
1: It is doubtful whether the patient is anxious.
2: The patient is moderately anxious.
3: The patient is clearly anxious.
4: The patient is overwhelmed by anxiety. E.g. shaking and trembling all over.

6.3 SCL-D_6

During the past week including today, how much were you bothered by:	Not at all	A little bit	Moderately	Quite a bit	Extremely
(30) Feeling blue	0	1	2	3	4

(26) Blaming yourself for things	0	1	2	3	4
(31) Worrying too much about things	0	1	2	3	4
(71) Feeling everything is an effort	0	1	2	3	4
(14) Feeling low in energy or slowed down	0	1	2	3	4
(32) Feeling no interest in things	0	1	2	3	4
Total score					

Standardization:
0 - 6 : no depression
7 - 11: mild depression
12 - 17: moderate depression
18 - 24: severe depression

6.4 SCL-A20 Anxiety scale

During the past week including today, how much were you bothered by:		Not at all	A little bit	Moderately	Quite a bit	Extremely
31	Worrying too much about things?	0	1	2	3	4
2	Nervousness or shakiness inside?	0	1	2	3	4
33	Feeling fearful?	0	1	2	3	4
57	Feeling tense or keyed up?	0	1	2	3	4
23	Suddenly scared for no reason?	0	1	2	3	4
17	Trembling?	0	1	2	3	4
72	Spells of terror or panic?	0	1	2	3	4
47	Feeling afraid to travel on buses, subways or trains?	0	1	2	3	4
25	Feeling afraid to go out of your house alone?	0	1	2	3	4

82	Feeling afraid you will faint in public?	0	1	2	3	4
55	Trouble concentrating?	0	1	2	3	4
42	Soreness of your muscles?	0	1	2	3	4
52	Numbness or tingling in parts of your body?	0	1	2	3	4
49	Hot or cold spells?	0	1	2	3	4
12	Pains in heart or chest	0	1	2	3	4
39	Heart pounding or racing?	0	1	2	3	4
48	Trouble getting your breath?	0	1	2	3	4
40	Nausea or upset stomach?	0	1	2	3	4
4	Faintness or dizziness?	0	1	2	3	4
78	Feeling so restless you can't sit still?	0	1	2	3	4
			Total score			

Standardization: A score between 20 and 29 is the risk zone of anxiety and a score of 30 or more is a clear clinical anxiety state

7. References

Allgulander, C., Dahl, A.A., Austin, C., Morris, P.L., Sogaard, J.A., Fayyad, R., Kutcher, S.P. & Clary, C.M. (2004), "Efficacy of sertraline in a 12-week trial for generalized anxiety disorder", *The American Journal of Psychiatry,* vol. 161, no. 9, pp. 1642-1649.

Angst, J., Bech, P., Boyer, P., Bruinvels, J., Engel, R., Helmchen, H., Hippius, H., Lingjaerde, O., Racagni, G., Saletu, B., Sedvall, G., Silverstone, J.T., Stefanis, C.N., Stoll, K. & Woggon, B. (1989), "Consensus Conference on the Methodology of Clinical Trials of Antidepressants.", *Pharmacopsychiatry,* vol. 22, pp. 3-7.

Bech, P. (2011), "Klinisk psykometri", *Munksgaard, Copenhagen Denmark,* .

Bech, P. (2007), "Dose-response relationship of pregabalin in patients with generalized anxiety disorder. A pooled analysis of four placebo-controlled trials", *Pharmacopsychiatry,* vol. 40, no. 4, pp. 163-168.

Bech, P. (1993), *Rating scales for psychopathology, health status and quality of life. A compendium on documentation in accordance with the DSM-III-R and WHO systems.* Springer, Berlin.

Bech, P., Bille, J., Lindberg, L., Waarst, S., Lauge, N. & Treufeldt, P. (2010), *Health of the Nation Outcome Scales (HoNOS). Ti år med HoNOS: 2000-2009,* Psykiatrisk Center Nordsjælland, Forskningsenheden. DK-3400 Hillerød, Hillerød.

Bech, P., Fava, M., Trivedi, M.H., Wisniewski, S.R. & Rush, A.J. (2011), "Factor structure and dimensionality of the two depression scales in STAR*D using Level 1 datasets", *Journal of Affective Disorders,* vol. in press.

Bech, P., Kastrup, M. & Rafaelsen, O.J. (1986), "Mini-compendium of rating scales for states of anxiety, depression, mania, and schizophrenia with corresponding DSM-III syndromes", *Acta psychiatrica Scandinavica.Supplementum,* vol. 326, pp. 1-37.

Child, D. (2006), *The essentials of Factor Analysis,* 3rd edn, Cassel Educational, London.

Cyr, J.J., McKenna-Foley, J.M. & Peacock, E. (1985), "Factor structure of the SCL-90-R: is there one?", *Journal of personality assessment,* vol. 49, no. 6, pp. 571-578.

de Bonis, M. (1974), "Content analysis of 27 anxiety inventories and rating scales" in *Psychological Measurements in psychopharmacology,* ed. P. Pichot, Karger, Basel, pp. 221-237.

Derogatis, L.R., Lipman, R.S., Rickels, K., Uhlenhuth, E.H. & Covi, L. (1974), "The Hopkins Symptom Checklist (HSCL) A measure of primary symptom dimension." in *Psychological measurements in psychopharmacology,* ed. P. Pichot, Karger, Basel, pp. 79-110.

Hamilton, M. (1969), "Diagnosis and rating of anxiety", *Br.J.Psychiatry,* vol. Special Publication 3, pp. 76-79.

Hamilton, M. (1959), "The assessment of anxiety states by rating", *The British journal of medical psychology,* vol. 32, no. 1, pp. 50-55.

Hotelling, H. (1933), "Analysis of a Complex of Statistical Variables with Principal Components", *Journal of Educational Psychology,* vol. 24, pp. 417-441.

Koponen, H., Allgulander, C., Erickson, J., Dunayevich, E., Pritchett, Y., Detke, M.J., Ball, S.G. & Russell, J.M. (2007), "Efficacy of Duloxetine for the Treatment of Generalized Anxiety Disorder: Implications for Primary Care Physicians", *Primary care companion to the Journal of clinical psychiatry,* vol. 9, no. 2, pp. 100-107.

Lipman, R.S., Covi, L. & Shapiro, A.K. (1977), "The Hopkins Symptom Checklist (HSCL): factors derived from the HSCL-90 [proceedings]", *Psychopharmacology bulletin,* vol. 13, no. 2, pp. 43-45.

Lydiard, R.B., Rickels, K., Herman, B. & Feltner, D.E. (2010), "Comparative efficacy of pregabalin and benzodiazepines in treating the psychic and somatic symptoms of generalized anxiety disorder", *The international journal of neuropsychopharmacology / official scientific journal of the Collegium Internationale Neuropsychopharmacologicum (CINP),* vol. 13, no. 2, pp. 229-241.

Meoni, P., Salinas, E., Brault, Y. & Hackett, D. (2001), "Pattern of symptom improvement following treatment with venlafaxine XR in patients with generalized anxiety disorder", *The Journal of clinical psychiatry,* vol. 62, no. 11, pp. 888-893.

Mitte, K., Noack, P., Steil, R. & Hautzinger, M. (2005), "A meta-analytic review of the efficacy of drug treatment in generalized anxiety disorder", *Journal of clinical psychopharmacology,* vol. 25, no. 2, pp. 141-150.

Mokken, R.J. (1971), *Theory and practice of scale analysis,* Mouton, Berlin.

Montgomery, S.A., Tobias, K., Zornberg, G.L., Kasper, S. & Pande, A.C. (2006), "Efficacy and safety of pregabalin in the treatment of generalized anxiety disorder: a 6-week, multicenter, randomized, double-blind, placebo-controlled comparison of pregabalin and venlafaxine", *The Journal of clinical psychiatry,* vol. 67, no. 5, pp. 771-782.

Parloff, M.B., Kelman, H.C. & Frank, J.D. (1954), "Comfort, effectiveness, and self-awareness as criteria of improvement in psychotherapy", *The American Journal of Psychiatry,* vol. 111, no. 5, pp. 343-352.

Pichot, P., Pull, C.B., von Frenckell, R. & Pull, M.C. (1981), "Une analyse factorielle de l'echelle d'appreciation de l'anxieté de Hamilton", *Psychiatria Fennica,* vol. 13, pp. 183-189.

Rasch, G. (1960), *Probalistic models for some intelligence and attainment tests,* Danish Institute for Educational Research, Copenhagen.

Rickels, K., Downing, R., Schweizer, E. & Hassman, H. (1993), "Antidepressants for the treatment of generalized anxiety disorder. A placebo-controlled comparison of imipramine, trazodone, and diazepam", *Archives of General Psychiatry,* vol. 50, no. 11, pp. 884-895.

Snaith, R.P., Baugh, S.J., Clayden, A.D., Husain, A. & Sipple, M.A. (1982), "The Clinical Anxiety Scale: an instrument derived from the Hamilton Anxiety Scale", *The British journal of psychiatry : the journal of mental science,* vol. 141, pp. 518-523.

Spearman, C. (1927), *The abilities of man: Their nature and measurement,* Macmillan, New York.

Spearman, C. (1904), "General intelligence objectively determined and measured", *American Journal of Psychology,* vol. 15, pp. 201-293.

Spielberger, C.D., Gorsuch, R. & Lushene, R.E. (1970), *The Stait-Trait Inventory: Test Manual,* Consulting Psychologist Press, Palo Alto, CA.

World Health Organization (1993), *International Statistical Classification of Diseases and Related Health Problems, 10th Revision (ICD-10). Diagnostic Criteria for Research.* World Health Organization, Geneva.

10

Social Anxiety Disorder, Fear of Public Speaking, and the Use of Assessment Instruments

Flávia de Lima Osório, José Alexandre S Crippa,
Jaime Eduardo C. Hallak and Sonia R.Loureiro
Ribeirão Preto Medical School, University of São Paulo
Brasil

1. Introduction

1.1 Social anxiety disorder

Social anxiety disorder (SAD) is considered to be the third most prevalent psychiatric disorder (Brunello, 2000; Moutier & Stein, 1999). The condition was officially recognized as a diagnostic category in the Diagnostic and Statistical Manual of Mental Disorders (DSM-III), in 1980 (American Psychiatric Association [APA], 1980), and currently, in the fourth edition of the manual (DSM-IV, APA, 1994), it is classified among anxiety disorders.

SAD is characterized by the fear and/or avoidance of public exposure and performance, in an attempt to avoid possible humiliation, shame or embarrassment, associated with significant subjective anxiety accompanied mainly by autonomic symptoms such as tachycardia, tremors, and sweating, with substantial psychic suffering and functional impairment (APA, 1994).

The most frequently feared and avoided situations include speaking, eating, drinking, and writing in public, interacting with strangers, people of the opposite sex, and authorities, and being the center of attention and/or the target of criticism (APA, 1994; Crippa et al., 2007). According to the situations avoided, SAD may be clinically classified as generalized (fear/avoidance of several performance situations and social interaction) or circumscribed (fear/avoidance of specific situations and events, the most frequent of which is public speaking) (APA, 1994; Raj & Sheehan, 2001).

The onset of SAD usually occurs in early adolescence (Crippa et al., 2007; Kessler et al., 1998). Although it is not considered a disabling condition, SAD causes severe impairment in such different areas of life as work, academic activities, family and loving relationships, and social and economic life (Furmark, 2000; Schneier et al., 1992; Stein et al., 2005). The level of comorbidity associated with SAD is significant - around 70% - and the most commonly associated conditions are depression, substance abuse (alcohol and drugs), dysthymia, suicidal ideation, and other anxiety disorders (Filho et al., 2010; Mohammadi et al., 2006; Raj &Sheehan, 2001; Wittchen & Fehm, 2003).

Despite its high prevalence rates (5-14%), the recognition of SAD as a pathological condition by patients and even by health professionals is low, around 3% (Davidson et al., 1993; Martin-Santos & Crippa, 2003). In a Brazilian study by Baptista (2006), only 0.8% out of 237

patients with SAD had been previously diagnosed, and none of them was aware, despite their experiences of impairment and limitations, that they suffered from an anxiety disorder. The under-diagnosis of SAD seems to be associated with its intrinsic characteristics, like the fear of seeking help due to the possibility of being criticized or negatively evaluated, as well as with the poor training of professionals in the field of mental health and others to recognize the condition (Crippa et al., 2008).
Although under-recognized, SAD is a treatable condition with good clinical response to pharmacological interventions, especially selective serotonin and noradrenalin reuptake inhibitors (Cordiolli, 2011), and to psychotherapy. Therefore, measures that favor the early and systematic recognition of SAD are important because they can bring relief to patients and prevent the onset of comorbid conditions and poor prognosis. In this context, assessment scales have a prominent role.

1.2 SAD assessment instruments

Instruments for the evaluation and measurement of symptoms are of great value for systematic diagnoses in Psychiatry, consisting of an excellent resource for the characterization of clinical signs and symptoms, prognosis, prediction of treatment response, and measurement of disorder severity in clinical and research settings (Ito & Ramos, 2000).
A number of resources to assess SAD are available today, from structured diagnostic interviews such as the Mini International Neuropsychiatric Interview (MINI – Amorin, 2000), the Composite International Diagnostic Interview (World Health Organization [WHO], 1997), the Anxiety Disorders Interview Schedule (ADIS – Di Nardo et al., 1983), and the Structured Clinical Interview for DSM-IV (SCID-IV – First et al., 1997), to self- and hetero-administered scales, of which there are many.
A literature review (Osório et al., 2009) concerning these instruments found 19 self-rated and three hetero-administered scales available in at least seven different languages, designed to assess from general aspects of SAD, such as the main feared and avoided situations (Social Phobia and Anxiety Inventory, Social Interaction Anxiety Scale, Social Phobia Scale, Liebowitz Social Anxiety Scale, Brief Social Phobia Scale), to specific features of the condition, including fear of public speaking (Personal Report of Confidence as a Speaker Questionnaire, Personal Report of Communication Apprehension), safety behaviors (Social Phobia Safety Behaviours Scale), negative beliefs (Social Thoughts and Beliefs Scale), and functional impairment (Liebowitz Self-Rated Disability Scale).

2. Studies involving different instruments for the assessment of SAD

As part of a broader investigation on different aspects of SAD, our research group in Brazil has adapted and assessed the psychometric properties of instruments aimed at improving the recognition of this condition, supporting clinical research on the efficacy of novel drugs for the treatment of SAD and furthering the understanding of its neurobiological substrates. The objective of this chapter is to present studies addressing (i) the adaptation and clinical validation of the module related to the diagnosis of SAD in the Structured Clinical Interview for DSM-IV (SCID-IV); (ii) the validation of the SAD screening instruments Social Phobia Inventory (SPIN) and its brief version (MINI-SPIN); and (iii) the validation of the Self-Statements during Public Speaking (SSPS) scale, used to assess cognitive aspects in SAD, and its adaptation to be used in the context of an experimental model of anxiety, the Simulated Public Speaking Test. These instruments have proven useful both in clinical practice and research settings. Additionally, they were shown to be easy and quick to apply and to require little training, thus having the potential to be established as important tools for researchers and clinicians involved with the study, diagnosis, and treatment of the many factors associated with SAD.

2.1 Structured clinical interview for DSM-IV (SCID-IV)

The objective of structured clinical interviews is to collect clinical and diagnostic data in a precise and exhaustive manner, especially for research purposes. Their use for the improvement of the validity and reliability of psychiatric diagnoses is also of unquestionable importance.

The SCID-IV was proposed in 1997 by First and colleagues. It is an instrument used for the elaboration of clinical psychiatric diagnoses based on DSM-IV criteria. The interview has a total of 10 modules that can be applied independently or in a combined manner, according to the objectives desired. Module F is the one used for the assessment of anxiety disorders in general and SAD in particular. Module F for SAD comprises 15 questions directed at establishing the diagnosis and five questions related to specificities of the disorder (subtype, onset, etc.). The interview is commonly conducted face-to-face and its duration varies as a function of the presence of symptoms to be investigated.

The accuracy of SAD diagnoses obtained through structured interviews has been evaluated, and the results obtained thus far show that the reliability of SAD diagnoses obtained with the original version of the SCID, as well as with versions adapted and translated into other languages, reaches satisfactory levels (Aziz & Kenford, 2004; Del-Ben et al., 2005; Lyneham & Rapee, 2005).

Although the SCID was developed to be used face-to-face, interviews in research settings (such as screening for epidemiological surveys) have also been carried out by telephone (Aziz & Kenford, 2004; Carlbring et al., 2007). Of the many advantages of telephone over in-person interviews, the following are worth mentioning: (a) cost efficiency, (b) simpler logistics, and (c) higher response rates (Carlbring et al., 2007; Lyneham & Rapee, 2005). As SAD may lead to the avoidance of social situations where there is potential for negative evaluation by others, most patients may indeed prefer telephone-administered diagnostic interviews, which makes them particularly suited for epidemiological surveys. The interviewer may represent authority to SAD patients; therefore, feelings of discomfort concerning exposure and scrutiny may be present, and this could, in turn, lead to refusal to participate, especially in the case of those more severely affected by the condition. Besides the clear implications for research, confirmation of the adequacy of data obtained by telephone may promote clinical advance. The use of telephone interviews for research and clinical purposes relies on the premise that the diagnosis made in such conditions is as valid as that obtained in person.

We have recently conducted a study to check the specific reliability of the SCID-IV for the diagnosis of SAD in face-to-face interviews in a sample of 100 university students (Crippa et al., 2008). Assessments were performed by five raters with different levels of clinical experience, and the agreement rates for positive and negative SAD diagnoses were 86% and 89%, with a Kappa index of 0.80, indicators considered to be excellent. We have also evaluated the reliability of the instrument for the diagnosis of SAD via telephone interviews,

and it also proved valid and reliable. When the reliability of the face-to-face and telephone interviews for the diagnosis of SAD was tested, an agreement of 89% was found for SAD cases, and of 95% for non-SAD cases. The Kappa value was 0.85, demonstrating the high correlation between these two forms of assessment (Crippa et al., 2008) and lending further support to the use of telephone interviews, which can be easily performed in around five minutes and have an excellent rate of acceptance (around 100%).
These findings support the acceptability of diagnostic interviews over the telephone, even when these are carried out by different mental health professionals. Therefore, telephone interviewing seems to be a useful tool for professionals in diagnosing SAD as the first stage of routine screening programs and epidemiological surveys. It allows an interview-based diagnosis to be made in situations where a face-to-face interview at the hospital or outpatient clinic is impossible.

2.2 Social phobia inventory (SPIN)

The Social Phobia Inventory (SPIN), elaborated by Connor and colleagues (2000), is a self-administered instrument proposed in order to satisfy the need for a brief and easily applied evaluation that conjointly assesses the physiological symptoms of fear and avoidance related to SAD. It consists of 17 items rated on a five-point Likert scale with a maximum total score of 68 (see Figure 1 for examples of SPIN items).

Social Phobia Inventory (SPIN)					
Instructions: *Please indicate how much the following problems have bothered you during the past week. Mark only one box for each problem, and be sure to answer all items*					
	not at all	a little	some what	very much	extre mely
2. I am bothered by blushing in front of people	(0)	(1)	(2)	(3)	(4)
10. Talking to strangers scares me	(0)	(1)	(2)	(3)	(4)
12. I would do anything to avoid being criticized	(0)	(1)	(2)	(3)	(4)
14. I am afraid of doing things when people might be watching	(0)	(1)	(2)	(3)	(4)

Fig. 1. Examples of SPIN items (adapted: Connor et al, 2000)

The psychometric qualities of the SPIN, demonstrated in the original study with samples of healthy individuals and subjects with SAD, were quite satisfactory, as indicated by the following properties: test-retest reliability, internal consistency (Cronbach's alpha), and convergent and discriminative validity. Factorial analyses of the instrument for the case sample indicated the extraction of five factors, namely: (1) talking to strangers and social situations; (2) criticism and embarrassment; (3) physiological changes; (4) authority figures; and (5) avoiding being the center of attention and public speaking. The SPIN and its subscales were also sensitive to identify the effects of pharmacological and psychotherapeutic treatments, proving to be an excellent instrument for the quantification of SAD symptoms and of the therapeutic effects of different treatment approaches.

Other studies were later conducted with the SPIN in order to determine its psychometric qualities in different settings. These studies were performed using three versions of the instrument in addition to the original one, applied to clinical and non-clinical samples of adults and to a non-clinical population of adolescents: a Brazilian (Osório et al., 2008a; 2010a), a Finnish (Ranta et al., 2007), and a French (Radomsky et al., 2006) version.

Our group performed a study using the Brazilian version of the SPIN with a sample of 2.314 university students, 88 SAD cases, and 90 SAD non-cases (Osório et al., 2009a; 2010a) to examine different parameters related to the validity of the scale.

Comparatively, SAD cases had significantly higher scores in all the items of the SPIN in relation to the general population sample, which in turn had higher scores than the non-case sample, demonstrating a higher prevalence of fear and avoidance behaviors in SAD cases and the lowest prevalence in non-cases. Among students from the general population and those diagnosed as SAD cases, the highest scores were seen in item 11, relative to the avoidance of public speaking (*"I avoid having to give speeches"*). Among SAD non-cases, the highest scores were found for item 5 (*"Being criticized scares me a lot"*).

In respect to the internal consistency of the SPIN in the three samples, the values obtained were quite similar and satisfactory (above 0.63). The total scale was the one with the best internal consistency, with values around 0.90, followed by the fear subscale, with values around 0.80. The avoidance and physiological symptoms subscales yielded values between 0.63 and 0.78. In general, the items had an adequate correlation with the total scale and contributed to increase its internal consistency.

Concerning the concurrent validity, the SPIN was initially compared to the Beck Anxiety Inventory (BAI), a self-rated instrument to assess general anxiety. For the general population of university students, the correlation between the two instruments was 0.63. For the sample of SAD cases and non-cases, the correlation values between the two scales were lower (0.42 and 0.25, respectively), as well as the correlations between the items. In general, these correlations were poorly defined, suggesting that although the two instruments may share common aspects, they have specificities that become clearer in samples of SAD cases and non-cases, in which diagnostic criteria ensure greater homogeneity.

These data indicate that a correlation exists, although weak and poorly defined, between the SPIN and the BAI, demonstrating the importance of specific instruments for the assessment of SAD. Screening instruments for general anxiety like the BAI are thought to cover some of the symptoms of SAD, but not its specificities, and this may result in the non-detection of the condition. Furthermore, screening with the BAI alone might attribute a prominent value to general anxiety symptoms that are common to many psychiatric disorders.

A concurrent validity analysis assessed the correlation between the SPIN and the Brief Social Phobia Scale (BSPS), a hetero-administered instrument to assess SAD. The values found were moderate (0.59 for SAD cases and 0.82 for non-cases), although the two scales were designed for the same purpose.

An explanation for this may be related to the different forms of assessing SAD. According to previous evidence, subjects completing self-rated instruments may underestimate their difficulties or fail to connect them with the disorder (Brunello et al., 2000; Figueira et al., 1994), whereas assessments performed by clinicians, especially those with specific training, tend to provide a more realistic symptom evaluation. In fact, studies on other anxiety disorders converge to this same point (Taylor et al., 1997). In the case of SAD, however, self-ratings are believed to have greater validity and reliability due to the intrinsic characteristics of the condition, which involve situations of social interaction and exposure.

In respect to the discriminative capacity of the SPIN, scores between 19 and 21 points were the ones that proved most adequate for the screening of SAD, with sensitivity of 0.86, specificity of 0.87, and diagnostic efficiency of 85%.
The factorial analysis also yielded a five-factor solution for the sample of SAD cases, accounting for 69.7% of the data variance, and a three-factor solution for the general population sample, explaining 54.1% of the variance.
The analysis of data related to construct validity revealed that the SPIN has a direct relationship with three of the ICD-10 (WHO, 1993) and DSM-IV (APA, 1994) diagnostic criteria for SAD. However, two other criteria that are also essential for the diagnosis, such as perception that the fear experienced is irrational (criterion C) and presence of significant occupational, social, and professional impairments (criterion E), are not covered by the scale, which further supports its use as a screening instrument but not as a diagnostic tool for SAD. Thus, the use of the SPIN as a diagnostic instrument may over-estimate the presence of SAD, since cases of sub-threshold SAD (presence of fear and avoidance without significant functional impairment [Ranta et al., 2007]) may be rated as SAD cases.
The values detected for all the psychometric qualities studied were quite close to the findings of the original study by Connor et al. (2000), supporting the adequacy of the SPIN for the evaluation of SAD in different languages, countries, and cultures.

2.3 Mini social phobia inventory (MINI-SPIN)

The MINI-SPIN is a reduced version of the SPIN proposed by the authors of the original study (Connor et al., 2001). It consists of three items of the original SPIN that proved indicative of SAD under empirical investigation (Figure 2).

Mini Social Phobia Inventory (MINI-SPIN)
1. Fear of embarrassment causes me to avoid doing things or speaking to people
2. I avoid activities in which I am the center of attention
3. Being embarrassed or looking stupid is among my worst fears

Fig. 2. Items of the Mini Social Phobia Inventory (adapted: Connor et al, 2001)

To develop this instrument, the authors identified those items of the SPIN that best discriminated between SAD patients and controls. Out of the 17 items of the original scale, a subset of three items with the highest sensitivity and specificity values for the screening of SAD were selected. This brief version was tested in a sample of 7.165 primary care patients, with a cut-off score of six points resulting in a sensitivity of 88.7%, specificity of 90%, positive predictive value of 52.6%, negative predictive value of 98.5%, and diagnostic efficacy of 89.9% (Connor et al., 2001).
Using the same sample of university students enrolled in the study of the SPIN, we investigated the psychometric properties of the MINI-SPIN (Osório et al., 2007; 2010b).
The study on the main discriminative items of the SPIN, which gave origin to the MINI-SPIN (Connor et al., 2001), was re-applied for the data of the SAD cases and non-cases sample, with significant correlations observed in both groups. To Connor and colleagues (2001), items 6, 9, and 15 were the ones with the highest discriminative power. In the

Brazilian setting, however, the items with the best discriminative capacities were items 11, 15, and 9, with item 6 yielding values quite close to the ones found for these three items.

Considering the information above, it can be stated that no differences were found in relation to the items with the best discriminative power, which shows that the feared situations remain the same regardless of the cultural context and sample studied (clinical or non-clinical). One second aspect to be highlighted is that, given the similarity of the four items in terms of discriminative power, a modification of the MINI-SPIN could be devised considering the inclusion of item 11. This proposition is further justified by the fact that item 11 refers to the fear of public speaking, the most common fear in SAD and the one that most often characterizes the non-generalized subtype of the disorder (Baptista, 2006; Furmark, 2000; Stein et al., 1994). However, the psychometric properties of the brief scale modified as suggested here have not yet been the object of research.

Despite the change proposed, the original form of the MINI-SPIN is adequate from the psychometric standpoint. Taking the SCID-IV as the gold standard, the cut-off score of six was associated with adequate sensitivity, specificity, and positive and negative predictive values. It is worth mentioning that the cut-off score of seven appears to be the most adequate for the sample of Brazilian university students (Osório et al., 2007).

In the sample studied, the MINI-SPIN had significant correlations with the SPIN (0.82 to 0.86) and presented other psychometric qualities that were quite similar to those found for the original scale, which endorses the use of the MINI-SPIN as a brief screening and triage instrument with advantages in relation to the SPIN, such as shorter administration and rating times. These properties favor the large-scale use of the reduced version, especially in primary healthcare settings. Also, the psychometric properties of the MINI-SPIN found in the Brazilian study were similar to those reported in the studies by Connor and colleagues (2001) and Weeks and colleagues (2007), the latter performed in Australia. This underscores the adequacy of the MINI-SPIN in different samples and cultural settings, with excellent indicators of diagnostic efficiency (Connor et al., 2001; Osório et al., 2007; 2010b; Weeks et al., 2007).

2.4 Self statements during public speaking scale (SSPS)

Epidemiological studies have shown that the fear of public speaking is the most prevalent fear in the general population (Geer, 1965; Furmark et al., 2000), irrespective of gender, ethnicity, or age (Phillips et al., 1997).

In a study performed by Stein and colleagues (1996) with a community sample, one third of the respondents reported that they experienced excessive anxiety when speaking to a large audience. In addition, subjects mentioned having anxious cognitions about public speaking, including the following fears: doing or saying something embarrassing (64%), one's mind going blank (74%), being unable to continue talking (63%), saying foolish things or not making sense (59%), and trembling, shaking, or showing other signs of anxiety (80%). In total, 10% of the respondents reported that public-speaking anxiety had resulted in a marked interference with their work (2%), social life (1%), or education (4%), or had caused them marked distress (8%). Twenty-three subjects (5%) had public-speaking anxiety alone (i.e., without evidence of additional social fears).

Public speaking has also been indicated as the most prevalent fear in the generalized subtype of SAD, and the most common symptom leading to diagnoses of the circumscribed or non-generalized subtype of the condition. In a study by Baptista (2006), 91.6% of subjects with SAD reported having this fear, compared to 24% of non-SAD subjects.

These facts have encouraged studies to examine this specific situation. However, a previous investigation (Osório et al., 2005) reported on the paucity of standardized and validated instruments to assess aspects related to circumscribed SAD or to the cognitive features of the disorder. One important exception is the Self Statements during Public Speaking (SSPS) scale, developed by Hofmann & DiBartolo in 2000. The SSPS is based on cognitive theories that assume that social anxiety is the result of a negative perception of self and of others in relation to self. It is a self-rated instrument comprising two subscales: positive self-assessment and negative self-assessment, each with five items rated on a scale from 0 to 5, with a maximum total score of 50. Figure 3 presents examples of items of this instrument.

Self-Statements During Public Speaking						
Instructions: *Please imagine what you have typically thought to yourself during any kind of public speaking situation. Imagining these situations, how much do you agree with the statements given below? Please rate the degree of your agreement on a scale between 0 (if you do not agree at all) to 5 (if you agree extremely with the statement)*						
1. What do I have to lose? It's worth a try	(0)	(1)	(2)	(3)	(4)	(5)
4. A failure in this situation would be more proof of my incapacity	(0)	(1)	(2)	(3)	(4)	(5)
8. I'll probably "bomb out" anyway	(0)	(1)	(2)	(3)	(4)	(5)

Fig. 3. Examples of SSPS items (adapted: Hofmann & DiBartolo, 2000)

The psychometric qualities of the SSPS were evaluated in a general population sample of healthy female university and non-university students and in SAD cases by Hofmann & DiBartolo (2000), who found quite adequate validity and reliability parameters. Later, the SSPS was translated and adapted into two languages: German (Gerlach et al., 2007) and Brazilian Portuguese (Osório et al., 2008b).

Our research group has assessed the validity of the Brazilian version of the SSPS (Osório et al., 2008b), which showed adequate internal consistency (Cronbach's alpha = 0.64 - 0.94) and concurrent validity with general (BAI: r = 0.22 - 0.53) and specific measures (SPIN: r = 0.22 – 0.65) of anxiety and social anxiety. The structure factor of the scale was also examined and found to explain 52% of the data variance.

Furthermore, we found that the scale was able to discriminate between SAD cases and non-cases ($p<0.001$), and that the higher the positive self-assessment, the fewer were the SAD-related symptoms, and the higher the negative self-assessment, the stronger were the symptoms of SAD. These data agree with the study by Stein and colleagues (1996).

These findings point to the existence of correlations between cognitive mechanisms and the etiology of the fear of public speaking and SAD. Nonetheless, it is important to highlight that such correlations are unspecific, and that the fear of public speaking is only one of the typical symptoms of SAD which, although being the most prevalent, might not be present in all subjects (especially in cases of non-generalized SAD, in which other fears such as drinking and eating in public can predominate).

2.5 Self statements during public speaking scale – state version (SSPS-S)

The need for systematic studies on the association between anxiety and public speaking has fostered the design of experimental procedures simulating real-life situations.

One important example of such procedures is described in the study by McNair and colleagues (1982), who developed a clinical-experimental model of anxiety named Simulated Public Speaking Test (SPST), later modified by Guimarães, Zuardi, and Graeff (1987). The test, initially used to measure the anxiolytic effects of diazepam, consists of asking the subject to prepare a speech and present it in front of a video camera that records his performance (see Figure 4).

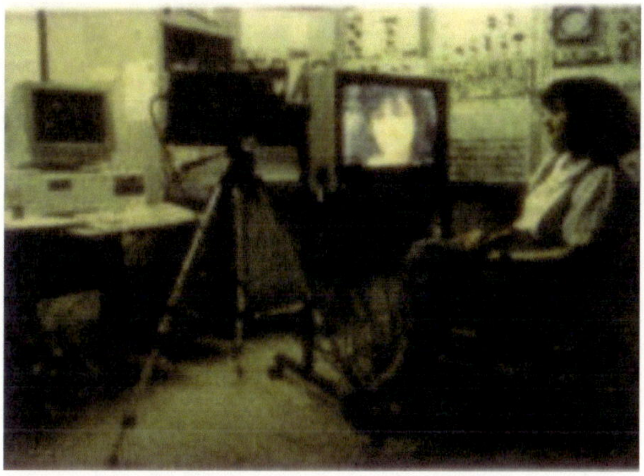

Fig. 4. Experimental Model: Simulated Public Speaking Test

The performance in the test is measured at seven phases: baseline (B), pre-stress (P), anticipatory (A), performance/speech (S), and post-stress/recovery (F0, F1, F2). Physiological measurements including heart rate, blood pressure, and skin conductance are recorded throughout the test, as well as subjective data related to the degree of tension, anxiety, and fatigue experienced in each phase of the experiment.

A literature review of studies using this experimental model (Osório et al., 2008c) revealed that instruments like the Visual Analogue Mood Scale (Folstein & Luria, 1973) and the State-Trait Anxiety Inventory (Spielberger et al., 1970) are often used to gauge subjective anxiety during the test, but that there are no standardized instruments available to assess cognitions associated with the experience.

Therefore, our group has proposed an adapted version of the SSPS, the Self Statements during Public Speaking Scale - state version (SSPS-S), to be used as a subjective measure of cognitive aspects in experimental models of anxiety, especially the SPST (Osório et al., 2010c).

The modification consisted of asking the subject to imagine what he would think about himself not in a hypothetical public speaking situation, as mentioned in the original instructions of the scale, but in the situation of talking in front of a camera. Therefore, the initial instructions were modified to: *"Imagine the things you are thinking now about yourself in this situation of talking in front of the camera. Keeping in mind this situation, to what extent do you agree with the statements given below? Please assign a note of 0 (if you fully disagree) to 5 (if you fully agree with the statement)".*

The SSPS-S proved sensitive to discriminate between SAD cases and non-cases throughout all the phases of the procedure, showing that cases make a lower positive assessment and a higher negative assessment of self and of their performance during public speaking as compared to non-cases. The negative subscale of the SSPS-S was the most sensitive and its indicators are shown in Figure 5.

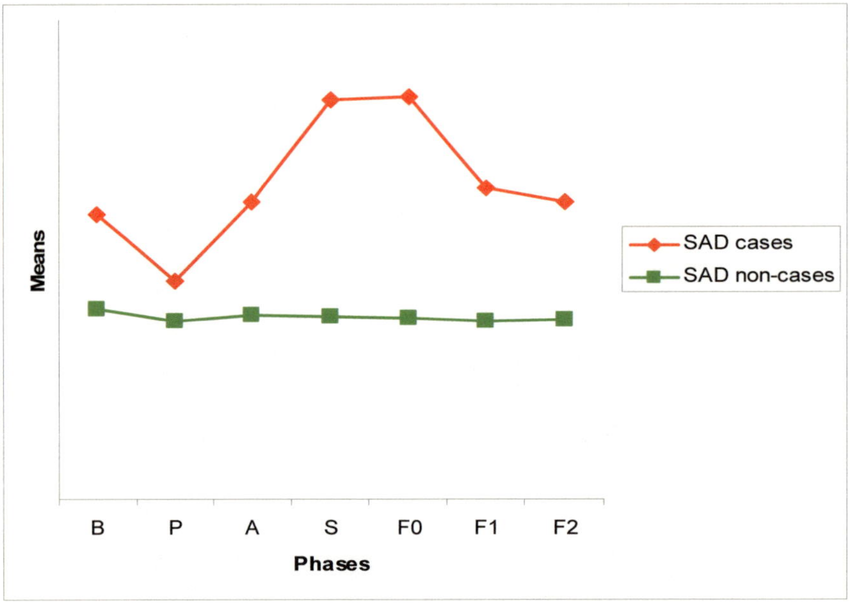

Fig. 5. Distribution of mean scores in the negative subscale of the Self- Statements during Public Speaking Scale - State version during the different phases of the Simulated Public Speaking Test

As the figure shows, the negative subscale bears positive correlations with the SPST for SAD cases, connected with the different levels of anxiety experienced: negative self-assessment decreases from baseline (B) to the pre-stress phase (P), increases from P to the anticipatory phase (A) and from this to the performance phase (S), tending to decrease in the post-stress phases (F0, F1, and F2). The same does not happen with non-cases, to whom measures remain stable during the experiment.

These data show that the SSPS-S is sensitive to assess the cognitive mechanisms associated with public speaking, and therefore with SAD.

3. Conclusion

This chapter describes studies concerning SAD screening instruments performed by our research group in Brazil. These studies are based on the premise that systematic assessment instruments have a crucial importance in Psychiatry, and particularly in the context of SAD, where a large percentage of under-diagnosis persists. This points to the need for actively seeking for individuals affected by SAD and for large-scale SAD screening in the community, where the use of scales is particularly valuable.

We have directed our efforts to the transcultural adaptation of previously validated instruments to the Brazilian context, filling an important gap in the national literature where such studies were scarce.

Our findings speak in favor of the adequacy of the instruments evaluated, regardless of the cultural setting in which they are used, which is of great importance especially for scientific research, fostering the conduction of multicenter studies.

The adaptations proposed in the forms of application of previously available instruments, such as the telephone administration of module F of the SCID-IV, might expand the use of the scale and increase its acceptance by subjects, since the contact by telephone is less frightening than face-to-face interactions for many people affected by SAD.

The adaptation of an instrument to assess cognition in an experimental model of anxiety may also foster a greater understanding of SAD and greatly contribute to treatment planning.

It is hoped that these studies shall contribute for the systematic assessment of SAD, especially in the Brazilian setting, encouraging clinicians and researchers to use the instruments now available.

4. References

American Psychiatric Association (1980). *Diagnostic and Statistical Manual of Mental Disorders* (3rd Edition), American Psychiatric Association, Washingtonn, DC.

American Psychiatric Association (1994). *Diagnostic and Statistical Manual of Mental Disorders* (4rd Edition), American Psychiatric Association, Washingtonn, DC.

Amorin, P. (2000). Mini International Neuropsychiatric Interview (MINI): validation of a short structured diagnostic psychiatry interview. *Revista Brasileira de Psiquiatria,* Vol.22, No 3, pp.106-115.

Aziz, M. A., & Kenford, S. (2004). Comparability of telephone and face-to-face interviews in assessing patients with posttraumatic stress disorder. *Journal of Psychiatric Practice,* Vol. 10, No. 5, pp.307–313.

Baptista, C.A. (2006). Estudo da prevalência do Transtorno de Ansiedade Social em estudantes universitários. *Dissertação (Mestrado),* Faculdade de Medicina, Universidade de São Paulo, Ribeirão Preto, 2006

Brunello, N.; Den Boer, J.A.; Judd, L.L.; Kasper, S.; Kelsey, J.E.; Lader, M.; Lecrubier,Y.; Lepine, J.P.; Lydiard, R.B.; Mendlewicz, J.; Montgomery, S.A.; Racagni, G.; Stein, M.B. & Wittchen, H.U. (2000). Social Phobia: diagnosis and epidemiology, neurobiology and pharmacology, comorbidity and treatment. *Journal of Affective Disordes,* Vol.60, pp.61-74.

Carlbring, P., Gunnarsdottir, M., Hedensjo, L., Andersson, G., Ekselius, L., & Furmark, T. (2007). Treatment of social phobia: Randomised trial of internet-delivered cognitive-behavioural therapy with telephone support. *British Journal of Psychiatry,* Vol. *190, pp.*123–128.

Connor, K.M.; Davidson J.R.; Churchill, L.E.; Sherwood, A.; Foa, E. & Weisler, R.H. (2000). Psychometric properties of Social Phobia Inventory (SPIN). *British Journal of Psychiatry,* London, Vol.176, pp. 379-386.

Connor, K.M.; Kobak, K.A.; Churchill, L.E.; Katzelnick, D. & Davidson, J.R. (2001). Mini-Spin: a brief screening assessment for generalized social anxiety disorder. *Depression and Anxiety,* Vol.14, pp. 137-140.

Cordioli, A.V. (2011). *Psicofármacos: consulta rápida.*Artmed, Porto Alegre.

Crippa, J.A.; Loureiro, S.R.; Baptista C.A. & Osório, F.L. (2007). Are there differences between early- and late-onset social anxiety disorder?. *Revista Brasileira de Psiquiatria*, Vol. 29, pp. 195-196.

Crippa, J.A.; Osório, F.L.; Del-Ben, C.M.; Filho, A.S.; Freitas, M.C.S. & Loureiro, S.R. (2008). Comparability Between Telephone and Face-to-Face Structured Clinical Interview for in Assessing Social Anxiety Disorder. *Perspectives in Psychiatric Care*, Vol. 44, pp. 241-247.

Davidson, J.R.; Hughes, D.L.; George, L.K. & Blazer, D.G. (1993). The epidemiology of social phobia: findings from the Duke Epidemiological Catchment Area Study. *Psychological Medicine*, Vol. 23, No. 3, pp. 709-718.

Del-Ben, C. M., Hallak, J. E., Sponholz, A. Jr., Marques, J. M., Labate, C. M., Contel, J. O., & Zuardi, A. W. (2005). Accuracy of psychiatric diagnosis performed under indirect supervision. *Revista Brasileira de Psiquiatria*, Vol. 27 , No.1, pp. 58–62.

Di Nardo, P.A.; Moraes, K.; Barlow, D.H.; Rapee, R.M. & Brow, T.A. (1993). Reliability of DSM-III-R Anxiety Disorder Categories. *Archives of General Psychiatry*,Vol. 50,pp. 251-256.

Figueira, I.; Coscarell, P.; Nardi, A.E.; Mendlowicz, M.; Marques, C.; Camisão, C.; Andrade, Y. & Versiani, M. (1994). Comparação entre fobia social e transtorno do pânico: psicopatologia geral e qualidade de vida. *Jornal Brasileiro de Psiquiatria*, Vol. 43, No. 5 , pp. 285-289.

Filho, A.S. ; Hetem, L.A.B. ; Ferrari, M.C.F.; Trzesniak, C. ; Martín-Santos, R. ; Borduqui, T.;

Osório, F.L. ; Loureiro, S. R. ; Busatto Filho, G. ; Zuardi, A.W. & Crippa, J.A.S. (2010). Social anxiety disorder: what are we losing with the current diagnostic criteria?. *Acta Psychiatrica Scandinavica*, Vol. 121, pp. 216-226.

First, M.B.; Spitzer, R.L.; Gibon, M. & Willians, J.B.W. (1997). *Structured Clinical Interview for DSM-IV Axis I Disorders - Clinican Version (SCID-CV)*, American Psychiatric Press, Washington, DC.

Folstein, M.F. & Luria R. (1973). Reliability, validity and clinical application of the Visual Analogue Mood Scale. *Psychological Medicine* , Vol 3, pp. 479-486.

Furmark, T. (2000). *Social Phobia – from epidemiology to brain function*. Dissertation (Doctor of Philosophy in Psychology), Uppsala University, 2000

Geer, J.H. The development of a scale to measure fear. (1965). *Behaviour Research and Therapy*, Vol.3, pp. 416-424.

Gerlach, A.L.; Heinrichs, N.; Bandl, C. & Zimmermann,T. (2007). SSPS- A German version of the questionnaire to assess the cognitive components of fear of public speaking. *Zeitschrift fur Klinische Psychologie und Psychotherapie: Forschung und Praxis*, Vol. 36, No. 2, pp.112-120.

Guimarães, F.S.; Zuardi, A.W. & Graeff, F.G. (1987). Effect of chlorimipramine and maprolitine on experimental anxiety in humans. *Journal of Psychoparmacology*, Vol. 1, pp. 184-192.

Hofmann, S.G. & Dibartolo, P.M. (2000) An instrument to assess self-statements during public speaking: scale development and preliminary psycometric properties. *Behaviour Therapy*, New York, Vol. 31, pp. 499-515.

Ito, L.M. & Ramos, R.T. (2000) Escalas de Avaliação Clínica Do Transtorno De Pânico. In: *Escalas de avaliação clínica em psiquiatria e psicofarmacologia*, Gorenstein, C.; Andrade, L.H.S.G.; Zuardi, A.W. , pp. 145-156, Lemos Editorial, São Paulo

Kessler, R.C.; Stein, M.B. & Berglund, P. (1998). Social phobia subtipes in national comorbitidy survey. *American Journal of Psychiatry, Hanover*, Vol. 155, No. 5, pp. 613-619, 1998.

Lyneham, H. J., & Rapee, R. M. (2005). Agreement between telephone and in-person delivery of a structured interview for anxiety disorders in children. *Journal of the American Academy of Child and Adolescent Psychiatry*, Vol. 44, No.3, pp. 274–282.

Martín-Santos, R. & Crippa, J.A.S. (2003). Transtornos de Ansiedad en Atención Primaria. In: *Abordaje de los problemas de salud mental en el ámbito extrahospitalario,* Solá, V.P., pp. 17-31, Profármaco, Barcelona.

Mcnair, D.M.; Frankenthaler, L.M.; Lzerlinsky, T.; White, T.W.; Sasson, S. & Fisher, S. (1982). Simulated public speaking as a model of clinical anxiety. *Psychopharmacology*, Vol. 77, pp. 7-10.

Mohammadi, M.R.; Ghanizadeh, A.; Mohammadi, M. & Mesgrpour, B. (2006). Prevalence of social phobia and its comorbitidy with psychiatric disorders in Iran. *Depression and Anxiety*, Vol.23, No.7, pp.405-411.

Moutier, C.Y. & Stein, M.B. (1999). The history, epidemiology, and differential diagnosis of social anxiety disorder. *Journal of Clinical Psychiatry*, Vol. 60, pp. 4-8.

Osório, F.L.; Crippa, J.A.C. & Loureiro, S.R. (2005). Instrumentos de avaliação do Transtorno de ansiedade social. *Revista de Psiquiatria Clínica*, Vol. 32, No. 2, pp. 73-83.

Osório, F., Crippa, J. A., & Loureiro, S. R. (2007). A study of the discriminative validity of a screening tool (MINI-SPIN) for social anxiety disorder applied to Brazilian university students. *European Psychiatry* Vol.22, No.4, pp.239–243.

Osório, F.L.; Crippa, J.A.S. & Loureiro, S.R. (2008a). Cross- cultural validation of the Brazilian Portuguese version of the Social Phobia Inventory (SPIN): study of the items and internal consistency. *Revista Brasileira de Psiquiatria*, Vol. 31, pp. 25-29.

Osório, F.L.; Crippa, J.A.S. & Loureiro, S.R. (2008b). Escala para auto-avaliação ao falar em público (SSPS): adaptação transcultural e consistência interna da versão brasileira. *Revista de Psiquiatria Clínica*, Vol. 35, pp. 207.

Osório, F.L.; Crippa, J.A.S. & Loureiro, S.R. (2008c). Experimental models for the evaluation of speech and public speaking anxiety: A critical review of the designs adopted. *The Journal of Speech - Language Pathology and Applied Behavior Analysis*, Vol. 2.4 - 3.1, pp. 97-121.

Osório, F.L.; Crippa, J.A.S. & Loureiro, S.R. (2009). Instruments for the Evaluation of Social Phobia. In: Social Phobia: Etiology, Diagnoses and Treatment. Hauppauge, Axelby, C.P., pp. 150-183, Nova Science Publishers.

Osório, F.L.; Crippa, J.A.S. & Loureiro, S.R. (2010a) Evaluation of the psychometric properties of the Social Phobia Inventory in university students. *Comprehensive Psychiatry*, Vol. 51, pp. 630-640.

Osório, F.L.; Crippa, J.A.S. & Loureiro, S.R. (2010b). Further Study of the Psychometric Qualities of a Brief Screening Tool for Social Phobia (MINI-SPIN) Applied to Clinical and Nonclinical Samples. *Perspectives in Psychiatric Care,* Vol. 46, pp. 266-278.

Osório, F.L. ; Crippa, J. A. S. & Loureiro, S. R. (2010c). Validação Trasncultural da versão estado de um instrumento de avaliação da ansiedade de falar em público. *Revista Brasileira de Psiquiatria*, Vol. 32, pp. S59.

Phillips, G.C.; Jones, G.E.; Rieger, E.R. & Snell, J.B. (1997). Normative data for the personal report of confidence as a speaker. *Journal of Anxiety Disorder*, Vol.11, pp. 215-220.

Radomsky, A.S.; Ashbaugh, A.R.; Saxe, M.L.; Ouimet, A.J.; Golden, E.R.; Lavoie, S.L. & O'connor, K.P. (2006). Psychometric properties of the French and English versions of the Social Phobia Inventory. *Canadian Journal of Behavioural Science*, Vol. 38, No. 4, pp. 354-360.

Raj, B.A. & Sheehan, D.V.(2001). Social anxiety disorder. *Medical Clinics of North America*, Vol. 85, No.3, pp. 711-733.

Ranta, K.; Kaltiala-Heino, R.; Rantanen, P.; Tuomisto, M.T. & Marttunen, M. (2007). Screening social phobia in adolescents from general population: the validity of the Social Phobia Inventory (SPIN) against a clinical interview. *European Psychiatry*, Vol. 22, No. 4, pp. 244-251.

Schneier, F.R.; Johnson, J.; Homig, C.D.; Liebowitz, M.R. & Weissman, M.M. (1992). Social phobia: comorbidity and morbidity in na epidemiologic sample. *Archives of General Psychiatry*, Vol. 49, No. 4, pp.282-288.

Spielberger, C.D.; Gorsuch, R.L. & Lushine, R.E.(1970). *Manual for the state-trait anxiety inventory*. Consulting Psychologists Press, Palo Alto, Califórnia.

Stein, M.B.; Walker, J.R. & Forde, D.R. (1994). Setting diagnostic thresholds for social phobia: considerations from a community survey of social anxiety. *American Journal of Psychiatry*, Vol.151, pp. 408-412.

Stein, M.B.; Walker, J.R. & Forde, D.R. (1996). Public speaking fears in a community sample. Prevalence, impact on functioning and diagnostic classification. *Archives of General Psychiatry*, Vol.53, pp.169-174.

Stein, M.B.; Roy-Byrne, P.P; Craske, M.G.; Bystritsky, A.; Sullivan, G.; Pyne, J.M.; Katon, W. & Sherbourne, C.D. (2005). Functional impact and health utility of anxiety disorders in primary care outpatients. *Medical Care, Philadelphia*, Vol. 43, No. 12, p. 1164-1170.

Taylor, S.; Woody, S.; Mclean, P.D. & Koch, W.J. (1997). Sensitivity of outcome measures for treatments of generalized social phobia. *Assessment*, Vol. 4, No.2, pp.181-191.

Weeks, J.W.; Spokas, M.E. & Heimberg, R.G. (2007). Psychometric evaluation of the Mini-Socal Phobia Inventory (Mini-Spin) in a treatment-seeking sample. *Depression and Anxiety*, Vol. 24, pp. 382-391.

Wittchen, H.U. & Fehm, L. (2003). Epidemiology and natural course of social fears and social phobia. *Acta Psychiatrica Scandinavica*, Vol. 417, pp. 4-18.

World Health Organization (1993). *Classificação de transtornos mentais e de comportamento da CID-10: descrições clínicas e diretrizes diagnósticas*. Artmed, Porto Alegre.

World Health Organization (1997). *The Composite International Diagnostic Interview (CIDI)*, World Health Organization, Genova, Switzerland.

11

The Measurement of Health-Related Quality of Life in a Population with Generalized Anxiety Disorder – Findings from the QUEST Study

Neesha Harnam[1], Kathleen W. Wyrwich[1], Dennis Revicki[1], Julie C. Locklear[2] and Jean Endicott[3]
[1]United BioSource Corporation, Bethesda, MD,
[2]AstraZeneca Pharmaceuticals LP, Wilmington, DE,
[3]New York State Psychiatric Institute, New York, NY,
USA

1. Introduction

The quality of life (QOL) of persons affected by generalized anxiety disorder (GAD), a condition characterized by periods of excessive anxiety and worry (American Psychiatric Association 1994), is significantly impaired, with an established link between GAD and impairment in a variety of areas (Henning et al. 2007). GAD is associated with increased self-reported disability days and impairments in psychosocial functioning, role functioning, work productivity, and QOL (Massion et al. 1993; Kessler et al. 1999; Wittchen et al. 2000; Kessler et al. 2001; Kessler and Wittchen 2002; Wittchen 2002). Consequently, comprehensive evaluations of treatment for GAD must include both clinical endpoints (i.e., Hamilton Anxiety Scale-Anxiety [HAM-A]) and assessments of patient-reported QOL and functioning. Moreover, it has been estimated that 92.1% of individuals with GAD also have another lifetime comorbid psychiatric disorder (Ruscio et al. 2007). Anxiety and depression often co-occur, and it has been proposed that a search for one condition should be accompanied by an assessment of the other (Kroenke et al. 2007). The inclusion of patient-reported outcomes (PROs) in clinical development programs for GAD treatments will provide useful information for clinicians and their patients about the benefits of treatment on patient functioning and well-being, and the relationship between GAD and depression.

The Quality of Life Enjoyment and Satisfaction Questionnaire (Q-LES-Q), in both the long and short form (Q-LES-Q(SF)), is a widely used instrument for measuring QOL and satisfaction. Originally developed for use in clinical trials and among trial participants with a wide variety of mental and medical diseases or disorders (Endicott et al. 1993), it has been shown to offer high internal consistency, validity and reproducibility in non-psychiatric populations and in patients with a range of psychiatric illnesses (Endicott et al. 1993; Ritsner et al. 2005; Rossi et al. 2005; Endicott et al. 2006; Schechter et al. 2007; Mick et al. 2008; Revicki et al. 2008). Thus, the Q-LES-Q(SF) is a PRO measure that has the potential to extend and complement clinical efficacy endpoints and demonstrate the impact of alleviating GAD symptoms on patients' everyday functioning. To date, few published studies have examined the validity of Q-LES-Q(SF) in GAD (Endicott et al. 2007; Demyttenaere et al. 2008; Revicki et al. 2008; Wyrwich et al. 2009; Matza et al. 2010; Wyrwich et al. 2011), and further studies are required to ascertain the sensitivity of the instrument to detect changes across the range of efficacy measures available to evaluate symptoms associated with GAD (including commonly observed co-occurring conditions). The availability of Q-LES-Q(SF) data from the Quality of life, Utilization of services and Effects of STress (QUEST) study (Revicki et al. 2008) provided the opportunity to contribute to existing evidence by further investigating the reliability, validity, and responsiveness of this instrument when administered via telephone as a measure of overall QOL and satisfaction related to various areas of functioning in patients with GAD.

2. Methods

This study was a post-hoc analysis of the QUEST study, which examined the treatment patterns, clinical and QOL outcomes, and direct and indirect costs associated with GAD in a US managed care organization; details of this study have been published elsewhere (Revicki et al. 2008). Briefly, this was a longitudinal study in which retrospective data were collected through an administrative claims database and prospective data were collected through telephone interviews. The study was approved by the institutional review board at Kaiser Permanente Northwest Region (KPNW Portland, Oregon), and complied with HIPAA requirements.

2.1 Study procedures

Patients who had 2 medical care encounters with diagnoses of GAD and/or anxiety state unspecified in the past 12 months (from 2003–2004) were recruited between June 2005 and June 2006. Eligible participants were identified through a review of the KPNW Data Warehouse. KPNW subsequently sent a memo and study fact sheet to the providers of each of these eligible participants asking for assistance in inviting their patients to participate. Interested potential participants, or those who did not invoke the initial refusal, were then contacted by telephone using a standardized screening script, during which time they were invited to participate in the study.

Other inclusion criteria included: a confirmed *DSM-IV* diagnosis of GAD (300.02) and/or anxiety state unspecified (300.00) based on the Structured Clinical Interview for *DSM-IV-TR;* age ≥18 years; the ability to speak and read English; and completion of a written informed consent. There were no treatment requirements; patients were assigned the standard of care. Patients with a diagnosis of psychosis, bipolar disorder, organic psychotic disorder or mental retardation within the past 12 months or who had current cognitive impairment (memory loss and temporal disorientation demonstrated during a telephone contact or reported by a family member) were excluded from the QUEST study. Retrospective data collection was conducted using administrative claims/encounter data to measure medical resource use and costs for the 12 months prior to the baseline survey, while prospective data were collected by following participants for a 6-month period, during which time 3 telephone interviews were conducted (at baseline, 3-month follow-up [10–14 weeks after baseline] and 6-month follow-up [22–26 weeks after baseline]) to administer several questionnaires. For purposes of this secondary analysis, the study population was limited to subjects with prospective data collected through the telephone interviews.

2.2 Measures administered

To evaluate overall QOL and satisfaction related to various areas of functioning, clinical symptoms associated with GAD, general health, fatigue, sleep, and disability, questionnaires administered in the study included the Q-LES-Q(SF), Patient Health Questionnaire Depression Questions (PHQ-8; (Kroenke and Spitzer 2002)), the Generalized Anxiety Disorder Questionnaire-IV (GAD-Q-IV (Newman et al. 2002)), the Structured Interview Guide for the Hamilton Anxiety Scale (SIGH-A (Hamilton 1959; Shear et al. 2001)), the Somatic Subscale of the Symptom Checklist (SCL-90 (Derogatis et al. 1974)), the Medical Outcomes Study 12-Item Short Form Health Survey, version 2 (SF-12v2 (Ware et al. 1996; Ware 2007)), Brief Fatigue Inventory (BFI (Mendoza et al. 1999)), Medical Outcomes Study Sleep Scale (MOS SS (Hays and Stewart 1992)), the Health Utilities Index Mark 2 (HUI2)/Mark 3 (HUI3 (Feeny et al. 1996; Horsman et al. 2003; Statistics Canada and US National Center for Health Statistics 2004)), the Sheehan Disability Scale (SDS (Leon et al. 1997)), and the Disability Days Questionnaire (DDQ (Broadhead et al. 1990; Revicki et al. 1994); Table 1). These were administered at baseline and at 3- and 6-month intervals, with the exception of the SIGH-A, which was only administered at baseline and 3 months.

Questionnaire	Characteristics	Scores
Q-LES-Q(SF)	• Participant-rated scale designed to measure the degree of enjoyment and satisfaction experienced by participants in their general activities of daily functioning • Composed of 14 general activity items (included in the score) and 2 additional items on medication satisfaction and overall life satisfaction item • Higher scores indicate greater enjoyment and satisfaction	0 to 100
PHQ	• 9-item scale consisting of the DSM-IV criteria used to diagnose MDD • Suicide item excluded in this study (PHQ-8) • Higher scores indicate greater depression severity	0 to 24
GAD-Q-IV	• 9-item self-reported revised diagnostic measure of GAD • Based on DSM-IV • Higher scores indicate greater anxiety severity	0 to 12
HAM-A (administered using SIGH-A)	• Developed to evaluate the severity of anxiety symptoms • Administered via the Structured Interview Guide for the [SIGH-A], the developer-approved interview guides for the HAM-A • Higher scores indicate greater anxiety severity	0 to 56
SCL-90	• Comprises 12 items that identify distress occurring from perceptions of bodily dysfunction • Higher scores indicate more somatic symptom distress	0 to 48

Questionnaire	Characteristics	Scores
SF-12 v2	• PCS and MCS scores used in this study • Scores < 50 represent below-average physical health or mental health	Norm-based scores with a mean of 50 and SD of 10*
BFI	• 9 items plus an introductory question used to measure fatigue in cancer patients • A single item on the BFI used in this study, which asks participants to rate their worst level of fatigue during the past 24 hours	0 (no fatigue) to 10 (as bad as you can imagine)
MOS SS	• 12-item self-reported questionnaire used to evaluate a participant's sleep disturbances over the past 4 weeks • Sleep Problem Index II was used in this study • Higher scores indicate more sleep problems	0 to 100
HUI2/HUI3	• Comprises the minimum number of questions (40 items) required to classify the health status of a broad range of participants (age 5 +) • Recall period for each item is the previous 4 weeks • Data on population norms are available for HU12 and HU13	0 (death) to 1.00 (best possible health)
SDS	• Patient-reported 3-item questionnaire • Assesses mental health-related functional impairment • In this study, for participants who selected "not applicable" for the work item, the mean value of their social and family items were substituted in for the work item when deriving the total scale score	0 to 30
DDQ	• Consists of 4 questions on missed work, late for work, bed disability and restricted activity days in the past 3 months due to GAD	0 to 92 days (each item)

BFI, Brief Fatigue Inventory; DDQ, Disability Days Questionnaire; GAD, Generalized Anxiety Disorder; GAD-Q-IV, Generalized Anxiety Disorder Questionnaire; HU12/HU13, Health Utilities Index; HAM-A, Hamilton Anxiety Scale; MDD, major depressive disorder; MOS SS, Medical Outcomes Study Sleep Scale; PHQ, Patient Health Questionnaire; Q-LES-Q(SF), Quality of Life Enjoyment and Satisfaction Questionnaire-Short Form; SIGH-A, Structured Interview Guide for the Hamilton Anxiety Scale; SCL-90, Symptom Checklist; SDS, Sheehan Disability Scale; SF-12, Short Form Health Survey.
*US-based population

Table 1. Questionnaires administered in the study (Hamilton 1959; Derogatis et al. 1974; Broadhead et al. 1990; Hays and Stewart 1992; Revicki et al. 1994; Feeny et al. 1996; Ware et al. 1996; Leon et al. 1997; Mendoza et al. 1999; Shear et al. 2001; Kroenke and Spitzer 2002; Newman et al. 2002; Horsman et al. 2003; Statistics Canada and US National Center for Health Statistics 2004; Ware 2007)

The Q-LES-Q(SF) total score was derived by summing scores from the first 14 Q-LES-Q(SF) items, each scored on a response scale ranging from 1 (very poor) to 5 (very good). The raw total score, which can range from 14 to 70, was then expressed as a percentage of the maximum (or % maximum) total score possible (ranging from 0–100) for ease of interpretation, with higher scores indicating greater enjoyment or satisfaction.

2.3 Statistical analyses

The eligible baseline sample (N = 296) was used for all baseline analyses. For 3- and 6-month analyses, those with at least 1 of these follow-up assessments were eligible for the respective analysis. Data analysis was conducted using SAS Version 9.1.3 (Copyright (c) 2002-2003 by SAS Institute Inc., Cary, NC, USA).

2.3.1 Reliability

Analyses of internal consistency from the baseline, 3-month, and 6-month data of the Q-LES-Q(SF) using Cronbach's alpha were conducted to ensure that the measure had strong internal consistency, where□ α >0.70 was indicative of a strong relationship among the measure's items (Cronbach 1951).

2.3.2 Validity

Convergent validity was examined by constructing and reporting the appropriate correlation coefficient (Pearson for continuous variables or Spearman for ordinal variables) between the Q-LES-Q(SF) with the PHQ-8, GAD-Q-IV, HAM-A, SCL-90, PCS, MCS, BFI, MOS SS, HUI2, HUI3, SDS, and the DDQ using the baseline data, and again using the 3- and 6-month data (with the exception of the HAM-A correlations calculated only at baseline and 3 months) to gauge the strength of the cross-sectional relationships as weak ($|r| < 0.30$), moderate ($0.30 \leq |r| < 0.60$), or strong ($|r| \geq 0.60$) (Hinkle et al. 1988). Moderate to strong relationships were hypothesized between the Q-LES-Q(SF) and all tested measures, except sleep and work-related measures, given the extreme nature of sleep and work when considered within overall QOL. The correlation of change scores across time (3 months - baseline and 6 months - baseline) were also analyzed to provide more support to the stability of the scale properties, and were hypothesized to be approximately the magnitude of the product of the cross-sectional correlations at each time point.

Analysis of variance (ANOVA) tests comparing the mean values on the Q-LES-Q(SF) scores between the participant groups listed below were conducted to examine discriminant (known groups) validity. Both unadjusted and adjusted comparisons were conducted using age, gender, and baseline Q-LES-Q(SF) as covariates when 3- and 6-month data were used, and statistical significance was set at the $P < .05$ level. Mean scores were compared for:

- Those with HAM-A scores ≤24 points and those with HAM-A scores >24 points (25–40) using the baseline scores (Matza et al. 2010).
- Those with GAD-Q-IV scores ≥5.70 and those with scores <5.70 cutoff (Newman et al. 2002).
- Those with total scores of ≥10 on the PHQ-8 and those with scores <10 (Kroenke et al. 2001).
- Those with SDS total scores ≥5 and those with SDS scores <5 (Leon et al. 1997).
- Those classified as asymptomatic (HAM-A ≤9); mild (HAM-A = 10–15), moderate (HAM-A = 16–24); or severe (HAM-A ≥25) using the baseline and 3-month data (Matza et al. 2010).

- Those with PHQ-8 total scores in the categories of 0–4 (minimal), 5–9 (mild), 10–14 (moderate), 15–19 (moderately severe) and 20–24 (severe) using the baseline, 3- and 6-month data (Kroenke et al. 2001).

Mean values for each of the groups were also compared to the Q-LES-Q(SF) norming values described in Schechter et al. (Schechter et al. 2007). In that investigation, controls were classified as never mentally ill (NMI); minor mental disorders only (MMD); currently not mentally ill (CNMI) with a history of mental illness that did not meet criteria for the MMD category; and currently mentally ill (CMI) with other than 1 specific phobia. Q-LES-Q(SF) mean scores were 81.8, 83.4, 78.4, and 72.7 for the NMI, MMD, CNMI, and CMI groups, respectively.

ANOVA tests were also conducted comparing the mean values on the Q-LES-Q(SF) change scores (3 months - baseline and 6 months - baseline) between the participant change groups listed below to assess responsiveness. Both unadjusted comparisons and adjusted comparisons were conducted using age, gender, and baseline Q-LES-Q(SF) as covariates when change scores were used, and statistical significance was set at the P <.05 level.

2.4 HAM-A change over time

Changes in anxiety were assessed using changes in HAM-A scores over the 3 months of the study. First, HAM-A responders (≥50% reduction in HAM-A scores at 3 months) were compared with HAM-A non-responders. Second, HAM-A remitters (HAM-A scores ≤7 at 3 months) were compared with HAM-A non-remitters.

2.5 PHQ-8 change over time

Changes in depression classification were assessed using changes in PHQ-8 levels over the 6 months of the study. The mean change scores were calculated for those who were at the minimal (0–4) level at baseline and stayed at minimal at 6 months, minimal at baseline and changed to mild depression (5–9) at 6 months, minimal to moderate (10–14), and mild at baseline to moderately severe (15–19), and minimal at baseline to severe (20–24) at 6 months. This same mean change scores analysis was executed among persons at the mild, moderate, moderately severe and severe levels at baseline and classified the change over the 6-month period to 1 of 5 PHQ-8 groupings (minimal, mild, moderate, moderately severe, and severe).

3. Results

Of the 296 participants in this study, 72.3% were female, with a mean age of 47.6 years (Table 2). The majority of participants identified themselves as white (92.9%), had at least some college education (75.3%), and most were employed on a full- or part-time basis (42.9 and 13.5%, respectively). At baseline, PHQ-8 mean scores corresponded with moderate depression, averaging 11.0 (possible range: 0–24; higher scores indicate greater depression severity), which is near the median of 12.5 reported in another GAD patient population (Kroenke et al. 2007). HAM-A scores indicated moderate levels of anxiety, averaging 16.7 (possible range: 0–56; higher scores indicate greater anxiety severity), which was lower than the range of 22.6–25.8 reported by Endicott et al. (Endicott et al. 2007) and the average of 25.54 reported by Wyrwich et al. in another GAD patient population (Wyrwich et al. 2009).

Mean SDS scores (13.7; possible range: 0–30; higher scores indicate greater impairment) were close to those seen in a primary care sample of GAD patients with an SDS score

Characteristic	N = 296
Age, y, mean (SD)	47.6 (13.7)
Female n (%)	214 (72.3)
White n (%)	275 (92.9)
Education n (%)	
Elementary/primary school	10 (3.4)
Secondary/high school	62 (20.9)
Some college	113 (38.2)
College degree	70 (23.6)
Postgraduate degree	40 (13.5)
Missing	1 (0.3)
Employment status n (%)	
Employed, full time	127 (42.9)
Employed, part time	40 (13.5)
Homemaker	20 (6.8)
Student	5 (1.7)
Unemployed	26 (8.8)
Retired	52 (17.6)
Disabled	19 (6.4)
Other	6 (2.0)
Missing	1 (0.3)
Baseline scores, mean (SD)	
PHQ-8	11.0 (5.6)
GAD-Q-IV	6.0 (3.0)
HAM-A	16.7 (7.2)
SCL-90	11.1 (7.3)
SF-12v2 - PCS	45.0 (10.3)
SF-12v2 - MCS	43.1 (8.3)
BFI	6.2 (2.3)
MOS SS (Sleep Quantity)	7.0 (1.8)
MOS SS (Sleep Problem Index II)	46.9(19.3)
HUI2	0.5 (0.2)
HUI3	0.5 (0.3)
SDS	13.7 (7.7)
DDQ (missed work days)	5.7 (13.8)
Q-LES-Q(SF)	55.8 (16.5)

Abbreviations: SD, standard deviation; PHQ-8, Patient Health Questionnaire; GAD-Q-IV, Generalized Anxiety Disorder Questionnaire-IV; HAM-A, Hamilton Anxiety Scale-Anxiety; SCL-90, Symptom Checklist; SF-12v2 – PCS, SF-12 Health Survey version 2 – Physical Component Summary; SF-12v2 – MCS, SF-12 Health Survey version 2 – Mental Component Summary; BFI, Brief Fatigue Inventory; MOS SS, Medical Outcomes Study Sleep Scale; HUI2/3, Health Utilities Indices, Mark 2/3; SDS, Sheehan Disability Scale; DDQ, Disability Days Questionnaire; Q-LES-Q(SF), Quality of Life Enjoyment and Satisfaction Questionnaire-Short Form

Table 2. Demographic characteristics for the generalized anxiety disorder patient sample

exceeding the cutoff of 5 or greater, which is an indicator of increased risk of mental health impairment (mean = 13.95) (Leon et al. 1997), and lower than the range of 14.3–17.5 seen at baseline in 3 independent studies among GAD patients (Endicott et al. 2007). Additionally, SF-12v2 PCS scores averaged 45.0 (possible range: 0–100; scores below 50 represent below average physical health), and SF-12v2 MCS scores averaged 43.1 (possible range: 0–100; scores below 50 represent below average mental health).

3.1 Reliability

Reliability of the Q-LES-Q(SF) at baseline, 3, and 6 months was excellent, with Cronbach's alphas of 0.88, 0.90, and 0.90, respectively. These reliability estimates 1) exceeded the recommended cutoff of 0.70; 2) demonstrated little change over time in the correlations of the Q-LES-Q(SF) items with each other; and 3) support the 1-factor structure of the Q-LES-Q(SF).

3.2 Validity

3.2.1 Construct validity

Using Pearson or Spearman correlations (as appropriate), convergent validity was examined between the Q-LES-Q(SF) and the PHQ-8, GAD-Q-IV, HAM-A, PCS, MCS, SDS, DDQ, MOS SS, SCL-90, BFI, HUI2, and HUI3 using the baseline data, and again using the 3- and 6-month data to gauge the strength and stability of the baseline relationships (Table 3). With the exception of correlations with the MOS SS at baseline, and the DDQ late for work at 3 months, all Q-LES-Q(SF) correlations were statistically significant at the $P<.05$ level. Measures of anxiety (GAD-Q-IV, HAM-A) demonstrated moderate correlations (with moderate defined as $0.30 < |r| < 0.60$) with values that were fairly consistent at baseline, 3 months and 6 months. The Q-LES-Q(SF) was most highly correlated with the PHQ-8, a measure of depression, with correlations of −0.69 at baseline, −0.73 at 3 months, and −0.72 at 6 months. Measures of general health (PCS, MCS) had moderate correlations and fairly consistent values at baseline, 3 months, and 6 months. As expected, the MCS had a higher correlation with the Q-LES-Q(SF) compared with the PCS. Measures of disability (SDS, DDQ bed days and kept from usual activity days) showed moderate correlations and consistency at baseline, 3 months, and 6 months. Sleep quantity, as measured through 1 MOS SS item, demonstrated a low correlation with the Q-LES-Q(SF) at baseline ($r = 0.08$), 3 months ($r = 0.17$), and 6 months ($r = 0.13$); however, the Sleep Problem Index II (also measured through the MOS SS) demonstrated moderate correlations of −0.49, −0.56, and −0.50 with the Q-LES-Q(SF) at baseline, 3 months, and 6 months, respectively. Distress due to perceptions of bodily dysfunction (SCL-90) and fatigue (BFI) also demonstrated moderate correlations and fairly consistent values at baseline, 3 months, and 6 months. Interestingly, data for measures of health utility (HUI2, HUI3) showed that the HUI3 demonstrated strong correlations ($r \geq 0.60$) with the Q-LES-Q(SF) at 3 and 6 months, while the HUI2 came close to, but did not achieve, this level of association with the Q-LES-Q(SF). Change score correlations supported the stability of the scale properties (data not shown), and slightly exceeded the hypothesized magnitude of the product of the cross-sectional correlations at each time point.

3.2.2 Known groups validity of the Q-LES-Q(SF)

Using a severe anxiety definition of HAM-A scores ≥ 24 (Matza et al. 2010), statistically significant ($P<.001$) differences in Q-LES-Q(SF) unadjusted mean scores between anxiety severity groups were observed at baseline and at 3 months (58.50 vs. 40.83 and 62.11 vs.

38.65, respectively), with higher Q-LES-Q(SF) mean scores observed in the less severe group (Table 4). Moreover, these differences between the mean scores were greater than 1 standard deviation (SD) at both time points. Analysis using adjusted scores demonstrated similar mean scores and differences between mean scores in these severity groups that were also greater than 1 SD.

Measure	Baseline		3 Months		6 Months	
	Correlation*	N	Correlation*	N	Correlation*	N
PHQ-8	–0.69	296	–0.73	246	–0.72	251
GAD-Q-IV	–0.43	296	–0.50	246	–0.48	251
HAM-A	–0.59	296	–0.60	246	[b]	[b]
SCL-90	–0.50	296	–0.54	246	–0.58	251
SF-12v2 - PCS	0.37	296	0.37	246	0.42	251
SF-12v2 - MCS	0.56	296	0.65	246	0.62	251
BFI	–0.45	295	–0.48	246	–0.50	251
MOS SS (Sleep Quantity)	0.08	296	0.17	246	0.13	251
MOS SS (Sleep Problem Index II)	–0.49	296	–0.56	246	–0.50	251
HUI2	0.48	262	0.59	209	0.59	223
HUI3	0.54	263	0.64	211	0.60	230
SDS	–0.54	296	–0.64	246	–0.55	251
DDQ[a]-Missed work	–0.25	172	–0.30	143	–0.27	147
DDQ[a]-Late for work	–0.25	171	–0.07	143	–0.26	147
DDQ[a]-Bed days	–0.32	294	–0.34	245	–0.31	251
DDQ[a]-Kept from usual activities	–0.36	296	–0.38	245	–0.52	250

*All correlations >0.08 were significant at the $p<0.05$ level.
[a]DDQ Recall period was over the past 4 weeks.
[b]HAM-A measured only at baseline and 3 months.
Abbreviations: Q-LES-Q(SF), Quality of Life Enjoyment and Satisfaction Questionnaire-Short Form; PHQ-8, Patient Health Questionnaire; GAD-Q-IV, Generalized Anxiety Disorder Questionnaire-IV; HAM-A, Hamilton Anxiety Scale-Anxiety; SCL-90, Symptom Checklist; SF-12v2 – PCS, SF-12 Health Survey version 2 – Physical Component Summary; SF-12v2 – MCS, SF-12 Health Survey version 2 – Mental Component Summary; BFI, Brief Fatigue Inventory; MOS SS, Medical Outcomes Study Sleep Scale; HUI2/3, Health Utilities Indices, Mark 2/3; SDS, Sheehan Disability Scale; DDQ, Disability Days Questionnaire

Table 3. Correlations of the Q-LES-Q(SF) with other clinician-reported and patient-reported outcomes in the QUEST study

Another known groups comparison of Q-LES-Q(SF) mean scores employed a different anxiety measure, the GAD-Q-IV, and a cutoff score of 5.70, a value that had previously been demonstrated to have optimal sensitivity and specificity for identifying individuals with GAD (Newman et al. 2002). Mean adjusted and unadjusted Q-LES-Q(SF) scores were similar (Table 4), with those above the 5.70 threshold reporting higher Q-LES-Q(SF) unadjusted mean scores of 61.12, 64.53 and 64.56 at baseline, 3 months, and 6 months, respectively, while those with scores below the threshold had unadjusted mean scores of 49.93, 49.66, and

49.48 at the baseline, 3-month and 6-month periods, with all differences between the 2 groups at the 3 time points nearing, if not exceeding, the 1 SD threshold. All of these groups' mean Q-LES-Q(SF) scores were much lower than NMI, MMD, CNMI, and CMI norming subgroups (Schechter et al. 2007), indicating the important burden on overall QOL and satisfaction related to various areas of functioning among patients with GAD.

Time	HAM-A ≤24 N, Mean (SD)	HAM-A >24 N, Mean (SD)	*P* Value[a]
Baseline	250, 58.50 (15.0)	46, 40.83 (16.4)	< .0001
3 month	216, 62.11 (15.5)	31, 38.65 (14.8)	< .0001
Time	**GAD-Q-IV <5.70 N, Mean (SD)**	**GAD-Q-IV ≥5.70 N, Mean (SD)**	***P* Value[a]**
Baseline	154, 61.12 (14.4)	142, 49.93 (16.6)	< .0001
3 month	156, 64.53 (14.8)	90, 49.66 (17.3)	< .0001
6 month	162, 64.56 (14.6)	88, 49.48 (16.1)	< .0001
Time	**PHQ-8 <10 N, Mean (SD)**	**PHQ-8 ≥10 N, Mean (SD)**	***P* Value[a]**
Baseline	132, 65.64 (11.9)	164, 47.79 (15.3)	< .0001
3 month	142, 67.54 (13.5)	105, 47.85 (15.3)	< .0001
6 month	159, 66.77 (13.1)	92, 46.22 (14.1)	< .0001
Time	**SDS <5.0 N, Mean (SD)**	**SDS ≥5.0 N, Mean (SD)**	***P* Value[a]**
Baseline	40, 68.98 (15.4)	256, 53.68 (15.7)	< .0001
3 month	56, 72.75 (14.4)	190, 55.06 (16.0)	< .0001
6 month	65, 71.38 (13.1)	185, 54.98 (15.8)	< .0001

[a]*P* Values for analysis of variance comparison.
Abbreviations: Q-LES-Q(SF), Quality of Life Enjoyment and Satisfaction Questionnaire-Short Form; HAM-A, Hamilton Anxiety Scale-Anxiety; GAD-Q-IV, Generalized Anxiety Disorder Questionnaire-IV; PHQ-8, Patient Health Questionnaire; SDS, Sheehan Disability Scale; SD, standard deviation

Table 4. Unadjusted Q-LES-Q(SF) mean scores for patients using recommended cutoff scores

Known groups analysis by severity group was also conducted using the PHQ-8. Using a minimal or mild depressive-state threshold of PHQ-8 scores <10, statistically significant (P<.0001) differences in Q-LES-Q(SF) unadjusted mean scores between those with minimal/mild depression compared with more severe depression were observed at baseline, 3 months, and 6 months (65.64 vs. 47.79, 67.54 vs. 47.85, and 66.77 vs. 46.22, respectively; P<.0001 for all comparisons), with higher Q-LES-Q(SF) mean scores consistently observed in the minimal/mild group (Table 4). Differences in mean scores between those with minimal/mild depression and those with more severe depression were greater than 1 SD at all 3 time points. Adjusted scores were similar to unadjusted scores and demonstrated equal levels of statistical significance. Again, all of these groups' mean Q-LES-Q(SF) scores were much lower that those found among any Q-LES-Q(SF) norming subgroups (Schechter et al. 2007).

Additional known groups validity of the Q-LES-Q(SF) was demonstrated when known groups based on disability status with an SDS cutoff score of 5.0 were evaluated. Subjects with SDS scores ≥5.0 were classified as at least moderately impaired, and had unadjusted mean Q-LES-Q(SF) scores of 53.68, 55.06, and 54.98 at the baseline, 3-month, and 6-month periods compared with subjects with less than moderate impairment, who had mean scores of 68.98, 72.75, and 71.38 for the same periods (Table 4). Differences in mean scores between those with moderate or greater impairment and those with less than moderate impairment exceeded 1 SD at the 3- and 6-month periods, with statistically significant differences at all 3 time points (*P*<.0001). Adjusted scores remained similar to the unadjusted scores, and demonstrated the same levels of statistical significance (*P*<.0001), and all of these groups' mean Q-LES-Q(SF) scores were much lower than any control subgroups (Schechter et al. 2007).

Unadjusted Q-LES-Q(SF) mean scores by 4 more refined HAM-A score severity groups (Fig. 1) and PHQ-8 severity levels (Fig. 2) were also similar to adjusted Q-LES-Q(SF) mean scores, with clear separation (>1/2 SD) of the sample in each score group for each time point when compared with adjacent groups (with the exception of the moderately severe vs. severe PHQ-8 comparison at 3 months). Statistically significantly (*P*<.0001) lower Q-LES-Q(SF) scores were observed as anxiety symptom severity increased, with pairwise comparisons that were statistically significant at baseline and 3-month follow-up (all unadjusted *P*<.01; all adjusted *P*<.001).

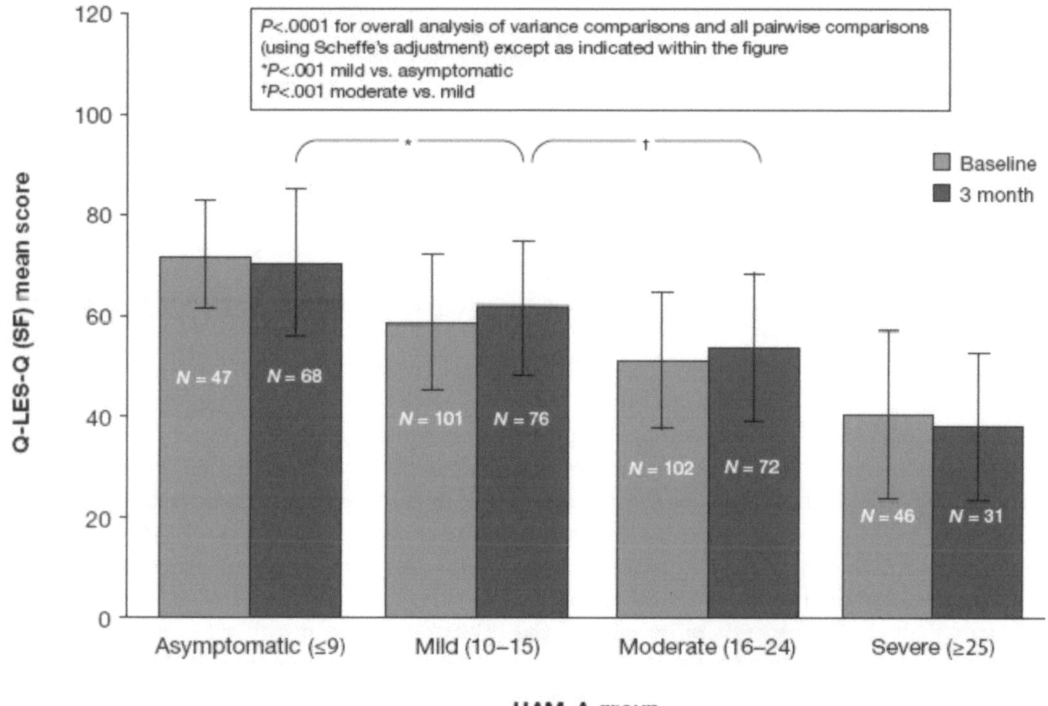

Abbreviations: Q-LES-Q(SF), Quality of Life Enjoyment and Satisfaction Questionnaire-Short Form; HAM-A, Hamilton Anxiety Scale-Anxiety

Fig. 1. Unadjusted Q-LES-Q(SF) mean scores by HAM-A score groups at baseline, month 3 – multiple comparisons between different HAM-A groups at each time point

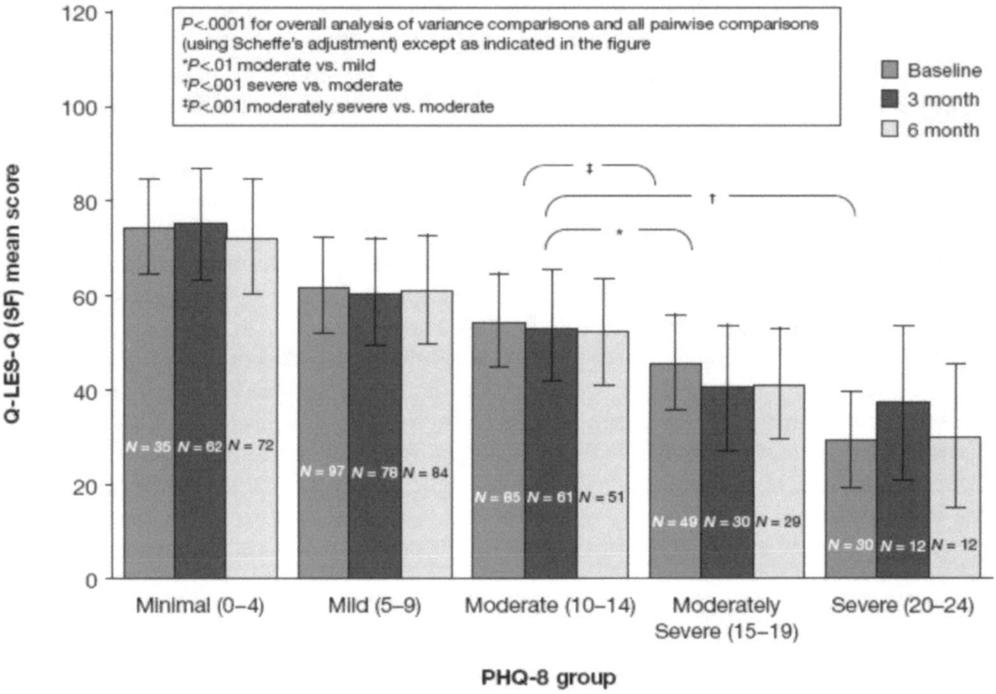

Abbreviations: Q-LES-Q(SF), Quality of Life Enjoyment and Satisfaction Questionnaire-Short Form; PHQ-8, Patient Health Questionnaire

Fig. 2. Q-LES-Q(SF) mean scores by PHQ-8 score groups at baseline, month 3 and month 6 – multiple comparisons between different PHQ-8 groups at each time point

3.2.3 Responsiveness of the Q-LES-Q(SF)

We conducted 3 different analyses to investigate the ability of the Q-LES-Q(SF) scores to detect important changes in this population of persons with GAD. T-tests compared responders with non-responders using 2 different criteria: HAM-A responders (patients who had at least a 50% reduction in their HAM-A scores between baseline and the 3-month follow-up), and HAM-A remitters (patients whose HAM-A scores decreased to levels at or below 7 points). In the HAM-A responders analysis, responders (n=229) had a mean level of improvement of 4.31 points on the Q-LES-Q(SF) over 3 months, compared with mean declines of 8.19 Q-LES-Q(SF) points for non-responders (n=16; P=.0011). HAM-A remitters (n=40) demonstrated a mean improvement of 10.85 points compared with the mean change of 2.06 points among non-remitters (n=205; P=.0006).

A third analysis tested the ability of the Q-LES-Q(SF) scores to detect a change over 6 months using change categories defined by PHQ-8 change scores (Table 5). The bolded values in this table represent the mean change scores for patients who remained in the same PHQ-8 depressive category over the course of the study; on average participants who remained in the minimal, mild, or moderate depression categories demonstrated very little change over time (≤2 points). For those who demonstrated a small improvement in depressive symptoms, as demonstrated by movement to a better adjacent category (italicized mean values), mean change levels ranged from 4.4 points (moderate → mild) to

10.8 points (severe → moderately severe). With few exceptions, all categories in Table 5 demonstrated a strong trend of decreasing Q-LES-Q(SF) mean change scores from baseline as depressive symptom categories worsened (left to right).

Baseline Depression Category (PHQ-8 Score)	Mean (SD), *N* 6-Month Depression Category (PHQ-8 Score)				
	Minimal (0–4)	Mild (5–9)	Moderate (10–14)	Moderately Severe (15–19)	Severe (20–24)
Minimal(0–4)	**-1.6** (10.1), 19	-4.3 (7.3), 11			-51.0 (n/a), 1
Mild (5–9)	*9.2* (13.7), 33	**-1.5** (11.5), 35	-0.2 (14.4), 14	-23.0 (12.7), 2	
Moderate (10–14)	18.4 (10.4), 11	*4.4* (12.3), 26	**-1.8** (14.6), 22	-21.3 (7.1), 4	-10.7 (5.0), 3
Moderately Severe (15–19)	20.8 (15.1), 5	16.0 (14.8), 13	*7.8* (12.6), 12	**-7.2** (16.0), 11	0.0 (12.7), 2
Severe (20–24)	39.3 (26.0), 4	36.0 (7.1), 2	11.0 (7.9), 3	*10.8* (12.3), 12	**3.7** (8.3), 6

Bolded values represent mean change levels for patient with GAD who stayed at the same depressive level over 6 months.
Italicized values represent mean change levels for patient with GAD who improved by 1 depressive level over 6 months.
Abbreviations: Q-LES-Q(SF), Quality of Life Enjoyment and Satisfaction Questionnaire-Short Form; PHQ-8, Patient Health Questionnaire

Table 5. Mean change Q-LES-Q(SF) scores, standard deviation and *N* by depression change categories over 6 months using PHQ-8 scores for classifying depression

4. Discussion

There is a critical need for psychometrically sound measures of mental health–related impairment (Leon et al. 1997). This study investigated the reliability, validity, responsiveness, and interpretation of the Q-LES-Q(SF) scores among the members of a group-model health care delivery system with GAD. Our findings strongly support the psychometric properties of the Q-LES-Q(SF) and give additional support for its use as a PRO in this mental health condition. Reliability was consistently robust, with Cronbach's alpha at 0.88 or higher at all time points (baseline, 3 months, and 6 months). High correlations (r ≥0.60) with other measures of anxiety and depression (PHQ-8 and HAM-A) at all time points, as well as the HUI3 at 3 and 6 months and SDS at the 3-month time point, support the construct validity of the measure. Although the Q-LES-Q(SF) scores demonstrated high correlations with these mental health severity measures, it is also important to note that the Q-LES-Q(SF) is not redundant with them; that is, there is at most 53% shared variance (-0.73^2) with the PHQ-8 at the 3-month measurement. Moreover, moderate ($0.30 < |r| < 0.60$) correlations with other measures associated with GAD (GAD-Q-IV, SCL-90, SF-12V2 PCS and MCS, BFI, HUI2, and disability days for missed work, bed days or kept from usual activities) were demonstrated at 1 or more of the time points.

In the current study, the Q-LES-Q(SF) mean baseline score was 55.8, and similar to the baseline mean score of 51.2 reported by participants across three GAD clinical trials (Wyrwich et al. 2009). A number of correlations between the Q-LES-Q(SF) and other outcomes detected in the current analysis are also consistent with previous studies, namely the low to moderate correlation with sleep measures, which mirrors that observed with the Pittsburgh Sleep Quality Index in other GAD samples (Wyrwich et al. 2009), and the moderate correlation between Q-LES-Q(SF) and HAM-A reported in 2 other studies (r = -0.45 (Endicott et al. 2007) and r = –0.36 (Wyrwich et al. 2009)).

Known groups validity found an effect size difference of 1 or more SDs between relevant groups using standard thresholds for classifying persons with GAD with HAM-A, PHQ-8, GAD-Q-IV, and SDS scores. Moreover, most of the relevant dichotomous cut points for the HAM-A (cut point of 24), PHQ (cut point of 10) and GAD-Q-IV (cut point of 5.70) yielded mean scores at similar levels, where the group with better health had a mean score of about 60–70 points, and the group with worst health averaged in the 40- to 50-Q-LES-Q(SF) point range. As seen earlier, all of these groups' mean Q-LES-Q(SF) scores were much lower than those found among any of the relevant subgroups of normal controls investigated by Schechter et al. (Schechter et al. 2007). Additional analyses comparing the change scores for HAM-A remitters and responders over 3 months, and PHQ-8 improvements in depressive states classifications over 6 months, yielded mean change scores in a consistent range corresponding to the responder threshold level established for persons with GAD in prior treatment studies.

In prior work we determined that the mean Q-LES-Q(SF) score change was 6.80 in patients experiencing minimal improvement reported by their clinicians using the Clinical Global Impressions-Improvement of Illness at 8 weeks (Wyrwich et al. 2009). In this post-hoc analysis, mean Q-LES-Q(SF) changes for the HAM-A responders and remitters were 4.31 and 10.85 points over 3 months, respectively. Similarly, small but possibly important changes on the PHQ-8 categories yielded mean change levels that ranged from 4.4–10.8 points over 6 months of observation, and these additional analyses appear to support the 6.80 point responder threshold using the novel anchors available in these data.

In considering potential methodological limitations of this study, it should be noted that retrospective data were collected through an administrative claims database, which may be subject to bias due to the inability to ensure coding accuracy. The fact that the Q-LES-Q(SF) does not represent a GAD-specific patient-reported measure of QOL is another potential limitation. However, the validity of the Q-LES-Q has been convincingly demonstrated across psychiatric disorders (Endicott et al. 1993; Ritsner et al. 2005; Rossi et al. 2005; Endicott et al. 2006; Schechter et al. 2007; Mick et al. 2008; Revicki et al. 2008). As an exploratory secondary data analysis, no method to control for the probability of family-wise type I error due to multiple comparisons planned was incorporated beyond Scheffe's method as mentioned for overall comparisons. Nonetheless, *P*-values were consistently less than .01 for all significant comparisons reported, and therefore, reduce the likelihood that any differences were the result of Type 1 error. Finally, questionnaires used in this study were administered via telephone. Previous psychiatric studies have successfully employed the telephone interview method for the administration of questionnaires (Larson et al. 2008; Kroenke et al. 2009; Simon et al. 2009). Cacciola et al. suggested caution in assuming comparability between telephone and in-person Structured Clinical Interview for DSM-III (SCID) Diagnosis based on telephone data collected from 41 college aged men with very limited psychiatric diagnoses (Cacciola et al. 1999); however, subjects in the QUEST study

were diagnosed with GAD by their physicians prior to study entry and the SIGH-A has demonstrated strong reliability among patients with GAD (Shear et al. 2001).
Although our focus in this investigation was on the psychometric properties of the Q-LES-Q(SF), it is important to note that these results also demonstrate the significant impairment to psychological well-being, physical functioning, work productivity, and additional disability associated with GAD. Despite estimated prevalence rates for GAD ranging from 2.7–5.4% in the general population in the United States and Europe (Massion et al. 1993; Kessler et al. 1999; Wittchen et al. 2000; Kessler et al. 2001; Henning et al. 2007), diagnosis and subsequent treatment are often missed (Kessler et al. 2005; Ruscio et al. 2007). Given the impact of this condition on health status and overall QOL (Revicki et al. 2008), this post-hoc study shows that Q-LES-Q(SF) constitutes a short, focused and psychometrically sound PRO that complements a range of outcome measures evaluating symptoms associated with patients with GAD seeking treatment for this condition.

5. Acknowledgments

The authors would like to acknowledge the editorial assistance of Eleanor Bull, PhD and Anusha Bolonna, PhD (PAREXEL). Financial support for this assistance was provided by AstraZeneca Pharmaceuticals LP.

6. Conflicts of interest

This study was supported by a research grant from AstraZeneca Pharmaceuticals LP, Wilmington, Delaware, USA.

7. References

American Psychiatric Association (1994). Diagnostic and Statistical Manual of Mental Disorders. Washington, DC, American Psychiatric Press.

Broadhead, W. E., Blazer, D. G., George, L. K. and Tse, C. K. (1990). "Depression, disability days, and days lost from work in a prospective epidemiologic survey." JAMA 264(19): 2524-8.

Cacciola, J. S., Alterman, A. I., Rutherford, M. J., McKay, J. R. and May, D. J. (1999). "Comparability of telephone and In-person structured clinical interview for DSM-III-R (SCID) diagnoses." Assessment 6(3): 235-42.

Cronbach, L. J. (1951). "Coefficient alpha and the internal structure of tests." Psychometrika 16: 297-334.

Demyttenaere, K., Andersen, H. F. and Reines, E. H. (2008). "Impact of escitalopram treatment on Quality of Life Enjoyment and Satisfaction Questionnaire scores in major depressive disorder and generalized anxiety disorder." Int Clin Psychopharmacol 23(5): 276-86.

Derogatis, L. R., Lipman, R. S., Rickels, K., Uhlenhuth, E. H. and Covi, L. (1974). "The Hopkins Symptom Checklist (HSCL): a self-report symptom inventory." Behav Sci 19(1): 1-15.

Endicott, J., Nee, J., Harrison, W. and Blumenthal, R. (1993). "Quality of Life Enjoyment and Satisfaction Questionnaire: a new measure." Psychopharmacol Bull 29(2): 321-6.

Endicott, J., Nee, J., Yang, R. and Wohlberg, C. (2006). "Pediatric Quality of Life Enjoyment and Satisfaction Questionnaire (PQ-LES-Q): reliability and validity." J Am Acad Child Adolesc Psychiatry 45(4): 401-7.

Endicott, J., Russell, J. M., Raskin, J., Detke, M. J., Erickson, J., Ball, S. G., Marciniak, M. and Swindle, R. W. (2007). "Duloxetine treatment for role functioning improvement in generalized anxiety disorder: three independent studies." J Clin Psychiatry 68(4): 518-24.

Feeny, D. H., Torrance, G. W. and Furlong, W. J. (1996). Health Utilities Index. Quality of Life and Pharmacoeconomics in Clinical Trials. B. Spilker. Philadelphia, Lippincott-Raven Press: 239-252.

Hamilton, M. (1959). "The assessment of anxiety states by rating." Br J Med Psychol 32(1): 50-5.

Hays, R. D. and Stewart, A. L. (1992). Sleep measures. Measuring Functioning and Well-Being: The Medical Outcomes Study Approach. A. L. Stewart and J. E. Ware. Durham, NC, Duke University Press: 235-259.

Henning, E. R., Turk, C. L., Mennin, D. S., Fresco, D. M. and Heimberg, R. G. (2007). "Impairment and quality of life in individuals with generalized anxiety disorder." Depress Anxiety 24(5): 342-9.

Hinkle, D. E., Jurs, S. G. and Wiersma, W. (1988). Applied Statistics for the Behavioral Sciences. Boston, Houghton Mifflin.

Horsman, J., Furlong, W., Feeny, D. and Torrance, G. (2003). "The Health Utilities Index (HUI): concepts, measurement properties and applications." Health Qual Life Outcomes 1: 54.

Kessler, R. C., DuPont, R. L., Berglund, P. and Wittchen, H. U. (1999). "Impairment in pure and comorbid generalized anxiety disorder and major depression at 12 months in two national surveys." Am J Psychiatry 156(12): 1915-23.

Kessler, R. C., Keller, M. B. and Wittchen, H. (2001). The epidemiology of generalized anxiety disorder. The Psychiatric Clinics of North America: Generalized Anxiety Disorder. O. Brawman-Mintzer. Philadelphia, W.B. Saunders: 19-40.

Kessler, R. C. and Wittchen, H. U. (2002). "Patterns and correlates of generalized anxiety disorder in community samples." J Clin Psychiatry 63 Suppl 8: 4-10.

Kessler, R. C., Brandenburg, N., Lane, M., Roy-Byrne, P., Stang, P. D., Stein, D. J. and Wittchen, H. U. (2005). "Rethinking the duration requirement for generalized anxiety disorder: evidence from the National Comorbidity Survey Replication." Psychol Med 35(7): 1073-82.

Kroenke, K., Spitzer, R. L. and Williams, J. B. (2001). "The PHQ-9: validity of a brief depression severity measure." J Gen Intern Med 16(9): 606-13.

Kroenke, K. and Spitzer, R. L. (2002). "The PHQ-9: a new depression diagnostic and severity measure." Psychiatric Annals 32: 509-521.

Kroenke, K., Spitzer, R. L., Williams, J. B., Monahan, P. O. and Lowe, B. (2007). "Anxiety disorders in primary care: prevalence, impairment, comorbidity, and detection." Ann Intern Med 146(5): 317-25.

Kroenke, K., Strine, T. W., Spitzer, R. L., Williams, J. B., Berry, J. T. and Mokdad, A. H. (2009). "The PHQ-8 as a measure of current depression in the general population." J Affect Disord 114(1-3): 163-73.

Larson, C. O., Schlundt, D., Patel, K., Beard, K. and Hargreaves, M. (2008). "Validity of the SF-12 for use in a low-income African American community-based research initiative (REACH 2010)." Prev Chronic Dis 5(2): A44.

Leon, A. C., Olfson, M., Portera, L., Farber, L. and Sheehan, D. V. (1997). "Assessing psychiatric impairment in primary care with the Sheehan Disability Scale." Int J Psychiatry Med 27(2): 93-105.

Massion, A. O., Warshaw, M. G. and Keller, M. B. (1993). "Quality of life and psychiatric morbidity in panic disorder and generalized anxiety disorder." Am J Psychiatry 150(4): 600-7.

Matza, L. S., Morlock, R., Sexton, C., Malley, K. and Feltner, D. (2010). "Identifying HAM-A cutoffs for mild, moderate, and severe generalized anxiety disorder." Int J Methods Psychiatr Res 19(4): 223-32.

Mendoza, T. R., Wang, X. S., Cleeland, C. S., Morrissey, M., Johnson, B. A., Wendt, J. K. and Huber, S. L. (1999). "The rapid assessment of fatigue severity in cancer patients: use of the Brief Fatigue Inventory." Cancer 85(5): 1186-96.

Mick, E., Faraone, S. V., Spencer, T., Zhang, H. F. and Biederman, J. (2008). "Assessing the validity of the Quality of Life Enjoyment and Satisfaction Questionnaire Short Form in adults with ADHD." J Atten Disord 11(4): 504-9.

Newman, M., Zuellig, A., Kachin, K., Constantino, M. J., Przeworski, A., Erickson, T. and et al. (2002). "Preliminary reliability and validity of the Generalized Anxiety Disorder Questionnaire-IV: a revised self-report diagnostic measure of Generalized Anxiety Disorder." Behavior Therapy 33: 215-233.

Revicki, D. A., Irwin, D., Reblando, J. and Simon, G. E. (1994). "The accuracy of self-reported disability days." Med Care 32(4): 401-4.

Revicki, D. A., Brandenburg, N., Matza, L., Hornbrook, M. C. and Feeny, D. (2008). "Health-related quality of life and utilities in primary-care patients with generalized anxiety disorder." Qual Life Res 17(10): 1285-94.

Ritsner, M., Kurs, R., Gibel, A., Ratner, Y. and Endicott, J. (2005). "Validity of an abbreviated quality of life enjoyment and satisfaction questionnaire (Q-LES-Q-18) for schizophrenia, schizoaffective, and mood disorder patients." Qual Life Res 14(7): 1693-703.

Rossi, A., Rucci, P., Mauri, M., Maina, G., Pieraccini, F., Pallanti, S. and Endicott, J. (2005). "Validity and reliability of the Italian version of the Quality of Life, Enjoyment and Satisfaction Questionnaire." Qual Life Res 14(10): 2323-8.

Ruscio, A. M., Chiu, W. T., Roy-Byrne, P., Stang, P. E., Stein, D. J., Wittchen, H. U. and Kessler, R. C. (2007). "Broadening the definition of generalized anxiety disorder: effects on prevalence and associations with other disorders in the National Comorbidity Survey Replication." J Anxiety Disord 21(5): 662-76.

Schechter, D., Endicott, J. and Nee, J. (2007). "Quality of life of 'normal' controls: association with lifetime history of mental illness." Psychiatry Res 152(1): 45-54.

Shear, M. K., Vander Bilt, J., Rucci, P., Endicott, J., Lydiard, B., Otto, M. W., Pollack, M. H., Chandler, L., Williams, J., Ali, A. and Frank, D. M. (2001). "Reliability and validity of a structured interview guide for the Hamilton Anxiety Rating Scale (SIGH-A)." Depress Anxiety 13(4): 166-78.

Simon, G. E., Ludman, E. J. and Rutter, C. M. (2009). "Incremental benefit and cost of telephone care management and telephone psychotherapy for depression in primary care." Arch Gen Psychiatry 66(10): 1081-9.

Statistics Canada and US National Center for Health Statistics (2004). "Joint Canada/United States Survey of Health, 2002-03: Joint Canada/United Status Survey of Health Statistics."

Ware, J., Jr., Kosinski, M. and Keller, S. D. (1996). "A 12-Item Short-Form Health Survey: construction of scales and preliminary tests of reliability and validity." Med Care 34(3): 220-33.

Ware, J. E., Jr. (2007). User's Manual for the SF-36v2™ Health Survey. Lincoln, RI, QualityMetric.

Wittchen, H. U., Carter, R. M., Pfister, H., Montgomery, S. A. and Kessler, R. C. (2000). "Disabilities and quality of life in pure and comorbid generalized anxiety disorder and major depression in a national survey." Int Clin Psychopharmacol **15**(6): 319-28.

Wittchen, H. U. (2002). "Generalized anxiety disorder: prevalence, burden, and cost to society." Depress Anxiety **16**(4): 162-71.

Wyrwich, K., Harnam, N., Revicki, D. A., Locklear, J. C., Svedsater, H. and Endicott, J. (2009). "Assessing health-related quality of life in generalized anxiety disorder using the Quality Of Life Enjoyment and Satisfaction Questionnaire." Int Clin Psychopharmacol **24**(6): 289-95.

Wyrwich, K. W., Harnam, N., Locklear, J. C., Svedsater, H. and Revicki, D. A. (2011). "Understanding the relationships between health outcomes in generalized anxiety disorder clinical trials." Qual Life Res 20(2): 255-62.

Part 4

Treatment: Dealing with Resistance

12

Treatment Resistant Generalized Anxiety Disorder

Nesrin Dilbaz, Serçin Yalcın Cavus and Aslı Enez Darcin
Ankara Numune Research and Training Hospital 2, Psychiatry Clinic
Turkey

1. Introduction

The *Diagnostic and Statistical Manual of Mental Disorders, Fourth Edition Text-Revision (DSM-IV-TR)* section on anxiety disorders includes several major disorders: generalized anxiety disorder (GAD), obsessive-compulsive disorder (OCD), panic disorder, specific phobia, social anxiety disorder (SAD), and posttraumatic stress disorder (PTSD) (DSM-IV-TR, 2000). Anxiety disorders are the most prevalent of all psychiatric disorders, with an estimated prevalence of 2% to 18% worldwide (Wittchen & Jacobi, 2005). Specific phobias have a lifetime prevalence of 12.5%; the lifetime prevalence for GAD, OCD, panic disorder, SAD, and PTSD are 5.7%, 1.6%, 4.7%, 12.1%, and 6.8%, respectively (Kessler et al., 2005).

Anxiety disorders mostly begin at an early age, significantly impair multiple areas of development and life, and are associated with numerous adverse consequences such as school failure, unemployment and underemployment, academic underachievement, interactional and marital problems, and excessive use of health care facilities (Demyttenaere et al., 2004; Wittchen & Jacobi, 2005). Although anxiety disorders are highly treatable disease the majority of the patients are underdiagnosed or do not receive adequate treatment.

The goal for the treatment of Anxiety disorders is achieving and sustaining remission complete resolution of symptoms and restoration of presymptomatic functioning level. However, a significant number of patients do not fully respond to an adequate trial of first line treatment with an serotonin reuptake inhibitors (SRIs) . For example, at least 40% to 60% of OCD patients still exhibit symptoms after treatment (Pallanti & Quercioli, 2006).

SRIs are currently the first-line pharmacotherapy for most anxiety disorders (Demyttenaere et al., 2004). Benzodiazepines are widely used for panic disorder, GAD, and SAD, but they are associated with unwanted cognitive side effects, a withdrawal syndrome, and potential for abuse. Use of tricyclic antidepressants and monoamine oxidase inhibitors is limited by their adverse side effect profiles. There are also new drugs that modify the γ-aminobutyric acid (GABA)-ergic, serotonergic, and glutamatergic receptor complexes and established drugs with anxiolytic properties such as antipsychotics and anticonvulsants. Approximately a few of the patients who receive treatment are fully symptomatic remitted (Wittchen & Jacobi, 2005; Craske et al., 2005).

Even in those who had response to treatment, remission cannot be achieved. There is no consensus on the operationalization of response, partial response, remission for each anxiety disorder (Ballenger, 2001). It remains important also to develop consensus on different

levels of non response ranging from failure respond to first line therapy to failure respond to complex procedures. The best definition for treatment resistance is still inadequate (Pallanti et al., 2002). A treatment-resistant patient could be defined as a patient who had a standard treatment with at least two antidepressants for a minimum of 6 weeks without response (Bandelow & Rüther, 2004).
This chapter presents a review of the current literature and issues related to GAD including definitions of response and remission, outcome measures and treatment strategies for treatment-resistant GAD.

2. Neurobiology of Generalized Anxiety Disorder (GAD)

Kessler and colleagues surveyed 5001 subjects and demonstrated that GAD and major depression are most likely to occur in the same year and this finding suggests that the disorders are probably linked in biologically, but certainly phenomenologically.(Kessler & Gruber 2008). The extensive overlap between depression and anxiety means that studying the neurobiology of GAD means also studying the neurobiology of depression. There is a variety of evidence implicating the dysfunction of GABA, noradrenergic and serotonerjic systems in the expression of GAD. (Ballenger,2001;Gorman and Hirschfeld, 2002).
Of all of the anxiety disorders, GAD has probably been the least well studied from a genetic perspective. In a recent study of more than 37000 twins from same-sex pairs examined the genetic interrelation among GAD, MDD, and neuroticism. The genetic correlation between major depression and GAD was very high, suggesting that the same genes influence major depression and GAD. The conclusion is that , genetically, MDD and GAD are strongly related and have a common connection to the personality trait neuroticism.(Kendler & Gardner, 2007)
Hettema and colleagues studied 2 subtypes of GAD genes, GAD1 and GAD2, and determined that variations in GAD1 account for a small proportion of the individual differences in neuroticism and may increase susceptibility for MDD and anxiety disorders. These preliminary findings are exciting, but replication is needed. (Hettema &An, 2006).
In neuroimaging studies of GAD, Mathew and colleagues compared GAD patients and the controls, the GAD subjects had higher ratios of N-acetylaspartate (NAA) to creatine in the right dorsolateral prefrontal cortex.(Mathew &Mao, 2004) In an other study, compared with the healthy subjects, individuals with GAD had increased activation in the right ventrolateral prefrontan cortex when viewing angry faces. (Monk &Nelson, 2006)
Available research has suggested that GAD is modestly heritable and shares substantial genetic variation with major depression and the personality trait neuroticism. Genetic association studies are starting to identify promising leads in the search for genes that may increase susceptibility to anxiety disorders. Neuroimaging studies in GAD suggest increased activity in the brain's fear circuitry, as well as increased activity in the prefrontal cortex, which appears to have a compansatory role in reducing GAD sypmtoms.

3. Assessment of GAD: Epidemiology, presentation, diagnosis and course

In the DSM-IV, the diagnostic features for GAD, include excessive anxiety and worry which is difficult to control and pertains to several events or activities. GAD is characterized by persistent and excessive anxiety and worry about a number of common events or situations (eg, finances, health of self or family, job performance or security) occurring on more days for 6 months or more (DSM-IV). The degree of anxiety is in excess of what would be considered reasonably warranted by the reality of the situation. Difficulty controlling worry is the cardinal feature of GAD and is associated with at least 3 additional symptoms from a list including restlessness or tension, easy fatigability, difficulty concentrating, irritability, muscular tension and sleep disturbance. (APA 1980). There are some diagnostic difficulties like high rates of comorbidity, confusion in defining the term "excessive" worry and duration requirement of 6 months. Because subthreshold cases that meet all GAD diagnostic criteria except for duration of symptoms has demostrated in researches, it is suggested that perhaps the duration requirement of 6 months should be revised downward. (Kessler & Brandenburg, 2005).

The main tool used in the clinical setting to assess the severity of symptoms of GAD is the Hamilton Anxiety Scale (HAM-A).(Hamilton, 1959). However, the HAM-A isa 14-item, clinician-rated scale and is quite time consuming to perform. Recently, scales useful for all anxiety disorders as GAD have been developed, such as the Anxiety Sensitivity Index, *(ASI)* b (Reiss et al 1986) Anxiety Sensitivity refers to a person's tendency to fear anxiety-related symptoms due to the belief that there will be some negative outcome as a result of having those symptoms. the ASI is a widely used measure that has been translated into many languages. The validity and the reliability of the Turkish version was also studied and used in clinical researches. (Dilbaz 2005)

Generalized anxiety disorder (GAD) is a relatively common condition (lifetime prevalence 5.7%,and the 12-month prevalence rate was reported to be 3.1%) with chronic course which is associated with suicidality, significant distress and disability. GAD is an adult onset disorder with an oldest median age (estimated 31 years among US population) at onset of any anxiety disorder. Approximately 25% of cases of GAD have an age onset of 20 years and an additional 50% have an age at onset between 20 and 47. (Kessler &Berglund, 2005). Prevalance is higher among female gender ,(twice as often in voman as it does in men) , older age , white adults, widowed, separated or divorced with a low income. (Grant &Hasin, 2005)

Individuals with GAD has a high risk of recurrence. Harvard Research Anxiety Disorders project (HARP) the probability of recovery was 0.58 and probability of recurrence among patients who had recovered was 0.45 over 12 years. Primary Care Anxiety Project's probability of recovery was 0.39 over 2 years that is a some higher than HARP study. Average amount of time that patients were ill during 12 years was %74 in HARP study. Comorbid Axis I disorders,(Bruce &Yonkers, 2005) substance use disorders, cluster C personality disorders(Yonkers &Dyck, 2000) and female gender(Yonkers& Bruce, 2003) have been found to be less likely to remit.

4. GAD and medical illness

Patients with GAD often have medical comorbidities such as migraine, rheumatoid arthritis, peptic ulcer, irritable bowel syndrome, coronary heart disease, hiperthyroidism, diabetes, asthma and cronic obstructive pulmonary disease that may influence treatment choice. Activation of the HPA axis and sympathetic pathways can lead to cardiac and metabolik alteration and chronic activation of stres response may play a role in the vulnerability to chronic medical illnesses in inmay not be dividuals with GAD. (Habib&Gold, 2002; Charney, 2004)

When treating patients with GAD and medical illness, GAD should be treated as an independent problem. Controlling GAD may not only improve the patient's quality of life, but may also improve the physical health which is mediated by the sympathetic nervous system and cortisol mechanism.

5. GAD and psychiatric comorbidities: Depression, bipolar disorder and substance abuse

GAD is frequently comorbid with several psychiatric disorders. 90% have likelihood of at least 1 psyhiatric disorder in their lifetime , 62.4% had a lifetime history of major depression, 37.6 % had a lifetime history of alcohol and substance use disorder and 23.5% to 35.1% had at least one other anxiety disorder. The highest comorbidities were major depressive disorder (MDD) and dysthymia, while alcohol abuse, social anxiety disorder were also common ((Wittchen & Hoyer, 2001).

Comorbidity may complicate the diagnosis, treatment and outcome, resulting with greater disability and impairment. (Wittchen & Hoyer, 2001; Goodwin & Gorman, 2002). In a recent meta-analysis it is compared the impact of pure GAD and GAD comorbide depression on functioning and quality of life. Because patients with comorbidity has more impairment overall, it is suggested that clinicians should use clinical interview structured to diagnose for the presence of comorbid conditions. (Hoffman &Dukes, 2008) The presence of anxiety comorbidity in patients with MDD has also been demonstrated to interfere with the treatment response in Sequenced Treatment Alternatives to Relieve Depression (STAR*D) study which eveluated 2,876 outpatients. Those who have comorbide anxiety and were given first-line pharmacotherapy treatment with citalopram had significantly lower remission rates (%22 versus %33) according to the Hamilton Rating Scale for Depression. (Fava & Rush, 2008)

As with MDD, anxiety comorbidity can worsen the course of bipolar disorder, having a greater lifetime risk of suicide attempts (with current GAD comorbidity it is reported %62; with lifetime GAD, %53) and greater risk of comorbide substance use disorder.(Simon &Otto, 2004) and higher impulsivity. (Taylor &Hisrshfeld, 2007).

Because patients with GAD and comorbid disorders are lekely to have more impairment, disability, suicidality, poorer functioning and quality of life, fort he best outcome careful treatment selection must be chosen. The choice of drug(s) will depend on the severity of GAD; other comorbidity; an assessment of the adverse effects; possible drug-drug interactions and other risks; and the need for an early onset of action

6. Treating GAD

6.1 First-line pharmacotherapy approaches for GAD

The aims of the treatment of GAD are to reduce the core symptoms of GAD (both the psychic and somatic), including restoration of sleep; to improve patient function and quality of life; to treat comorbid disorders—present at the time of diagnosis and those that appear over the long term; and to continue treatment for long enough to produce remission and, where possible, prevent relapse. Many patients with GAD do not receive adequate treatment. Benzodiazepines, selective serotonine reuptake inhibitors (SSRIs), serotonine-norepinephrine reuptake inhibitors (SNRIs) and cognitive therapy are consistantly effective as a first-line treatment. Dose ranges may need to be individualized according to the age, medical comorbidity , psychiatric comorbidity and other medications of the patients.

6.1.1 SSRIs

Several analyses have shown similar efficacy among antidepressant agents in the management of GAD.(Baldwin&Anderson,2005) Of these, SSRIs and SNRIs are generally preferred as first-line therapy, as the evidence supporting their efficacy is more robust, and they are usually better tolerated than the other classes of antidepressants. More recently, sertraline (Dahl &Ravindran, 2005) and paroxetine has been shown to be efficacious in GAD ,and citalopram has demonstrated efficacy in older patients (≥ 60 years of age) with GAD (Lenze&Mulsant, 2005).Because of the prevalence of sexual dysfunction has been estimated to be as high as 40% during treatment with SSRIs, it is a common reason for treatment discontinuation.

The SSRIs escitalopram (10–20 mg/day) and paroxetine (20–50 mg/day) have also been shown to be effective in the long-term treatment of GAD. (Bielski & Bose, 2005) Relapse prevention studies have been reported for both drugs. (Allgulander & Florea, 2006; Stocchi &Nordera, 2003). Escitalopram reduced the risk of relapse compared with placebo during 24 to 72 weeks of randomized treatment following 12 weeks of open-label treatment. Similar results were found with paroxetine versus placebo in a shorter study.Essitalopram was also showen to exceed the effects of plasebo in an other study , and citalopram was effective in a geriatric population with GAD. (Goodman &Bose, 2005; Lenze &Mulsant,2005)

6.1.2 SNRIs (venlafaxine, duloksetin)

Venlafaxine, which affects both serotonin and norepinephrine systems, was the first drug that is approved fort he treatment of GAD and also has been showen to be effective in treating depression. Two placebo-controlled studies have demonstrated the efficacy of venlafaxine XR in GAD and have provided that both the psychic and somatic manifestations of anxiety can be controlled. One of these study compared venlafaxine (75 mg/da yor 150 mg/day fixed dose) with buspirone (30 mg7day) treatment for 8 weeks in 365 patients with GAD. A significantly higher response rate as measured on the CGI was seen for venlafaxine 75 mg/day, compared with either buspirone or placebo after week 1. The mean HAM-A anxious mood and tension scores were significantly lower for both doses of venlafaxine XR at week 8 compared with placebo , however, the mean total HAM-A scores for all the treatment groups compared with placebo were not significant. (Davidson&Dupont, 1999)

In the second study the efficacy of venlafaxine XR (75 to 225 mg/day) assessed by the HAM-A anxiety subscale was statistically higher than placeboin 238 patients with GAD, over a 28-week maintenance period.(Gelenberg& Lydiard, 2000) The results from these studies demonstrate the efficacy of venlafaxine XR in both the short- and long-term treatment of GAD, but the optimal dose was not defined. In an 8-week study of 349 patients with GAD , venlafaxine at 225 mg/doses was found to have more efficacy than placebo, in reducing HAM-A total scores. (Rickels &Pollack, 2000).

The efficacy of duloksetin, another SNRI, was approved in 2007 for the treatment of GAD. In two studies flexible doses of duloksetin (60-120 mg/day) was compared with placebo , found significantly greater improvement for both doses on HAM-A total scores.(Koponen&Allgulander, 2007). Duloxetine has also been shown to have long-term efficacy among patients with GAD who responded to 26 weeks of open-label treatment; administration of duloxetine for a further 26 weeks reduced the risk of relapse compared with placebo. (Davidson &Wittchen ,2008).

6.1.3 Benzodiazepines

Although benzodiazepines diazepam, alprazolam and lorazepam have showen efficacy in controlled trials and were commonly used in GAD; they must be used with caution because of modest abuse potential (Fraser, 1998) interactions with other drugs, including hypnotics sedating antidepressants, opiate analgesics, antihistamines, anticonvulsants and alcohol, particularly in older patients, falls, memory impaierment, incoordination, drowsiness and confusion (Petrovic & Mariman 2003)

Although benzodiazepines have a rapid onset of action on improving the core symptoms of GAD, they are not recommended as monotherapy for depression, dysthymia, obsessive-compulsive disorder, and posttraumatic stress disorder, which commonly occur with GAD.(Ballenger &Davidson,2001; Kessler &Chiu,2005).

Benzodiazepines are generally recommended only for short-term use and are not recommended for first-line long-term treatment of GAD,(Swinson & Anthony 2006) although they have a role in the management of acute anxiety (Bandelow B, Zohar,2008; Ballenger JC, Davidson,2001) and may have a role in some cases in which somatic symptoms are more prominent than psychic symptoms.

6.1.4 Nonpharmacological treatments (cognitive behavioral therapy-CBT)

CBT has been used in GAD as a psychological treatment strategy. However, comparisons between standard drugs for GAD and psychotherapy are lacking. Although CBT is the most effective of the psychological treatments available for GAD, clinical response occurs in less than 50% of people receiving this form of therapy (46% versus 14% for control), so unmet needs still remain (Hunot &Churchill R, 2007). When GAD is comorbid with depression, which is very common, pharmacotherapy with antidepressants is increasingly indicated (Ballenger et al., 2001).

6.2 Treatment comorbidity

Comorbidity is a critical factor that influence the treatment choice of GAD. Rickels and collegues found that, for GAD patients with significant depressive symptoms, an antidepressant drug is more useful than a benzodiazepine. In another study,MDD patients with a comorbidity of GAD, venlafaxine XR was found to be more effective than placebo and flouksetine.(Silverstone&Salinas, 2001). The data to support appropriate choices in the comorbide GAD and bipolar disorder is lacking. Risk of mania with an antidepressant and risk of SUD about using benzodiazepines are the likely reasons for inadequate treatments.

6.3 Treatment in children, adolescents and pregnancy

For children and adolescents, there are published studies of the treatment of GAD, evaluating the SSRIs sertraline, fluoxetine, fluvoxamine (Walkup & Labellarte 2001;Rynn & Siqueland 2001) and venlafaxine XR. (Sheehan & Keene 2008) These data suggest that these agents may be effective in treating the symptoms of GAD in children and adolescents. The SSRIs are generally well tolerated in this population. Guidelines from the British Association for Psychopharmacology recommend that, in children, pharmacologic treatments should be reserved for individuals who have not responded to psychological therapies and careful consideration of dosage is also necessary because of the adverse effects.

In addition, the risk of possible suicidal thoughts or behaviors should be considered and these potential adverse effects monitored when any antidepressants are administered in this age group.(FDA ,2008).

In pregnancy nonpharmacologic treatment such as cognitive-behavioral therapy or interpersonal psychotherapy should be employed whenever possible. But it is equally important to discuss the risks of the untreated illness to both mother and the infant. So if medication is required, the use of SSRIs in the lowest effective dosage for the minimum amount of time is preferable in the first-line treatment because of the data supporting their efficacy, minimal need for dose titration and favorable side effect profile. Paroxetine has been shown to be efficacious in GAD; however, the US Food and Drug Administration (FDA) labeling for its use in pregnancy was reclassified to category D due to possible risk of congenital malformations, especially septal defects, when used during the first trimester of pregnancy. Newer antidepressants such as venlafaxine XR and mirtazapine are options for patients unresponsive or intoleran to SSRIs. Benzodiazepines should be avoided because of physiological dependence and withdrawal in the newborn.

7. Other potentially effective agents

7.1 Bupropion

In a recent double-blind, randomized study, which performed on a small sample sizeof GAD patients , bupropion XL (150-300mg/day) compared with essitalopram (10-20 mg/day) for 12 weeks.The primary efficacy measures were the Clinical Global Impression of Improvement (CGI-I) and the Hamilton Anxiety Rating Scale (HARS).Bupropion XL is found to be demonstrated comparable anxiolytic efficacy to escitalopram in outpatients with GAD. These preliminary results needs to be improved further.

7.2 Atypical antipsychotics

Several preliminary reports of monotherapy trials of quetiapine versus placebo have described efficacy at doses in the range of 50–150 mg/day, (Chouinard & Ahokas A, 2008 ; Khan & Joyce 2008) but quetiapine cannot yet be recommended as a routine GAD treatment. However the use of quetiapine could be considered after other classes of drugs have proved ineffective orwhen certain types of symptoms are present. In the studies by Chouinard, quality of life was measured using the Quality of Life Enjoyment and Satisfaction Questionnaire (Q-LES-Q)., and the highest score were seen with quetiapine XR 150 mg and paroxetine compared with placebo at week 8 (Chouinard et al 2008) . The efficacious application of quetiapine in MDD and GAD ranges from quetiapine monotherapy to adjunctive therapy with antidepressants for shortterm and maintenance treatment at a dose range between 50–300 mg/day. Despite the often benefi cial sedative effects of quetiapine on clinically relevant sleep problems in psychiatric patients, quetipaine is not recommended soley as a sleeping agent. Overall, the most recently available evidence on quetiapine suggests that it can play a signifi cant role in the management of MDD and GAD.For olanzapine or risperidone, it is suggested that the results have been obtained in partialresponders to antidepressants rather than as monotherapy in all patients (Pollack &Simon, 2006; Brawman& Knapp, 2005).

7.3 Antihistamines

Efficacy of the antihistamines in GAD was established in two studies. (Llorca& Spadone, 2002; Lader &Scotto, 1998).The antihistamine hydroxyzine appears to have higher anxiolytic efficacy than placebo in controlled studies. Because of the side effects (sedation, anticholinergic effects) , slow onset of action, and lack of efficacy for comorbid disorders, hydroxyzine was not recommended to be used as first-line therapy in some guidelines. (IPAP,2008; Bandelow& Zohar,2008).

7.4 TCAs

The tricyclic drug imipramine is effective in GAD but is associated with the usual range of tricyclic antidepressant side effects, which limits its use for those who have not responded to an SSRI or SNRI.(Baldwin & Anderson ,2005 ; Ballenger &Davidson 2001). Another possible second-line antidepressant includes trazodone (Rickels & Downing ,1993).

7.5 Buspirone

The 5HT-1 receptor partial agonist buspirone is found to be effective in the treatment of GAD according to controlled studies (Goa &Ward 1986), but less effective than the benzodiazepines, (Laakmann & 1998) venlafaxine or hydroxyzine. Because of side effects like dizziness, drowsiness and nause, slow onset of action lack of effectivity on comorbid conditions, buspiron is not recommended as first-line treatment for GAD. (Bandelow&Zohar,2008)

7.6 $\alpha_2\delta$ Ca ++ channel modulators, pregabaline

The $\alpha_2\delta$ Ca++ channel modulator pregabalin was shown to have greater efficacy than placebo, nearly equal to benzodiazepines and venlafaxine both in the first week and maintenance of 6 months in several placebo controlled studies (Pande&Crockatt,2003; Montgomery,2006; Montgomery&Tobias, 2006; Owen,2007). The long-term efficacy of pregabalin has also been demonstrated in patients with GAD that it reduced the risk of relapse compared with placebo, during 24 weeks of randomized treatment following 8 weeks of open-label treatment. (Feltner & Wittchen, 2008)

7.7 Tiagabine

The selective GABA reuptake inhibitor tiagabin has been studied in 3 large placebo-controlled trials in 1830 patients with GAD and no significant difference from placebo was showen, moreover side effects were too high that %47 of patients were drop out. It seem hard to justify the use of tiagabine for GAD. (Pollack& Tiller ,2008)

7.8 Agomelatine

Agomelatine a novel agent that acts on melatonergic and serotonergic receptors was assessed on a randomized, double-blind, placebo-controlled trial on one hundred twenty-one patients with GAD with no comorbid disorders.The patients were randomized to agomelatine (25-50 mg/d) or placebo for 12 weeks. The primary outcome measure was the Hamilton Anxiety Rating Scale, whereas secondary outcome measures included the Clinical Global Impression scales. Analysis of covariance of change in the last Hamilton Anxiety Rating Scale total score from baseline demonstrated significant superiority of agomelatine 25 to 50 mg as compared with placebo.Safety analysis indicated that agomelatine was tolerated as well as placebo and was devoid of discontinuation emergent symptoms. This study suggests that agomelatine is effective in the treatment of GAD and is well tolerated (Stein & Ahokas,2008).

8. Adequate and poor response to pharmacotherapy: Switching medication and augmentation strategies

In most studies, response is commonly defined as a ≥50% reduction on the commonly used standard scales. This definition is also arbitrary, because that cannot be applied for all disorders. Assessment of changes on disease-specific rating scales and measures of global illness severity and improvement, social, occupational, and academic functioning, and quality of life should be performed. Remission implies not only the relief of symptoms but also restoration of patients to their premorbid high level of functioning, including resumption of family, social, and work-related role.

Treatment resistance patient could be defined as a patient who had a standard treatment for a minimum of 6 weeks without showing response. Before a treatment is considered as failure it should be ascertained that the diagnosis is correct, the patient is compliant with therapy, the dosage prescribed is therapeutic and there has been an adequate trial period. Comorbid personality disorders such as borderline personality disorder, depression and substance abuse may be associated with poor outcome. Coocurrence of GAD with medical disorders such as heart disease and gastrointestinal and chronic pain disorders causes an extended clinical course and poorer outcome than patients with GAD alone (Harter et al., 2003; Bowen et al., 2000; McWilliams et al., 2003; Roy-Byrne et al., 2008).

If partial response is not seen after 4–6 weeks, there is still a chance that the patient will respond after another 4–6 weeks of therapy with increased dose. When initial treatment fails,the psychiatrist can either *augment* the current treatment by adding another agent (in the case of pharmacotherapy) or another modality (i.e., add CBT if the patient is already receiving pharmacotherapy, or add pharmacotherapy if the patient is already receiving CBT) , or they can decide to *switch* to a different medication or therapeutic modality. Augmentation is generally a reasonable approach if some significant benefits were observed with the original treatment . On the other hand, if the original treatment failed to provide any significant alleviation of the patient's symptoms, a switch in treatment may be more useful. Treatment resistance are usually based on clinical judgment , "augmentation and switching studies" are lacking. Low doses of risperidone have been shown to improve in anxiety symptoms when added to initial treatment in patients who had not responded to first-line anxiolytic drugs. (Brawman& Knapp ,2005) A study of quetiapine augmentation of paroxetine did not provide evidence as an augmenting agent in GAD.(Simon & Connor,2008). Olanzapine has shown similar augmentation effects when added to fluoxetine in patients with refractory GAD, although this efficacy was achieved at the expense of substantial weight gain.(Pollack&Simon, 2006). Other augmentation strategies might include addition of a benzodiazepine or other GABAergic drug to an antidepressant. Augmentation of medication with cognitive-behavioral therapy (CBT) has not been studied meaningfully in GAD, and its benefit still awaits adequate evaluation.

9. Maintenance treatment

Because GAD is a chronic illness, maintenance treatment is required and it is showen that stopping acute treatment with anxiolytic after 4 weeks, %60 to 80 patients led to relapse within a year. (Rickels &Schweizer, 1990). In a study, even after 6 months of buspirone treatment for GAD, stopping treatment led to relapse of %25 within a month. (Rickels &Schweizer, 1988) After treating with essitalopram for 12 weeks, the patients randomized to essitalopram or placebo up to 76 weeks and the relapse rates were %19 and %56, respectively. (Allgulander&Florea, 2006). Likely, After 8 weeks of treatment with paroxetine, the patients were randomized for 24 weeks and the relapse rates were%10,9 and %39,9. (Davidson&Wittchen, 2008). GAD requires long-term treatment that remission can take several moths and stopping medication increases the risk of relapse within the first year of initiating treatment.

10. Conclusion

It is recommended that the first-line treatment for patients with GAD should consist of an antidepressant, such as SSRI (paroxetine and essitalopram) or SNRI (venlafaxine and duloksetine). On the other hand they have efficacy limitations, including lack of response, lack of full remission, risk of relapse and adverse effects. This means that there is a need for alternative treatment options. Following the first-line treatment in case of inappropriate response; 1) increasing the dose of the SSRI/SNRI, 2)switching to a same class or different class agent or 3) augmentation therapy may be considered.The strategy of augmentation SSRIs/SNRIs with atypical antipsychotics may be useful in improving the rates of remission but randomized controlled studies are needed.

11. References

Allgulander C, Florea I, Huusom AK. Prevention of relapse in generalized anxiety disorder by escitalopram treatment. Int J Neuropsychopharmacol. 2006;9(5):495–505.

American Psychiatric Association. Diagnostic and Statistical Manual of Mental Disorders, Fourth Edition. Washington, DC:American Psyciatric Association;1994.

American Psychiatric Association. Diagnostic and Statistical Manual of Mental Disorders, Fourth Edition.Text revised. Washington, DC:American Psyciatric Association; 2000.

Baldwin DS, Anderson IM, Nutt DJ, et al. Evidence-based guidelines for the pharmacological treatment of anxiety disorders: recommendations from the British Association for Psychopharmacology. J Psychopharmacol. 2005;19(6):567–596.

Ballenger JC. Overview of different pharmacotherapies for attaining remission in generalized anxiety disorder. J Clin Psychiatry 2001; 62 Suppl. 19; 11-9.

Ballenger JC, Davidson JRT, Lecrubier Y, et al. Consensus statement on generalized anxiety disorder from the international consensus group on depression and anxiety. *J Clin Psychiatry.* 2001;62(suppl 11):53-58.

Bandelow B, Rüther E. Treatment resistant panic disorder. *CNS Spectr. 2004;9(10):725-730, 732-739.*

Bandelow B, Zohar J, Hollander E, et al. World Federation of Societies of Biological Psychiatry (WFSBP) Guidelines for the Pharmacological Treatment of Anxiety, Obsessive-Compulsive and Post-Traumatic Stress Disorders: First Revision. World J Biol Psychiatry. 2008;9(4):248–312.

Bielski RJ, Bose A, Chang CC. A double-blind comparison of escitalopram and paroxetine in the long-term treatment of generalized anxiety disorder. Ann Clin Psychiatry. 2005;17(2):65–69.

Brawman-Mintzer O, Knapp RG, Nietert PJ. Adjunctive risperidone in generalized anxiety disorder: a double-blind, placebo-controlled study. J Clin Psychiatry. 2005;66(10):1321–1325

Bruce SE, Yonkers KA, Otto MW, et al. Influence of psychiatric comorbidity on recovery and recurrence in generalized anxiety disorder, social phobia, and panic disorder:a 12 year prospective study. Am J Psychiatry. 2005;162:1179-1187.

Bystritsky A, Kerwin L, Feusner JD, Vapnik T.A Pilot Controlled Trial of Bupropion XL Versus Escitalopram in Generalized Anxiety Disorder. Psychopharmacol Bull. 2008;41(1):46-51.

Charney DS. Psycobiological mechanisms of resilience and vulnerability: implications for successful adaptation to extreme stres. Am J Psychiatry. 2004;161(2):195-216.

Chouinard G, Ahokas A, Bandelow B, et al. Extended release quetiapine fumarate (quetiapine XR) once-daily monotherapy in generalized anxiety disorder (GAD). Presented at the 27th Annual Meeting of the Anxiety Disorders Association of America; March 6–9, 2008; St Louis, MO.

Craske MG, Edlund MJ, Sullivan G, Roy-Byrne PP, Sherbourne CD, Bystritsky AS. M.B. Perceived unmet need for mental health and barriers to among care patients with panic disorder. Psychiatric Services 2005;56:988–94.

Dahl AA, Ravindran A, Allgulander C, et al. Sertraline in generalized anxiety disorder: efficacy in treating the psychic and somatic anxiety factors. *Acta Psychiatr Scand.* 2005;111(6):429–435.

Davidson JTR, Dupont RL, Hedges D, et al. Efficacy, safety, and tolerability of venlafaxine extended release and buspirone in outpatients with generalized anxiety disorder. J Clin Psychiatry 1999 ;60 :528-535.

Davidson JR, Wittchen HU, Llorca PM, et al. Duloxetine treatment for relapse prevention in adults with generalized anxiety disorder: a double-blind placebo-controlled trial. Eur Neuropsychopharmacol. 2008;18(9):673–681.

Demyttenaere K, Bruffaerts R, Posada-Villa J, et al. Prevalence, severity and unmet need for treatment of mental disorders in the World Health Organization World Mental Health (WMH) Surveys. Journal of the American Medical Association 2004;291:2581–90.

Dilbaz N. Turkish Anxiety Sensitivity Index: Psychometric properties. Presented at National Anxiety Disorders Congress in Tunusia, in 2005

Fava M, Rush AJ, Alpert JE, et al. Difference in treatment outcome in patients with anxious versus nonanxious depression: a STAR*D report. Am J Psychitry. 2008;165(3):342-351.

Feltner D, Wittchen HU, Kavoussi R, et al. Long-term efficacy of pregabalin in generalized anxiety disorder. Int Clin Psychopharmacol. 2008;23(1):18–28.

Fraser AD. Use and abuse of the benzodiazepines. Ther Drug Monit. 1998;20(5):481–489.

Food and Drug Administration. Revisions to product labeling: suicidality and antidepressant drugs; 2007. Accessed November 2008.

Gelenberg AJ, Lydiard RB, Rudolph RL, et al. Efficacy of venlafaxine extended-release capsules in nondepressed outpatients with generalized anxiety disorder: a 6-month randomized controlled trial. JAMA 2000;283:3082-3088.

Goa KL, Ward A. Buspirone: a preliminary review of its pharmacological properties and therapeutic efficacy as an anxiolytic. Drugs. 1986;32(2):114–129.

Gorman JM, Hirschfeld RM. Ninan PT. New developments in the neurobiological basis of anxiety disorders. Psychopharmacol Bull 2002; 36 Suppl. 2; 49-67

Goodman WK, Bose A, Wang Q. Treatment of generalized anxiety disorder with escitalopram: pooled results from double-blind, placebo-controlled trials. J Affect Disord. 2005;87(2-3):161-167.

Goodwin RD, Gorman JM. Psychopharmacologic treatment of generalized anxiety disorder and the risk of major depression. Am J Psychiatry. 2002;159(11):1935–1937.

Grant BF, Hasin DS, Stinson FS, et al. Prevalence, correlates, comorbidity, and comperative disability of DSM-IV generalized anxiety disorder in the USA:results from the National Epidemiologic Survey on Alcohol and Related Conditions. Psychol Med. 2005;35(12):747-759.

Habib KE, Gold PW, Chrousos GP. Neuroendocrinology of stres. Endocrinol Metab Clin North Am. 2001;30(3):695-728.

Hettema JM. What is the genetic relationship between anxiety and depression? Am J Med Genet C Semin Med Genet. 2008;148(2):140-146.

Hettema JM, An SS, Neale MC, et al. Association between glutamic acid decarboxylase genes and anxiety disorders, major depression, and neuroticism. Mol Psychiatry. 2006;11(8):752-762. Correction in 2006;11(8):794.

Hoffman DL, Dukes EM, Wittchen HU. Human and economic burden of generalized anxiety disorder. Depress Anxiety. 2008;25(1):72-90.

Hunot V, Churchill R, Silva de Lima M, et al. Psychological therapies for generalised anxiety disorder. Cochrane Database Syst Rev. 2007;(1):CD001848

International Psychopharmacology Algorithm Project. IPAP General Anxiety Disorder (GAD) Algorithm Notes. http://www.ipap.org/gad/index.php. Accessed November 2008.

Khan A, Joyce M, Eggens I, et al. Extended release quetiapine fumarate (quetiapine XR) monotherapy in the treatment of generalized anxiety disorder (GAD). Presented at the 27th Annual Meeting of the Anxiety Disorders Association of America; March 6–9, 2008; St Louis, MO.

Kendler KS, Gardner CO, Gatz M, et al. The sources of co-morbidity between major depression and generalized anxiety disorder in a Swedish national twin sample. Psychol Med. 2007;37(3):453-462.

Kessler RC, Brandenburg N, Lane M, et al. Rethinking the duration requirement for generalized anxiety disorder: evidence from the National Comorbidity Survey Replication. Psychol Med. 2005;35(7):1073-1082.

Kessler RC, Berglund P, Demler O, Jin R, Walters EE. Lifetime prevalence and age-of-onset distributions of DSM-IV disorders in the National Comorbidity Survey Replication. *Arch Gen Psychiatry*. 2005;62:593-602.

Kessler RC, Chiu WT, Demler O, et al. Prevalence, severity, and comorbidity of 12-month DSM-IV disorders in the National Comorbidity Survey Replication. Arch Gen Psychiatry. 2005;62(6):617–627.

Koponen H, Allgulander C, Erikson J, et al. Efficacy of duloksetine fort he treatment of generalized anxiety disorder: implications for primary care phsicians. Prim Care Companion J Clin Psychiatry. 2007;9(2):100-107.

Laakmann G, Schule C, Lorkowski G, et al. Buspirone and lorazepam in the treatment of generalized anxiety disorder in outpatients. Psychopharmacology (Berl). 1998;136(4):357–366.

Lader M, Scotto JC. A multicentre double-blind comparison of hydroxyzine, buspirone, and placebo in patients with generalized anxiety disorder. Psychopharmacology (Berl):1998;139(4):402-406.

Lenze EJ, Mulsant BH, Shear MK, et al. Efficacy and tolerability of citalopram in the treatment of late-life anxiety disorder:results from an 8-week randomized, placebo-controllled trial. Am J Psychiatry. 2005;162(1):146-150.

Llorca PM, Spadone C, Sol O,et al. Efficacy and safety of hydroxyzine in the treatment of generalized anxiety disorder: a 3-month double-blind study. J Clin Psychiatry. 2002;63(11):102-1027.

Mathew SJ, Mao X, Coplan JD, et al. Dorsolateral prefrontal cortical pathology in generalized anxiety disorder:a proton magnetic resonance spectroscopic imaging study. Am J Psychiatry. 2004;161(6):1119-1121.

Monk CS, Nelson EE, McClure EB, et al. Ventrolateral prefrontal cortex activation and attentional bias in response to angry faces in adolescents with generalized anxiety disorder. Am J Psychiatry. 2006;163(6):1091-1097.

Montgomery SA. Pregabaline fort he treatment of generalized anxiety disorder. Expert Opin Pharmacother. 2006;7(15):2139-2154.

Montgomery SA, Tobias K, Zomberg GL, et al. Efficacy and safety of pregabalin in the treatment of generalized anxiety disorder:a 6- week, multicenter, randomized, double-blind, placebo-controlled comparison of pregabalin and venlafaxine. J Clin Psychiatry. 2006;67(5):771-782.

Owen RT. Pregabalin:its efficacy, safety and tolerability profile in generalized anxiety disorder. Drugs Today (Barc). 2007;43(9):601-610.

Pallanti S, Hollander E, Bienstock C, et al. Treatment non-response in OCD: methodological issues and operational definitions. Int J Neuropsychopharmacol. 2002;5:181-191.

Pallanti S, Quercioli L. Treatment-refractory obsessive-compulsive disorder: methodological issues, operational definitions and therapeutic lines. Prog Neuropsychopharmacol Biol Psychiatry. 2006;30(3):400-412.

Pande AC, Crockatt JG, Feltner DE, et al.Pregabaline in generalized anxiety disorder: a placebo-controlled trial. Am J Psychiatry. 2003;160(3):533-540.

Petrovic M, Mariman A, Warie H, et al. Is there a rationale for prescription of benzodiazepines in the elderly? review of the literature. Acta Clin Belg. 2003;58(1):27–36.

Pollack MH, Simon NM, Zalta AK, et al. Olanzapine augmentation of fluoxetine for refractory generalized anxiety disorder: a placebo-controlled study. Biol Psychiatry. 2006;59(3):211–215. PubMed doi:10.1016/j.biopsych.2005.07.005.

Pollack MH, Tiller J, Xie F, et al. Tiagabine in adult patients with generalized anxiety disorder: results from 3 randomized, double-blind, placebo-controlled, parallel-group studies. J Clin Psychopharmacol. 2008;28(3):308–316

Pollack MH, Simon NM, Zalta AK, et al. Olanzapine augmentation of fluoxetine for refractory generalized anxiety disorder: a placebo-controlled study. *Biol Psychiatry.* 2006;59(3):211–215.

Rickels K, Pollack MH, Sheehan DV, et al. Efficacy of extended-release venlafaxine in nondepressed outpatients with generalized anxiety disorder. Am J Psychiatry. 2000;157(6):968-974.

Rickels K, Downing R, Schweizer E, et al. Antidepressants for the treatment of generalized anxiety disorder: a placebo-controlled comparison of imipramine, trazodone, and diazepam. Arch Gen Psychiatry. 1993;50(11):884–895

Rickels K, Schiweizer E. The clinical course and long-term management of generalized anxiety disorder. J Clin Psychopharmacol. 1990;10(suppl 3):101S-110S.

Rickels K, Schiweizer E, Csanalosi I, et al. Long-term treatment of anxiety and risk of withdrawal. Prospective comparison of clorazepate and buspirone. Arch Gen Psychiatry. 1988;45(5):444-450.

Rynn MA, Siqueland L, Rickels K. Placebo-controlled trial of sertraline in the treatment of children with generalized anxiety disorder. Am J Psychiatry. 2001;158(12):2008–2014.

Sheehan DV, Keene MS, Eaddy M, et al. Differences in medication adherence and healthcare resource utilization patterns: older versus newer antidepressant agents in patients with depression and/or anxiety disorders. CNS Drugs. 2008;22(11):963–973.

Silverstone PH, Salinas e. Efficacy of venlafaxine extended release in patients with major depressive disorder nd comorbid generalized anxiety disorder. J Clin Psychiatry.2001:62(7):523-529.

Simon NM, Connor KM, LeBeau RT, et al. Quetiapine augmentation of paroxetine CR for the treatment of refractory generalized anxiety disorder: preliminary findings. Psychopharmacology (Berl). 2008;197(4):675–681.

Simon NM, Otto MW, Wisniewski SR, et al. Anxiety disorder comorbidity in bipolar disorder patients: data from the first 500 participants in the Systematic Treatment Enhancement Program for Bipolar Disorder (STEP-BD). Am J Psychiatry. 2004;161(12):2222-2229.

Stein DJ, Ahokas AA, de Bodinat C. Efficacy of agomelatine in generalized anxiety disorder: a randomized, double-blind, placebo-controlled study. J Clin Psychopharmacol. 2008 Oct;28(5):561-6.

Stocchi F, Nordera G, Jokinen RH, et al. Efficacy and tolerability of paroxetine for the long-term treatment of generalized anxiety disorder. J Clin Psychiatry. 2003;64(3):250–258.

Swinson RP, Anthony MM, Bleau P, et al. Clinical practice guidelines: management of anxiety disorders. Can J Psychiatry. 2006;51(suppl 2):9S–91S

Taylor CT, Hirshfeld-Becker DR, Ostacher MJ, et al. Anxiety is associated with impulsivity in bipolar disorder. J Anxiety Disord. 2007;22(5):868-876.

Walkup JT, Labellarte MJ, Riddle MA, et al, for the Research Unit on Pediatric Psychopharmacology Anxiety Study Group. Fluvoxamine for the treatment of anxiety disorders in children and adolescents. N Engl J Med. 2001;344(17):1279–1285.

Wittchen HU, Hoyer J. Generalized anxiety disorder: nature and course. J Clin Psychiatry. 2001;62(suppl 11):15–19.

Wittchen H-U, Jacobi F. Size and burden of mental disorders in Europe: a critical review and appraisal of 27 studies. European Neuropsychopharmacology 2005;15(4):357–67.

Yonkers KA, Dyck IR, Warshaw M, et al. Factors predicting the clinical sourse of generalized anxiety disorder. Br J Psychiatry. 2000;176:544-549.

Yonkers KA, Bruce SE, Dyck IR, et al. Chronicity, relapse and illness:course of panic disorder, social phobia and generalized anxiety disorder: findings in men and women from 8 years of follow-up. Depress Anxiety. 2003;17(3):173-179.

13

The Treatment of Obsessive-Compulsive Disorder and the Approaches to Treatment Resistance

Stefano Pallanti[1,2,3], Giacomo Grassi[2] and Andrea Cantisani[2]
[1]*Department of Psychiatry, Mount Sinai School of Medicine, New York;*
[2]*Department of Psychiatry, University of Florence,*
[3]*Institute of Neuroscience, Florence,*
[1]*USA*
[2,3]*Italy*

1. Introduction

Obsessive-compulsive disorder (OCD) is characterized by recurrent intrusive ideas, impulses, or urges (obsessions) along with overt or covert behaviors (compulsions) aimed at reducing the distress (DSM-IV-TR). Patients have either obsessions, compulsions, or, most commonly, both. Obsessions are defined as recurrent and persistent thoughts, impulses, or images that are experienced as intrusive and inappropriate and cause anxiety. The obsessions are not simply excessive worries about real-life problems and the affected individual usually recognizes that these thoughts, impulses or images are excessive, unreasonable and a product of their own mind (DSM-IV-TR). In order to naturalize the obsessions, other thoughts or actions are performed (compulsions). Examples of obsessions include, among others, contamination (concern with dirt or germs, fear of blood) symmetry (concern about order, exactness), obsessions about safety and harm (fear of harm due to carelessness, fear of being responsible for terrible events) hoarding, pathological doubt (after completing a routine activity the affected individual wonders whether he or she performed it correctly or did it at all), numbers with special significance, etc.
Compulsions are repetitive behaviors (e.g. hand washing, ordering, checking) or mental acts (e.g. praying, counting, repeating words silently) that patients with OCD feel compelled to do in response to an obsession, or according to rules which must be applied rigidly (e.g. checking that a light switch is turned off by switching it on and off without any interruption). The behaviors or mental acts are aimed at preventing or reducing distress or preventing some dreaded event or situation; however, these behaviors are either not connected in a realistic way with what they are designed to neutralize or prevent, or are clearly unreasonable or excessive. Examples of compulsive activities are washing hands until they are raw, repeatedly checking the locked door, arranging and rearranging items in a set order, counting, asking, repeating reassurance questions etc.
The diagnosis is made by clinical interview, with a specific and detailed focus on OCD. To diagnose the disorder according to the DSM-IV criteria, the patient must suffer from either obsessions or compulsions that cause great distress, are time-consuming (more then 1 hour

per day), or substantially interfere with normal function, and that, at some point of the disorder, are recognized as excessive or unreasonable. The Yale-Brown obsessive-compulsive scale (Y-BOCS) is regarded as the gold standard measure of obsessive-compulsive symptom severity and is used in most treatment trials (Goodman et al., 1989).

2. OCD treatment: First-line treatments and first-line treatments choice

The first case report indicating that the tricyclic antidepressant (TCA) clomipramine might have some benefit in patients with OCD was published more than 40 years ago (Fernandez et al., 1967), but more than 20 years passed before clomipramine was approved for the treatment of OCD (Thorén et al. 1980).

Since then, a wide number of researchers have been working in order to find effective pharmacological treatments, and despite treatment resistance still being a core issue in the therapeutic process, many goals have been achieved. Nowadays the clinician has the possibility of choosing a variety of treatment strategies that are effective in about the half of the patients (Pallanti et al. 2002). Both cognitive-behavioral therapy (CBT) and serotonin reuptake inhibitors (SRI) are considered valuable and safe first-line treatments for obsessive-compulsive disorder (Koran et al., 2007).

A broad range of factors may have an influence on the choice of the treatment strategy adopted by the clinician. Some of them are the severity of the symptoms, the characteristics of psychiatric or medical comorbidity and the relative treatment, the possibility to get a CBT, past and actual treatment and patient's preference. Given the fact that most of the trials are based on 3-4 months long observations, there are no reliable data concerning the best options for long-term therapies.

Behavioral therapy seems to be the most effective kind of psychotherapy, in particular exposure and response prevention (ERP) techniques (Abramowitz, 1998; Eddy et al., 2004; Fisher et al., 2005; Meyer, 1966). Also cognitive approaches, aiming at the identification and modification of dysfunctional beliefs and thoughts are considered appropriate strategies if coupled to the behavioral ones: in fact, only a small amount of data supports the efficacy of the cognitive techniques alone.

CBT with ERP is indicated as first-line treatment for patients without particular depressive or anxious symptoms, for those whose disorder's severity does not interfere with the therapeutic process, and in those who refuse a pharmacological treatment (Koran et al., 2007).

Although there are no sufficiently controlled trials to provide solid evidence, the experts agree on the optimal duration of the treatment, which should at least consist of 13-20 sessions (Koran et al., 2007).

The use of a SRI without CBT intervention is indicated for those patients who were already treated in the past with a drug with good results or that prefer an exclusive pharmacological treatment. However, an initial approach with a SRI may be helpful in comprehensively increasing the compliance of the patient to all the components of the treatment, as an effect of the reduction of the symptoms' severity. Therefore, the use of a SRI alone is indicated also for the patients who are not eligible for a CBT intervention because of their scarce compliance and collaboration or when psychotherapy is not available (Koran et al., 2007).

The Food and Drug Administration (FDA) have approved clomipramine, fluoxetine, fluvoxamine, paroxetine and sertraline for the treatment of obsessive-compulsive disorder. There are sufficient evidences that support the efficacy of citalopram and escitalopram, although the FDA still does not approve them.

Citalopram is the most selective serotonin reuptake inhibitor. Its efficacy and safety as first line treatment or in case of treatment-resistance for OCD has been proved in various single and double blind trials (Marazziti et al, 2001; Pallanti et al, 1999; Pidrman et al., 1997; Stengler-Wenzke et al., 2006).
Montgomery et al. (Montgomery et al., 2001) confronted in a double-blind trial the efficacy of different citalopram dosages (20, 40, 60 mg/die) and placebo; the Authors reported the effectiveness of all of the three dosages, with a slight advantage for the higher one, particularly in terms of rapidity of response.
Escitalopram is the left enantiomer of citalopram; due to the fact that the right enantiomer (that contrasts the effect of citalopram on serotonin) is not included in the drug, escitalopram has a greater re-uptake blocking efficacy.
A series of open and retrospective studies supports the potential efficacy of citalopram in OCD (Dougherty et al., 2009; Galvao-de Almeida et al., 2007; Rabinowitz et al., 2008; Shim et al., 2008). These results have been confirmed by two double-blind placebo controlled trials (Kahn et al., 2007; Stein et al., 2007). Stein et al. recruited 466 patients with a diagnose of OCD that were randomly treated with escitalopram 10 or 20 mg/die, paroxetine 40 mg/die, or placebo for 24 weeks. After 12 weeks of therapy, the mean Y-BOCS score reduction in comparison with placebo was of 3.21 points ($p<0.1$) for escitalopram 20 mg and 2.47 point ($p<0.5$) for paroxetine 40 mg. After 24 weeks there was a statistically significant difference for all the groups in comparison with placebo ($p<0.5$ for escitalopram 10 mg, $p<0.1$ for escitalopram 20 mg and paroxetine); the mean Y-BOCS score reduction was of 3.10 points for escitalopram 10 mg, 3.12 for escitalopram 20 mg and 4.24 for paroxetine 40 mg. Escitalopram was better tolerated when compared with paroxetine, as proved by the smaller number of treatment withdrawals caused by adverse effects, although this difference was not statistically significant. Moreover, escitalopram has been proved to be effective in the long-term treatment and in the prevention of the exacerbation of the obsessive-compulsive symptoms after treatment discontinuation (Fineberg et al., 2007).
With regards to the supposed superiority of Clomipramine (CMI) over SSRIs clear evidences are still lacking. Nevertheless, the experts agree on the fact that SSRIs have to be considered first-choice treatments because of their more favorable side-effects profile (Koran et al., 2007). The efficacy of the different SSRIs does not differ in a critical way from one to another, but the response may be patient-specific. The reasons of this issue are still not clear and accurate predictors of response to be used in the clinical practice are still lacking.
Important aspects to be considered when choosing a SSRI are the tolerability for the individual patient of the specific side-effects of the drug, previous treatments and relative responses to them, the presence of psychiatric or medical comorbidities (i.e. paroxetine should never be prescribed to patients suffering from diabetes or neurologic bladder, as it is the SSRI most frequently associated with weight gain and anticholinergic effects (Koran et al., 2007).
The duration of the therapy and the dosage of the chosen drug represent two features of primary importance in the treatment of OCD. In fact, in order to obtain a clinical response in OCD the usual settings fixed for depression or other anxiety disorders are not functional.
Most of the patients do not achieve particular symptomatology improvements before 4-6 weeks of treatment, but some of them don't obtain it even before 10-12 weeks from the beginning of the therapy.
Thus, 12 weeks is the minimal duration of treatment necessary to correctly estimate the efficacy of a drug and plan long-term strategies. Instead, in order to obtain the full response

6 months are necessary: consequently, the treatment of the acute phase of the disorder should be administered for at least 6 months at full dose (Zohar et al., 2007).
With regards to the dosages, these are considerably higher that the ones used for depression and other anxiety disorder and often is necessary to prescribe the maximal dose in order to obtain a good response (Koran et al., 2007). In the following table (Table 1) the dosage details of the most commonly used SRIs are illustrated.

SRI	Starting dose (mg/day)	Usual target dose (mg/day)	Maximum dose (mg/day)
Citalopram	20	40-60	120
Escitalopram	10	20	60
Fluoxetine	20	40-60	120
Fluvoxamine	50	200	450
Paroxetine	20	40-60	100
Sertraline	50	200	400
Clomipramine	25	100-250	300

Table 1. (Modified by that of Koran et al. (Work group on obsessive-compulsive disorder): Practice guideline for the treatment of patients with obsessive-compulsive disorder. 2007) (American Psychiatric Association)

In case of adequate response to the first-choice drug, the duration of the maintaining phase of the treatment should last not less than 2 years at the dose necessary to elicit the clinical response. After this period, if relapse and symptom exacerbation have not occurred, is possible to slowly reduce the dose over some months, strictly monitoring the course of the disorder, otherwise the treatment should be continued.
A careful planning of long term treatment should consider the possibility of using lower doses of that used in the acute phase of the disorder. If many authors suggest keeping the dosage always at the same level, others state that is possible to greatly reduce it after the acute phase. In this perspective, it seems sensible to consider the efficacy and the tolerability of the therapy during the previous stages of the illness as the main guidance criteria, reducing the daily dose only in patients that achieve a complete, stable and long-lasting recovery after the treatment of the acute phase or in that patients that do not well tolerate high dosages of SRIs.
Other drugs have been proposed as first-line treatment in the acute phase of OCD, even if no clear evidence about their efficacy is available.
Increasing attention has been paid to the possible role of serotonin–norepinephrine reuptake inhibitors (SNRIs) in patients with OCD. The first evidence of the effectiveness of these compounds came from the observation that clomipramine is an inhibitor of the reuptake of serotonin as well as of norepinephrine (Dell'Osso et al., 2006). Venlafaxine is a 2-phenyl-2 ethylamine derivate that is chemically unrelated to tricyclic, tetracyclic or other available antidepressant. It shows different degrees of serotonin, norepinephrine and dopamine reuptake inhibition, as a function of the dosage (at higher dosis, the action on the noradrenergic and dopamine system becomes more marked) (Dell'Osso et al., 2006). Although mostly not placebo-controlled, the majority of venlafaxine short and intermediate-

term trials suggests the efficacy of this drug in both treatment-naïve and treatment-resistant OCD patients (Dell'Osso et al., 2006). Venlafaxine was as effective as paroxetine and clomipramine, and it was generally well tolerated by patients. However, due to the absence of double-blind placebo-controlled trials, venlafaxine should not be considered a first line medication treatment for patients with OCD at this time. Perhaps venlafaxine might be considered in specific clinical situations such as OCD with comorbid attention/deficit/hyperactivity disorder (ADHD) (Dell'Osso et al., 2006).

One placebo-controlled trial supports the efficacy of phenelzine (MAO inhibitor) (Vallejo et al., 1992). However, another one that compared phenelzine both to fluoxetine and to placebo demonstrated superiority over placebo for fluoxetine but not for phenelzine (Jenike et al., 1997).

Mirtazapine is an antidepressant that does not enhance 5-HT neurotransmission directly, but disinhibits the norepinephrine activation of 5-HT neurons and thereby increases 5-HT neurotransmission by a mechanism that does not require a time dependent desensitization of receptors (unlike SSRIs). The treatment of OCD patients has been tested in a single-blind study, which compared citalopram alone to a combination of mirtazapine and citalopram. This study indicated that the responses were faster (after four weeks) but that there was no difference between the groups after eight weeks and twelve weeks (Pallanti et al., 2004). Another open study showed the superiority of mirtazapine to placebo (Koran et al., 2005).

3. Approaches to treatment resistance and pharmacological strategies in resistant-OCD

Even if SSRIs have brought to a significant progress in the treatment of OCD, clinical evidence suggests that a high percentage of patients, ranging from about 40% to 60%, does not reach satisfying clinical improvement and does not "respond" properly to therapy (CMI-group, 1991; Goodman et al., 1992; Jenike and Rauch, 1994; McDougle et al., 1993; Piccinelli et al., 1995; Pigott et al., 1999; Rasmussen et al., 1993), with a strong impact on their quality of life, both in terms of disability and morbidity (Hollander et al., 1996).

We introduced operational criteria for the evaluation of the different "stages of response" in order to provide to the clinician a template to organize the best treatment strategy (Pallanti et al., 2002). The response to treatment is seen as a continuum of steps that ranges from the worse outcome, the refractoriness to all type of therapies, to the best outcomes, "remission" and "recovery".

Some terminological issues need to be clarified in order to avoid misunderstandings.

The term "resistant" should be used in case of a fail of one trial of therapy with a first choice treatment (at least 10-12 weeks with full dose of an SRI), whereas "refractory" only after at least three trials with SRI agents (one of them with Clomipramine), two augmentation trials with atypical antipsychotics, and at least 20-30 hours of cognitive-behavioral therapy.

Also the concept of "recovery" is different from that of "remission", although in OCD this last one seems to be a rare event; episodic course has been described in adults (Perugi et al., 1998; Ravizza et al., 1997) and because of this, the introduction of these two different definitions in the staging of illness seems to be rational and practical, as proposed by Frank et al. (1991) for depression.

"Recovery" should be used in case of complete absence of symptoms after treatment, corresponding to a Y-BOCS score of less than 8. Unfortunately, full recovery concerns only the 5% of patients with an episodic course of OCD (Rasmussen and Eisen 1997). The most probable result in a case of non-episodic courses is instead "remission", that indicates a reduction of the symptoms after treatment to the lower limit, which corresponds to a Y-BOCS score of 16 or less (see Table 2).

The presence of comorbid conditions also influences the course of the response to treatment. Non-responsive patients are more likely to meet criteria for comorbid psychiatric disorders and the presence of a specific comorbid condition could be a distinguishing feature in OCD, with influence on the treatment adequacy and outcome (Pallanti & Quercioli, 2006). For example, conditions such as bipolar disorder and ADHD (attention deficit hyperactivity disorder) are common in treatment-resistant patients, but there are only few studies investigating their impact on treatment resistance (Magalhães et al., 2010; Sheppard et al., 2010).

The majority of the proposed treatment-resistance therapeutic options are not FDA approved, but they are strongly recommended on the basis of preclinical and clinical evidences.

Stage of response	Stage	Description
I	Recovery	Not at all ill; less than 8 on Y-BOCS
II	Remission	Less than 16 on Y-BOCS
III	Full Response	35% or greater reduction of YBOCS and CGI 1 or 2
IV	Partial Response	Greater than 25% but less than 35% YBOCS reduction
V	Non-response	Less than 25% YBOCS reduction, CGI 4
VI	Relapse	Symptoms return (CGI 6 or 25% increase in Y-BOCS from remission score) after 3+ months of "adequate" treatment
VII	Refractory	No change or worsening with allavailable therapies

Table 2. Stages of response

3.1 Switching

Switching consists in replacing a serotoninergic agent with another one, or with a molecule of another class of drugs. The successfulness of this strategy in resistant patients is suggested by a number of studies (Ackerman et al., 1998; Denys et al., 2004; Goodman et al., 1997; Hollander et al., 2002; Koran et al., 2006; Rasmussen et al., 1997), but is not possible to predict the response of the patient to another drug. As suggested by clinical experience, the response rate to a successive treatment is around 50%, but it also declines with an inverse relationship to the number of failed trials (Koran et al., 2007).

The majority of the authors suggest switching from a SSRI to clomipramine (CMI) or vice versa, while the advantages of shifting from a SSRI to another one still remain unclear (Bogetto et al., 2003; Koran et al., 2007). The only data available are that of an open-label trial showing that a non-response to a SSRI does not imply the non-response to other molecules of the same class: 18 non-responders patients to at least two SSRI trials were treated with citalopram 40 mg/die and a response rate of 77% was obtained (Marazziti et al., 2001). In a case series, switching from SSRIs to the SNRI duloxetine was successful in a number of treatment-resistant patients (Dell'Osso, 2008). Some other trials have been performed with venlafaxine and mirtazapine. The switch from venlafaxine to paroxetine showed an improvement in 56% of the cases after the treatment, while from paroxetine to venlafaxine the rate was only 19% (Denys et al., 2004). The switch to mirtazapine is supported by one open pilot study and a double blind discontinuation trial (Koran et al., 2005).

So, considering the fact that there are no double blind studies that confirm the efficacy of switching a SSRI with another one, the rationale of this strategy derives from pharmacokinetic and side-effects issues. Citalopram and sertraline are for example poor inhibitors of the cit. P-450, which is involved in the metabolism of largely prescribed drugs, and could be therefore used in cases of complex pharmacological interactions. Instead, fluoxetine and paroxetine significantly inhibit the enzymes CYP2D6, that metabolize tricyclic antidepressants, antipsychotics, antiarrhythmic drugs and beta-blockers; fluvoxamine inhibits CYP1A2 and CYP3A4, which are implicated respectively in the elimination of warfarin and tricyclic antidepressants, benzodiazepines and antiarrhythmic drugs. Fluoxetine has a long half-life and an active metabolite that reduces the effects of abstinence, and this could result useful in patients with a low compliance (Pallanti & Koran, 2003).

3.2 Augmentation

3.2.1 SRIs

This augmentation strategy consists of the combination of two serotoninergic drugs, usually clomipramine or SSRIs, depending on which was the initial agent. Sertraline and citalopram represent first choice SSRIs augmentation molecules to clomipramine, due to the fact that they have a minor inhibitor effect on cit P-450 (Bogetto et al., 2003). The efficacy of clomipramine as augmentation agent to SSRIs is supported by a number of studies (Pallanti et al., 1999; Ravizza et al., 1996; Szegedi et al., 1996) and by a large expert-consensus (Koran et al., 2007). It's recommended to check the plasmatic concentration of clomipramine and of his metabolite desmethyl-clomipramine during an augmentation therapy and keep it below 500 ng/ml, because of cardiac and CNS toxic side effects. Fluvoxamine seems to be the SSRI that primarily has such an increasing effect (Koran et al., 2007).

With regards to the efficacy of SSRI augmentation during clomipramine treatment, research has focused on sertraline and fluoxetine. In an open trial a 20-40 mg dose of fluoxetine was effective in clomipramine-resistant patients (Simeon et al., 1990) and sertraline augmentation was more effective when compared to the dosage increase of the first choice treatment (Ravizza et al., 1996).

Besides SSRIs, a number of studies have been performed in the last years to investigate the usefulness of other serotoninergic drugs, but the results are not clear and need further investigations before being considered as standard treatments.

3.2.2 Dopaminergic agents

The dopaminergic system has a central role in the pathophysiology of OCD, as supported by pre-clinical and clinical evidences. Experimental studies in animals, using dopaminergic drugs (amphetamine, bromocriptine, apomorphine and L-dopa), have provided evidence for the dopamine involvement in compulsive behaviors such as grooming and repetitive checking behaviors, which are commonly considered animal models of OCD (Denys et al

2004; Pitman 1989; Tizabi 2002). Several evidences of dopamine dysregulation in OCD have also been found in humans. An indirect strong evidence of the role of dopamine in OCD is provided by some neurological diseases associated with dopaminergic dysfunction such as Tourette's syndrome, Sydenham's chorea and Parkinson disease, which often show obsessive-compulsive symptoms in their clinical presentation (Lochner et al., 2005; Pauls et al., 1986, 1995); in addition, Tourette's Syndrome and OCD are supposed to share common neurobiological underpinnings and genetic factors, due to the fact that they are described as comorbid, mainly in the childhood-onset forms (Perani et al. 2008). Moreover, the increase in synaptic dopamine levels due to the effect of drugs such as cocaine and amphetamines have been reported to exacerbate or induce as well as to improve OCD symptoms (Westemberg et al. 2007). Also neuroimaging studies provide interesting data about the dopamine involvement in OCD. Recently Perani et al. (Perani et al. 2008) conducted a positron emission tomography (PET) study in drug-naïve OCD patients, measuring both serotonin (5HT2A) and dopamine (D2) receptors distribution in vivo. The observed reduction of D2 receptors binding potential suggests a dopaminergic dysfunction, in particular in the ventral portion of striatum.

3.2.2.1 Antipsychotics

The effectiveness of antipsychotics augmentation in OCD treatment-resistant patients has been tested in many studies. Evidences of the efficacy of haloperidol and risperidone are provided by some randomized double-blind placebo-controlled studies; nevertheless, data regarding the effectiveness of quetiapine and olanzapine are still open to question. The effect of antipsychotics augmentation on OCD symptoms is relative quick, and patients are unlike to improve if they have not responded after one month of intervention (Bloch et al. 2006). The reason of the greater haloperidol and risperidone effectiveness is probably that they have a greater D2-dopamine receptor affinity. Preliminary available data highlight interesting perspectives regarding the use of new agents such as aripiprazole, although they do not provide yet sufficient basis for their wide use in OCD. The identification of predictors of antipsychotics response would represent a relevant progress in the treatment of resistant patients but unfortunately at the moment there is no reliable evidence regarding this issue. However, several data show that the subgroup of OCD patients with comorbid tics have particularly beneficial response to this intervention (especially to haloperidol) as well as those with poor insight (Hollander et al. 2003) and co-occurring schizotypal personality disorder (Bogetto et al. 2000; McDougle et al., 1990).

Until recently, mainly short-term response data were produced with regards to antipsychotics augmentation. Matsunaga et al. (2009) conducted the only available trial concerning the effectiveness and safety of long-term atypical antipsychotics augmentation. SRI-resistant patients responded to augmentation with atypical antipsychotics but showed a significantly higher rate of body mass index, as well as a significantly higher level of fasting blood sugar or elevated levels of triglycerides and total cholesterol, when compared to SRI-responders. These data are consistent with previous findings from short-term clinical trials and emphasize the importance to assess the metabolic and nutritional aspects in the management of OCD treatment-resistant patients.

3.2.2.2 Dextroamphetamine and caffeine

A single 30 mg dose of dextroamphetamine (d-amphetamine) was superior to placebo in immediately relieving OC symptoms in two small double blind placebo-controlled studies conducted before the introduction of SSRI for OCD treatment (Insel et al., 1983; Joffe et al., 1991). Methylphenidate monotherapy was effective in two cases of comorbid attention-deficit/hyperactivity disorder (ADHD) and OCD (van der Feltz-Cornelis, 1999). Nevertheless, in another open-label study, methylphenidate (40 mg) had no significant effect on OCD symptoms (Joffe et al., 1987).

Recently Koran et al. (2009) conducted a 5-week, double-blinded, caffeine controlled study of d-amphetamine augmentation in treatment-resistant OCD. Caffeine appeared to be slightly more effective, in both terms of number of responders (33% for d-amphetamine and 50% for caffeine) and degree of response (mean Y-BOCS score decrease was 48% for d-amphetamine and 55% for caffeine). The OC symptoms improvement associated with both drugs was maintained or increased over all the duration of the study. A possible explanation for the mechanism of this therapeutic effect could be that the increased release of dopamine induced by both drugs may increase D1 receptor stimulation in the prefrontal cortex; this enhancement is associated with improved attention regulation and working memory in patients with ADHD (Arnsten, 2006) that could lead to fewer obsessive intrusions, increased ability to shift attention away from them, and thus, decreased urges to perform compulsions (Koran et al., 2009).

3.2.3 Opioids

A remarkable number of studies (both preclinical and clinical) suggest the involvement of the opioid system in the pathophysiology of OCD (Amiaz et al., 2008; Koran et al., 2005b; McDougle et al., 1999; Roy et al., 1994; Urraca et al., 2004, Warneke et al., 1997). At the moment the results of the clinical trials concerning the use of opioid drugs as augmentation strategy in treatment-resistant OCD are controversial and there is no sufficient evidence supporting its use. Morphine, lorazepam and placebo were compared in a double blind study (Koran et al., 2005b) but only one patient had a sufficient response to morphine. Shapira and colleagues provided a report of the efficacy of the opioid agonist tramadol (26% reduction of the Y-BOCS score after 2 weeks of treatment) (Shapira et al., 1997). The opioid antagonist naltrexone did not improve OCD symptomatology and caused a worsening of anxiety and depressive symptoms in a double blind trial (Amiaz et al., 2008).

3.3 Infusion therapy

Infusion therapy is widely considered as a valid therapeutic strategy for treatment-resistant cases; clomipramine and citalopram are the drugs currently available for this kind of treatment.

The absorption of an intravenous administered drug is rapid, constant, and complete and is not affected by gastrointestinal variables, simultaneous administration of other drugs and first pass metabolism. Moreover, from a clinical point of view infusion therapy may improve treatment compliance, reinforce the therapeutic alliance and reduce the frequency of adverse events.

A greater efficacy of clomipramine i.v. versus placebo was reported in a double-blind placebo controlled study on 54 non-responders patients (in a previous 8 weeks-long trial with clomipramine per os) (Fallon et al., 1998). This could be explained considering the fact that the metabolite desmethyl-clomipramine has a weaker serotoninergic effect than clomipramine and intravenous administration may therefore increase the plasmatic clomipramine/desmethyl-clomipramine ratio and enhance the therapeutic effect.

Koran et al. (1998) compared clomipramine gradual increase administration and "pulse loading" administration. The results suggest a faster response with pulse loading administration. "Pulse loading" strategy consists in the application 150 mg i.v. at the first day, 200 mg i.v. at the second day, no administration for four consecutive days and then oral administration.

At the present time citalopram is the only SSRI available for infusion therapy. Our group administered for three weeks intravenous citalopram (followed by oral administration for other 9 weeks) to treatment-resistant OCD patients that were non-responders in at least two adequate trials with SSRI but not citalopram: 59% of the patients showed a reduction of at least 25% of the initial Y-BOCS score after the first 3 weeks of therapy, and improved more at the end of the 12 weeks (Pallanti et al., 2002b).

4. Physical therapies

4.1 Deep brain stimulation (DBS)

Another option to the neurosurgical interventions performed as last resource in treatment-resistant patients with extremely disabling symptoms is represented by deep brain stimulation. In deep brain stimulation (DBS) procedures, stimulation electrodes are implanted into specific brain regions and continuous electrical high frequency stimulation is delivered from a pulse generator. DBS is externally programmable and reversible, in that the stimulator can be turned on or off and controlled at the discretion of the clinician. The targets that have shown to provide the best results are both the anterior limbs of the internal capsule. The stimulation of this area seems to disrupt the activity in the loop fibers that connect the cortex with the thalamus and therefore interrupt the pathological circuit of this area (Shah et al., 2008). DBS in this site was successful in several case series (Abelson et al., 2005; Anderson and Hamed, 2003; Gabriels et al., 2003; Nuttin et al., 1999, 2003, 2008). In an open study, DBS was still effective after three years from the implantation (Greenberg et al., 2006). A multicenter randomized sham-controlled crossover study based on the stimulation of the subthalamic nucleus on 16 patients with severe OCD showed interesting results (Mallet et al., 2008). After 10 months of active stimulation 10 patients had a significant improvement of the symptoms and 4 recovered (Y-BOCS of 6 or less). However, the good results of this study are limited by the onset of some major adverse events (including a brain hemorrhage) and several minor adverse events.

4.2 Repetitive transcranial magnetic stimulation (rTMS)

There is no clear evidence regarding the use of rTMS in the treatment of OCD due to the fact that the design of the few studies performed differs in many important aspects such as site stimulation, parameters, and treatment duration. In double-blind sham-controlled studies, rTMS was ineffective both over the left dorsolateral prefrontal cortex was ineffective (Prasko et al. 2006; Sachdev et al. 2007) and over the right prefrontal rTMS (Alonso et al., 2001). Finally, interesting results were provided by two recent studies concerning the stimulation of the orbitofrontal cortex (Ruffini et al., 2009) and of the supplementary motor area (Mantovani et al., 2010) that showed a significant reduction of Y-BOCS score when compared to sham stimulation.

4.3 Electroconvulsive therapy (Ect)

Experts agree on the fact that ECT has a very limited role in OCD treatment, as there is no relevant evidence of benefits regarding the control of core symptoms of OCD (Bandelow et al., 2008) even if some case reports suggest the efficacy of it (Fukuchi et al., 2003; Strassnig et al., 2004;). Anyway, it may represent a useful tool for the treatment of OCD comorbidities such as depression, catatonia, etc. (Casey & Davis, 1994; Hanisch et al., 2009).

5. Conclusions and future perspectives

In conclusion, the range of therapeutic options for treatment-resistant patients is wide, and a number of them seem to have a quite good efficacy. Current research on animal and human models suggests that the discovery of more precise and distinctive neurofunctional targets is possible and that may successfully lead to a patient-tailored treatment algorithm. Identifying the different groups of patients and basing the treatment on reliable and easily detectable neurodysfunctional targets is one of the most desirable and exciting goals that in the next future may be achieved, in order to offer a highly specific treatment for each single patient.

6. References

Abelson, J.L., Curtis, G.C., Sagher, O., Albucher R.C., Harrigan M., Taylor S.F., Martis B., & Giordani B. (2005). Deep brain stimulation for refractory obsessive-compulsive disorder. *Biol Psychiatry*, 57, 510-516.

Abramowitz, J. (1998). Does cognitive-behavioral therapy cure obsessive-compulsive disorder? A meta-analytic evaluation of clinical significance. *Behavior Therapy*, 29, 355.

Alonso, P., Pujol, J., Cardoner, N., Benlloch, L., Deus, J., & al. (2001). Right prefrontal repetitive transcranial magnetic stimulation in obsessive-compulsive disorder: a double-blind, placebo-controlled study. *Am J Psychiatry*, 1143-1145.

Anderson, D., & Ahmed, A. (2003). Treatment of patients with intractable obsessive-compulsive disorder with anterior capsular stimulation. Case report. *J Neurosurg*, 98, 1104-1108.

Arnsten, A.F.T. (2006). Fundamentals of attention-deficit/hyperactivity disorder: circuits and pathways. *J Clin Psychiatry*, 67, 7-12.

American Psychiatric Association. (2000). *Diagnostic and Statistical Manual of Mental Disorders. 4th edition, text rev*. Washington DC.

Amiaz, R., Fostick, L., Gershon, A., & al. (2008). Naltrexone augmentation in OCD: a double-blind placebo-controlled cross-over study. *Eur Neuropsychopharmacol*, 18, 455-461.

Bandelow, B., et al. (2008). World Federation of Societies of Biological Psychiatry (WFSBP) guidelines for the pharmacological treatment of anxiety, obsessive-compulsive and post-traumatic stress disorders - first revision. *World J Biol Psychiatry*, 9, 248-312.

Bloch, M.H., Landeros-Weisenberger, A., Kelmendi, B., Coric, V., Bracken, M.B., & Leckman, J.F. (2006). A systematic review: antipsychotic augmentation with treatment refractory obsessive-compulsive disorder. *Mol Psychiatry*, 11, 622-632.

Bogetto, F., Bellino, S., Vaschetto, P., & Ziero, S. (2000). Olanzapine augmentation of fluvoxamine-refractory obsessive-compulsive disorder (OCD): a 12-week open trial. *Psychiatry Res*, 96, 91-98.

Bogetto, F., Maina, G., Locatelli, M., & Lucca, A. (2003). Terapie biologiche nel DOC. In *Il disturbo ossessivo-compulsivo e il suo spettro,* Smeraldi, E., et al., 336-366, Masson, Milano.

Casey, D.A., Davis, M.H. (1994). Obsessive-compulsive disorder responsive to electroconvulsive therapy in an elderly woman. *South Med J*, 87, 862-4.

CMI-group. (1991). Clomipramine in the treatment of patients with obsessive-compulsive disorder. The clomipramine collaborative study group. *Arch Gen Psychiatry*, 48, 730-738.

Cottraux, J., Note, I., Yao, S., Lafont, S., et al. (2001). A randomized controlled trial of cognitive therapy versus intensive behavior therapy in obsessive-compulsive disorder. *Psychother Psychosom*, 70, 288-297.

Dell'Osso, B., Nestadt, G., Allen, A., & Hollander, E. (2006). Serotonin-norepinephrine reuptake inhibitors in the treatment of obsessive-compulsive disorder: A critical review. *J Clin Psychiatry*, 67, 600-10.

Dell'Osso, B., Mundo, E., Marazziti, D., & Altamura, A. (2008). Switching from serotonin reuptake inhibitors to duloxetine in patients with resistant obsessive-compulsive disorder: a case series. *J Psychopharmacol* , 22, 210-213.

Denys, D., van Megen, H., van der Wee, N., & Westenberg, H. (2004). A double-blind switch study of paroxetine and venlafaxine in obsessive compulsive disorder. *J Clin Psychiatry* , 65, 37-43.

Dougherty, D.D., Jameson, M., Deckersbach, T., Loh, R., Thompson-Hollands, J., Jenike, M., & Keuthen, N.J. (2009). Open-label study of high (30 mg) and moderate (20 mg) dose escitalopram for the treatment of obsessive-compulsive disorder. *Int Clin Psychopharmacol*, 24, 306-11.

Eddy, K., Dutra, L., Bradley, R., & Westen, D. (2004). A multidimensional meta-analysis of psychotherapy and pharmacotherapy for obsessive-compulsive disorder. *Clin Psychol Rev*, 24, 1011-1030.

Fallon, B., Liebowitz, M., Campeas, R., Schneier, F., Marshall, R., Davies, S., et al. (1998). Intravenous clomipramine for obsessive-compulsive disorder refractory to oral clomipramine: a placebo-controlled study. *Arch Gen Psychiatry*, 55, 918-924.

Fernandez, C.E., & Lopez-Ibor, J.J. (1967) Monochlorimipramine in the treatment of psychiatric patients resistant to other therapies. *Actas Luso Esp Neurol Psiq Ciec Afines*, 26, 119-147.

Fineberg, N., Tonnoir, B., & al. (2007). Escitalopram prevents relapse of obsessive-compulsive disorder. *European Neuropsychopharmacology* , 17, 430-439.

Fisher, P., & Welles, A. (2005). How effective are cognitive and behavioral treatments for obsessive-compulsive disorder? A clinical significance analysis. *Behav Res Ther*, 43, 1543-1558.

Frank, E., Prien, R., Jarret, R., Keller, M., Kupfer, D., Lavori, P., et al. (1991). Conceptualization and rationale for consensus definitions of terms in major depressive disorder. Remission, recovery, relapse, and recurrence. *Arch Gen Psychiatry*, 48, 851-855.

Freeston, M., & al. (1996). Correcting faulty appraisals of obsessional thoughts. *Beh Res Ther* , 34, 433-446.

Fukuchi, T., Okada, Y., Katayama, H., Nishijima, K., Kato, S., Netsu, S., & Fukuda, H. (2003). A case of pregnant woman with severe obsessive-compulsive disorder successfully treated by modified-electroconvulsive therapy. *Seishin Shinkeigaku Zasshi*, 105, 927-32.

Gabriels, L., Cosyns, P., Nuttin, B., Demeulemeester, H., & Gybels, J. (2003). Deep brain stimulation for treatment-refractory obsessive-compulsive disorder: psychopathological and neuropsychological outcome in three cases. *Acta Psychiatr Scand*, 107, 275-282.

Galvao-de Almeida, A., Quarantini, L., Gois, C., & al. (2007). Obsessive-compulsive disorder: an open-label pilot trial of escitalopram. *CNS Spectrum*, 12 , 519-524.

Goodman, W., Price, L., Rasmussen, S., Mazure, C., Delgado, P., Heninger, G., & Charney, D. (1989). The Yale Brown obsessive compulsive scale: validity. *Arch gen psychiatry*, 46, 1012-16.

Goodman, W., McDougle, C., & Price, L. (1992). Pharmacotherapy of obsessive-compulsive disorder. *J Clin Psychiatry*, 43, 29-37.

Goodman, W., Ward, H., Kablinger, A., & al. (1997). Fluvoxamine in the treatment of obsessive-compulsive disorder and related conditions. *J Clin Psychiatry*, 58, 32-49.

Greenberg, B.D., Malone, D.A., Friehs, G.M., Rezai, A.R., Kubu, C.S., Malloy, P.F., Salloway, S.P., Okun, M.S., Goodman, W.K, & Rasmussen, S.A. (2006). Three-year outcomes in deep brain stimulation for highly resistant obsessive-compulsive disorder. *Neuropsychopharmacology*, 31, 2384-2393.

Hanisch, F., Friedemann, J., Piro, J., & Gutmann, P. (2009). Maintenance electroconvulsive therapy for comorbid pharmacotherapy-refractory obsessive-compulsive and schizoaffective disorder. *Eur J Med Res*, 14, 367-8.

Hollander, E., Kwon, J., Stein, D., Broatch, J., Rowland, C., & Himelein, C. (1996). Obsessive-compulsive and spectrum disorders: overview and quality of life issues. *J Clin Psychiatry*, 57, 3-6.

Hollander, E., Baldini Rossi, N., Sood, E., & Pallanti, S. (2003). Risperidone augmentation in treatment-resistant obsessivecompulsive disorder: a double-blind, placebo-controlled study. *Int J Neuropsychopharmacol*, 6, 397-401.

Insel, T.R., Hamilton, J.A., Guttmacher, L.B., et al. (1983). D-amphetamine in obsessive-compulsive disorder. *Psychopharmacology*, 80, 231-235.

Jenike, M.A., Baer, L., Minichiello, W.E., Rauch, S.L., & Buttolph, M.L. (1997). Placebo-controlled trial of fluoxetine and phenelzine for obsessive-compulsive disorder. *Am J Psychiatry*, 154, 1261-4.

Jenike, M., Rauch, S., & al. (1994). Managing the patients with treatment resistant obsessive-compulsive disorder: current strategies. *J Clin Psychiatry*, 55, 11-17.

Joffe R.T., & Swinson, R.P. (1987) Metylphenidate in primary obsessive-compulsive disorder. *J Clin Psychopharmacol*, 7, 420-422.

Joffe, R.T., Swinson, R.P., & Levitt, A.J. (1991). Acute psychostimulant challenge in primary obsessive-compulsive disorder. *J Clin Psychopharmacol*, 11, 237-241.

Khan, M.N., Hotiana, U.A., & Ahmad, S. (2007). Escitalopram in the treatment of obsessive-compulsive disorder: a double blind placebo control trial. *J Ayub Med Coll Abbottabad*, 19, 58-63.

Koran, L., Pallanti, S., Quercioli, L., & Paiva, R. (1998). Pulse loading versus gradual dosing of intravenous clomipramine in obsessive-compulsive disorder. *Eur Neuropsychopharmacol*, 8, 121-126.

Koran, L.M., Gamel, N.N., Choung, H.W., Smith, E.H., & Aboujaoude, E.N. (2005). Mirtazapine for obsessive-compulsive disorder: an open trial followed by double-blind discontinuation. *J Clin Psychiatry*, 66, 515-20.

Koran, L., Aboujaoude, E., Bullok, K., et al. (2005)b. Double-blind treatment with oral morphine in treatment resistant obsessive-compulsive disorder. *J Clin Psychiatry*, 66, 353-359.

Koran, L., Aboujaoude, E., Ward, H., Shapira, N., Sallee, F., Gamel, N., et al. (2006). Pulse-loaded intravenous clomipramine in treatment-resistant obsessive compulsive disorder. *J Clin Psychopharmacol*, 26, 79-83.

Koran, L., Hanna, G., Hollander, E., Nestadt, G., & al. (2007). American Psychiatry Association. Practice guideline for the treatment of patients with obsessive-compulsive disorder. *Am J Psychiatry*, 164, 1-56.

Koran, L.M., Aboujaoude, E., & Gamel, N.N. (2009). Double-blind study of dextroamphetamine versus caffeine augmentation for treatment-resistant obsessive-compulsive disorder. *J Clin Psychiatry*, 70, 1530-1535.

Lochner, C., Hemmings, S.M., Kinnear, C.J., Niehaus, D.J., Nel, D.G., Corfield, V.A., Moolman-Smook, J.C., Seedat, S., & Stein, D.J. (2005). Cluster analysis of obsessive-compulsive spectrum disorders in patients with obsessive-compulsive disorder: clinical and genetic correlates. *Compr. Psychiatry*, 46, 14–19.

Magalhães, P.V., Kapczinski, N.S., & Kapczinski, F. (2010). Correlates and impact of obsessive-compulsive comorbidity in bipolar disorder. *Compr Psychiatry*, 51, 353-6.

Mallet, L., Polosan, M., Jaafari, N., Baup, N., Welter, M.L., Fontaine, D., du Montcel, S.T., Yelnik, J., Chereau, I., Arbus, C., et al. (2008). Subthalamic nucleus stimulation in severe obsessive-compulsive disorder. *N Engl J Med*, 359, 2121-2134.

Mantovani, A., Simpson, H.B., Fallon, B.A., Rossi, S., & Lisanby, S.H. (2010). Randomized sham-controlled trial of repetitive transcranial magnetic stimulation in treatment-resistant obsessive-compulsive disorder. Int J Neuropsychopharmacol, 13, 217-227.

Marazziti, D., Dell'Osso, L., Gemignani, A., & al. (2001). Citalopram in refractory obsessive-compulsive disorder: an open study. *Int Clin Psychopharmacol*, 16, 215-219.

Matsunaga, H., Nakata, T., Hayashida, K., Ohya, K., Kiriike, N., & Stein, D.J. (2009). A long term trial of effectiveness and safety of atipica antipsychotic agents in augmenting SSRI-refractory obsessive-compulsive disorder. *J Clin Psychiatry*, 70, 863-868.

McDougle, C.J., Goodman, W.K., Price, L.H., Delgado, P.L., Krystal, J.H., Charney, D.S., et al. (1990). Neuroleptic addition in fluvoxamine- refractory obsessive-compulsive disorder. *Am J Psychiatry*, 147, 652-654.

McDougle, C., Goodman, W., Leckman, J., & Price, L. (1993). The psychopharmacology of obsessive-compulsive disorder. Implications for treatment and pathogenesis. *Psych Clinics of North America*, 15, 749-766.

McDougle, C., Barr, L., Goodman, W., & Price, L. (1999). Possible role of neuropeptides in obsessive compulsive disorder. *Psychoneuroendocrinology*, 24, 1-24.

Meyer, V. (1966). Modifications of expectations in cases of obsessional rituals. *Behavior Res Ther*, 4, 273-280.

Montgomery, S., Kasper, S., Stein, D., et al. (2001). Citalopram 20 mg, 40 mg and 60 mg are all effective and well tolerated compared with placebo in obsessive-compulsive disorder. *Int Clin Psychopharmacol*, 16, 75-86.

Nuttin, B., Cosyns, P., Demeulemeester, H., Gybels, J., & Meyerson, B. (1999). Electrical stimulation in anterior limbs of internal capsules in patients with obsessive-compulsive disorder. *Lancet*, 354, 1526.

Nuttin, B.J., Gabriels, L.A., Cosyns, P.R., Meyerson, B.A., Andreewitch, S., Sunaert, S.G., Maes, A.F., Dupont, P.J., Gybels, J.M., Gielen, F., Demeulemeester, H.G. (2003). Long-term electrical capsular stimulation in patients with obsessive-compulsive disorder. *Neurosurgery*, 52, 1263-1272.

Nuttin, B.J., Gabriels, L.A., Cosyns, P.R., Meyerson, B.A., Andreewitch, S., Sunaert, S.G., Maes, A.F., Dupont, P.J., Gybels, J.M., Gielen, F., & Demeulemeester, H.G. (2008). Long-term electrical capsular stimulation in patients with obsessive-compulsive disorder. *Neurosurgery*, 62, 966-977.

Pallanti, S., Quercioli, L., & Paiva, R. (1999). Citalopram for treatment-resistant obsessive-compulsive disorder. *Eur Psychiatry*, 14, 101-106.

Pallanti, S., Hollander, E., Bienstock, C., et al. (2002). Treatment non-response in OCD: methodological issues and operational definitions. *Int J Neuropsychopharmacol*, 5, 181-191.

Pallanti, S., Quercioli, L., & Koran, L.M. (2002b). Citalopram intravenous infusion in resistant obsessive-compulsive disorder: an open trial. *J Clin Psychiatry*, 63, 796-801.

Pallanti, S., & Koran, L. M. (2003). *La cura del paziente con disturbo ossessivo compulsivo resistente*. Airon Edizione, Milano.

Pallanti, S., Quercioli, L., Bruscoli, M. (2004). Response acceleration with mirtazapine augmentation of citalopram in obsessive-compulsive disorder patients without comorbid depression: a pilot study. *J Clin Psychiatry*, 65, 1394-9

Pallanti, S., & Quercioli, L. (2006). Treatment-refractory obsessive-compulsive disorder: methodological issues, operational definitions and therapeutic lines. *Prog Neuropsychopharmacol Biol Psychiatry*, 30, 400-412.

Pauls, D.L., Alsobrook II, J.P., Goodman, W., Rasmussen, S., & Leckman, J.F. (1995). A family study of obsessive-compulsive disorder. *Am J Psychiatry*, 152, 76–84.

Pauls, D.L., Towbin, K.E., Leckman, J.F., Zahner, G.E., & Cohen, D.J., (1986). Gilles de la Tourette's syndrome and obsessive-compulsive disorder. Evidence supporting a genetic relationship. *Arch Gen Psychiatry*, 43, 1180–1182.

Perani, D., Garibotto, V., Gorini, A., Moresco, R.M., Henin, M., Panzacchi, A., Matarrese, M., Carpinelli, A., Bellodi, L., Fazio, F. (2008). In vivo PET study of 5HT2A serotonin and D2 dopamine dysfunction in drug-naive obsessive-compulsive disorder. *Neuroimage*, 42, 306-314.

Perugi, G., Akiskal, H.S., Gemingnani, A., Pfanner, C., Presta, S., Milanfranchi, A., et al. (1998). Episodic course in obsessive-compulsive disorder. *Eur Arch Psychiatry Clin Neurosci*, 248, 240-4.

Piccinelli, M., Pini, S., Bellantuono, C., et al. (1995). Efficacy of drug treatment in obsessive-compulsive disorder: a meta-analityc review. *Br J Psychiatry*, 166, 242-243.

Pigott, T., & Seay, S. (1999). A review of the efficacy of selective serotonin reutake inhibitors in obsessive-compulsive disorder. *J Clin Psychiatry*, 608, 101-106.

Pidrman, V., & Tuma, I. (1997). Fenfluramine challenge test in obsessive-compulsive disorder: first results. *Acta Medica*, 40, 99-102.

Pitman, R.K. (1989). Animal models of compulsive behavior. *Biol. Psychiatry* 26, 189–198.

Prasko, J., Paskova, B., Zalesky, R., Novak, T., et al. (2006). The effect of repetitive transcranial magnetic stimulation (rTMS) on symptoms in obsessive compulsive disorder. A randomized, double blind, sham controlled study. *Neuro Endocrinol Lett* , 27, 327-332.

Rabinowitz, I., Baruch, Y., & Barak, Y. (2008). High-dose escitalopram for the treatment of obsessive-compulsive disorder. *Int clin Psychopharmacol*, 23, 49-53.

Rasmussen, S.A., Eisen, J.L., & Pato, M.T. (1993). Current issues in the pharmacological management of obsessive-compulsive disorder. *J Clin Psychiatry*, 54, 4-9.

Rasmussen, S.A., & Eisen, J.L. (1997). Treatment strategies for chronic and refractory obsessive-compulsive disorder. *J Clin Psychiatry*, 58, 9-13.

Ravizza, L., Barzega, G., Bellino, S., Bogetto, F., & Maina, G. (1996). Drug treatment of obsessive-compulsive disorder: long-term trial with clomipramine and selective serotonin reuptake inhibitors (SSRIs). *Psychopharmacol Bull*, 32, 167-173.

Ravizza, L., Maina, G., & Bogetto, F. (1997). Episodic and chronic obsessive-compulsive disorder. *Depress Anxiety*, 6, 154–158.

Roy, B., Benkelfalt, C., Hill, J., Pierce, P., Dauphin, M., Kely, T., et al. (1994). Serum antibody for somatostatin-14 and prodynorphine in patients with obsessive-compulsive disorder, schizophrenia, Alzheimer's disease, multiple sclerosis, and advance HIV infection. *Biol Psychiatry*, 35, 335-344.

Ruffini, C., Locatelli, M., Lucca, A., Benedetti, F., Insacco, C., & Smeraldi, E. (2009). Augmentation effect of repetitive transcranial magnetic stimulation over the orbitofrontal cortex in drug-resistant obsessive-compulsive disorder patients: a controlled investigation. *J Clin Psychiatry*, 11, 226-230.

Sachdev, P.S., Loo, C.K., Mitchell, P.B., et al. (2007). Repetitive transcranial magnetic stimulation for the treatment of obsessive-ompulsive disorder: a double-blind controlled investigation. *Psychol Med*, 37, 1645–1649.

Shah, D.B., Pesiridou, A., Baltuch, G.H., Malone, D.A., & O'Reardon, J.P. (2008) Functional neurosurgery in the treatment of severe obsessive compulsive disorder and major depression: overview of disease circuits and therapeutic targeting for the clinician. *Psychiatry*, 5, 24-33.

Shapira, N., Keck, P., Goldsmith, T., et al. (1997). Open-label pilot study of tramadol hydrochloride in treatment-refractory obsessive-compulsive disorder. *Depress Anxiety*, 6, 170-173.

Sheppard, B.A., Chavira, D., Azzam, A., Grados, M.A., Umana, P., Garrido, H., & Mathews, C.A. (2010). ADHD prevalence and association with hoarding behaviors in childhood-onset OCD. *Depress Anxiety*, 27, 667–674.

Shim, G., Kang, D., & Kwon, J. (2008). High-dose escitalopram treatment in patients with obsessive-compulsive disorder: a naturalistic case series. *J Clin Psychopharmacol*, 28, 108-110.

Simeon, J., Thatte, S., & Wiggins, D. (1990). Treatment of adolescent obsessive-compulsive disorder with a clomipramine-fluoxetine combination. *Psychopharmacol Bull*, 26, 285-290.

Stengler-Wenzke, K., Muller, U., Barthel, H., Angermeyer, M., & al. (2006). Serotonin transporter imaging with (123 I)-CIT SPECT before and after one year of citalopram treatment of obsessive-compulsive disorder. *Neuropsychobiology*, 53, 40-45.

Strassnig, M., Riedel, M., & Müller, N. (2004). Electroconvulsive therapy in a patient with Tourette's syndrome and co-morbid Obsessive Compulsive Disorder. *World J Biol Psychiatry*, 5, 164-6.

Szegedi, A., Wetzel, H., Leal, M., Hartter, S., et al. (1996). Combination treatment with clomipramine and fluvoxamine: drug monitoring, safety and tollerabity data. *J Clin Psychiatry*, 57, 257-264.

Tizabi, Y., Louis, V.A., Taylor, C.T., Waxman, D., Culver, K.E., & Szechtman, H. (2002). Effect of nicotine on quinpirole-induced checking behavior in rats: implications for obsessive-compulsive disorder. *Biol Psychia*try, 51, 164–171.

Thorén, P., Asberg, M., Cronholm, B., Jörnestedt, L., & Träskman, L. (1980). Clomipramine treatment of obsessive-compulsive disorder. A controlled clinical trial. *Arch Gen Psychiatry*, 37, 1281-5.

Urraca, N., Camarena, B., Gomez-Caudillo, L., et al. (2004). Mu opioid receptor gene as a candidate for the study of obsessive compulsive disorder with and without tics. *Am J of Med Genet Neuropsychiatr Genet*, 127B, 94-96.

Vallejo, J., Olivares, J., Marcos, T., Bulbena, A., & Menchón, J.M. (1992). Clomipramine versus phenelzine in obsessive-compulsive disorder. A controlled clinical trial. *Br J Psychiatry*, 161, 665-70.

Van Balkom, A., De Hann, E., Van Hoppen, P., et al. (1998). Cognitive and behavioral therapies alone versus in combination with fluvoxamine in the treatment of obsessive-compulsive disorder. *J Nerv Ment Dis*, 186, 492-499.

Van der Feltz-Cornelis, C.M. (1999). Intractable obsessive-compulsive disorder: comorbidity with unrecognized adul attention-deficit hyperactivity disorder? *Nerv Ment Dis*; 187: 243-245.

Warneke, L. (1997). A possible new treatment approach to obsessive-compulsive disorder [letter]. *Can J Psychiatry*, 42, 667-668.

Westemberg, H.G.M., Fineberg, N.A., & Denys, D. (2007). Neurobiology of obsessive-compulsive disorder: serotonin and beyond. *CNS Spectrum*, 12, 14-27.

Whittal, M., Thordarson, D., & McLean, P. (2005). Treatment of obsessive-compulsive disorder: cognitive behavior therapy vs exposure and response prevention. *Behav Res Ther*, 43, 1559-1576.

14

A Review of Interventions for Treatment-Resistant Posttraumatic Stress Disorder

Cara Katz[1], Murray Stein[2], J. Don Richardson[3], Soraya Seedat[4] and Jitender Sareen[1]
[1]University of Manitoba;
[2]University of California San Diego;
[3]University of Western Ontario;
[4]University Stellenbosch
[1,3]Canada
[2]United States
[4]South Africa

1. Introduction

A traumatic experience evokes a stress response and increased anxiety in those who witness or experience the event. In most, the stress symptoms will alleviate with time. However, within a significant proportion of individuals, the effects of the trauma will not diminish. Rather, residual symptoms will remain and will surface as Posttraumatic Stress Disorder (PTSD). PTSD is an anxiety disorder that can develop after one experiences or witnesses a traumatic event involving actual or threatened death or harm, or when one learns of someone else's threat of actual harm (APA Diagnostic and Statistical manual, 1994).

According to DSM-IV, PTSD manifests itself through clusters of three symptoms: re-experiencing; avoiding and numbing; and hyper-arousal. Re-experiencing the traumatic event includes recurring nightmares; flashbacks; intrusive memories or images; extreme emotional or physical responses and dissociation. The symptoms of re-experiencing the trauma can be enhanced by olfactory, visual or auditory sensory information that act as a reminder to the event. Avoidance and numbing symptoms are expressed through efforts to avoid thoughts, feelings, activities or memories associated with the trauma; alienating oneself; loss of interest in and avoidance of activities; and the inability to have loving feelings. The hyper-arousal cluster of symptoms includes increased startle responses; insomnia, in addition to other sleep issues; difficulties in concentrating; and outbursts of anger (Pivac & Kozaric-Kovacic, 2006). A positive diagnosis for PTSD includes the presence of these symptoms for at least one month accompanied with functional impairment, often including occupational and social difficulties (Bandelow et al., 2008). When symptoms last more than three months, PTSD is considered chronic (Berger et al., 2009). PTSD is often comorbid with substance abuse, major depression, other anxiety disorders and suicidality. In more severe cases, often seen in veteran populations, psychotic features and increased resistance to treatment is evident (Pivac & Kozaric-Kovacic, 2006). The present chapter will focus on the literature on the interventions for Treatment Resistant PTSD (TR-PTSD).

2. Standard first line of treatment

The goal of treating PTSD is to reduce symptom severity and frequency, fear responses, and functional impairment, to treat concurrent disorders, to prevent relapse and to build resilience capacity and improve quality of life (Berger et al., 2009).

2.1 Psychotherapy

Meta-analytic studies have demonstrated that trauma-focused cognitive behavioral therapies have large effect sizes in treating PTSD (Otto et al., 2003). Exposure therapy is useful in treating characteristic features of PTSD and is considered the best psychotherapy for PTSD treatment (Ballenger et al., 2004). This technique helps patients confront thoughts and situations related to their trauma in a safe environment in order to reduce anxiety and fear responses. Other techniques include stress inoculation training to teach anxiety management in order to cope with fear; cognitive therapy, designed to modify irrational interpretations of the trauma that are often the root of the negative emotions; and eye movement desensitization, the process of stimulating rapid eye movements simultaneous to image exposure. Trauma-focused cognitive behavioral therapy (CBT) uses some elements of these treatments (Seedat, Stein, & Carey, 2005). As discussed in the psychotherapy methods for TR-PTSD, refugees resistant to treatment often respond well to this form of treatment (see section 4.7).

2.2 Pharmacotherapy

Antidepressants are the standard first-line pharmacological approach in treating PTSD. Selective serotonin reuptake inhibitors (SSRIs) are the most studied family of antidepressant for the treatment of PTSD, with fluoxetine, sertraline and paroxetine being the most examined for this purpose. Sertraline and paroxetine have been approved by Federal Drug Administration (FDA) for the treatment of PTSD. These SSRIs have demonstrated short-term (6-12 weeks) effects in PTSD treatment, and if continued for longer (6-12 months) also reduce relapse rates (Asnis, Kohn, Henderson, & Brown, 2004). SSRIs block the serotonin transporter, thereby preventing the re-uptake of serotonin, increasing the amount of serotonin in the synapse. However, the mechanism(s) by which SSRIs achieve their beneficial effect in PTSD is not well understood.

Selective serotonin and norepinephrine reuptake inhibitors (SNRIs) have also been indicated in the treatment of PTSD (Asnis et al., 2004). One of the SSRIs, venlafaxine extended release (ER), has been evaluated in two randomized controlled trials (Davidson, Baldwin et al., 2006; Davidson, Rothbaum et al., 2006), and was well tolerated and effective for treating PTSD.

3. Definition of PTSD-treatment resistance

Although considered the first line of treatment, response rates to treatment with SSRIs are usually no higher than 60% and fewer than 30% of people achieve full relief (Berger et al., 2009). Response to antidepressant treatment is currently defined as a greater than 30% reduction in Clinician Administered PTSD Scale (CAPS) scores or a score of 1 (very much improved) or 2 (much improved) on the Clinical Global Impressions scale-Improvement item (CGI-I). Therefore, even those who respond partially to treatment may still meet the criteria for PTSD at the end of treatment (Berger et al., 2009). The ultimate goal of treatment is remission.

Remission in PTSD can be defined as a CAPS score ≤20. When determining if a patient is resistant to treatment, the initial diagnosis should be reviewed. Medication compliance, dosage, and duration of trial should be assessed (Bandelow et al., 2008). If after eight to 12 weeks the patient has not responded to the optimized dose, the medication should be changed. If the patient experiences a partial response, they may respond within another four to six weeks on the medication. In patients who are still unresponsive, trauma-focused cognitive-behavior therapy should be added (Bandelow et al., 2008).

Unfortunately, at this point, many patients are still refractory to treatment. An individual who, despite adequate treatment with antidepressants and cognitive behavioral therapy, still meets the criteria for PTSD is considered treatment-resistant. Additionally, some patients who experience partial response to treatment can still meet the criteria for a diagnosis of PTSD and are therefore also considered treatment-resistant. The definition of treatment resistance may vary across studies, but is generally the failure to fully respond or to respond at all to previous treatment, such as antidepressants and psychotherapy, after an appropriate trial period. There is little consensus on the next step in treatment.

Resistance to PTSD treatment can be associated with more severe cases of PTSD, the experience of multiple traumas, the type of trauma, other comorbid psychiatric disorders and gender, among other factors (Hamner, Robert, & Frueh, 2004). The additive effect of such factors manifests itself differently in civilian, combat-veteran and refugee populations. For example, civilian populations are most often responsive to antidepressants (Hamner et al., 2004), whereas, combat-veterans often have co-morbid psychiatric disorders (Hamner, 1997; Pivac & Kozaric-Kovacic, 2006), which can increase the severity of PTSD symptoms and the likelihood of treatment-resistance. Refugees commonly suffer from extreme forms of PTSD, often co-morbid with panic disorder. Among refugees, the prevalence of PTSD is estimated to range from 10-86%, a prevalence rate much higher than that of the general population. The nature of PTSD in refugee populations is often more severe due to prolonged exposure to traumatic events, pre-, post- or during migration (Boynton, Bentley, Strachan, Barbato, & Raskind, 2009). As such, refugees often have forms of PTSD that are not responsive to standard treatment with SSRIs.

Due to additional cultural issues and barriers with refugees, cognitive behavioral therapy is recommended for treatment refractoriness and can be adjusted to meet the specific needs of different cultures (Hinton et al., 2005; Hinton, Hofmann, Rivera, Otto, & Pollack, 2011; Hinton et al., 2004; Otto et al., 2003).

4. Pharmacotherapy and psychotherapy for TR-PTSD

After treatment-resistance is determined, there are several proposed pharmacotherapuetic and psychotherapeutic approaches. Though the literature base is small, several randomized controlled trials (RCTs), open-label trials and case series exist that evaluate the efficacy of alternative treatments. As noted above, the criteria for response can be based on the CAPS score or the CGI-I score. Previous studies have differed in use of drug treatments for monotherapy or as add-on therapy, trial duration and goals of treatment. This section reviews each class of drug and the evidence-base (or lack thereof) for efficacy in TR-PTSD.

4.1 Antidepressants

SSRIs and SNRIs are considered to be first line treatments for PTSD. Only SNRIs have demonstrated preliminary efficacy in treatment specific to cases of treatment-resistance. Duloxetine is another SNRI that has been evaluated for its efficacy in treating refractory-PTSD. In an open-label trial, duloxetine has demonstrated efficacy for treating TR-PTSD in mostly male and military samples; however, further investigation is still required.

4.1.1 Duloxetine

As a dual reuptake inhibitor and approved treatment for major depressive disorder (MDD), duloxetine was evaluated for its efficacy for treatment of PTSD. In an eight-week open label trial, Walderhaug et al (2010) treated 21 male patients with both refractory PTSD and comorbid MDD. Duloxetine was administered as monotherapy with a dose of 60-120mg/day. All patients were deemed treatment-resistant by having failed at least two previous treatments with antidepressants. On the primary outcome measure, PCL-C, scores improved significantly. Scores also improved on the HAM-A, MADRS and CGI-S. At the end of the eight weeks, 42% of the patients (N=8/21) responded to treatment and 21% (N=4/21) were considered to have reached remission criteria. Overall, duloxetine was found to decrease PTSD and concurrent MDD symptoms, and improve upon quality of sleep.

4.1.2 Other antidepressants

Only a small literature exists about the use of other antidepressants such as TCAs and MAOIs for non-refractory PTSD, and with no consistent positive results. The only antidepressant to be tested in a treatment-resistant sample was nefazodone (Gillin et al., 2001; Zisook et al., 2000). While positive effects were seen in the nefazodone evaluations, it was taken off the market in Canada and the United States due to adverse effects on the liver.

4.2 Atypical antipsychotics

Psychotic symptoms can be quite prevalent in those with PTSD, especially in veterans with combat exposure (Stein, Kline, & Matloff, 2002). The prevalence of psychosis in veterans with PTSD is estimated to range from 30-40% (M. B. Hamner, 1997). Psychotic symptoms are often associated with more severe symptoms that are not affected by the standard treatment with SSRIs or other antidepressants (Pae et al., 2008; Sareen, Cox, Goodwin, & Asmundson, 2005). It is suggested that PTSD affects serotonergic and dopaminergic pathways, both of which can be acted on by atypical antipsychotics (M. B. Hamner, Faldowski et al., 2003). There is also some indication that PTSD can affect alpha-adrenergic receptors as well, which can also be acted on by some atypical antipsychotics. Some activities of these drugs include, D_2, 5-HT_2 and $alpha_1$ adrenergic receptor antagonism. Certain drugs also have an antihistaminic role, helping with some of the sleep-disturbances accompanying PTSD (Ravindran & Stein, 2009). As such, atypical antipsychotics have been utilized as a monotherapy and as adjunctive treatment for PTSD, with or without psychotic symptoms, with most evidence supporting the use of them as an adjunctive therapy.

Three RCTs (see Table 1), eight open-label trials and multiple case series were identified for the use of atypical antipsychotics in the treatment of TR-PTSD. The following is a summary of the studies on atypical antipsychotics:

Name of Anti-psychotic		Definition of treatment-resistance	Dose (mg/day) [mean]	Trial (wks)	Existing therapy	Outcomes	Findings (as compared to control groups)
Olanzapine	Stein *et al.*, 2002 (n=19)	Only minimal response to 12 weeks of SSRIs	10 [15]	8	SSRIs	1. CAPS total score 2. CES-D 3. PSQI 4. CGI -I	- Improved on CAPS, CES-D, PSQI - No significant differences between control and treatment group on CGI-I
Risperidone	Hamner *et al.*, 2003 (n=37)	Only partially responsive to current medication	1-6 [Final dose: 2.5 ± 1.25]	5	Antide-pressants	1. PANSS total score 2. PANSS subscale scores 3. CAPS total score 4. CAPS subscale scores	- Modest results in treatment of psychotic and re-experiencing symptoms - Decrease in PANSS
	Bartzokis *et al.*, 2004 (n=65)	Patients deemed "probably treatment resistant"	1-3	16	Antide-pressants	1. CAPS total score 2. CAPS subscale scores 3. PANSS-P 4. HAM-A 5. HAM-D	- significant improvement on all measures - reduced PTSD symptoms, symptoms clusters (anxiety, psychosis, depression)
	Rothbaum *et al.*, 2008 (n=20)	Unresponsive to SSRIs over the past year	0.5-2 mg/day.	8	SSRIs	1. PANSS 2. CAPS total score 3. CAPS subscale score 4. DTS 5. CGI	- Improved on DTS scores -improved on CGI-I scores -No change in CAPS

Table 1. **Summary of RCTs of atypical antipsychotics for treatment of TR-PTSD.** CAPS: Clinician Administered PTSD Scale; CGI: Clinical Global Improvement Scale; PNASS: Positive and Negative Syndrome Scale; CES-D: Center for Epidemiologic Studies Depression Scale; PSQI: Pittsburgh Sleep Quality Index; DTS: Davidson Trauma Scale

4.2.1 Olanzapine

Olanzapine has high affinity for D_2 dopamine receptors and 5-HT_2 serotonin receptors (Jakovljevic, Sagud, & Mihaljevic-Peles, 2003) as well as affinities for adrenergic, histaminergic and muscarinic receptors (Butterfield et al., 2001). Olanzapine, with its sedative activities, has the potential to treat sleep disturbances accompanied with PTSD (Stein et al., 2002).
One RCT (Stein et al., 2002) shows beneficial results for the use of olanzapine in treating refractory PTSD over an 8-week trial. 19 patients who only minimally responded to 12 weeks of SSRIs were considered treatment-resistant. Stein et al. (2002) found that when using olanzapine (mean dose 15 mg/day) in conjunction with previously indicated SSRIs at a maximally tolerated dose, scores on CAPS, CES-D and PSQI measures significantly improved as compared to individuals who were given a placebo in conjunction with SSRIs. Based on the CGI-I measure, the percentage of responders was not significantly different between the treatment (30%) and placebo (11%) groups. Although a small RCT, this study shows olanzapine to be effective in treating individuals with TR-PTSD, and in particular, treatment-resistant sleep symptoms. One open-label trial (Pivac, Kozaric-Kovacic, & Much-Seler, 2004) shows the efficacy of olanzapine in reducing PTSD symptoms. Pivac et al., (2004) defined treatment resistance as those patients who were unresponsive with SSRIs for six to 12 months prior to the study. In a series of case reports (Jakovljevic et al., 2003), five patients who had been given various psychotropic medications for years were treated additionally with olanzapine. Sleep disturbance symptoms in these patients were much improved with adjunctive olanzapine treatment. Olanzapine appears to be an effective adjunctive treatment for refractory PTSD.

4.2.2 Risperidone

Risperidone has affinity for 5-HT_{2A}, 5-HT_7, D_2, and alpha-1 and 2 receptors. As such, risperidone has the capacity to reduce positive and negative symptoms of PTSD, such as, delusions, hallucinations, thought disorder, hostility, social and emotional withdrawal and aggression, among others (Kozaric-Kovacic, Pivac, Muck-Seler, & Rothbaum, 2005). Two RCTs (Hamner, Faldowski et al., 2003; Bartzokis et al., 2004) and two open-label trials (David, De Faria, & Mellman, 2006; Kozaric-Kovacic et al., 2005) demonstrate the positive effect of risperidone in the treatment of refractory PTSD. However, Rothbaum et al (2005) failed to find any benefit of risperidone on the primary CAPS outcome. Treatment resistance includes criteria such as, unresponsive to SSRIs over the past year (Bartzokis et al., 2004; Kozaric-Kovacic et al., 2005; Rothbaum et al., 2008) and as only partially responsive to current medications (David et al., 2006; M. B. Hamner, Faldowski et al., 2003). Risperidone is evaluated in conjunction with participants' regular doses of either SSRIs (Rothbaum et al., 2008) or all antidepressants (M. B. Hamner, Faldowski et al., 2003). Average daily doses of risperidone ranged between 1.9-2.5mg/day for 5-16 weeks. The percentage of responders to risperidone compared to the placebo was not recorded. Modest results were found for the combination of antidepressants and risperidone in treatment of the psychotic and re-experiencing symptoms of PTSD. (Hamner, Faldowski et al., 2003). The open label trials were consistent in showing the benefit of adjunctive treatment and monotherapy treatment with risperidone. One study in particular (David et al., 2006) specifically showed risperidone to be effective in treating the sleep symptoms accompanying PTSD. In summary, risperidone has shown some promise for TR-PTSD, but larger, more rigorous RCTs are needed for confirmation.

4.2.3 Quetiapine

Quetiapine demonstrates alpha-1 blocking activity and has low side effects (Kozaric-Kovacic & Pivac, 2007). Quetiapine use for treating refractory PTSD is shown to be effective in three open-label trials (Ahearn, Mussey, Johnson, Krohn, & Krahn, 2006; M. B. Hamner, Deitsch, Brodrick, Ulmer, & Lorberbaum, 2003; Kozaric-Kovacic & Pivac, 2007). Two studies examine quetiapine as an adjunctive therapy to antidepressants or other psychotropics (Hamner, Deitsch et al., 2003) or with SSRIs (Ahearn et al., 2006), whereas Kozaric-Kovacic and Pivac (2007) examine quetiapine as a monotherapy. Resistance to treatment was defined as no change in CAPS scores after two 8-week trials with different antidepressants (Kozaric-Kovacic & Pivac, 2007), incomplete responsiveness to treatment (Hamner, Deitsch et al., 2003) or as still experiencing PTSD symptoms despite being on a stable dose of SSRIs (Ahearn et al., 2006). The CAPS total and subscores are used as primary outcomes in all open label studies. Before treatment, CAPS scores, on average were above 80. All studies demonstrated a significant reduction in CAPS total scores and CAPS subscale scores (avoidance, re-experiencing and hyperarousal). Ahearn et al. (2006) found an average final CAPS score of 46, representing a 42% decrease in symptom severity. All three subscales, B, C and D, showed significant reduction as well (23 to 10, 27 to 23 and 26 to 14, respectively). Treatment doses across all three trials ranged from 25 mg per day to 400 mg per day (mean dose ranging from 100 ± 70 mg/day to 335.75 mg/day). The open-label trials indicate the efficacy of quetiapine for TR-PTSD; however, larger and more rigorous studies are required for conclusive results.

4.2.4 Fluphenazine

One open label study reports on the effectiveness of fluphenazine as a treatment for refractory PTSD as compared to olanzapine (Pivac et al., 2004). Patients included were all unresponsive to six to 12 months of prior treatment with SSRIs. The six-week trial using 5-10 mg/day of fluphenazine as a monotherapy showed effectiveness of the drug in reducing re-experiencing, avoidance and hyperarousal symptoms; however, olanzapine had a greater effect on both avoidance and hyperarousal symptoms. Fluphenazine was effective in treating the cluster symptoms of PTSD in a treatment resistant sample. However, to date, there is not enough evidence to be conclusive as to the utility of fluphenazine or other typical antipsychotics in TR-PTSD.

4.2.5 Clozapine

One open-label study indicates that clozapine may be effective in treating PTSD with psychotic symptoms (Wheatly, Plant, Reader, Brown, & Cahill, 2004). Six participants, whose psychotic features were resistant to at least two conventional antipsychotics, were given between 600 and 800 mg/day of clozapine. Four participants responded either significantly or moderately to the treatment, whereas two others remained uncertain of the effect. Due to the open-label design and small sample size, there is not yet enough evidence to conclude that clozapine is effective for treatment refractory PTSD.

4.2.6 Aripiprazole

Aripiprazole is a 5-HT_{2A} antagonist with partial agonist effects on the 5-HT_{1A} and D_2 receptors contributing to a reduction in anxiety. Two open-label trials demonstrate the potential effectiveness of aripiprazole in treating refractory-PTSD. In a 12-week trial, participants were given a mean dose of 12.95 mg/day of the drug as a monotherapy treatment (Villarreal et al., 2007). Of the 22 participants, 15 of them (68%) had previously been unresponsive to two or more antidepressants. By the end of the trial, 14 people (64%) responded to treatment, defined as a minimum of 20% improvement on the CAPS scale, and two participants remitted. Of the 14 responders, twelve participants had a CGI-I score of very much, or much improved. In a second 12-week trial, a flexible dose (15-30 mg/day) of the drug was given adjunctively to the 20 participants (Robert, Hamner, Durkalski, Brown, & Ulmer, 2009). Of these 20 participants, 85% of them had previously been treated with an average of 1.5 antidepressants trials, but were still experiencing significant PTSD symptoms. Based on the response criteria of a minimal decrease in CAPS score by 20%, 53% of the sample responded to treatment. In addition, a recent chart review of veterans with both PTSD and comorbid depression that received this drug in an open-label fashion for 12 weeks experienced a reduction in both PTSD and depression severity. Treatment resistance was defined as being minimally or partially responsive to previous medication (Richardson, Fikretoglu, Liu, & McIntosh, 2011). These findings suggest that aripiprazole may be effective in treating PTSD in those who are considered treatment resistant; however, further and more rigorous evaluation of the drug is required.

Based on the evidence, it appears that olanzapine and risperidone are the most effective atypical antipsychotics for the treatment of refractory PTSD. The study of atypical antipsychotics in treatment of refractory PTSD is promising, however more research is needed, including larger sample sizes and more double blind randomized controlled trials.

4.3 Anti-adrenergic agents

Prolonged duration of adrenergic activation heightens the risk of developing PTSD. Often those with PTSD have an altered regulation of their adrenergic system. Anti-adrenergic agents may therefore be able to reverse or minimize the development and/or symptoms of PTSD (Marmar, Neylan, & Schoenfeld, 2002).

The following drugs have been evaluated in relation to PTSD. Three RCTs (see Table 2), four open-label trials and two case series have examined anti-adrenergic agents in the context of reducing sleep disturbances, preventing PTSD development and reducing hyper-arousal symptoms.

4.3.1 Prazosin

Nightmares and other sleep disturbance symptoms are common in combat-related traumas, and are often symptoms that are resistant to treatment. Prazosin is an anti-adrenergic agent that has been specifically evaluated in such individuals where nightmare symptoms are not responding (Raskind et al., 2002). Prazosin is a selective alpha-1 antagonist. It is proposed that alpha-1 receptor stimulation is associated with sleep disturbances and stress-linked disruptions in cognitive processing, both evident in PTSD. Therefore, prazosin, with its blocking effects, might be useful in reducing the sleep-related symptoms of PTSD (Ravindran & Stein, 2009).

Two RCTs test the efficacy of prazosin as augmentative therapy for reducing sleep disturbance symptoms associated with PTSD in combat veterans (Raskind et al., 2007; Raskind et al., 2003). Ten combat veterans with refractory PTSD participated in the 20-week, double blind crossover design (Raskind et al., 2003). Refractory PTSD symptoms were defined by frequent and severe trauma- related nightmares (>6 on CAPS), despite treatment

Name of Anti-adrenergic		Definition of Treatment Resistance	Dose (mg/day) [Mean}	Trial (wks)	Existing Therapy	Outcomes	Findings (as compared to control groups)
Prazosin	Raskind et al., 2003 (n=10)	Frequent and severe trauma-related nightmares (>6 on CAPS), despite treatment with a stable dose of psychoactive medications.	1-10 [9.5]	20	Augmentation	1. CAPS 2. CGI-C	- Improved sleep and nightmare symptoms - Improved CGI-C score
	Raskind et al., 2007 (n=40)	Frequent and severe trauma-related nightmares (>6 on CAPS), despite treatment with a stable dose of psychoactive medications.	1-15 [13.3± 3]	8	Augmentation	1. CAPS 2. CGI 3. PSQI	- Reduced trauma-related nightmares and improved sleep - Improved Global Clinical Status
Guanfacine	Neylan et al., 2006 (n=63)	Participants taking no medication, or continued to meet the criteria for PTSD even though they were on a stable dose of medication	1-3 [2.4]	8	Augmentation	1. CAPS 2. IES-R 3. SQI	- No effect on PTSD symptoms, sleep quality or general mood

Table 2. **Summary of RCTs of antiadrenergics for treatment of Post-traumatic Stress Disorder.** CAPS: Clinician Administered PTSD Scale; CGI: Clinical Global Improvement Scale; PSQI: Pittsburgh Sleep Quality Index; PCL-C: Posttraumatic Stress Disorder checklist-civilian version; IES-R: Impact event scale revised; SQI: subjective sleep quality.

with a stable dose of psychoactive medications. A mean dose of 9.5mg/day of prazosin or placebo was given before bed. On outcome measures, sleep disturbances, nightmares and CGI-C, those taking prazosin showed more improvement as compared to the control group. The drug group also showed reduced symptoms in all three PTSD symptom clusters. In their eight-week RCT (Raskind et al., 2007), a mean dose of 13.3mg/day of prazosin or placebo was administered. All participants had chronic nightmares that were unresponsive or only partially responsive to prior treatment. Prazosin greatly improved PTSD-related nightmares, sleep quality and CGI-C scores, as compared with the placebo. The drug group experienced a decrease of 50% in recurring, distressing dreams, whereas the placebo group only experienced a decrease in 15%. These two studies show prazosin to be effective in treating the sleep disturbance and nightmare symptoms associated with PTSD in combat veterans. Three open label studies are also consistent in demonstrating the effectiveness of prazosin in treating sleep disturbance symptoms associated with PTSD (Peskind, Bonner, Hoff, & Raskind, 2003; Taylor & Raskind, 2002; Taylor et al., 2006). Taylor et al (2006) demonstrated that in those civilians that continued to experience daytime PTSD symptoms even though on a stable dose of nighttime prazosin, it was beneficial to add a daytime dose (mean dose 3.2mg/day) as well. Raskind et al (2002) retrospectively examined combat veterans with PTSD who had been treated with prazosin. All participants had chronic trauma-related nightmares (score of 5-8 on CAPS recurrent distressing dreams item), despite treatment with stable dose of medication. Primary outcome measures were CAPS and CGI-C scores. In those who completed at least eight-weeks of prazosin (mean dose 9.6mg/day), recurring, distressing dreams were significantly reduced. In those that were prescribed prazosin but did not comply, there was no such change. There is a good level of evidence to support the use of prazosin in TR-PTSD patients with sleep disturbance and nightmare symptoms.

4.3.2 Guanfacine

Guanfacine acts as an alpha-2 adrenergic agonist (Ravindran & Stein, 2009), and as such is proposed as a mechanism for reducing hyper-arousal symptoms associated with PTSD. In an eight-week double blind, randomized controlled trial, 63 veterans with TR-PTSD received either an average dose of 2.4mg/day of guanfacine or of placebo (Neylan et al., 2006). Included participants were either taking no medication, or continued to meet the criteria for PTSD even though they were on a stable dose of medication. Guanfacine showed a small but statistically significant effect in reducing CAPS scores, as compared to the placebo group, as well as a decrease in the average total IES-R score. After eight weeks, the drug was no more effective than the placebo in reducing PTSD symptoms. In addition, those who were given guanfacine experienced high rates of adverse effects, such as dry mouth, light-headedness and a drop in blood pressure. Based on the results of this trial, guanfacine is not suggested to benefit individuals with PTSD.

4.3.3 Clonidine

Similar to the effect of guanfacine, clonidine, an alpha-2 adrenergic agonist, blocks the alpha-2 receptors in areas with high concentrations of norepinephrine, thus reducing symphathetic tone. As such, it is hypothesized that the drug can have beneficial effects on the hyper-arousal symptoms exhibited in PTSD (Ravindran & Stein, 2009). In an open-clinical trial (Harmon & Riggs, 1996), pre-school children with PTSD were treated with clonidine (average dose, once stabilized, 0.1-0.105mg/day). Children were only included in this study if they had been unresponsive to at least one, but often several months of behavioral treatment. Based on teacher and physician opinion, all children experienced a decrease in aggressive behavior, and 71% of the children exhibited decreased impulsivity, hypervigilance, anxiety, temper-tantrums, oppositional behavior and sleep disturbances. After trying out many different drugs, Kinzie and Leung (1989) found TCAs most effective in relieving PTSD symptoms. Cambodian refugees (N=12) with PTSD were treated with a combination of imipramine (maximum dose 150mg/day) and clonidine (0.1-0.6mg/day). Only two patients showed enough improvement to no longer meet the criteria of PTSD, however most showed reduced symptoms, such as, improved sleep, startle reactions and avoidance. This study indicates the usefulness of the TCA-clonidine combination in reducing PTSD symptoms; however, further RCTs are needed to investigate.

Prazosin has been the most rigorously evaluated anti-adrenergic agent that has shown benefit in treating refractory-PTSD patients. Further evaluation of clonidine in the future may provide additional insight into its use.

4.4 Anticonvulsants

Kindling, the process whereby repeated sub threshold stimulation to the central nervous system (CNS), makes the nerves more sensitive to stimuli. This phenomenon has been shown to occur in the amygdala and limbic regions of the CNS, areas linked to fear and stress. Anticonvulsants, known for their anti-kindling properties, are therefore proposed as a possible treatment for PTSD (Berger et al., 2009).

There have been numerous studies, including, one RCT, three open label trials and several case studies, examining the potential efficacy of anticonvulsants in treating refractory PTSD. Such anticonvulsant drugs include, topiramate, valproic acid, tiagabine and levetiracetam. The following is a summary of the existing literature on anticonvulsants in the treatment of TR-PTSD.

4.4.1 Topiramate

Topiramate has several different mechanisms of operation. Topiramate blocks calcium and sodium channels, increasing the activity of GABA, inhibiting the activity of carbonic anhydrase enzyme and blocking the AMPA receptor. Topiramate's anti-kindling properties may block certain pathways involved in PTSD (Andrus & Gilbert, 2010).

One RCT testing the efficacy of topiramate in treating PTSD shows potential benefit. In a 12-week adjunctive therapy, double blind, randomized control trial, 67 patients who were being treated with psychotropic medications, but experiencing no response were included. There was a significant improvement between those combat veterans receiving the drug (50-500mg/day) and those receiving the placebo (Akuchekian & Amanat, 2004). PTSD symptoms of re-experiencing, sleep disturbances, irritability, anger, difficulty recalling, and startle reaction were reduced in the experimental group. In a case series (Berlant, 2001), when previous medications were ineffective, topiramate was reported to help with re-experiencing symptoms, such as nightmares and intrusive flashbacks. There is suggestion that topiramate, as an anticonvulsant agent, may be effective in treatment-resistant individuals with PTSD; however, the findings of the RCT need to be replicated and additional investigation is required.

4.4.2 Valproic acid (Valproate and Divalproex)

Valproic acid and its derivatives (valproate and divalproex) have been commonly studied as treatments for refractory PTSD. Valproic acid increases the amount of GABA, a neurotransmitter (Adamou, Puchalska, Plummer, & Hale, 2007) and enhances the inhibition of gamma-aminobutyric acid. Through these mechanisms, it is hypothesized that valproic acid reduces intrusion and hyperarousal symptoms associated with PTSD (Otte, Wiedemann, Yassouridis, & Kellner, 2004).

One open label study has been conducted examining the use of valproate as an effective treatment for PTSD. Otte et al (2004) treated ten civilians with valproate monotherapy in an eight-week open label trial. The average duration of PTSD for the participants was 8.6 ± 8.7 years, and previous, ineffective treatments included, antidepressants, antipsychotics and CBT. The drug was initiated at 250mg/day and was titrated incrementally up to 2000mg/day, as tolerated (mean dose 1400 ± 380mg/day). This trial found no significant improvement in PTSD symptoms in the civilian population.

The use of divalproex in treating refractory PTSD has shown beneficial results. One open label study (Goldberg, Cloitre, Whiteside, & Han, 2003) supports the use of divalproex in treating patients with PTSD related to childhood abuse. All participants in this study were considered treatment-resistant on the basis of continued PTSD symptoms in the past three months, regardless of receiving treatment. A mean dose of 1500mg/day was given to each of the seven participants. Significant improvement was seen in all clusters of PTSD symptoms as well as in general symptom severity.

The mixed results of the evaluations of the valproic acid derivatives warrant further research, including larger studies.

4.4.3 Tiagabine

Tiagabine is a selective GABA reuptake inhibitor, and as such, increases the extracellular supply of GABA (Connor, Davidson, Weisler, Zhang, & Abraham, 2006). The increased availability of GABA in the neural cleft interacts with postsynaptic GABA receptors, producing quick inhibition, resulting in a potential treatment mechanism for PTSD.

In a case series, women whose PTSD was still symptomatic despite treatment with a stable dose of medication, were treated with an adjunctive dose of tiagabine(Taylor, 2003). Within two weeks of the treatment, six out of seven of the patients showed improvement when given a mean dose of 8mg/day of the drug. However, in a 12-week RCT Davidson et al (2007) administered between four and 16mg/day of tiagabine or placebo to 232 patients. No significant differences were found between the treatment and control group on the CAPS scale or on other measures. This study demonstrates that tiagabine was clearly ineffective in reducing PTSD symptoms. This study however, excluded individuals who were unresponsive to at least two or more previously pharmacological treatments for PTSD. Therefore, it is unlikely for this treatment to be effective in a treatment resistant sample; however, this has not been investigated.

4.4.4 Levetiracetam

Levetiracetam reduces signal transmission through high voltage calcium channels. This drug might also effect the functioning of the SV2A synaptic vesicle protein. Animal models show that levetiracetam may reduce the anxiety induced by withdrawal from benzodiazepines (Kinrys, Wygant, Pardo, & Melo, 2006).

In a retrospective study, Kinrys et al (2006) treated non-responding PTSD patients with levetiracetam in an adjunctive therapy fashion. A mean dose of 1967 ± 650 mg/day was given to patients for an average of 9.7 ± 3.7 weeks. Significant improvements were seen in PCL-C, CGI-S and HAM-A scores. Thirteen patients (56%) were characterized as responders, and 6 patients (26%) were characterized as remitters. No patients discontinued treatment due to adverse effects. These findings are inconclusive pending further research that must include RCTs.

Based on the literature to date, there is not enough evidence to recommend the use of anticonvulsants for treating TR-PTSD.

4.5 Mood stabilizers

4.5.1 Lithium carbonate

Lithium stimulates serotonin synthesis and increases the sensitivity of pre- and post-synaptic receptors to serotonin. These mechanisms may be responsible for the ability of lithium to reduce aggression (Forster, Schoenfeld, Marmar, & Lang, 1995).

In a case series Kitchner and Greenstein (1985) reported on the effect of low dose lithium carbonate (300-600 mg/day) in treating the PTSD-related anger, irritability, anxiety and sleep disturbance symptoms in individuals who were resistant to other treatment (tranquilizers, antidepressants, hypnotics and psychotherapy). Over three to 12 months, adjunctive treatment with lithium was effective in treating these treatment-resistant symptoms. No further and more up-to-date studies on lithium treatment of refractory PTSD patients were found in the literature. As a result, lithium may be an effective treatment for specific symptoms of TR-PTSD, but more rigorous evaluation is necessary.

4.6 Anxiolytics

Benzodiazepines exert their effect on the GABA benzodiazepine receptor, further increasing the activity of inhibitory neurotransmitter, GABA. Generally, this results in sedation, anxiolysis, muscle relaxation, as well as decreased arousal (Ravindran & Stein, 2009). Benzodiazepines have not been evaluated in a treatment-resistant sample. On the other hand, buspirone, a non-benzodiazepine anxiolytic acts similarly and is evaluated for efficacy in treating refractory PTSD.

Only one clinical series was identified in the literature to deal with treatment-resistant individuals specifically.

4.6.1 Buspirone

In a clinical series (Hamner, Ulmer, & Horne, 1997), patients who were completely unresponsive or only partially responsive to prior medication were additionally treated with buspirone. Of the participants, 73%(N= 11/14) responded positively to buspirone augmentation (mean dose 40mg/day). Randomized trials are needed to further examine the effectiveness of buspirone.

4.7 Cognitive Behavioral Therapy (CBT)

Several studies have found cognitive behavioral therapy (CBT) to be effective for treatment-resistant refugees. Otto et al (2003) randomly assigned ten women to either receive sertraline (mean dose 125mg/day) or sertraline (mean dose 100mg/day) plus CBT. All women had previously failed to respond to a combination of clonazepam (0.5-1mg/day) plus an SSRI other than sertraline. CBT focused on information, exposure and cognitive modification. The combination of sertraline and CBT was more effective than sertraline alone. Hinton et al (2004) randomly assigned Vietnamese refugees with PTSD and concurrent panic attacks to two different cohorts, one to receive treatment immediately, and the other to be on the waitlist. All included participants still met criteria for PTSD diagnosis despite treatment with a stable dose of SSRIs and supportive counseling. CBT was adapted to be culturally appropriate. Significant improvements were seen on all outcome measures, demonstrating the efficacy of culturally adapted CBT. A trial with Cambodian refugees with TR-PTSD and comorbid panic attacks (Hinton et al., 2005) likewise found benefit of a culturally adapted CBT program. In the randomized controlled trial, Hinton et al (2009) studied the mechanism behind the efficacy for CBT in Cambodian refugees. Patients receiving the treatment showed much greater improvement on one physiological measure and on all psychometric measures. In addition, those in the waitlist group significantly improved once they too received treatment. The study found the severity of PTSD to be mediated by orthostatic panic and emotion regulation. The vagal tone and emotional regulation ability is improved by CBT, suggesting a decrease in vagal tone to be associated with PTSD and orthostatic panic among refugees, as well as with emotional regulation ability. In a culturally adapted, 14-week, CBT trial of Latino women with TR-PTSD (Hinton et al., 2011), significant reduction in PTSD symptoms was again demonstrated. Treatment resistance was defined as still meeting PTSD criteria despite receiving supportive therapy and a maximally tolerated dose of SSRIs for at least six months. These few studies demonstrate the ability of culturally adapted CBT to be an effective treatment for refuges with PTSD who are not responding to first line treatment.

4.8 Alternative treatments

Multiple alternative treatments have been evaluated for their uses in treating refractory PTSD. Two RCTs have been performed looking at different methods for treatment.

Kaplan et al (1996) evaluated the use of inositol in a double-blind randomized, controlled cross-over trial. Inositol is a second messenger that exerts its effect over neurotransmitters such as serotonin. It has been shown to have antidepressant and anti-panic properties, and is therefore proposed to also help alleviate PTSD symptoms. Included participants were those who had no response or only partial response to a trial of antidepressants or other treatment, or had refused treatment with medication. Participants were treated with either 12g/day of inositol or of placebo only. Response to treatment was based on the IES, and its two subscales for avoidance and intrusion. Overall, no significant differences were found between treatment and placebo groups in overall IES score, either subscale or on the Hamilton depression and anxiety scales. This study shows inositol to have no effect on TR-PTSD.

A second RCT evaluated the use of ±3,4-methylendioxymethamphetamine (MDMA) for TR-PTSD (Mithoefer, Wagner, Mithoefer, Jerome, & Doblin, 2010). In the past, MDMA has been shown to reduce fear, while maintaining a state of alertness and is therefore proposed to be helpful in conjunction with psychotherapy. Individuals who were resistant to both psychotherapy and psychopharmacology were randomized to receive either MDMA or placebo in two 8-hour experimental psychotherapy sessions. The CAPS was used to indicate response to treatment. In the treatment-group, 83% (N= 10/12) individuals responded, whereas, only 25% (N=2/8) in the placebo-group responded. No serious adverse effects were seen. This is an interesting proof-of-concept and the role of this drug in the treatment of PTSD remains to be determined.

Abramowitz and Lichtenberg (2010) conducted a prospective open study on the efficacy of a new hypnotic technique for TR-PTSD. The new technique, hypnotherapeutic olfactory conditioning (HOC), consists of six 1.5 hour sessions per week where the patient is taught to use a pleasant-smelling scent to help them re-enter and remain calm in situations that trigger anxiety and panic. All participants in this study had continual PTSD symptoms and olfactory trigger components despite prior treatment. The IES-R, BDI and Dissociative Experiences Scale were used to assess the treatment. At the end of the six weeks, a significant reduction was seen in PTSD symptoms, depression and dissociative experiences. Response to treatment was indicated by a 50% decrease in in IES-R scores. Of the participants, 58% responded. In those who have olfactory trigger components to their PTSD, HOC may be an effective treatment.

Nabilone, a synthetic cannabinoid substance was also evaluated as a potential treatment for individuals whose PTSD-related nightmares were resistant to treatment for at least two years (Fraser, 2009). In this open label clinical trial, nabilone (mean dose 0.5mg/day) was added to the medication regiment of 47 patients. Thirty-four of the patients (72%) experienced complete or significant reductions in their nightmares. Nabilone may be effective for treatment-resistant nightmares, but its role in treatment of TR-PTSD is cautioned as it is still inconclusive.

5. Implications for clinicians

While SSRIs and cognitive behavioral therapy have been deemed the prime treatment for PTSD, many do not respond. There are many different factors contributing to treatment-resistance and it varies between individuals. As such, there is limited evidence-based research on the obvious next step for treatment of these patients. As evidenced by the array of pharmacological and psychotherapeutic methods for treatment, little consensus exists. Further research is required on the better strategies for treating individuals with refractory-PTSD.

Although there is no treatment algorithm for the management of TR-PTSD, since PTSD commonly presents with comorbidities it is essential that the clinician confirms the diagnosis and assesses treatment adherence in order to confirm treatment resistance. For example, to aggressively treat the comorbidities that are often present in TR-PTSD, such as treating major depression and addiction.

A clinician can also make use of current guidelines to aggressively treat and manage specific comorbidity, which might have contributed to the treatment resistance. According to updated guidelines for treating PTSD (VA/DoD, 2010), the choice of treatment should be based on symptom severity and all treatments should be evidence-based and within the clinician's capabilities to provide. When beginning pharmacotherapy for PTSD, clinicians should initiate a monotherapy trial with an optimized dose of first-line medication. An optimized dose takes into account the outcomes of the medication, the dose and the time until response. If the patient exhibits some response, the medication should be continued, unless the drug is not well tolerated. However, if the patient exhibits no response by approximately eight weeks, the dose should be increased, or the medication should be changed or augmented. The patient's adherence to the medication should be consistently assessed.

Based on the available evidence, when a first-line treatment (SSRI, SNRI) is not effective, switching to another antidepressant or another class of medication should be considered. The use of the anti-adrenergic agent, guanfacine, and anticonvulsants are not recommended as a monotherapeutic treatment for PTSD.

If switching medications does not elicit a response, augmenting the first-line treatment with another class of medication has demonstrated effectiveness. There is at present limited evidence that augmentation with atypical antipsychotics, risperidone, olanzapine or quetiapine can be effective for TR-PTSD; these agents can be tried when appropriate. The evidence for treatment with adjunctive anticonvulsant therapy is mixed and therefore not conclusive at this time.

When choosing which medication to switch to or to augment with, it is important to consider which PTSD symptoms the patient is experiencing. For those patients experiencing TR-PTSD sleep disturbances, prazosin has demonstrated effectiveness, particularly in a combat-veteran population where these symptoms are common. Psychotic features are also often associated with combat-related PTSD, for which augmenting with atypical antipsychotics may be efficacious.

While only two drugs (sertraline and paroxetine) are FDA approved for treating PTSD, many other drugs have evidence in treating specific symptoms of PTSD or commonly comorbid conditions. Some of the drugs discussed in this chapter, such as, olanzapine, risperidone and prazosin have been have been rigorously tested and demonstrated positive effects on PTSD symptoms. Other drugs have shown some benefit for PTSD symptoms, yet lack the rigorous evaluation needed for a recommendation at this time.

Due to the limited literature base and multitude of options, it may be difficult for the clinician to determine the best course of action. Today, we are still unable to draw a conclusion. Although remission is not always possible, it is important to maintain and promote hope in patients who continue to be symptomatic as significant symptom reduction and improve quality of life are possible with treatment. A better understanding of the physiological and neurobiological underpinnings of PTSD will be essential to developing new and better treatments for PTSD. This greater understanding may also help us to prevent treatment-resistance by treating the PTSD earlier and more effectively. We can also do this by addressing not only those affected with PTSD, but those who have higher risk factors for being exposed to trauma and developing treatment-resistance.

6. References

Abramowitz, E. G., & Lichtenberg, P. (2010). A new hyptonic technique for treating combat-related Posttraumatic Stress Disorder: A prospective open study. *International Journal of Clinical and Experimental Hypnosis, 58*(3), 316-328.

Adamou, M., Puchalska, S., Plummer, W., & Hale, A. S. (2007). Valproate in the treatment if PTSD: systematic review and meta analysis. *Current Medical Research and Opinion, 23*(6), 1285-1291.

Ahearn, E. P., Mussey, M., Johnson, C., Krohn, A., & Krahn, D. (2006). Quetiapine as an adjunctive treatment for post-traumatic stress disorder: an 8-week open-lbel study. *International Clinical Psychopharmacology, 21*, 29-33.

Akuchekian, S., & Amanat, S. (2004). The Comparison of Topiramate and Placebo in the Treatment of Posttraumatic Stress Disorder: A Randomized, Double-Blind Study. *Journal of Research in Medical Sciences, 5*, 240-244.

Andrus, M. R., & Gilbert, E. (2010). Treatment of civilian and combat-related Posttraumatic Stress Disorder with Topiramate. *The Annals of Pharmacotherapy, 44*, 1810-1816.

Asnis, G. M., Kohn, S. R., Henderson, M., & Brown, N. L. (2004). SSRIs versus Non-SSRIs in Post-traumatic Stress Disorder. *Drugs, 64*(4), 383-404.

Ballenger, J. C., Davidson, J. R. T., Lecrubier, Y., Nutt, D. J., Marshall, R. D., Nemeroff, C. B., et al. (2004). Consensus Statement Update on Posttraumatic Stress Disorder From the International Consensus Group on Depression and Anxiety. *Journal of Clinical Psychiatry, 65*(Suppl 1), 55-62.

Bandelow, B., Zohar, J., Hollander, E., Kasper, S., Moller, H. J., & Disorders., W. T. F. o. T. G. f. A. O.-C. P.-t. S. (2008). World Federation of Societies of Biological Psychiatry (WFSBP) Guidelines for the Pharmacological Treatment of Anxiety, Obsessive-Compulsive and Post-Traumatic Stress Disorders First Revision. *The World Journal of Biological Psychiatry, 9*(4), 248-312.

Bartzokis, G., Lu, P.H., Turner, J., Mintz, J., Saunders, C.S. (2004) Adjunctive risperidone in the treatment of chronic combat-related posttraumatic stress disorder. *Biological Psychiatry*, 57: 474-479.

Berger, W., Mendlowicz, M. V., Marquez-Portella, C., Kinrys, G., Fontenelle, L. F., Marmar, C. R., et al. (2009). Pharmacologic alternatives to antidepressants in posttraumatic stress disorder: A systematic review. *Progress in Neuro-Psychopharmacology & Biological Psychiatry, 33*, 169-180.

Berlant, J. L. (2001). Topiramate in Posttraumatic Stress Disorder: Preliminary Clinical Observations. *Journal of Clinical Psychiatry, 62*(Suppl 17), 60-63.

Boynton, L., Bentley, J., Strachan, E., Barbato, A., & Raskind, M. (2009). Preliminary findings concerning the use of prazosin for the treatment of posttraumatic nightmares in a refugee population. *Journal of Psychiatric Practice, 15*(6), 454-459.

Butterfield, M. I., Becker, M. E., Conner, K. M., Sutherland, S., Churchill, L. E., & Davidson, J. R. T. (2001). Olanzapine in the treatment of post-traumatic stress disorder: a pilot study. *International Clinical Psychopharmacology, 16*, 197-203.

Connor, K. M., Davidson, J. R. T., Weisler, R. H., Zhang, W., & Abraham, K. (2006). Tiagabine for posttraumatic stress disorder: effects of open-label and double-blind discontinuation treatment. *Psychopharmacology, 184*, 21-25.

David, D., De Faria, L., & Mellman, T. A. (2006). Adjunctive Risperidone Treatment and Sleep Symptoms in Combat Veterans with Chronic PTSD. *Depression and Anxiety, 23*, 489-491.

Davidson, J., Baldwin, D., Stein, D. J., Kuper, E., Benattia, I., Ahmed, S., et al. (2006). Treatment of posttraumatic stress disorder with venlafaxine extended release: a 6-month randomized controlled trial. *Archives of General Psychiatry, 63*, 1158-1165.

Davidson, J., Rothbaum, B. O., Tucker, P., Asnis, G., Benattia, I., & Musgnung, J. J. (2006). Venlafaxine extended release in posttraumatic stress disorder: a sertraline and placebo-controlled study. *Journal of Clinical Psychopharmacology, 26*(3), 259-267.

Forster, P. L., Schoenfeld, F. B., Marmar, C. R., & Lang, A. J. (1995). Lithium for Irritability in Post-Traumatic Stress Disorder. *Journal of Traumatic Stress, 8*(1), 143-149.

Fraser, G. A. (2009). The Use of a Synthetic Cannabinoid in the Management of Treatment-Resistant Nightmares in Posttraumatic Stress Disorder (PTSD). *CNS Neuroscience and Therapeutics, 15*, 84-88.

Gillin, J. C., Smith-Vaniz, A., Schnierow, B., Rapaport, M. H., Kelsoe, J., Raimo, E., et al. (2001). An Open-Label, 12-Week Clinical and Sleep EEG Study of Nefazodone in Chronic Combat-Related Posttraumatic Stress Disorder. *Journal of Clinical Psychiatry, 62*(10), 789-796.

Goldberg, J. F., Cloitre, M., Whiteside, J. E., & Han, H. (2003). An Open-Label Pilot Study of Divalproex Sodium for Posttraumatic Stress Disorder Related to Childhood Abuse. *Current Therapeutic Research, 64*(1), 45-54.

Hamner, M. B., Ulmer, H., & Horne, D. (1997). Buspirone Potentiation of Antidepressants in the Treatment of PTSD. *Depression and Anxiety, 5*, 137-139.

Hamner, M. B. (1997). Psychotic Features and Combat-Associated PTSD. *Depression and Anxiety, 5*, 34-38.

Hamner, M. B., Deitsch, S. E., Brodrick, P. S., Ulmer, H. G., & Lorberbaum, J. P. (2003). Quetiapine Treatment in Patients with Posttraumatic Stress Disorder: An Open Trial of Adjunctive Therapy. *Journal of Clinical Psychopharmacology, 23*(1), 15-20.

Hamner, M. B., Faldowski, R. A., Ulmer, H. G., Frueh, B. C., Huber, M. G., & Arana, G. W. (2003). Adjunctive risperidone treatment in post-traumatic stress disorder: a preliminary controlled trial of effects on comorbid psychotic symptoms. *International Clinical Psychopharmacology, 18*(1), 1-8.

Hamner, M. B., Robert, S., & Frueh, B. C. (2004). Treatment-Resistant Posttraumatic Stress Disorder: Strategies for Intervention. *CNS Spectrums, 9*(10), 740-752.

Harmon, R. J., & Riggs, P. D. (1996). Clonidine for Posttraumatic Stress Disorder in Preschool Children. *Journal of the American Academy of Child and Adolescent Psychiatry, 35*(9), 1247-1249.

Hinton, D. E., Chhean, D., Pich, V., Safren, S. A., Hofmann, S. G., & Pollack, M. H. (2005). A randomized Controlled Trial of Cognitive-Behavior Therapy for Cambodian Refugees with Treatment-Resistant PTSD and Panic Attacks: A cross-over design. *Journal of Traumatic Stress, 18*(6), 617-629.

Hinton, D. E., Hofmann, S. G., Pollack, M. H., & Otto, M. W. (2009). Mechanisms of Efficacy of CBT for Cambodian Refugees with PTSD: Improvement in Emotion Regulation and Orthostatic Blood Pressure Response. *CNS Neuroscience & Therapeutics, 15*, 255-263.

Hinton, D. E., Hofmann, S. G., Rivera, E., Otto, M. W., & Pollack, M. H. (2011). Culturally adapted CBT (CA-CBT) for Latino women with treatment-resistant PTSD: A pilot study comparing CA-CBT to applied muscle relaxation. *Behaviour Research and Therapy*([Epub ahead of Print]).

Hinton, D. E., Pham, T., Tran, M., Safren, S. A., Otto, M. W., & Pollack, M. H. (2004). CBT for Vietnamese Refugees with treatment-resistant PTSD and Panic Attacks: A Pilot Study. *Journal of Traumatic Stress, 17*(5), 429-433.

Jakovljevic, M., Sagud, M., & Mihaljevic-Peles, A. (2003). Olanzapine in the treatment-resistant combat-realted PTSD- a series of case reports. *Acta Psychiatrica Scandinavica, 107*(394-396).

Kaplan, Z., Amir, M., Swartz, M., & Levine, J. (1996). Inositol treatment of Post-Traumatic Stress Disorder. *Anxiety, 2*, 51-52.

Kinrys, G., Wygant, L. E., Pardo, T. B., & Melo, M. (2006). Levetiracetam for Treatment-Refractory Posttraumatic Stress Disorder. *Journal of Clinical Psychiatry, 67*(2), 211-214.

Kinzie, J. D., & Leung, P. (1989). Clonidine in Cambodian Patients with Posttraumatic Stress Disorder. *The Journal of Nervous and Mental Disease, 177*(9), 546-550.

Kitchner, I., & Greenstein, R. (1985). Low Dose Lithium Carbonate in the Treatment of Post Traumatic Stress Disorder: Brief Communication. *Military Medicine, 150*, 378-381.

Kozaric-Kovacic, D., & Pivac, N. (2007). Quetiapine treatment in an open trial in combat-related post-traumatic stress disorder with psychotic features. *International Journal of Neuropsychopharmacology, 10*, 253-261.

Kozaric-Kovacic, D., Pivac, N., Muck-Seler, D., & Rothbaum, B. O. (2005). Risperidone in Psychotic Combat-Related Posttraumtic Stress Disorder: an open trial. *Journal of Clinical Psychiatry, 66*(7), 922-927.

Marmar, C. R., Neylan, T. C., & Schoenfeld, F. B. (2002). New Direction in the Pharmacotherapy of Posttraumatic Stress Disorder. *Psychiatric Quarterly, 73*(4), 259-270.

Mithoefer, M. C., Wagner, M. T., Mithoefer, A., Jerome, I., & Doblin, R. (2010). The safety and efficacy of 3,4-methylenedioxymethamphetamine-assisted psychotherapy in subjects with chronic, treatment-resistant posttraumatic stress disorder: the first randomized controlled pilot study. *Journal of Psychopharmacology* ([Epub ahead of Print]).

Neylan, T. C., Lenoci, M., Samuelson, K. W., Metzler, T. J., Henn-Haase, C., Hierholzer, R. W., et al. (2006). No Improvement of Posttraumatic Stress Disorder Symptoms with Guanfacine Treatment. *American Journal of Psychiatry, 163*(12), 2186-2188.

Otte, C., Wiedemann, K., Yassouridis, A., & Kellner, M. (2004). Valproate Monotherapy in the Treatment of Civilian Patients With Non-combat-related Posttraumatic Stress Disorder: An Open-Label Study [Letter to the Editor]. *Journal of Clinical Psychopharmacology, 24*(1), 106-108.

Otto, M. W., Hinton, D., Korbly, N. B., Chea, A., Ba, P., Gershuny, B. S., et al. (2003). Treatment of pharmacotherapy-refractory posttraumatic stress disorder among Cambodian refugees: a pilot study of combination treatment with cognitive-behavior therapy vs sertraline alone. *Behavior Research and Therapy, 41*, 1271-1276.

Pae, C. U., Lim, H. K., Peindl, K., Ajwani, N., Serretti, A., Patkar, A., et al. (2008). The atypical antipsychotics olanzapine and risperidone in the treatment of posttraumatic stress disorder: a meta-analysis of randomized, double-blind, placebo-controlled clinical trials. *International Clinical Psychopharmacology 23*(1), 1-8.

Peskind, E. R., Bonner, L. T., Hoff, D. J., & Raskind, M. A. (2003). Prazosin Reduces Trauma-Related Nightmares in Older Men with Chronic Posttraumatic Stress Disorder. *Journal of Geriatric Psychiatry and Neurology, 16*, 165-171.

Pivac, N., & Kozaric-Kovacic, D. (2006). Pharmacotherapy of Treatment-Resistant Combat-related Posttraumatic Stress Disorder with Psychotic Features. *Croatian Medical Journal, 47*, 440-451.

Pivac, N., Kozaric-Kovacic, D., & Much-Seler, D. (2004). Olanzapine versus fluphenazine in an open trial in patients with psychotic combat-related post-traumatic stress disorder. *Psychopharmacology, 175*, 451-456.

Raskind, M. A., Peskind, E. R., Hoff, D. J., Hart, K. L., Holmes, H. A., Warren, D., et al. (2007). A parallel group placebo controlled study of prazosin for trauma nightmares and sleep disturbance in combat veterans with post-traumatic stress disorder. *Biological Psychiatry, 61*, 928-934.

Raskind, M. A., Peskind, E. R., Kanter, E. D., Petrie, E. C., Radant, A., Thompson, C. E., et al. (2003). Reduction of Nightmares and Other PTSD Symptoms in Combat Veterans by Prazosin: a placebo controlled study. *American Journal of Psychiatry, 160*(2), 371-373.

Raskind, M. A., Thompson, C., Petrie, E. C., Dobie, D. J., Rein, R. J., Hoff, D. J., et al. (2002). Prazosin Reduces Nightmares in Combat Veterans with Posttraumatic Stress Disorder. *Journal of Clinical Psychiatry, 63*(7), 565-568.

Ravindran, L. N., & Stein, M. B. (2009). Pharmacotherapy of PTSD: Premises, principles and priorities. *Brain Research, 1293*, 24-39.

Richardson, J.D., Fikretoglu, D., Liu, A., McIntosh, D. (2011). Aripiprazole Augmentation in the Treatment of Military-Related PTSD with Major Depression: a retrospective chart review. *BMC Psychiatry*, 11(1), 86.

Robert, S., Hamner, M. B., Durkalski, V. L., Brown, M. W., & Ulmer, H. G. (2009). An open-label assessment of Aripiprazole in the treatment of PTSD. *Psychopharmacology Bulletin, 42*(1), 69-80.

Rothbaum, B. O., Killeen, T. K., Davidson, J. R. T., Brady, K. T., Connor, K. M., & Heekin, M. H. (2008). Placebo-Controlled Trial of Risperidone Augmentation for Selective Serotonin Reuptake Inhibitor-Resistant Civilian Posttraumatic Stress Disorder. *Journal of Clinical Psychiatry, 69*, 520-525.

Sareen, J., Cox, B. J., Goodwin, R. D., & Asmundson, G. (2005). Co-occurrence of posttraumatic stress disorder with positive psychotic symptoms in a nationally representative sample. *Journal of Traumatic Stress, 18*(4), 313-322.

Seedat, S., Stein, D. J., & Carey, P. D. (2005). Post-Traumatic Stress Disorder in Women: Epidemiological and Treatment Issues. *CNS Drugs, 19*(5), 411-427.

Stein, M. B., Kline, N. A., & Matloff, J. L. (2002). Adjunctive Olanzapine for SSRI-Resistant Combat-Related PTSD: A Double-Blind, Placebo-Controlled Study. *American Journal of Psychiatry, 159*, 1777-1779.

Taylor, F. B., & Raskind, M. A. (2002). The alpha-1 Adrenergic Antagonist Prazosin Improves Sleep and Nightmares in Civilian Trauma Posttraumatic Stress Disorder. *Journal of Clinical Psyhcopharmacology, 22*(1), 82-85.

Taylor, F. B. (2003). Tiagabine for Posttraumatic Stress Disorder: A Case Series of 7 Women. *Journal of Clinical Psychiatry, 64*(12), 1421-1425.

Taylor, F. B., Lowe, K., Thompson, C., McFall, M. M., Peskind, E. R., Kanter, E. D., et al. (2006). Daytime Prazosin Reduces Psychological Distress to Trauma Specific Cues in Civilian Trauma Posttraumatic Stress Disorder. *Biological Psychiatry, 59*, 577-581.

VA/DoD. (2010). *VA/DoD Clinical Practice Guideline for Management of Post-traumatic Stress: Guideline Summary*.

Villarreal, G., Calais, L. A., Canive, J. M., Lundy, S. L., Pickard, J., & Toney, G. (2007). Prospective study to evaluate the efficacy of Aripiprazole as a monotherapy in patients with severe chronic posttraumatic stress disorder: an open trial. *Psychopharmacology Bulletin, 40*(2), 6-18.

Walderhaug, E., Kasserman, S., Aikins, D., Vojvoda, D., Nishimura, C., & Neumeister, A. (2010). Effects of Duloxetine in Treatment-Refractory Men with Posttraumatic Stress Disorder. *Pharmacopsychiatry, 43*, 45-49.

Wheatly, M., Plant, J., Reader, H., Brown, G., & Cahill, C. (2004). Clozapine Treatment of Adolescents with Posttraumatic Stress Disorder and Psychotic Symptoms. *Journal of Clinical Psychopharmacology, 24*(2), 167-173.

Zisook, S., Chentsova-Dutton, Y. E., Smith-Vaniz, A., Kline, N. A., Ellenor, G. L., Kodsi, A. B., et al. (2000). Nefazodone in Patients with treatment-refractory Posttraumatic Stress Disorder. *Journal of Clinical Psychiatry, 61*(3), 203-208.

Part 5

Treatment: Alternative Approaches

15

Herbal Remedies to Treat Anxiety Disorders

Bhagya Venkanna Rao[1], Bettadapura N. Srikumar[2] and
Byrathnahalli S. Shankaranarayana Rao[1]
[1]Department of Neurophysiology, National Institute of Mental Health and Neuro Sciences, Deemed University, Bengaluru,
[2]Laboratoire "Physiologie Cellulaire de la Synapse", UMR 5091 CNRS, Université Bordeaux 2, Institut François Magendie, Bordeaux Cedex
[1]India
[2]France

1. Introduction

Anxiety, fear and worry are all completely natural human feelings. If these feelings occur and endure for an extended period, it affects both physical and mental health. This leads to clinical anxiety disorders. There are many types of treatment available to treat anxiety disorders. This article outlines more common herbal remedies to treat anxiety disorders.

Anxiety is an aversive emotional state, in which the feeling of fear is disproportionate to the threat (Weinberger, 2001). Anxiety is implicated in a number of psychiatric disorders, such as depression, panic attacks, phobias, generalized anxiety disorder, obsessive-compulsive disorder and post-traumatic stress disorder (Gross and Hen, 2004). Anxiety disorders are the most common class of neuropsychiatric disorders in USA (Kessler et al., 2005) and many other countries (Alonso and Lepine, 2007). The life time prevalence of panic attacks (a form of anxiety disorder) is around 7-9% in most countries and 1% alone in India with the prevalence of generalized anxiety disorder is very high i.e. 8.5% in the general population (WHO, 2001). Anxiety disorders affect 16.6% of population worldwide (Somers et al., 2006) and numerous efforts have been made to understand the pathophysiology of the disease and treatments.

According to the Diagnostic and Statistical Manual of Mental Disorders (DSM-IV-TR), anxiety is characterized by a feeling of persistent worry that hinders an individual's ability to relax [Diagnostic and Statistical Manual of Mental Disorders Washington D.C.: American Psychiatric Association, 4 2000]. Anxiety disorders are described and classified in DSM and several anxiety disorders share common clinical symptoms such as widespread anxiety, physiological anxiety symptoms, and behavioral disturbances.

2. Common anxiety disorders

2.1 Generalized anxiety disorders (GAD)

Generalized anxiety disorder is a syndrome of ongoing anxiety and worry about many events or feelings that the patient generally recognizes as extreme and inappropriate (DSM-IV-TR). Individuals manifest both physical and psychological symptoms leading to significant distress or impairment.

2.2 Obsessive-compulsive disorder (OCD)

People suffering from OCD tend to have bothersome and intrusive thoughts that generate anxiety (obsession) and perform repetitive actions (compulsion). Obsessions include unwanted thoughts, impulses, or images that cause great anxiety. Compulsions include repetitive behaviors or mental acts that those affected feel driven to perform.

2.3 Panic disorder

People suffering from panic disorders often have panic attacks, defined as discrete periods of sudden symptom onset usually peaking in 10 minutes and can occur with most anxiety disorders.

2.4 Post-traumatic stress disorder (PTSD)

Individuals with PTSD avoid stimuli associated with the trauma and feel an extreme amount of fear and anxiety after presenting stimuli. Stress is a condition which affects physiological and psychological homeostasis. Evidence indicates that chronic repeated stress precipitates neuropsychiatric disorders like anxiety and depression (Holsboer, 1988; McEwen and Stellar, 1993; McEwen, 2000; Vyas et al., 2002; Veena et al., 2009b; 2011). Previous work in an animal model of stress revealed that chronic stress impairs learning in the T-maze (Sunanda et al., 2000a) and radial arm maze (Srikumar et al., 2006; 2007; Veena et al., 2009a) tasks in addition to inducing anxiety-like behavior (Adamec et al., 1999; Vyas et al., 2002; Govindarajan et al., 2006). Stress-induced behavioral impairments are associated with structural (Ramkumar et al., 2008; Shankaranarayana Rao et al., 2001; Shankaranarayana Rao & Raju, 2004; 2005; 2007), biochemical (Sunanda et al., 2000b), molecular (Bennur et al., 2007; Pawlak et al., 2005; Veena et al., 2011) and electrophysiological (Hegde et al., 2008) alterations in the hippocampus and amygdala regions. Recent studies have clearly demonstrated the abnormal synaptic plasticity is responsible for cognitive deficits including enhanced anxiety in fragile X mental retardation and autism (Dolen et al., 2007; Hayashi et al., 2007). Induction of progressive plasticity is known to be responsible for amelioration of stress-induced cognitive deficits and depression-like behavior by enriched environment and brain stimulation rewarding experience (Asha Devi et al., 2011; Ramkumar et al., 2008; Shankaranarayana Rao, 2009; 2010; Veena et al., 2009a).

Anxiety and other psychiatric conditions are one of the most frequent conditions seen by clinicians and often require long-term treatment with medications. Selective serotonin reuptake inhibitor (SSRI) and benzodiazepines are important class of drugs used to treat generalized anxiety disorders (Davidson, 2001; Davidson, 2009) and depression (Bhagya et al., 2008; Bhagya et al., 2011). With the increasing cost of anti-anxiety medications and their increased side effects like suicidal ideation, decreased alertness, sexual dysfunction and dependency (Hu et al., 2004; Gunnell et al., 2005; O'brien, 2005; Lader et al., 2009), drugs of natural origin are promising alternatives to treat neuropsychiatric disorders (Kienzle-Horn, 2002; Carlini, 2003).

3. Common herbal remedies for anxiety

Ayurveda, the Indian traditional system of medicine uses herbs and their preparations to treat various neuropsychiatric disorders. Numerous herbs have been used for centuries in folk and other traditional medicine to calm the mind and positively enhance mood. Herbal medicine which plays an important role in developing countries, are once again becoming popular throughout developing and developed countries. Study by Sparreboom et al. (2004) revealed that use of herbal medicine is increasing enormously in the Western world. In spite of the large number of animal studies evaluating the potential anxiolytic effects of plant extracts, very few controlled studies have been conducted in a clinical setup. The efficacy and safety of utilizing these natural drugs to treat anxiety, has only just begun to be exactly tested in clinical trials within the last 10 to 15 years (Saeed et al., 2007; Garcia-Garcia et al., 2008; Kinrys et al., 2009). For instance, both Kava-kava (*Piper methysticum*) and St. John's wort (*Hypericum perforatum*) showed beneficial effectiveness in double blind, randomized placebo controlled trials to treat anxiety and depression (Ernst, 2002). Also, extracts of valerian, hops, lemon balm and passion flower preparations have been employed for the prevention and treatment of psychiatric disorders such as anxiety, sleep disorders, convulsions, cognitive impairment and depression (Beaubrun and Gray, 2000). The commonly used herbal remedies for treating anxiety disorders are described below.

3.1 Passion flower

Passiflora incarnata is a folk remedy for anxiety. The anxiolytic effects of passionflower are well documented in rodents (Dhawan et al., 2001; Dhawan et al., 2002). In randomized double-blind study, passion flower extract was effective in 18 generalised anxiety disorder (GAD) out-patients as compared to oxazepam. Also, impairment in the job performance was increased in oxazepam group as compared to Passiflora extract treated group (Akhondzadeh et al., 2001). In another double-blind placebo-controlled study, preoperative oral *Passiflora incarnata* reduces anxiety in ambulatory surgery patients (Movafegh et al., 2008).

3.2 Kava kava (*Piper methysticum*)

There is substantial evidence that kava has a positive effect on the symptoms of anxiety disorders. Animal studies have demonstrated anti-anxiety activity of kava (Garrett et al., 2003; Bruner and Anderson, 2009). Several randomized double-blind clinical studies in GAD patients showed beneficial effect of kava-kava in reducing anxiety (Watkins et al., 2001; Connor and Davidson, 2002; Boerner et al., 2003; Sarris et al., 2009). Kava-kava was used in numerous controlled clinical studies to treat anxiety disorders, but the subjects included in these studies were heterogeneous i.e., they were diagnosed with agoraphobia, specific phobia, social phobia, adjustment disorder with anxiety (Volz and Kieser, 1997; Malsch and Kieser, 2001; Gastpar and Klimm, 2003; Lehrl, 2004). In the study by Connor & Davidson, kava extract was compared with placebo in GAD patients (2002). In another 8-week randomized, double-blind multi-center clinical trial, the efficacy of *Piper methysticum* was compared with two anxiolytic drugs opipramol and buspirone in GAD patients (Boerner et al., 2003). Meta-analysis study by Pittler and Ernst reinforced the anxiolytic effect of kava in generalized anxiety patients and indicated a significant reduction in anxiety parameters evaluated by the Hamilton Anxiety (HAMA) scale (Pittler and Ernst, 2000; 2002).

3.3 St. John's wort (*Hypericum perforatum*)

St. John's wort is a popular supplement for treating depression but is much less popular for treating anxiety disorders. Studies conducted by Flausino et al. and Singewald et al. have shown that chronic administration of *Hypericum perforatum* induced an antidepressant-like effect in Magnesium-depleted mice in the forced swim test and anxiolytic effect in the elevated T-maze and the light/dark transition test (Flausino, Jr. et al., 2002; Singewald et al., 2004). St. John's wort administration resulted in anti-anxiety effect in animal models of restraint stress and sleep deprivation (Flausino, Jr. et al., 2002; Singewald et al., 2004; Kumar and Singh, 2007; Kumar et al., 2010). *Hypericum perforatum* inhibits the reuptake of serotonin, noradrenaline, dopamine (Wonnemann et al., 2000) and modulates neuronal excitability via glutamatergic and GABAergic mechanisms (Langosch et al., 2002).

Studies specifically testing the effects of St. John's wort on patients with anxiety are extremely limited. The evidence of positive effects of St. John's wort on anxiety disorders is weak. No placebo-controlled, randomized, double-blind trials have shown St. John's wort to be effective in treating generalized anxiety disorder, post-traumatic stress disorder, obsessive-compulsive disorder (OCD), or phobias. Volz et al. (2002) showed that Hypericum extract to 149 out patients diagnosed with somatization disorder, undifferentiated somatoform disorder, or somatoform autonomic dysfunctions, significantly reduced anxiety scores in HAMA scale. Another open-label uncontrolled observation with 500 subjects showed beneficial effect of St. John's wort extract in reducing anxiety disorder symptoms in patients diagnosed with depression comorbid with anxiety (Muller et al., 2003). However, stronger evidence is needed before St. John's wort should be considered as a treatment option for patients with diagnosable anxiety disorders.

3.4 *Valeriana officinalis*

Valerian is one of the most popularly used herbal medicines for insomnia (Donath et al., 2000) and is also used to treat anxiety. Hydroalcoholic and aqueous extracts of valerian roots have shown affinity for the GABA-A receptor in the brains of rats (Benke et al., 2009). In humans, valerian has been successful in the treatment of insomnia and tension (Schmidt-Voigt, 1986; Vorbach, 1996; Leathwood, 1985; Donath et al., 2000; Stevinson and Ernst, 2000; Ziegler, 2002). Andreatini et al. (2002) compared the extract of *Valeriana officinalis* L. (81mg of valepotriates as active ingredients) with placebo and diazepam (6.5 mg) in patients with GAD (DSM-III-R, 12 patients per group). Only the diazepam and valepotriates groups showed a significant reduction in the psychic factor of HAMA scale and the preliminary data obtained in the present study suggest that the valepotriates may have a potential anxiolytic effect on the psychic symptoms of anxiety. The limitations of this study are small sample size and a low dose of diazepam, such studies should be replicated with improved methodological design.

3.5 *Ginkgo biloba*

Extract of *Ginkgo biloba* (EGb 761) significantly reduced the detrimental effect of learned helplessness in a subsequent conditioned avoidance task. In the elevated plus maze, senescent mice treated with EGb 761 spent more time in open arms than those treated with vehicle control (Ward et al., 2002). Woelke et al. (2007) compared a standardized extract of *Ginkgo biloba* L. (EGb 761) in doses of 480mg and 240mg with placebo for four weeks, involving patients with GAD and adjustment disorder with anxious mood (DSM-III-R). The two doses of EGb 761 showed a greater reduction in HAMA scores compared to placebo, as well as a statistically significant reduction in somatic symptoms compared to baseline (which was not observed in the placebo group).

3.6 *Galphimia glauca*

Galphimia glauca Cav. is a plant used in Mexican traditional medicine as a "nerve tranquilizer". Previous studies have demonstrated anxiolytic effect of methanolic extract from this plant species. Herrera-Arellano et al. (2007) conducted a controlled study comparing the extract *Galphimia glauca* Cav. with lorazepam in patients with GAD with 72 and 80 patients per group, respectively. Both groups of patients showed a significant reduction in scores of HAMA, without any difference between treatments.

3.7 *Matricaria recutita* (chamomile)

Chamomile is one of the most popular single ingredient of herbal teas, or tisanes. Chamomile tea, brewed from dried flower heads is used traditionally for several medicinal purposes like gastrointestinal tract ailments. Other uses include allergic rhinitis, attention deficit-hyperactivity disorder (ADHD), restlessness, insomnia, dysmenorrhea, mastitis and varicose ulcers. Chamomile contains flavonoids, which exert benzodiazepine-like activity (Avallone et al., 2000) and also has a phosphodiesterase inhibitory action, which leads to increased cAMP levels (Kuppusamy and Das, 1992). A recent study evaluated the efficacy of a standardized extract of *Matricaria recutita* (L), compared with placebo for eight weeks in patients with mild to moderate GAD (DSM-IV). There was a statistically significant reduction in the scores of HAMA in the group treated with extract compared to placebo-treated group (Amsterdam et al., 2009).

3.8 *Astragalus membranaceus*

Astragalus membranaceus (AM) is a useful Korean herb that has been clinically prescribed for stress-related illness. AM significantly restores learning and memory deficits in chronically stressed rats. In the elevated plus maze, AM treatment significantly increases the time spent in the open arms compared to control group. It also enhanced choline acetyltransferase (ChAT) expression in stressed rats (Park et al., 2009). No clinical data is available for its anxiolytic effect. But one clinical study demonstrated the protective effect of astragalous on oxidative stress status in maintenance of hemodialysis patients (Qu et al., 2008).

4. Indian traditional herbs

4.1 *Centella asiatica (Mandookaparni* or Gotu Kola)

Centella asiatica is reputed for its beneficial effects in various neurological disorders. Gotu Kola has been used for centuries in Ayurvedic and traditional Chinese medicine to alleviate symptoms of depression and anxiety. Recent studies in the rat have shown that long-term pretreatment with Gotu Kola decreases locomotor activity, enhance elevated-plus maze performance and attenuate acoustic startle response (Chen et al., 2006; Wijeweera et al., 2006). In a double-blind, placebo-controlled study, the anxiolytic activity of *Centella asiatica* in healthy subjects was undertaken and compared to placebo, Gotu Kola significantly reduced peak acoustic startle response amplitude 30 and 60 minutes after treatment (Bradwejn et al., 2000). In another clinical study, 70% hydro-ethanolic extract of *Centella asiatica* was given to 33 participants for two months and Hamilton's Brief Psychiatric Rating Scale (BPRS) was used to screen the subjects. The results show that, *Mandookaparni* significantly attenuated anxiety related disorders (Jana et al., 2010). These preliminary findings suggest that *Centella asiatica* has anxiolytic activity in humans and it remains to be seen whether this herb has therapeutic efficacy in the treatment of anxiety syndromes in large population.

4.2 *Bacopa monnieri (Brahmi)*

In Indian traditional medicine, several herbs have been used as nerve tonics. The most popular of these herbs is *brahmi*, a well known memory booster. This herb is used by Ayurvedic medical practitioners for almost 3000 years. The traditional use of *brahmi* as an anti-anxiety remedy in Ayurvedic medicine is supported by both animal and clinical studies. *Brahmi* is used in Indian tradition medicine in treatment of number of brain disorders namely anxiety and poor memory (Singh and Dhawan, 1997). Pharmacologically, *Bacopa monnieri* comprises of five major saponins: bacoside A3, bacopaside II, bacopasaponin C isomer, bacopasaponin C and bacopaside I (Phrompittayarat et al., 2007). *Bacopa monniera* extract or its constituent bacosides showed anxiolytic activity in animals (Bhattacharya and Ghosal, 1998: Shankar and Singh, 2000; Singh et al., 1979: Singh and Singh, 1980) and Singh et al. (1996) suggest an involvement of the GABA-ergic activity in *brahmi*'s action on central nervous system . *Brahmi* not only enhances memory, it also shows an anti-stress effect. Pretreatment with Bacosides resulted in decrease Hsp expression in the hippocampus; it restored P450 enzyme activity and increased superoxide dismutase activity in the stressed rats. *Brahmi* modulates the activities of Hsp70, P450 and SOD and thereby protects the brain from deleterious effect of stress (Kar Chowdhury et al., 2002). In another study, pretreatment with *brahmi* restored both acute and chronic immobilization stress-induced changes in ulcer index, adrenal gland weight, creatine kinase, and aspartate aminotransferase (Rai et al., 2003). Treatment with *Bacopa monnieri* extract 40 mg/kg/day effectively reversed behavioral deficits of PCAPP mice in open field tests compared with non-transgenic controls (Holcomb et al., 2006).

Previous clinical study demonstrated that administration of *brahmi* syrup to 35 patients diagnosed with anxiety neurosis resulted in significant decrease in anxiety symptoms and level of anxiety (Asthana et al., 1996). In a recent randomized, double-blind, placebo controlled clinical trial, effect of standardized *Bacopa monniera* extract in healthy elderly patients on anxiety, depression and recall memory was evaluated. *Bacopa* participants had enhanced delayed word recall memory scores in Rey Auditory Verbal Learning Test (AVLT) compared to placebo. Affective measures like depression scores, anxiety scores, and heart rate decreased in due course for the *Bacopa* group but increased for the placebo group (Calabrese et al., 2008). In a study by Stough et al., the chronic effects of *brahmi* extract were examined on memory function in forty six healthy human subjects aged between 18 to 60 years. The study was a double-blind placebo-controlled independent group design in which subjects were randomly allocated to one of the two treatment conditions, i.e., *brahmi* extract (300 mg) or placebo. Neuropsychological tests were conducted pre-baseline and at 5 and 12 weeks post-drug administration. *Brahmi* extract significantly improved speed of visual information processing measured by the Inspection Time, learning rate and memory consolidation measured by Auditory Verbal Learning Test, and state anxiety examined using Strait-Trait Anxiety Inventory. The results of the clinical trial suggested that *brahmi* extract improved higher order cognitive processes that are critically dependent on the input of information from our environment such as learning and memory (Stough et al., 2001). Another study to measure the effect of *brahmi* extract on human memory was conducted by Roodenrys et al. (2002). Seventy six adults aged between 40 and 65 years volunteered for the double-blind randomized, placebo control study in which various memory functions were tested and levels of anxiety measured in three testing sessions: one prior to the trial, one after three months on the trial, and one six weeks after the completion of the trial. The results showed a significant effect of *brahmi* on the test for the retention of new information. In the follow-up tests it was found that the rate of learning was unaffected, suggesting that *brahmi* decreases the rate of forgetting of newly acquired information.

4.3 *Withania somnifera (ashwagandha)*

This has been an important herb in use within Ayurvedic and indigenous medical systems for over 3000 years. Both preclinical and clinical studies demonstrate the use of *ashwagandha* for anxiety, inflammation, Parkinson's disease, cognitive and neurological disorders. It is also used therapeutically as an adaptogen in nervous exhaustion, insomnia, debility due to stress (Mishra et al., 2000; Withania, Monograph 2004). Preclinically, the extract of *Withania somnifera* (WS) root exhibited anxiolytic activity in the elevated plus-maze, social interaction and feeding latency in an unfamiliar environment (Bhattacharya et al., 2000). Chronic stress-induced hyperglycemia, cognitive deficits, immunosupression and depression was attenuated by *ashwagandha*. The results indicate that *ashwagandha* has significant antistress adaptogenic activity, confirming the clinical use of the plant in Ayurveda (Bhattacharya and Muruganandam, 2003). A recent study has demonstrated the anxiolytic potential of a compound natural health product which had *Withania* as the main herb in an open label human trial (Seely and Singh, 2007). Also, studies have demonstrated that WS possesses GABA-mimetic properties (Kulkarni and Verma, 1993a; Mehta et al., 1991). Since GABA agonism has been linked to anxiolysis (Stahl, 1998), the extracts of WS may have beneficial effect in anxiety and related disorders. A double blind placebo control study in patients with ICD-10 anxiety disorders, 6 weeks treatment with ethanolic extract of *W. somnifera* showed anxiolytic activity over placebo. The extract was well tolerated and did not cause more adverse effects than placebo. So, it was concluded that the ethanolic extract of WS has useful anxiolytic potential (Andrade et al., 2000).

5. Polyherbal formulations

In Ayurveda, compound formulations are generally used in the therapy as the combination of many drugs provides a synergistic therapeutic effect and also includes ingredients which help to minimize the adverse effects of few other major drugs. A recent study demonstrated adaptogenic potential of a compound natural health product which had *Withania* as the main herb in an open label human trial. An open-label and uncontrolled clinical trial evaluated the impact of OCTA© on known parameters of stress (OCTA©, an aqueous-based liquid herbal preparation consisting of eight herbs as follows: *W. somnifera, Lagerstroemia speciosa, Bacopa monniera, Zizyphus jujuba, Morinda citrifolia, Punica granatum, Shisandrae chinensis* and *Lycium barbarum*) (Seely and Singh, 2007). Another herbal formulation, Sumind is (Ayurvedic nomenclature and the quantity of each ingredient are given in parentheses), *Nardostachys atamans* (*Jatamansi*), *Acorus calamus* (*Vacha*), *Celastrus paniculata* (*Jyotishmati*), *Convolvulus microphyllus* (*Shankapushpi*), *Bacopa monnieri* (*Brahmi*), *Withania somnifera* (*Ashwagadha*), *Valerian wallichii* (*Tagara*), *Eclipta alba* (*Bhringaraja*). Sumind showed antidepressant activity as indicated by reduced immobility time in rats subjected to swim stress. It also restored biogenic amine levels to normal levels and reduced corticosterone levels in stressed rats (Nanjappa et al., 2007).

Mentat (BR-16A) is an herbal medication contains 20 different ingredients. The main herbs present in the mentat are *Brahmi* (*Bacopa monnieri*), *Mandookparni* (*Centella asiatica*).

Ashwagandha (*Withania somnifera*), *Jatamansi* (*Nardostachys jatamansi*), *Shankhapuspi* (*Evolvulus alsinoides*), *Tagar* (*Valeriana wallichi*). *Vach* (*Acorus calamus*), *Guduchi* (*Tinospora cordifolia*), *Malkangni* (*Celastrus paniculatus*), Kuth (*Saussurea lappa*) Amla (*Embelica officinalis*), *Terminalia chebula* and *Terminalia belerica*. Some of these plants namely, *B. monnieri, C. asiatica, W. somnifera, N. jatamansi, E. alsinoides, V. wallichi, A. calamus, T. cordifolia* and *C. paniculatus*, have been classified in Ayurveda as Medharasayanas and claimed to improve memory and intellect (Sharma, 1978). Polyherbal formulations are generally used in Ayurveda, based on the concept that such combinations provide synergistic therapeutic effect. Mice show a natural aversion to open and high spaces and therefore, spend more time in enclosed arms. Mice receiving chronic treatment with BR-16A-Mentat (100 mg/kg) followed by ethanol failed to show any withdrawal-induced anxiety. There was a significant decrease in the time spent in closed arms. The duration and the number of entries in open arms increased significantly as compared with the ethanol withdrawn group (Kulkarni and Verma, 1993b). Also, the anti-stress effect of mentat was evident against social isolation-induced stress in mice (Kumar and Kulkarni, 2006).

Agrawal et al. (1990a,b) reported that BR-16A improves memory parameters and decreases anxiety parameters in normal volunteers. Also, mentat (BR-16) brought about marked improvement in memory in all age groups and caused decrease in anxiety level and neuroticism index (Agrawal et al., 1991). Mentat in the form of syrup was given to patients of anxiety neurosis and depression in a placebo controlled study. Both anxiety and depressive patients showed memory impairment and also increased fatiguability. 3 month treatment with Mentat improved memory and decreased fatiguability in these patients (Sharma et al., 1990). Psychological problems like stress, anxiety and depression play an important role in the prognosis, quality of life as well as the survival rate of cancer patients. Treatment with mentat in cancer patients reduced stress, anxiety and depressive symptoms (Durgesh Kumar, 2000).

Another polyherbal formulation Geriforte showed significant anxiolytic effect in clinical studies. Geriforte contains Chyavanprash concentrate and the extracts of *Asparagus adscendens, Withania somnifera, Glycyrrhiza glabra, Centella asiatica, Mucuna pruriens*, Shilajeet, *Asparagus racemosus, Terminalia arjuna*, Makardhwaj and *Piper longum*, besides some others. An earlier open study demonstrated the beneficial effects of Geriforte in anxiety patients as per DSM III R criteria. There was significant reduction in the total Hamilton Anxiety Rating Scale (HARS) score at the end of four weeks (Boral et al., 1989; Shah et al., 1990). Another double-blind, placebo-controlled study authors have observed improvement in HARS scores in patients of mixed anxiety-depression following 4 weeks of Geriforte treatment in comparison with placebo (Shah et al., 1993; Upadhyaya et al., 1990). Preclinical studies show that Geriforte stimulates antioxidant defense system in both mice and rats (Vandana et al., 1998). Various studies have demonstrated the efficacy of Geriforte as an anti-stress adaptogen. The prolongation of survival time and prevention of stress-induced changes in adrenals, prevention of stress-induced ulcers and milk-induced leucocytosis, indicate the anti-stress properties of Geriforte (Singh et al., 1978).

Another common polyherbal formulation Euphytose, which is a combination of six extracts: Crataegus, Ballota, Passiflora and Valeriana, which have mild sedative effects, and Cola and Paullinia, which mainly act as mild stimulants. Euphytose reduced HAMA scores in outpatients with adjustment disorder with anxious mood in multicenter, double-blind, placebo-controlled study (Bourin et al., 1997).

Recent preclinical studies have shown anxiolytic activity of several herbal drugs. *Securidaca longepedunculata* is a savannah shrub commonly used by traditional medicine practitioners in Nigeria. The aqueous root extract of *Securidaca longepedunculata* showed anxiolytic activity in the elevated plus maze (EPM) by significantly increasing time spent in the open arms as compared to control (Adeyemi et al., 2010). Another herbal medicine yokukansan improved age related anxiety in the open filed and EPM (Mizoguchi et al., 2010). *Petiveria alliacea* L has been traditionally used in South America and Brazil for anxiety and whole plant extract of *Petiveria alliacea* caused anxiolytic-like effects in mice subjected to the EPM (Blainski et al., 2010). *Cirsium rivulare* (Jacq.) All. (Asteraceae) is an herbaceous perennial plant traditionally used in Polish folk medicine to treat anxiety. In a recent study, methanolic extracts from flowers and leaves of *Cirsium rivulare* produced anxiolytic activity in the EPM. Extract from flowers in addition to its anxiolytic effects, improves memory of the appetitively and aversively motivated tasks (Walesiuk et al., 2010). In Brazil, *Erythrina mulungu* and *Erythrina velutina* (Fabaceae) are widely used as a tranquilizer and/or sedative, and their extract exerts an anxiolytic-like effect profile in animal models. In herbal medicine, a leaf or bark decoction or tincture from mulungu is considered to calm agitation and other disorders of the nervous system, including insomnia and depression. Chronic *Erythrina mulungu* exerted anxiolytic effect in the elevated T maze inhibitory avoidance and in the light/dark transition model (Onusic et al., 2003). *Erythrina velutina* administration increased the percentage of open arm entries in the elevated plus maze (Raupp et al., 2008). No clinical data is available to substantiate anxiolytic effect of these herbs.

Our own studies have demonstrated the role of different herbs and herbal formulations namely *Euphorbia hirta, Celastrus paniculatus* Willd and Sumind in amelioration of anxiety, depression, cognitive deficits and associated neurodegeneration in these disorders (Anuradha et al., 2008; 2010; Nanjappa et al., 2007). Recent studies have shown that treatments with the crude extract of *Astragalus membranaceus* reduced repeated stress induced anxiety and memory loss (Park et al., 2009). In similar lines, our previous work demonstrated that *Euphorbia hirta* (Eh) reverses chronic immobilization stress-induced anxiety behavior in elevated plus maze and open field test. Extracts of Eh Linn have been found to possess central analgesic, antipyretic, anti-inflammatory properties in addition to its central antidepressant, sedative and anxiolytic effects (Lanhers et al., 1990; Lanhers et al., 1991; Johnson et al., 1999). The anxiolytic activity of this drug has been established in mice subjected to two-compartment, staircase and light/dark choice situation tests (Lanhers et al., 1990). *Euphorbia hirta* produces its anxiolytic effect in an animal model of chronic stress through $GABA_A$ receptor-benzodiazepine receptor-Cl^- channel complex. Eh also appears to mediate its anxiolytic action through this complex since all of the three antagonists, flumazenil, bicuculline and picrotoxin inhibited Eh-induced increase in open arm exploration and also recovered the acetylcholinesterase (AChE) activity in discrete regions of the brain (Anuradha et al., 2008; 2010).

Celastrus paniculatus Willd has been known for centuries as "the elixir of life". Ayurveda describes drug the *Jyotishmati* (*Celastrus paniculata*) as early as 1500BC in Charaka samhita (the most ancient and authoritative text book of ayurveda) for diseases of the brain and as *buddhiprada* (enhancing intellect), *smritiprada* (enhancing memory). *Jyotishmati* translates as *Jyoti* and *mati* (enlightens intellect). *Celastrus paniculatus* (CP), a plant belonging to Celastraceae was in use from time immemorial to treat brain related disorders and to enhance learning and memory. CP treated rats exhibited a significantly increased learning curve compared with vehicle treated animals in the avoidance paradigm (Karanth et al., 1980). In another study, rats treated daily with 850 mg/kg of CP oil for 15 days exhibited a significant improvement in their retention time in a two-way passive avoidance task. CP also produced a significant decrease in the content of norepinephrine, dopamine and serotonin and certain of their respective metabolites in the brain (Nalini et al., 1995). Previous findings indicate that the aqueous extract of CP seed has cognitive-enhancing properties and an antioxidant effect might be involved (Kumar and Gupta, 2002). CP enhanced learning and memory in naïve rats when tested in a partially baited radial arm maze task by altering acetyl cholinesterase activity in the hippocampus and frontal cortex (Lekha et al., 2010a). Acute and chronic immobilisation-induced oxidative stress was restored back to normal after CP oil treatment (Lekha et al., 2010b). Recently we have demonstrated that chronic stress-induced learning impairment in radial arm maze task was restored by chronic CP oil treatment. The behavioural recovery was associated with restoration of both hippocampal long-term potentiation and cholinergic activity. This opens up the possibility of developing novel agents from nature to enhance synaptic plasticity as a means of treating a variety of psychiatric diseases, including depression (Unpublished data). An *in vitro* study has demonstrated neuroprotective effect of CP water extract in forebrain primary neuronal cell cultures. Pre-treatment of neuronal cells with CP-water extract significantly attenuated glutamate-induced neuronal death. Also, CP significantly and reversibly inhibited whole-cell NMDA currents (Godkar et al., 2004).

6. Conclusion

Despite a large number of animal studies evaluating the potential anxiolytic effects of herbal drugs, very few controlled clinical studies have been conducted. These studies have methodological problems like small number of subjects, lack of placebo and control groups, and inclusion of heterogeneous subjects and short treatment duration, which hinders consistent conclusion about these herbal preparations. Some herbs like kava-kava, gingko showed promising results with substantial clinical significance when compared with benzodiazepines, buspirone and antidepressants. Although evidence of effectiveness of herbs and their preparations in treating neuropsychiatric disorders is increasing, translating these results to treat patients effectively is slowed down by the limited knowledge regarding chemical composition of the products, lack of standardization of these preparations and the paucity of well controlled studies. Preliminary evidence suggests that herbal medicines may have a role in the treatment of anxiety disorders and warrants further research. However, we would like to clearly warn that most of the remedies are not approved for clinical use and herbal remedies are not solely alternatives of clinical treatment regimens. Also some of the herbal remedies may interact with other medicines leading to drug-drug interactions, which may cause severe side effects and in some cases it may be fatal. Accordingly, it is advised to use herbal drugs under strict supervision of qualified ayurvedic physicians with periodic follow-ups.

7. Acknowledgement

We acknowledge the financial support from the Council of Scientific and Industrial Research (CSIR), New Delhi, India through a Senior Research Associate fellowship to BV, Research grants from Department of Biotechnology (DBT) and Department of Science and

Technology (DST), Government of India to BSS, Fondation pour la recherche médicale (FRM) fellowship to BNS.

8. References

Adamec RE, Burton P, Shallow T & Budgell J. (1999). NMDA receptors mediate lasting increases in anxiety-like behavior produced by the stress of predator exposure-implications for anxiety associated with posttraumatic stress disorder. *Physiology & Behavior* 65: 723-737

Adeyemi OO, Akindele AJ, Yemitan OK, Aigbe FR & Fagbo FI. (2010). Anticonvulsant, anxiolytic and sedative activities of the aqueous root extract of Securidaca longepedunculata Fresen. *Journal of Ethnopharmacology* 130: 191-195

Agrawal A, Dubey ML & Dubey GP. (1990a). Effects of "mental" on memory and anxiety scores of normal subjects in three age groups. *Pharmacopsychoecologia* 3:43-45

Agrawal A, Dubey ML & Dubey GP. (1990b). Effects of "Mentat" on memory span, attention, galvanic skin resistance (GSR) and muscle action potential (EMG) among normal adults. *Pharmacopsychoecologia* 3: 39-42

Agrawal A, Dubey ML & Dubey GP. (1991). Effect of mentat on memory, anxiety scores and neuroticism index in normal subjects in three age groups. *Probe* 3: 257

Akhondzadeh S, Naghavi HR, Vazirian M, Shayeganpour A, Rashidi H & Khani M. (2001). Passionflower in the treatment of generalized anxiety: a pilot double-blind randomized controlled trial with oxazepam. *Journal of Clinical Pharmacy & Therapeutics* 26: 363-367

Alonso J & Lepine JP. (2007). Overview of key data from the European Study of the Epidemiology of Mental Disorders (ESEMeD). *Journal of Clinical Psychiatry* 68: 3-9

Amsterdam JD, Li Y, Soeller I, Rockwell K, Mao JJ & Shults J. (2009). A randomized, double-blind, placebo-controlled trial of oral Matricaria recutita (chamomile) extract therapy for generalized anxiety disorder. *Journal of Clinical Psychopharmacology* 29: 378-382

Andrade C, Aswath A, Chaturvedi SK, Srinivasa M & Raguram R. (2000). A double-blind placebo-controlled evaluation of anxiolytic efficacy of an ethanolic extract of Withania somnifera. *Indian Journal of Psychiatry* 42: 295–30

Andreatini R, Sartori VA, Seabra ML & Leite JR. (2002). Effect of valepotriates (valerian extract) in generalized anxiety disorder: a randomized placebo-controlled pilot study. *Phytotherapy Research* 16: 650-654

Anuradha H, Srikumar BN, Shankaranarayana Rao BS & Lakshmana M. (2008). Euphorbia hirta reverses chronic stress-induced anxiety and mediates its action through the GABA(A) receptor benzodiazepine receptor-Cl(-) channel complex. *Journal of Neural Transmission* 115: 35-42

Anuradha H, Srikumar BN, Deepti N, Shankaranarayana Rao BS & Lakshmana M. (2010). Restoration of acetylcholinesterase activity by Euphorbia hirta in discrete brain regions of chronically stressed rats. *Pharmaceutical Biology* 48: 499-503

Asha Devi S, Manjula KR & Shankaranarayana Rao BS. (2011). Healthy brain and well-being: Sedentary lifestyle can impact cognitive ability adversely. *in* Bergin MG (ed.), *Sedentary Behavior: Physiology, Health risks & Interventions*. Nova Science Publishers, Inc., New York, USA. In Press.

Asthana OP, Srivastava JS, Ghatak A, Gaur SPS & Dhawan BN. (1996). Safety and tolerability of bacosides A and B in healthy human volunteers. *Indian Journal of Pharmacology* 28: 37

Avallone R, Zanoli P, Puia G, Kleinschnitz M, Schreier P & Baraldi M. (2000). Pharmacological profile of apigenin, a flavonoid isolated from Matricaria chamomilla. *Biochemical Pharmacology* 59: 1387-1394

Beaubrun G & Gray GE. A review of herbal medicines for psychiatric disorders. (2000). *Psychiatric Services* 51: 1130-1134

Benke D, Barberis A, Kopp S, Altmann KH, Schubiger M, Vogt KE, Rudolph U & Mohler H. (2009). GABA A receptors as in vivo substrate for the anxiolytic action of valerenic acid, a major constituent of valerian root extracts. *Neuropharmacology* 56: 174-181

Bennur S, Shankaranarayana Rao BS, Pawlak R, Strickland S, McEwen BS & Chattarji S. (2007). Stress-induced spine loss in the medial amygdala is mediated by tissue-plasminogen activator. Neuroscience 144: 8-16

Bhagya V, Srikumar BN, Raju TR & Shankaranarayana Rao BS. (2008). Neonatal clomipramine induced endogenous depression in rats is associated with learning impairment in adulthood. Behavioral Brain Research 187: 190–194

Bhagya V, Srikumar BN, Raju TR & Shankaranarayana Rao BS. (2011). Chronic escitalopram treatment restores spatial learning, monoamine levels, and hippocampal long-term potentiation in an animal model of depression. Psychopharmacology. 214: 477-494

Bhattacharya SK & Ghosal S. (1998). Anxiolytic activity of a standardized extract of Bacopa monniera: an experimental study. *Phytomedicine* 5: 77-82

Bhattacharya SK, Bhattacharya A, Sairam K & Ghosal S. (2000). Anxiolytic-antidepressant activity of Withania somnifera glycowithanolides: an experimental study. *Phytomedicine* 7: 463-469

Bhattacharya SK & Muruganandam AV. (2003). Adaptogenic activity of Withania somnifera: an experimental study using a rat model of chronic stress. *Pharmacology Biochemistry & Behavior* 75: 547-555

Blainski A, Piccolo VK, Mello JC & de Oliveira RM. (2010). Dual effects of crude extracts obtained from Petiveria alliacea L. (Phytolaccaceae) on experimental anxiety in mice. *Journal of Ethnopharmacology* 128: 541-544

Boerner RJ, Sommer H, Berger W, Kuhn U, Schmidt U, & Mannel M. (2003). Kava-Kava extract LI 150 is as effective as Opipramol and Buspirone in Generalised Anxiety Disorder--an 8-week randomized, double-blind multi-centre clinical trial in 129 out-patients. *Phytomedicine* 10: 38-49

Boral GC, Gautam Bandopadyaya, Anjan Boral Das NN & Nandi PS. (1989). Geriforte in anxiety neurosis. *Indian Journal of Psychiatry* 31: 258-260

Bourin M, Bougerol T, Guitton B & Broutin E. (1997). A combination of plant extracts in the treatment of outpatients with adjustment disorder with anxious mood: controlled study versus placebo. *Fundamental and Clinical Pharmacology* 11: 127-132

Bradwejn J, Zhou Y, Koszycki D & Shlik J. (2000). A double-blind, placebo-controlled study on the effects of Gotu Kola (Centella asiatica) on acoustic startle response in healthy subjects. *Journal of Clinical Psychopharmacology* 20: 680-684

Bruner NR & Anderson KG. (2009). Discriminative-stimulus and time-course effects of kava-kava (Piper methysticum) in rats. *Pharmacology Biochemistry & Behavior* 92: 297-303

Calabrese C, Gregory WL, Leo M, Kraemer D, Bone K & Oken B. (2008). Effects of a standardized Bacopa monnieri extract on cognitive performance, anxiety, and depression in the elderly: a randomized, double-blind, placebo-controlled trial. *The Journal of Alternative & Complementary Medicine* 14: 707-713

Carlini EA. (2003). Plants and the central nervous system. *Pharmacology Biochemistry & Behavior* 75: 501-512

Chen SW, Wang WJ, Li WJ, Wang R, Li YL, Huang YN & Liang X. (2006). Anxiolytic-like effect of asiaticoside in mice. *Pharmacology Biochemistry & Behavior* 85: 339-344

Connor KM & Davidson JR. (2002). A placebo-controlled study of Kava kava in generalized anxiety disorder*International Clinical Psychopharmacology* 17: 185-188

Davidson JR. (2001). Pharmacotherapy of generalized anxiety disorder. *Journal of Clinical Psychiatry* 62: 46-50

Davidson JR. (2009). First-line pharmacotherapy approaches for generalized anxiety disorder. *Journal of Clinical Psychiatry* 70: 25-31

Dhawan K, Kumar S & Sharma A. (2001). Anti-anxiety studies on extracts of Passiflora incarnata Linneaus. *Journal of Ethnopharmacology* 78: 165-170

Dhawan K, Kumar S & Sharma A. (2002). Comparative anxiolytic activity profile of various preparations of Passiflora incarnata linneaus: a comment on medicinal plants' standardization. *The Journal of Alternative & Complementary Medicine* 8: 283-291

Diagnostic and Statistical Manual of Mental Disorders. (2000). 4th ed. Text Revision. Washington, DC: American Psychiatric Association 429-430

Dölen G, Osterweil E, Shankaranarayana Rao BS, Smith GB, Auerbach BD Chattarji S & Bear MF. (2007). Correction of fragile X syndrome in mice. Neuron 56:955-962

Donath F, Quispe S, Diefenbach K, Maurer A, Fietze I & Roots I. (2000). Critical evaluation of the effect of valerian extract on sleep structure and sleep quality. *Pharmacopsychiatry* 33: 47-53

Durgesh Kumar A. (2000). Effects of psychological imbalances in cancer patients and its management. *The Antiseptic* 97: 234

Ernst E. (2002). The risk-benefit profile of commonly used herbal therapies: Ginkgo, St. John's Wort, Ginseng, Echinacea, Saw Palmetto, and Kava. *Annals of Internal Medicine* 136: 42-53

Flausino OA, Jr., Zangrossi H, Jr., Salgado JV & Viana MB. (2002). Effects of acute and chronic treatment with Hypericum perforatum L. (LI 160) on different anxiety-related responses in rats. *Pharmacology Biochemistry & Behavior* 71: 251-257

Garcia-Garcia P, Lopez-Munoz F, Rubio G, Martin-Agueda B & Alamo C. (2008). Phytotherapy and psychiatry: bibliometric study of the scientific literature from the last 20 years. *Phytomedicine* 15: 566-576

Garrett KM, Basmadjian G, Khan IA, Schaneberg BT & Seale TW. (2003). Extracts of kava (Piper methysticum) induce acute anxiolytic-like behavioral changes in mice. *Psychopharmacology (Berl)* 170: 33-41

Gastpar M & Klimm HD. (2003). Treatment of anxiety, tension and restlessness states with Kava special extract WS 1490 in general practice: a randomized placebo-controlled double-blind multicenter trial. *Phytomedicine* 10: 631-639

Godkar PB, Gordon RK, Ravindran A & Doctor BP. (2004). Celastrus paniculatus seed water soluble extracts protect against glutamate toxicity in neuronal cultures from rat forebrain. *Journal of Ethnopharmacology* 93: 213-219

Govindarajan A, Shankaranarayana Rao BS, Nair D, Trinh M, Mawjee N, Tonegawa S & Chattarji S. (2006). Transgenic brain-derived neurotrophic factor expression causes both anxiogenic and antidepressant effects. *Proceedings of the National Academy of Sciences (United States of America)* 103: 13208-13213

Gross C & Hen R. (2004). The developmental origins of anxiety. *Nature Reviews Neuroscience* 5: 545-552

Gunnell D, Saperia J & Ashby D. (2005). Selective serotonin reuptake inhibitors (SSRIs) and suicide in adults: meta-analysis of drug company data from placebo controlled, randomised controlled trials submitted to the MHRA's safety review. *British Medical Journal* 330: 385

Hayashi ML, Shankaranarayana Rao BS, Seo JS, Choi HS, Dolan BM, Choi SY, Chattarji S, Tonegawa S. (2007). Inhibition of p21-activated kinase rescues symptoms of fragile X syndrome in mice. Proceedings of National Academy of Sciences (United States of America) 104:11489-11494

Hegde P, Singh K, Chaplot S, Shankaranarayana Rao BS, Chattarji S, Kutty BM & Laxmi TR. (2008). Stress-induced changes in sleep and associated neuronal activity in rat hippocampus and amygdala. *Neuroscience* 153:20-30

Herrera-Arellano A, Jimenez-Ferrer E, Zamilpa A, Morales-Valdez M, Garcia-Valencia CE & Tortoriello J. (2007). Efficacy and tolerability of a standardized herbal product from Galphimia glauca on generalized anxiety disorder. A randomized, double-blind clinical trial controlled with lorazepam. *Planta Medica* 73: 713-717

Holcomb LA, Dhanasekaran M, Hitt AR, Young KA, Riggs M & Manyam BV. (2006). Bacopa monniera extract reduces amyloid levels in PSAPP mice. *Journal of Alzheimer's Disease* 9: 243-251

Holsboer F. (1988). Implications of altered limbic-hypothalamic-pituitary-adrenocortical (LHPA)-function for neurobiology of depression. *Acta Psychiatr Scand Suppl* 341: 72-111

Hu XH, Bull SA, Hunkeler EM, Ming E, Lee JY, Fireman B & Markson LE. (2004). Incidence and duration of side effects and those rated as bothersome with selective serotonin reuptake inhibitor treatment for depression: patient report versus physician estimate. *Journal of Clinical Psychiatry* 65: 959-965

Jana U, Sur TK, Maity LN, Debnath PK & Bhattacharyya D. (2010). A clinical study on the management of generalized anxiety disorder with Centella asiatica. *Nepal Medical College Journal* 12: 8-11

Johnson PB, Abdurahman EM, Tiam EA, bdu-Aguye I & Hussaini IM. (1999). Euphorbia hirta leaf extracts increase urine output and electrolytes in rats. *Journal of Ethnopharmacology* 65: 63-66

Kar Chowdhury P, Parmar D, Kakkar P, Shukla R, Seth PK & Srimal RC. (2002). Anti-stress effect of bacosides of Bacopa monniera: Modulation of Hsp 70 expression, superoxide dismutase and cytochrome P450 activities in rat brain. *Phytotherapy Research* 16: 639-645

Karanth KS, Haridas KK, Gunasundari S & Guruswami MN. (1980). Effect of Celastrus paniculatus on learning process. *Aroyga Journal of Health. Science* 6: 137-139

Kessler RC, Berglund P, Demler O, Jin R, Merikangas KR & Walters EE. (2005). Lifetime prevalence and age-of-onset distributions of DSM-IV disorders in the National Comorbidity Survey Replication. *Archives of General Psychiatry* 62: 593-602

Kienzle-Horn S. (2002). Herbal medicines for neurological diseases. *Current Opinion in Investigational Drugs* 3: 763-767

Kinrys G, Coleman E & Rothstein E. (2009). Natural remedies for anxiety disorders: potential use and clinical applications. *Depression & Anxiety* 26: 259-265

Kulkarni SK & Verma AV. (1993a). GABA receptor mediated anticonvulsant action of Withania somnifera root extract. *Indian Drugs* 30: 305–312

Kulkarni SK & Verma AV. (1993b). Protective effect of BR-16A (Mentat), a herbal preparation on alcohol abstinence-induced anxiety and convulsions. *Indian Journal of Experimental Biology* 31:435-9

Kumar A, Garg R & Prakash AK. (2010). Effect of St. John's Wort (Hypericum perforatum) treatment on restraint stress-induced behavioral and biochemical alteration in mice. *BMC Complementary and Alternative Medicine* 10: 18

Kumar A & Kulkarni SK. (2006). Protective effect of BR-16A, a polyherbal preparation against social isolation stress: possible GABAergic mechanism. *Phytotherapy Research* 20: 538-541

Kumar A & Singh A. (2007). Protective effect of St. John's wort (Hypericum perforatum) extract on 72-hour sleep deprivation-induced anxiety-like behavior and oxidative damage in mice. *Planta Medica* 73: 1358-1364

Kumar MH & Gupta YK. (2002). Antioxidant property of Celastrus paniculatus willd.: a possible mechanism in enhancing cognition. *Phytomedicine* 9: 302-311

Kuppusamy UR & Das NP. (1992). Effects of flavonoids on cyclic AMP phosphodiesterase and lipid mobilization in rat adipocytes. *Biochemical Pharmacology* 44: 1307-1315

Lader M, Tylee A & Donoghue J. (2009). Withdrawing benzodiazepines in primary care. *CNS Drugs* 23: 19-34

Langosch JM, Zhou XY, Heinen M, Kupferschmid S, Chatterjee SS, Noldner M & Walden J. (2002). St John's wort (Hypericum perforatum) modulates evoked potentials in guinea pig hippocampal slices via AMPA and GABA receptors. *European Neuropsychopharmacology* 12: 209-216

Lanhers MC, Fleurentin J, Cabalion P, Rolland A, Dorfman P, Misslin R & Pelt JM. (1990). Behavioral effects of Euphorbia hirta L.: sedative and anxiolytic properties. *Journal of Ethnopharmacology* 29: 189-198

Lanhers MC, Fleurentin J, Dorfman P, Mortier F & Pelt JM. (1991). Analgesic, antipyretic and anti-inflammatory properties of Euphorbia hirta. *Planta Medica* 57: 225-231

Leathwood PD & Chauffard F. (1985). Aqueous extract of valerian reduces latency to fall asleep in man. *Planta Medica* 51: 144–148

Lehrl S. (2004). Clinical efficacy of kava extract WS 1490 in sleep disturbances associated with anxiety disorders. Results of a multicenter, randomized, placebo-controlled, double-blind clinical trial. *The Journal of Affective Disorders* 78: 101-110

Lekha G, Bhagya PK, Shankaranarayana Rao, Arockiasamy I & Mohan K. (2010a). Cognitive enhancement and Neuroprotective effect of Celastrus paniculatus Willd. seed oil (Jyothismati oil) on male Wistar rats. *Journal of Pharmaceutical Science & Technology* 2: 130-138

Lekha G, Mohan K & Arockiasamy I. (2010b). Effect of Celastrus paniculatus seed oil (Jyothismati oil) on acute and chronic immobilisation stress induced in swiss albino mice. *Pharmacognosy Research* 2: 169-174

Malsch U & Kieser M. (2001). Efficacy of kava-kava in the treatment of non-psychotic anxiety, following pretreatment with benzodiazepines. *Psychopharmacology (Berl)* 157: 277-283

McEwen BS. (2000). The neurobiology of stress: from serendipity to clinical relevance. *Brain Research* 886: 172-189

McEwen BS & Stellar E. (1993). Stress and the individual. Mechanisms leading to disease. *Archives of Internal Medicine* 153: 2093-2101

Mehta AK, Binkley P, Gandhi SS & Ticku MK. (1991). Pharmacological effects of Withania somnifera root extract on GABAA receptor complex. *Indian Journal of Medical Research* 94: 312–5

Mishra LC, Singh BB & Dagenais S. (2000). Scientific basis for the therapeutic use of Withania somnifera (ashwagandha): a review. *Alternative Medicine Review* 5: 334-346

Mizoguchi K, Tanaka Y & Tabira T. (2010). Anxiolytic effect of a herbal medicine, yokukansan, in aged rats: involvement of serotonergic and dopaminergic transmissions in the prefrontal cortex. *Journal of Ethnopharmacology* 127: 70-76

Monograph. (2004). Withania somnifera. *Alternative Medicine Review* 9: 211-214

Movafegh A, Alizadeh R, Hajimohamadi F, Esfehani F & Nejatfar M. (2008). Preoperative oral Passiflora incarnata reduces anxiety in ambulatory surgery patients: a double-blind, placebo-controlled study. *Anesthesia & Analgesia* 106: 1728-1732

Muller D, Pfeil T, & von dD V. (2003). Treating depression comorbid with anxiety--results of an open, practice-oriented study with St John's wort WS 5572 and valerian extract in high doses. *Phytomedicine* 10: 25-30

Nalini K, Karanth KS, Rao A, & Aroor AR. (1995). Effects of Celastrus paniculatus on passive avoidance performance and biogenic amine turnover in albino rats. *Journal of Ethnopharmacology* 47: 101-108

Nanjappa KN, Md. Shalam, Harish MS, Prabhu BM, Shankaranarayana Rao BS & Kutty BM. (2007). Pharmacological and neurobiochemical evidence for antidepressant-like effect of Sumind - A herbal product in animals. *The Internet Journal of Nutrition and Wellness* 4: 1. Available from http://www.ispub.com/ostia/index.php?xmlFilePath =journals/ijnw/vol4n1/Sumind .xml.

O'brien CP. (2005). Benzodiazepine use, abuse, and dependence. *Journal of Clinical Psychiatry* 66: 28-33

Onusic GM, Nogueira RL, Pereira AM, Flausino Junior OA & Viana MB. (2003). Effects of chronic treatment with a water-alcohol extract from Erythrina mulungu on anxiety-related responses in rats. *Biological & Pharmaceutical Bulletin* 26: 1538-1542

Park HJ, Kim HY, Yoon KH, Kim KS & Shim I. (2009). The Effects of Astragalus Membranaceus on Repeated Restraint Stress-induced Biochemical and Behavioral Responses. *Korean Journal of Physiology and Pharmacology* 13: 315-319

Pawlak R, Shankaranarayana Rao BS, Melchor JP, Chattarji S, McEwen BS & Strickland S. (2005). Tissue plasminogen activator and plasminogen mediate stress-induced decline of neuronal and cognitive functions in the mouse hippocampus. Proceedings of National Academy of Sciences (United States of America) 102: 18201-18206

Phrompittayarat W, Putalun W, Tanaka H, Jetiyanon K, Wittaya-Areekul S & Ingkaninan K. (2007). Determination of pseudojujubogenin glycosides from Brahmi based on immunoassay using a monoclonal antibody against bacopaside I. *Phytochemical analysis* 18: 411-418

Pittler MH & Ernst E. (2000). Efficacy of kava extract for treating anxiety: systematic review and meta-analysis. *Journal of Clinical Psychopharmacology* 20: 84-89

Pittler MH, & Ernst E. (2002). Kava extract for treating anxiety. *Cochrane Database System Review*: CD003383

Qu XL, Dai Q, Qi YH, Tang YH, Xu DH, Wu ZH & Wang XX. (2008). Effects of Astragalous Injection on oxidative stress status in maintenance hemodialysis patients. *Journal of Chinese Integrative Medicine* 6: 468-472

Rai D, Bhatia G, Palit G, Pal R, Singh S & Singh HK. (2003). Adaptogenic effect of Bacopa monniera (Brahmi). *Pharmacology Biochemistry & Behavior* 75: 823-830

Ramkumar K, Srikumar BN, Shankaranarayana Rao BS & Raju TR. (2008). Self-stimulation rewarding experience restores stress-induced CA3 dendritic atrophy, spatial memory deficits and alterations in the levels of neurotransmitters in the hippocampus. Neurochemical Research 33: 1651-1662

Raupp IM, Sereniki A, Virtuoso S, Ghislandi C, Cavalcanti E Silva EL, Trebien HA, Miguel OG & Andreatini R. (2008). Anxiolytic-like effect of chronic treatment with Erythrina velutina extract in the elevated plus-maze test. *Journal of Ethnopharmacology* 118: 295-299

Roodenrys S, Booth D, Bulzomi S, Phipps A, Micallef C & Smoker J. (2002). Chronic effects of Brahmi (Bacopa monnieri) on human memory. *Neuropsychopharmacology* 27: 279-281

Saeed SA, Bloch RM & Antonacci DJ. (2007). Herbal and dietary supplements for treatment of anxiety disorders. *American Family Physician* 76: 549-556

Sarris J, Kavanagh DJ, Byrne G, Bone KM, Adams J & Deed G. (2009). The Kava Anxiety Depression Spectrum Study (KADSS): a randomized, placebo-controlled crossover trial using an aqueous extract of Piper methysticum. *Psychopharmacology (Berl)* 205: 399-407

Schmidt-Voigt J. (1986). Treatment of nervous sleep disorders and unrest with a sedative of purely vegetable origin [Die Behandlung nervoser schfstorungen und innerer unruhe mit einem rein pflanzlichen sedativum]. *Therapiewoche* 36:663–667

Seely D & Singh R. (2007). Adaptogenic potential of a polyherbal natural health product: report on a longitudinal clinical trial. *Evidence Based Complementary Alternative Medicine* 4: 375-380

Shah LP, Mazumdar K, Nayak PR, Shah Anjali, Shah N & Parker SR. (1990). Clinical Evaluation of Geriforte in Patients of Generalized Anxiety Disorders. *Bombay Hospital Journal* 3: 29

Shah LP, Nayak PR & Anureet Sethi. (1993). A Comparative Study of Geriforte in Anxiety Neurosis and Mixed Anxiety-Depressive Disorders. *Probe* 3: 195-201

Shankar G & Singh HK. (2000). Anxiolytic profile of standardized brahmi extract. *Indian Journal of Pharmacology* 32: 152

Shankaranarayana Rao BS, Madhavi R, Sunanda & Raju TR. (2001). Complete reversal of dendritic atrophy in CA3 neurons of the hippocampus by rehabilitation in restraint stressed rats. *Current Science* 80: 653-659

Shankaranarayana Rao BS & Raju TR. (2004). Neuronal plasticity and brain remodelling. *in* Raju TR, Kutty BM, Sathyaprabha TN & Shankaranarayana Rao BS (ed.), *Brain and*

Behavior. National Institute of Mental Health and Neuro Sciences, Bangalore, India pp. 1-13

Shankaranarayana Rao BS & Raju TR. (2005). Neuronal plasticity in developing and adult nervous system. *in* Thakur MK & Prasad S (ed.), *Molecular & Cellular Neurobiology,* Narosa Publishing House Pvt. Ltd, New Delhi, India pp. 3-17

Shankaranarayana Rao BS & Raju TR. (2007). Neuronal plasticity and biological basis of rehabilitation., *in* Prabhakar S & Taly AB (ed.), *Reviews in Neurology,* Indian Academy of Neurology, India pp. 210-249

Shankaranarayana Rao BS. (2009). Cellular and molecular basis of stress-induced cognitive deficits: implications for treating neurological and psychiatric disorders. *in Proceedings of Continuing Education Programme on Oxidative Stress in Health & Disease,* Defence Institute of Physiology and Allied Sciences, Delhi, India. 2009: pp. 11-15

Shankaranarayana Rao BS. (2010). Recent trends in understanding brain plasticity. *in* Md Basha Mohidden, Gaythrammma K & Ponnamma SU (ed.). *Proceedings of the Transdisciplinary National Conference on Recent trends in Biomedical Research.* Presidency College, Bangalore, India. pp 8-29

Sharma AK, Agrawal A, Agrawal U & Dubey GP. (1990). Influence of mentat on memory and mental fatigue in cases of anxiety neurosis and depression. *Indian. Journal of Cancer & Biology Research* 3: 27-30

Singewald N, Sinner C, Hetzenauer A, Sartori SB & Murck H. (2004). Magnesium-deficient diet alters depression- and anxiety-related behavior in mice--influence of desipramine and Hypericum perforatum extract. *Neuropharmacology* 47: 1189-1197

Singh HK, Shanker G & Patnaik GK: (1996). Neuropharmacological and anti-stress effects of bacosides: A memory enhancer. *Indian Journal of Pharmacology* 28: 47

Singh HK & Dhawan BN. (1997). Neuropsychopharmacological effects of the Ayurvedic nootropic Bacopa Monniera Linn. (Brahmi). *Indian Journal of Pharmacology* 29: 359–365

Singh RH, Singh L & Sen SP. (1979). Studies on the anti-anxiety effect of the Medhya Rasayana drug Bahmi (Bacopa monniera Linn) - Part II (experimental studies). *Journal of Research in Indian Medicine of Yoga & Homeopathy.* 14: 1-6

Singh RH & Singh L. (1980). Studies on the anti-anxiety effect of the Medhya Rasayana drug Brahmi (Bacopa monniera Wettst) - Part I. *Journal of Research in Ayurveda & Siddha* 1: 133-148

Somers JM, Goldner EM, Waraich P & Hsu L. (2006). Prevalence and incidence studies of anxiety disorders: a systematic review of the literature. *Canadian Journal of Psychiatry* 51: 100-113

Sparreboom A, Cox MC, Acharya MR & Figg WD. (2004). Herbal remedies in the United States: potential adverse interactions with anticancer agents. *Journal of Clinical Oncology* 22: 2489-2503

Srikumar BN, Raju TR & Shankaranarayana Rao BS. (2006). The involvement of cholinergic and noradrenergic systems in behavioral recovery following oxotremorine treatment to chronically stressed rats. *Neuroscience* 143: 679-688

Srikumar BN, Raju TR, & Shankaranarayana Rao BS. (2007). Contrasting effects of bromocriptine on learning of a partially baited radial arm maze task in the presence and absence of restraint stress. *Psychopharmacology (Berl)* 193: 363-374

Veena J, Shankaranarayana Rao BS & Srikumar BN. (2011). Regulation of adult neurogenesis in the hippocampus by stress, acetylcholine and dopamine. *Journal of Natural Science, Biology & Medicine*. 2:26-37

Stahl SM. (1998). *Essential psychopharmacology*. New Delhi Cambridge University Press

Stevinson C & Ernst E. (2000). Valerian for insomnia: a systematic review of randomized clinical trials. *Sleep Medicine* 1: 91-99

Stough C, Lloyd J, Clarke J, Downey LA, Hutchison CW, Rodgers T & Nathan PJ. (2001). The chronic effects of an extract of Bacopa monniera (Brahmi) on cognitive function in healthy human subjects. *Psychopharmacology (Berl)* 156: 481-484

Sunanda, Shankaranarayana Rao BS & Raju TR. (2000a). Chronic restraint stress impairs acquisition and retention of spatial memory task in rats. *Current Science* 79: 1581-1584

Sunanda, Shankaranarayana Rao BS & Raju TR. (2000b). Restraint stress- induced alterations in the levels of biogenic amines, aminoacids and AChE activity in the hippocampus. Neurochemical Research 25: 1547-1552

Upadhyaya L, Tiwari AK., Agrawal A & Dubey GP. (1990). Role of an indigenous drug geriforte on blood levels of biogenic amines and its significance in the treatment of anxiety neurosis. *Activ. Nerv. Super., Czechoslovakia* 32: 1

Veena J, Srikumar BN, Mahati K, Bhagya V, Raju TR & Shankaranarayana Rao BS. (2009a). Enriched environment restores hippocampal cell proliferation and ameliorates cognitive deficits in chronically stressed rats. *Journal of Neuroscience Research* 87: 831-843

Veena J, Srikumar BN, Raju TR & Shankaranarayana Rao BS. (2009b). Exposure to enriched environment restores the survival and differentiation of new born cells in the hippocampus and ameliorates depressive symptoms in chronically stressed rats. *Neuroscience Letters* 455: 178-182

Veena J, Shankaranarayana Rao BS & Srikumar BN. (2011). Regulation of adult neurogenesis in the hippocampus by stress, acetylcholine and dopamine. *Journal of Natural Science, Biology & Medicine*. 2:26-37

Veena J, Srikumar BN, Mahati K, Raju TR & Shankaranarayana Rao BS. (2011). Oxotremorine treatment restores hippocampal neurogenesis and ameliorates depression-like behavior in chronically stressed rats. *Psychopharmacology* DOI 10.1007/s00213-011-2279-3 *In Press.*

Volz HP & Kieser M. (1997). Kava-kava extract WS 1490 versus placebo in anxiety disorders--a randomized placebo-controlled 25-week outpatient trial. *Pharmacopsychiatry* 30: 1-5

Volz HP, Murck H, Kasper S & Moller HJ. (2002). St John's wort extract (LI 160) in somatoform disorders: results of a placebo-controlled trial. *Psychopharmacology (Berl)* 164: 294-300

Vorbach EU, Gortelmeyer R & Bruning J. (1996). Therapy of insomnia. The efficacy and tolerability of valerian [Therapie von Insomnien. Wirksamkeit und Vertraglichkeit eines Baldrianpraparats]. *Psychopharmakotherapie* 3: 109–15

Vyas A, Mitra R, Shankaranarayana Rao BS & Chattarji S. (2002). Chronic stress induces contrasting patterns of dendritic remodeling in hippocampal and amygdaloid neurons. *Journal of Neuroscience* 22: 6810-6818

Walesiuk A, Nazaruk J & Braszko JJ. (2010). Pro-cognitive effects of Cirsium rivulare extracts in rats. *Journal of Ethnopharmacology* 129: 261-266

Ward CP, Redd K, Williams BM, Caler JR, Luo Y & McCoy JG. (2002). Ginkgo biloba extract: cognitive enhancer or antistress buffer. *Pharmacology Biochemistry & Behavior* 72: 913-922

Watkins LL, Connor KM & Davidson JR. (2001). Effect of kava extract on vagal cardiac control in generalized anxiety disorder: preliminary findings. *Journal of Psychopharmacology* 15: 283-286

Weinberger DR. (2001). Anxiety at the frontier of molecular medicine. *New England Journal of Medicine* 344: 1247-1249

Wijeweera P, Arnason JT, Koszycki D & Merali Z. (2006). Evaluation of anxiolytic properties of Gotukola--(Centella asiatica) extracts and asiaticoside in rat behavioral models. *Phytomedicine* 13: 668-676

Woelk H, Arnoldt KH, Kieser M & Hoerr R. (2007). Ginkgo biloba special extract EGb 761 in generalized anxiety disorder and adjustment disorder with anxious mood: a randomized, double-blind, placebo-controlled trial. *Journal of Psychiatric Research* 41: 472-480

Wonnemann M, Singer A & Muller WE. (2000). Inhibition of synaptosomal uptake of 3H-L-glutamate and 3H-GABA by hyperforin, a major constituent of St. John's Wort: the role of amiloride sensitive sodium conductive pathways. *Neuropsychopharmacology* 23: 188-197

World Health Organization. (2001). *Composite International Diagnostic Interview (CIDI) 2.1.* Geneva, Switzerland, WHO

Ziegler G, Ploch M, Miettinen-Baumann A & Collet W. (2002). Efficacy and tolerability of valerian extract LI 156 compared with oxazepamin the treatment of non-organic insomnia, a randomized double blind comparative clinical study. *European Journal of Medical Research* 7: 480–6

16

A Context-Aware System for Anxiety Disorders

Theodor Panagiotakopoulos[1], Maria-Anna Fengou[1],
Panagiotis Malliaris[2] and Dimitrios Lymberopoulos[1]
[1]*Wire Communication Laboratory, Electrical & Computer Engineering Department, University of Patras, GR 265 04 Panepistimioupoli – Rion*
[2]*Psychiatric Department of the General University Hospital of Patras, Greece*

1. Introduction

Recent advances in ICT technologies have led to a new generation of systems and services with potentials to play very important role in the healthcare domain. Ubiquitous technologies and context-aware computing have drawn huge attention as they enable the delivery of personalized healthcare services at any time and any place. Context-awareness is a concept first described around the early 90s along with the introduction of ubiquitous computing (Weiser, 1991). It has emerged as the key concept in order to realize ubiquitous applications, encompassing several ICT technologies and supporting seamless integration of activities between communicating entities. The term context-awareness has received many definitions, which do not meet a consensus among researchers. It is a rather general concept that refers to the capability of a system to be aware of its physical and logical environment (i.e. its context) and to intelligently react according to this awareness (Dey & Abowd, 1999).
Along with the introduction of these technologies in healthcare, the clinical practices are changing too, requiring healthcare professionals to collaborate across disciplines and organizational boundaries. Contemporary health systems provide a more protective (proactive self-care), reachable (i.e. at home, at work, while travelling abroad) and high-quality health advice and assistance. Modern healthcare services are available around the clock, seven days a week and systems with ubiquitous access are becoming indispensable. During the last decade ubiquitous technologies and context-awareness facilitated the design and development of many prototype systems and applications in the healthcare domain, addressing, among others, dementia (Bharucha, 2006), diabetes (Pentland, 2004), Parkinson (Sung et al., 2005) and physical fitness (Buttussi & Chittaro, 2008). Little effort has so far been put into the investigation of context-awareness as the enabling technology for assisting the treatment of anxiety disorders.
Anxiety disorders are a group of major psychiatric disorders, characterized by disproportional anxiety, compared with the stimulus which provoked the anxiety response. Anxiety is a natural physiological reaction that helps individuals to cope with situations that require increased level of performance (e.g. during exams). But, when anxiety becomes disproportionately excessive to the provoking stimulus and persistent, even in the absence

of the corresponding stimulus, it can lead to specific anxiety disorders. They include several stress - related disorders, such as panic disorder with or without agoraphobia; agoraphobia with or without panic disorder; specific phobias, social phobia, posttraumatic stress disorders and acute stress disorders, among others. Anxiety disorders are associated with significant morbidity and are often chronic and resistant to treatment (Merikangas & Swanson, 2010). Their impact is huge both in personal level (e.g. low self-esteem and isolation) and social level (e.g. family problems and low productivity).

The chronic aspect of these disorders, as well as the high possibility of recurrence, indicate the need of a persistent monitoring of patients suffering from anxiety disorders. For instance, panic disorder has a high rate of recurrences, the presentation of which is a significant factor in the treatment decision's procedure (Kessler et al., 2010) In addition, high stress level is not always worrying since many situations of increased stress are normal (e.g. professional meetings). All these suggest that patients suffering from anxiety disorders should be continuously monitored for disorders' progress assessment, treatment evaluation and adjustment, stress level assessment and provision of proper medical assistance.

From a technological perspective, anxiety disorders' treatment has been mainly addressed through teleconference (Himle et al., 2006) and virtual reality (Parsons & Rizzo, 2008; Wood et al., 2008), while other solutions include e-mail support (Andersson, 2009) and internet-based treatment (Shandley et al., 2008). Teleconference is mainly used when patients are not able or willing to visit the medical expert at his physical space. It saves patients from transportation costs and time but it provides only subjective data as these are given by the patient during the teleconference sessions. On the other hand, virtual reality approaches require co-existence of patients and medical experts at the same physical space, providing objective data for the patients' medical condition. Virtual reality is mainly used for exposure-based therapies and aims at creating virtual environmental settings where the patients' attitude is monitored.

Nevertheless, the aforementioned technological approaches are not used as means for persistent monitoring that anxiety disorders require. Towards this direction, we propose a context-aware tele-monitoring system, for patients diagnosed with anxiety disorders, which will provide persistent health monitoring services and additional support to therapists for decision making, assessment of treatment efficiency and treatment personalization to the needs of the individual. Since this system is not yet fully integrated, and therefore evaluated, its design is hypothetical. The main target of the proposed system is the provision of a comfortable and safe environment, for daily living and mobility of patients diagnosed with anxiety disorders. This is achieved through: (a) health tele-monitoring services for continuous assessment of patient condition and provision of feedback to authorized persons, and (b) self-help services assisting patients to identify and change the harmful and unhelpful attitudes that strengthen their disorders.

2. Context-aware computing in healthcare

Context-awareness in healthcare implies the capability of a system to adapt to changes in its environment and patient preferences in order to deliver personalized health-related services. The most fundamental contextual elements for medical context-aware systems are the physiological parameters, based on which the patient's medical condition is assessed. The values of several contextual parameters (e.g. location) are further collected and the overall patient's context is obtained. The final step is the service provision and personalization according to the identified context and the patient's needs and preferences. Thus, in general terms, context is mainly used to achieve two goals: a) medical condition assessment and b) personalized healthcare services provision.

The first context-aware systems in healthcare are tracked in the beginning of the 2000-2010 decade focusing on professional work settings. Their target is to assist the daily tasks of the medical staff through seamless ICT services, supporting their direct and uninterrupted communication, as well as immediate access to medical data regardless of location and time. Characteristic examples of such systems include the *Qos Dream* platform (Mitchel et al., 2000), the *"Hospital of the Future"* prototype (Bardram, 2004) and the *MobileWard* prototype (Kjeldskov & Skov, 2007). The Qos Dream platform provides seamless context-sensitive communications, through strategically placed terminals at the emergency department of the Royal London Hospital, which can adapt to the user's location. When a video call is requested by one clinician, the individual being called is located through appropriate tracking technologies and this call is put through to the terminal closest to him. The *"Hospital of the Future"* prototype includes a context-aware bed, a context-aware pill container and a context-aware Electronic Patient Record (EPR). The bed is able to identify who and what lies in its proximity displaying relevant medical information according to this context. The *MobileWard* prototype supports the daily morning procedure tasks of nurses providing patient lists and patient-related information based on their location and the time of the day.

Apart from the systems focusing in professional work environments, there have been developed several context-aware solutions for home-based healthcare provision. The context-aware systems focusing on providing healthcare services at home, aim at keeping patients' autonomy, improving their quality of life and at the creation of a safe environment where patients are constantly monitored for abnormal situations, while being able to perform their daily activities. For example, in the context of the *INHOME* project (Korhonen et al., 2003), several technologies were developed for the management of the domestic environment and the enhancement of security and autonomy of elders living at their homes. Furthermore, the *House_n* project (Intille et al., 2004) deployed a proactive context-aware medical system that uses wearable biometric sensors and cameras, aiming at identifying potential symptoms of congestive heart failures. If the system identifies any abnormal symptoms (e.g. weight changes), it produces alerts and suggests interventions for minimizing the risk of a congestive heart failure occurrence.

A different category of context-aware systems in healthcare consists of the so called wearable systems. These systems provide persistent monitoring and healthcare service provision to patients while ensuring their mobility and independence. One of the major systems developed in this application area is the wearable system *MIThril* (Pentland, 2004) that offers the capability of collecting and processing real-time data provided by various sources, such as biosensors, accelerometers and Global Positioning System (GPS). These data are used to assess the patients' medical condition based on which the system either delivers feedback and notifications to the patients or to other authorized people. Similarly, the wearable system *LiveNet* (Sung et al., 2005) is able to continuously monitor a wide range of physiological signals, through various wearable biosensors, together with the user's activity and context, developing a personalized, data-rich health profile of a patient over time. This profile is used to provide objective information to patients so as to promote better behavior, as well as to medical staff in order to evaluate the treatment progress. The *LiveNet* system is designed to support the monitoring of several disorders, such as epilepsy and depression.

3. Context-awareness and anxiety disorders

While context-awareness has been barely used in anxiety disorders, several factors indicate that its implementation has the potentials to offer an integrated and effective technological solution for the support of their treatment. The most important factor is that situations that provoke anxiety highly depend on specific attributes, such as location, noise, temperature, visibility, activity and time. These attributes form the context of a patient and determine the environmental situation a patient finds himself in. In addition, these attributes (i.e. the patient's context) strongly affect the way anxiety is expressed, kind of presented symptoms and their tension and the duration of critical episodes. For this reason, we propose the use of context-awareness for the inference of various attributes related to anxiety disorders and their treatment support.

A common feature of the majority of the disorders being addressed by context-aware systems is that context itself does not affect any of their basic attributes, such as manifestation triggers and symptoms. It is simply used to assess the patients' medical status and determine the appropriate actions to be performed in case of an emergency. On the contrary, when it comes for anxiety disorders, the patient's context plays a very important role in a number of attributes directly related to these disorders, as mentioned above. The following example will illustrate this difference between anxiety and some other disorders. Let's consider the following context: "Peter is at a bar with friends on Sunday". If Peter suffers from diabetes, his location, or the day do not play any role in a potential critical episode. On the other hand, these contextual parameters may be strongly related with a critical episode if Peter suffers from anxiety disorders. For example, when Peter finds himself in a crowded place like a bar he may feel overstressed. Due to the above, the acquisition of semantically enriched contexts is required in order to create a rich knowledge base regarding stress-provoking situations, symptoms occurrence and other stress-related attributes.

Moreover, anxiety disorders have a really dynamic nature and require persistent and long-term monitoring in order to verify several attributes, such as symptoms and stress-provoking situations. For example, Generalized Anxiety Disorder (GAD) diagnostic criteria require persistent specific anxiety symptoms for at least 6 months while some disorders occur along with other mental or physical disorders (Brawman-Mintzer et al., 2007). This means that a collection and analysis of a series of contexts should be performed, aiming to provide efficient objective data to expertized medical staff in order to make a diagnosis and then establish, direct and adjust (if necessary) the offered treatment accordingly. To achieve this, two things are needed: a storage mechanism where the identified contexts will be kept and appropriate algorithms for their processing.

In summary, anxiety disorders raise two fundamental research and technological challenges in the implementation of context-awareness. First, the acquisition of semantically enriched contexts that will describe with the highest possible expressivity the situation a patient is or was. Second, the integration of a mechanism that will store and process the acquired patient contexts. One approach that addresses both challenges is the use of user profiles, which will actively participate in the context reasoning process and then store the acquired contexts for future process and analysis. Structure and content of these profiles is discussed in detail in Section 5.

3.1 Context information

Similarly to context-awareness, the term context has received numerous definitions that are most likely tailored to the specific research needs for which context is used. According to the

most cited definition that provides an abstract view of this term, context is "any information that can be used to characterize the situation of entities (i.e. a person, a place or an object) that are considered relevant to the interaction between a user and an application, including the user and the application themselves. Context is typically the location, identity and state of people, groups and computational and physical objects" (Dey & Abowd, 1999).
One of the initial steps while designing context-aware systems is to identify the context parameters to be monitored. Concerning anxiety disorders, we consider six primary categories of the patient's context, as illustrated in Fig. 1.

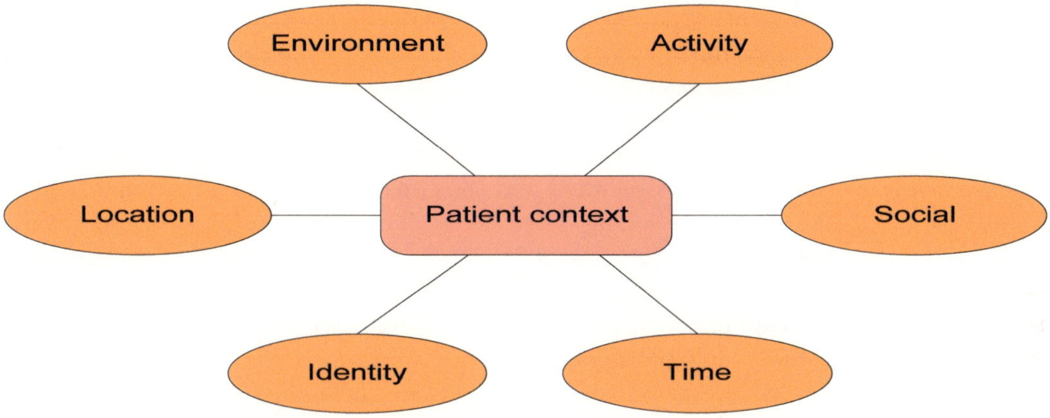

Fig. 1. Context information for anxiety disorders

Location context captures the current location of a patient and correlates it (if possible) with a social arena (e.g. home, office, etc.). Specific locations may cause increased stress (e.g. office) while others may be more relaxing (e.g. home).
Environment context refers to physical conditions such as humidity, noise and luminance. These conditions are strongly related with stress as increased noise, temperature and luminance may result to increased stress.
Activity context describes the current task the patient performs. A sub-context of activity could be the patient's role in the performed task. Some activities may be highly relaxing (e.g. hobbies), while others may be overstressing (e.g. social activities).
Social context provides information regarding the people interacting with the patient in a given patient context. These people have a strong influence in stress as the presence of family members and friends give the patient a feeling of safety making him less vulnerable to critical episodes.
Time context captures the day of the week and the time of the day. Time is highly correlated with stress, as specific points in time and/or specific days of the week may be associated with increased (e.g. morning hours) or decreased stress.
Identity context consists of three sub-contexts: personal context, stress context and symptoms context. Personal context contains the demographic data of the patient, while stress and symptoms context keep track of the patient's stress level and symptoms respectively.
Identity context is used to assess the patient's medical condition, as well as the way stress is expressed (through symptoms). All the other contexts are exploited for the creation of a rich knowledge base (i.e. patient profiles) that will associate context parameters with several

disorder-related attributes. This knowledge will be used for the provision of self-help services to the patients (e.g. suggestions for improving their lifestyle) and several treatment supportive services to medical staff (e.g. stress-provoking situations pattern detection service (Panagiotakopoulos et al., 2010a)).

3.2 Context modeling

Context modeling is a key feature in context-aware systems in order to describe context information in a semantic level and obtain an interoperable representation of diverse data coming from heterogeneous sources. It provides context in a structured form for the development of intelligent services, where information is situation dependent. The fundamental role of context modeling is to describe the relationship between the vocabulary and the concept of knowledge in a domain.

Ontologies are widely used in ubiquitous computing environments and context-aware systems for the representation of context information. They provide a uniform representation of context data, a structured and semantically rich way to model a domain and enable rule-based context reasoning. They also facilitate knowledge reuse and sharing among system components and count classes, inheritance, relationships between classes and instances as some of their major components. Due to the above, we developed an ontology-based context model written in OWL (Ontology Web Language), which shows an increased expressivity against other ontology languages.

Based on the context classification illustrated in Fig.1, we considered the Patient Ontology, which is comprised of the following parts:

- Person Ontology: it describes information of the personal context of the patient.
- Medical Condition Ontology: it contains the values of the physiological parameters measured by biosensors that determine the stress level of the patient (an excerpt of the Medical Condition ontology is illustrated in Fig.2).
- Symptoms Ontology: It describes the symptoms of a patient in defined stress levels.
- Environmental Ontology: it represents information regarding time, location, activity, physical conditions and people interacting with the patient.
- Social Ontology: Represents the members of the care provision chain as well as their context information (e.g. availability).

4. System architecture

From the architectural point of view the proposed system (Fig. 3) will be composed by three main parts, the Body Area Network (BAN), the Health Care Center (HCC) and the Network of Third Authorized People (NTAP). Each part is described in detail in the following subsections.

4.1 Body Area Network (BAN)

The BAN is located at the patient's body and includes the following components:

- Bio-sensors acquiring essential implicit information concerning the patient's medical situation,
- sensors acquiring essential context data,
- a gateway.

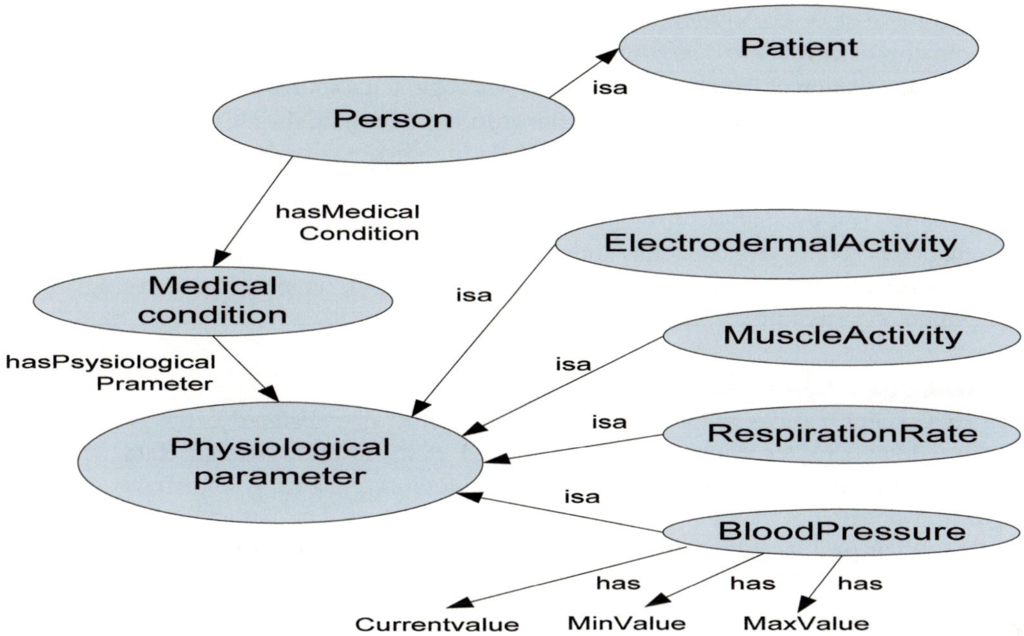

Fig. 2. An excerpt of the Medical Condition Ontology

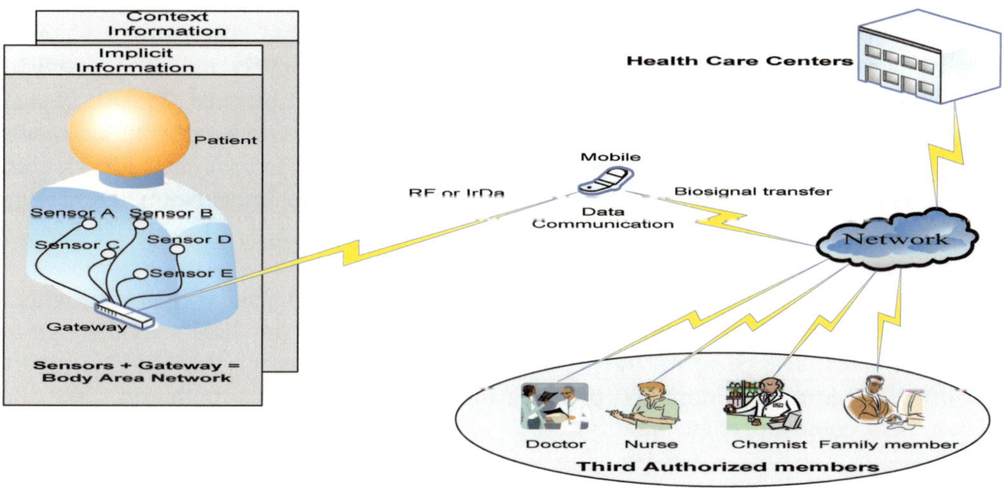

Fig. 3. Overall System Architecture

The gateway is the core element of the proposed system and can be implemented on a personal digital assistant (PDA), cell phone, or home personal computer. It controls the sensor network handling the sensor registration (type and number of sensors), initialization (e.g., specify sampling frequency and mode of operation), customization (e.g., run user specific calibration or user-specific signal processing procedure upload) as well as the dynamical configuration of the sensor network according to the service's needs. It also has the responsibility to communicate the acquired information to the HCC, as well as the actions that must be fulfilled by the system, so that the delivered service adapts to the context and the requirements of the patient. The BAN's gateway encapsulates a variety of processes, such as:

- data acquisition of the above mentioned heterogeneous sources,
- local storing and communicating of the acquired data with the HCC,
- local evaluation of the acquired data and deduction of the patient's medical condition in case of interruption of the communication connection,
- patients' self-evaluation through a proper GUI (Graphical Unit Interface), as well as channelling of advices or commands from the HCC, and
- determination of a group of events (within the BAN), which occurrence indicates the patient's current medical condition.

4.2 Health Care Center (HCC)

The HCC keeps the Electronic Medical Records (EMR) of registered users as well as their profiles. User profiles contain gateway related data, location related data, application specific data, user preferences, physician preferences, alerting thresholds of values regarding physiological data, user specific data and so on. The patient does not have any access to their profiles while the authorized physicians have full access and the opportunity to check the context history of the patients, forward new instructions to the patients (e.g. prescribed exercises) and alter the thresholds of the measured values that indicate some kind of anomaly. Patients interact with their profiles in an indirect manner, initially discussing with the respective physician, reaching to an agreement for the changes to be performed and authorizing the physician to make these changes.

Furthermore, the HCC performs a group of functions based on the information provided by the BAN's gateway (e.g. context information) and the patients' user profiles. More specifically, the functions performed at the HCC include context modeling, context reasoning and continuous patients' medical condition assessment (normal state, increased stress state, emergency state, etc.). Moreover, it offers medical decision support mechanisms that process context and profile information in a proactive manner, to provide feedback both to patients and medical experts. Based on context and profile information, HCC also provides medical decision support mechanisms that facilitate reactive healthcare service execution in case of emergencies.

Finally, the Network of Third Authorized People (NTAP) is established at the HCC, where patients and medical staff collaborate to determine its members (medical staff belongs to NTAP as well). HCC also performs the process of selecting the appropriate NTAP members to be notified, based on the identified patient's medical condition, his preferences and the NTAP members' context (e.g. availability).

4.3 Network of Third Authorized People (NTAP)

The NTAP consists of several groups of people that form a caregiving support network providing both medical and social assistance. A single NTAP is established for each patient. This network includes an additional group of people (e.g. relatives) apart from expertized medical staff and paramedicals. These people are authorized to participate in the patient's treatment process and are requested to play a specific and well-defined role according to the identified patient's medical condition and the treatment guidelines set by the expertized medical staff (Panagiotakopoulos, 2010b). Potential members include relatives, close friends, co-workers and volunteers. Their role, training, capabilities, way of engagement and context information is described in their user profiles, parts of which are integrated in the patient's profile.

5. Context-aware framework

This section presents the context-aware framework architecture that we have developed to offer the required functionality for the implementation of context-aware healthcare services for patients suffering from anxiety disorders. Furthermore, it provides further insight to some core functions of this framework, such as context processing, user profile structuring and event-based notification of NTAP members.

5.1 Framework architecture

The proposed framework architecture is depicted in Fig.4. The framework is deployed at the patient's side, the HCC's side and the NTAP's side, consisting of several modules and components described in detail in the following sub sections.

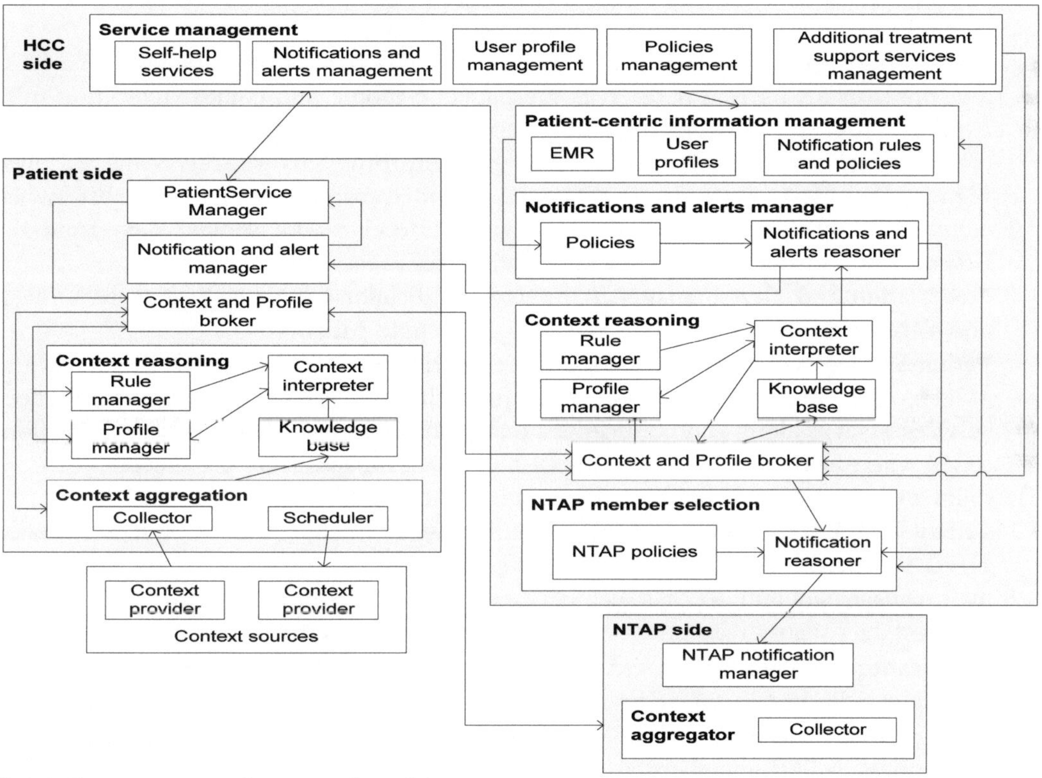

Fig. 4. Context-aware framework architecture

The patient's side includes the following modules and components implemented in the BAN's gateway:

- **Context aggregation.** It consists of two components, the *Collector* and the *Scheduler*. The *Collector* gathers all the context data from the context providers, pre-processes the collected data creating low level contexts and reasons about the redundant and the useful data. The *Scheduler* allocates corresponding timers and pointers triggering data acquisition.

- **Context reasoning.** It consists of four components, the *Rule manager*, the *Profile manager*, the *Knowledge base* and the *Context interpreter*. The *Rule manager* is responsible of maintaining and updating subscribed rules and transforming them into rules that can be handled by the *Context interpreter*. The *Profile manager* downloads, stores and keeps the patient's user profile updated, in order to deliver it to the *Context interpreter*. The *Knowledge base* contains the ontology context models and instances, which are stored in a local database Based on ontology context instances, rules and profile information, the *Context interpreter* provides the high level contexts interpreting the low level ones that come from the context aggregation module and assesses the patient's medical condition, through rule-based reasoning techniques.
  It has to be mentioned that this module is activated only when communication with HCC is unavailable and processes locally the collected context information. In this case, the reasoned high level contexts are then transmitted back to the *Profile manager* that sends them to the HCC (through the patient's *context and profile broker*) when the communication is re-established for archiving purposes.
- **Context and profile broker.** It essentially comprises the mediator between the HCC and the BAN's gateway. It receives the patient's profile and context reasoning rules from the HCC and provides them to the context reasoning module, while periodically checking their consistency. In case of connectivity problems it receives the reasoned high level contexts from the *Profile manager* and transmits them to the HCC when communication is re-established. Otherwise, it receives the context data from the *Collector* and transmits them to the HCC for further processing.
- **Notification and alert manager.** It receives notifications (e.g. medication reminders) and alerts originated by the HCC and delivers them to patients.
- **PatientService manager.** This component comprises the interface between patient and system. The patient may access and request the delivery of several patient-centric services, such as alerts and notifications management and self-help services. It includes a GUI where alerts, notifications and self-help services content are presented.

The following modules and components are part of the HCC's side:

- **Patient-centric information management.** It stores the patient's EMR and user profile, NTAP's members' user profiles, as well as several policies regarding the notification and alert management and NTAP's members' selection process. It also has the responsibility to collect the patients' reasoned contexts and store them for further processing.
- **Notifications and alerts manager.** Based on the identified patient's context, his inferred medical condition and specific policies, it determines potential notifications and alerts to be pushed to patients, as well as to NTAP's members. It also initially defines the appropriate NTAP members that have to be notified and requests their context information through the HCC's context and profile broker.
- **Context and profile broker.** This module communicates both with the BAN's gateway and the NTAP. Concerning the patient's side, it provides user profile instances as well as context-related information (e.g. context reasoning rules, context acquisition scheduling etc.) to the BAN's gateway, while it constantly (unless communication is broken) receives the collected context data. Regarding the NTAP it requests the

collection of specific NTAP members' context data through the HCC's *context and profile broker*, which provides them to the NTAP member selection module.

- **Context reasoning.** It performs exactly the same actions with the respective module located at the BAN's gateway. It receives the context data from the HCC's *context and profile broker* and provides the reasoned contexts back to it, in order to be archived in the patient's user profile and used by other modules and components that lie at the HCC. It also provides the reasoned contexts to the *notifications and alerts reasoner* for the determination of the actions that have to be performed according to the identified high level context.
- **NTAP member selection.** Based on information provided by the *notification and alert reasoner*, the identified NTAP members' context information, and NTAP-related policies, it determines the appropriate member to be notified when assistive healthcare actions are required.
- **Service management.** It hosts the service logic of the context-aware healthcare services, including patient-centric services (e.g. self-help services) and medical staff-centric services (e.g. user profile management and policies management).

Finally, the NTAP's side includes the:

- **Context aggregation module.** It is responsible for collecting the requested context information of the initially identified NTAP members and providing them to the HCC's *context and profile broker*.
- **NTAP notification manager.** It sends notifications to the selected NTAP members, along with information concerning the specific actions they have to perform.

The developed context-aware framework addresses the two challenges that anxiety disorders raise in the implementation of context-aware computing, as mentioned in Section 3. The context reasoning module actively engages user profiles in the context interpretation process aiming at producing semantically enhanced high level contexts. In addition, the patients' reasoned contexts (including his medical condition while being at this context) are always archived in their respective user profiles. The archived contextual information is further processed through various data mining algorithms for the delivery of additional personalized treatment supportive services to medical staff. The kind of these services along with the potential algorithms for their implementation are out of scope of this study and are comprehensively presented in (Panagiotakopoulos et al., 2010a).

5.2 User profiling

Each patient has an individual user profile (patient profile), which contains information organized in distinct sections. The patient profiles are used as data storage mechanisms and as means of providing personalized healthcare services. They consist of various types of information summarized in the following list:

- Demographic data
- Medical history
- Disorder-related data (e.g. guidelines for providing medical care and conditions that cause reduced/increased levels of stress)
- Context-related information (e.g. normal and abnormal values of measured physiological parameters, social arenas and scheduled activities)
- NTAP-related data (e.g. list of persons, contact numbers and roles)

- Preferences (e.g. hierarchies of notifications and alerts priorities in a NTAP group basis and service-related preferences)

Some of that information stored in the patient profile is quite static while other is rather dynamic as a user moves from place to place interacting with diverse entities. Personal information (i.e. demographic data and preferences) and medical history are predominantly static and defined at the patient profile creation. This information can be considered permanent in the sense that it does not change so often, and its attributes are not affected by external factors. The other types of information are highly dynamic, changing according to the patient's context and treatment needs.

Similarly, each NTAP member has an individual user profile (NTAP member profile) that contains the following types of information:

- Personal information (e.g. status and role)
- Preferences (e.g. visual or sound alerts and notifications)
- Context-related information (e.g. location and availability)
- Device capabilities

For the provision of timely-critical and accurate healthcare services, NTAP members need access to information hosted by patient profiles. However, patient profiles contain sensitive information which patients do not want to be accessible by everyone and especially by the people they do not know (e.g. volunteers). This leads to the need for degraded access to patient profiles. Therefore, NTAP members (e.g. paramedical staff) should have access only to those parts of the patient profile that provide the necessary information for the fulfilment of their role in the treatment process. For example, when a volunteer is called to provide his services, there is no need to access the patient's preferences or the complete list of his demographic data, but has to receive knowledge upon disorder-related data and context-related information. Fig. 5 depicts the parts of the patient profile that each NTAP group has access to.

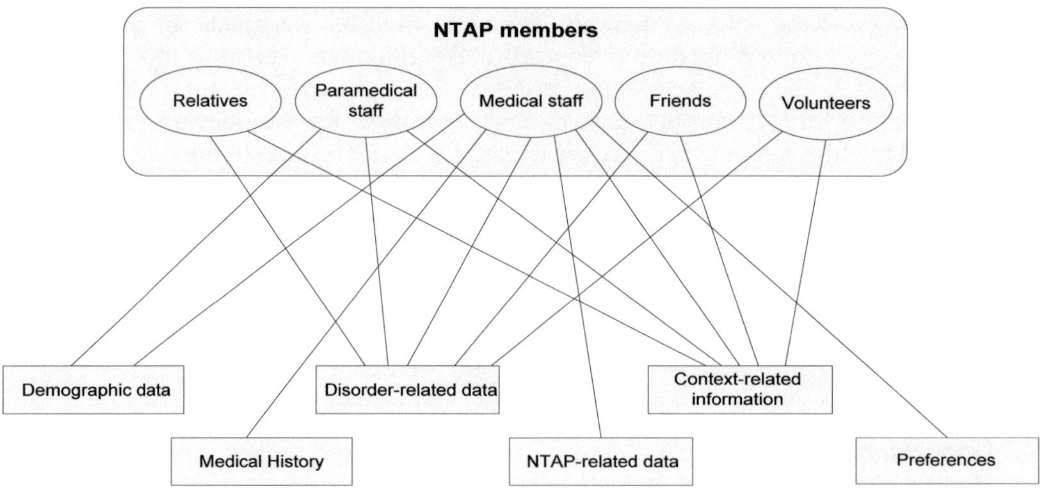

Fig. 5. Degradation of access rights to the patient profile for the NTAP members

5.3 Context reasoning

The context reasoning process converts sensor readings to meaningful context information. Sensor readings are considered to be low level contexts, which on their own do not provide

rich information on a semantic level. The processing of low level contexts by using the context ontology instances, several inferential rules and user profile information, produces the high level contexts. For instance, the values of physiological parameters, such as blood pressure, are considered low level contexts, while an alert of "critical medical condition" that may be deduced from the processing of these physiological parameters consists a high level context.
The proposed system addresses the need of high level contexts acquisition through a rule-based approach performed by the "Context reasoning" module (see Fig. 4). Several user-defined rules are used to reason about the patients' medical condition, as well as the notifications and alerts that have to be triggered. Regarding the medical condition assessment, rule-based reasoning over the "Medical Condition Ontology" instances is performed. Due to the fact that the patients' medical condition is tightly connected to the stress level they might present, we used a four valued scale to represent their medical condition through their stress level: low, medium, high and very high. For example, the following rule shows that if the heart rate frequency is higher than 50% and blood pressure is higher than 40% of their respective average values then the stress level is "very high":

$$\mathit{IF}\ \left\{\begin{array}{l}\text{HeartRateFrequency} > 1{,}5*\text{HRFavg} \\ \text{AND BloodPressure} > 1{,}4*\text{BPavg}\end{array}\right\}\ \mathit{THEN}\ \{\text{STRESS LEVEL} = \text{'VERY HIGH'}\}$$

Where:
HRFavg is the average value of the heart rate frequency
BPavg is the average value of the blood pressure
When the patient's stress level is assessed, the "Notifications and alerts manager" module (see Fig. 4) initiates a rule-based reasoning process to determine the actions that have to be performed based on the identified stress level. These actions consist of alerts and notifications that have to be sent at the appropriate NTAP members. The rules that determine whether an alert or a notification will be sent, as well as the respective NTAP recipients, are represented by specific policies, illustrated in Table 1.

Stress level	Notifications and alerts policy
Low	-
Medium	Notification to relatives
High	Notification to relatives and notification to paramedical staff
Very high	Alert to relatives and paramedical staff, notification to medical expert

Table 1. Notifications and alerts policies for the patients' stress levels

Examining the case where the stress level is "very high", the actions that the system has to perform are the following:
- First, it has to send alerts to the patient's relatives along with information regarding his/her stress level.
- Second, the paramedical staff is alerted, being responsible to communicate with the patients' relatives to gain awareness of the incident. In order to do so, the system has to

inform the alerted paramedical of the patients' relatives engaged in the treatment procedure of the current incident. In addition, the system has to inform the paramedical whether a medical expert is available or not, in order to determine his/her further actions.
- Third, the system has to notify the medical expert for the ongoing incident.

Apart from the deduction of their medical condition (i.e. stress level) that is constantly performed by the system, patients might request to receive alerts (self-help services) in case of abnormal environmental conditions (e.g. increased environmental temperature), in order to perform proactive actions. This would initiate a context-monitoring process, where rule-based reasoning is performed over the "Environmental Ontology" instances, to identify a potential abnormal situation and produce the respective alert messages. Alert messages are determined through specific policies (contained in patient profiles) similar to those presented in table 1.

5.4 NTAP's members' selection

The previous sub-section described the reasoning process that determines the NTAP members that have to be alerted or notified based on the identified stress level a patient presents. For instance, when the patient's stress level is "Very high" the patients' relatives have to be alerted. Nevertheless, alerting all of the relatives would be inconvenient as some of them might be engaged with important activities not wanting to be interrupted (e.g. professional meeting), while other might be unavailable to provide their assistance (e.g. enjoying a family trip). For this reason, a selection process must be performed to define the appropriate relative that has to be alerted.

The proposed framework uses rule-based reasoning over the "Social Ontology" instances to deduce the exact members that have to be alerted or notified. The selection process is performed by the "NTAP member selection" module (see Fig. 4), which utilizes the following information:

- NTAP group that have to be alerted/notified
- Availability the NTAP group's members
- Location of the NTAP group's members
- NTAP member selection policies

Continuing our example, the system has to select the appropriate relative that will be alerted. At first, the availability of each relative is checked. Next, the distance of each available relative from the patient is inferred by comparing their respective locations. Finally, according to the NTAP member selection policies (representing the rules), the appropriate relative is selected. The NTAP member selection policies may vary on a per patient basis. For example, one patient may designate a special relative who should be alerted regardless of location, unless he/she is unavailable. In this case, the system checks the availability of this relative and if he/she is available it immediately sends an alert without checking the availability and the location of the rest relatives. If this relative is unavailable, the system performs the selection process as described above to find an appropriate relative to be alerted.

5.5 Alerts and notifications subsystem

There are two modes through which NTAP members interact with the system (European Telecommunications Standards Institute [ETSI], 2009). In the first mode (polling mode), they can explicitly perform queries to get information about specific context information. The second mode (subscription mode) allows them to subscribe specifying what they are interested in receiving (e.g. patient's medical condition). The subscription is followed by a notification which confirms the subscription and informs the NTAP members about the current value of the subscribed context information. After their subscription, the NTAP members are asynchronously notified about changes in the subscribed context information when these occur.

The mode of interaction depends on the application requirements for context distribution, as well as the nature and characteristics of the context information. Due to the fact that in the proposed context-aware system for anxiety disorders the context information is highly dynamic, the subscription mode is preferred, which reduces the overhead created by polling as well. The polling mode is usually used used when subscription is not supported or when the information is seldom variable.

To enable efficient and scalable content delivery to different NTAP members, and at the same time offer content filtering, we suggest the use of SIP (Session Initiating Protocol) and more specifically the SIP/SIMPLE protocol (SIP for Instant Messaging and Presence Leveraging Extensions) (Roach, 2002; Niemi, 2004). SIP is a simple, scalable, text-based protocol that offers a number of benefits including extensibility and provision for call/session control. In addition, SIP has been adopted by several organizations and is the foundation for session initiation for presence support in desktop, mobile and server platforms. SIP has been extended by IETF's SIMPLE (SIP for Instant Messaging and Presence Leveraging Extensions) Working Group to enhance the basic protocol with Instant Messaging and Presence (IMP) functionalities. The SIMPLE extensions to the SIP protocol enable it to exchange messages inside a SIP session and provide an event package mechanism for notification of presence information.

The alerts and notifications subsystem involves two types of users: publishers and subscribers. Publishers (patients) "offer" the content that is submitted to the service for the subsequent delivery to subscribers. Subscribers (NTAP members) define subscriptions that describe the type of content they are interested in receiving. The infrastructure enables publishers to publish the information through content provider (Presence SIP Server), and allows subscribers to declare interest in certain types of information (Devlic & Podnar, 2009). The content provider stores the subscription (Fig. 6), checks if there is a publication to match it, and in the case of successful match it delivers the published content to the subscribed user. The notification of the user can be synchronous or asynchronous.

6. Anxiety-related context-aware services

The proposed context-aware system is able to provide differentiated context-aware healthcare services both to patients and medical experts. These services are based either on the identification of the patient's current context and execution of the respective reactive actions, or on the processing of a series of contexts stored in the patient profiles aiming to provide objective data for several disorder-related features. Concerning medical experts, offered services include, among others, lifestyle and habits pattern detection, context and stress level pattern detection and stress level prediction, which are comprehensively described in (Panagiotakopoulos et al., 2010a). Regarding patients, the proposed system provides several services focusing both on proactive and reactive aspects of anxiety disorders. The most important patient-oriented healthcare services are the self-evaluation service and the stress monitoring service.

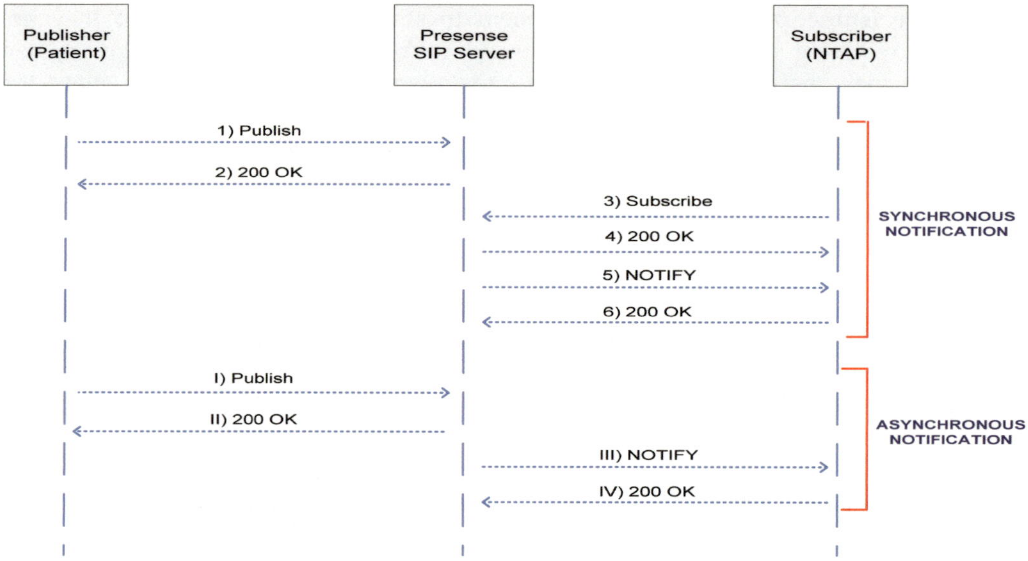

Fig. 6. Notification of NTAP members

The self-evaluation service offers patients the capability to check their stress levels within specific periods of time (e.g. one week) in specific environmental settings (e.g. at work). This way they receive an overview of the behavior of their stress at specific days and hours of a day and can try on their own to understand the exact situations that lead to increased or reduced stress levels. Next, they can experiment on alternative lifestyles and behavioral patterns evaluating their impact on their stress levels. Thus, patients become more familiar with their disorder by gaining knowledge on important features relative to its manifestation and are motivated to actively participate in their treatment process. In a similar way, patients have the ability to gain knowledge on the correlation of the symptoms that they suffer from and the stress level that has provoked them. This feature increases the patients' self-awareness on the way that stress is physically expressed to them helping them identify increased stress level conditions (through specific symptoms manifestation) and perform the appropriate actions for its reduction.

Regarding the stress monitoring service, the patients' stress level is constantly monitored for the execution of the appropriate actions with respect to their healthcare needs, as described in section 5.3. This service has a huge impact both for patients and their close environment (e.g. relatives and close friends). As for patients they feel safer to perform daily actions knowing that they will receive the required support whenever and wherever this will be needed. Concerning the members of a patient's close environment, they do not have to always be in the same physical space with the patient for the provision of the appropriate healthcare assistance that dramatically limits their social activities. Having the ability to get informed of the patient's medical condition either on demand, or whenever their intervention is needed without time and space restrictions, they ensure a better quality of life.

7. Conclusions and future work

This chapter presented a context-aware system for the support of patients suffering from anxiety disorders. The proposed system facilitates the persistent tele-monitoring of patients' medical condition and administrates the collaboration of a network of third authorized people for the provision of timely-critical and accurate health assistance in case of emergencies. Based on the analysis of context information, it provides several healthcare services to patients for self-help purposes, as well as to medical experts for the selection, evaluation and adaptation of the offered treatment to the patients' needs. The ultimate objectives are the creation of a safe and comfortable daily living environment for the patients and the better coordination and collaboration between caregivers in the treatment process.

Our research is now proceeding in several directions. We will examine several physiological signals to produce an optimum model that will assess the patients' stress level as accurately as possible. Furthermore, we will introduce further adaptation capabilities by allowing patients to explicitly state their stress level estimations through an adaptive interactive interface located at the BAN's gateway. This information will be considered for the optimization of the stress level assessment process through appropriate machine learning algorithms.

Moreover, we will focus on security and privacy issues regarding the patient profiles aiming to define specific policies that will determine the access rights of third authorized people according to various features, such as their roles. Finally, we will implement the SIP/SIMPLE based alerts and notifications subsystem and conduct an experimental evaluation of its performance.

8. References

Andersson, G. (2009). Using the Internet to provide cognitive behaviour therapy. *Behaviour Research and Therapy*, Vol. 47, No. 3, pp. 175-180, ISSN 0005-7967

Bardram, J. (2004). Applications of context-aware computing in hospital work—examples and design principles. *Proceedings of ACM symposium on Applied computing*, ISBN:1-58113-812-1, Nicosia, Cyprus, March 14 -17, 2004

Bharucha, A. J. "CareMedia: Automated video and sensor analysis for geriatric care," *19th Annual Meeting of the American Association for Geriatric Psychiatry*, San Juan, Puerto Rico, March 10-13, 2006

Brawman-Mintzer, O.; Lydiard, R. B.; Emmanuel, N.; Payeur, R.; Johnson, M.; Roberts, J.; Jarell, M. P.; Ballenger, J. C. (1993). Psychiatric comorbidity in patients with generalized anxiety disorder. *American Journal of Psychiatry*, Vol. 150, pp. 1216-1218, ISSN: 1535-7228

Buttussi, F. & Chittaro, L. (2008). MOPET: A context-aware and user-adaptive wearable system for fitness training. *Artificial Intelligence in Medicine*, Vol. 42, No. 2, pp. 153—163, ISSN: 0933-3657

Devlic, A. & Podnar, I. (2003). Location-aware Content Delivery Service Using Publish/Subscribe. *Proceedings of the* Telecommunications and Mobile Computing *(tcmc 2003), Workshop on Nomadic Data Services and Mobility*, ISBN: 3-85133-029-3 Graz, Austria, March 11-12, 2003

Dey, A. & Abowd, G. (1999). Towards a Better Understanding of Context and Context-Awareness. *1st International Symposium on Handheld and Ubiquitous Computing*, pp. 304-307, ISBN: 3-540-66550-1, Karlsruhe, Germany, September 27-29, 1999

ETSI (2009). Human Factors (HF); Personalization and User Profile Management; Architectural Framework. TS 102 747 V0.0.32

Himle, J.; Fischer, D.; Muroff, J.; Van Etten, M.; Lokers, L.; Abelson, J. & Hanna G. (2006). Videoconferencing-based cognitive-behavioral therapy for obsessive-compulsive disorder. *Behaviour Research and Therapy*, Vol. 44, No. 12, pp. 1821-1829, ISSN 0005-7967

Intille, S. S. ; Bao, L.; Munguia Tapia, E. & Rondoni, J. (2004). Acquiring in situ training data for context-aware ubiquitous computing applications. *Proceedings of CHI 2004*

Connect: Conference on Human Factors in Computing Systems, pp. 1-9, ISBN: 1-58113-702-8, Vienna, Austria, April 24-29, 2004

Kessler, R.C.; Ruscio, A.M.; Shear, K, & Wittchen, H.U. (2010). Epidemiology of anxiety disorders. *Behavioral Neurobiology of Anxiety and its Treatment*, Stein, M. & Steckler, T. (Eds.), pp. 21-36, Springer, e-ISBN: 978-3-642-02911-0

Kjeldskov, J. & Skov, B. (2007). Exploring context-awareness for ubiquitous computing in the healthcare domain. *Personal and Ubiquitous Computing, Vol. 11, No.* 7, pp. 549-562, ISSN: *1617-4917*

Korhonen, I.; Paavilainen, P. & Särela, A. (2003). Application of ubiquitous computing technologies for support of independent living of the elderly in real life settings. *2nd International Workshop on Ubiquitous Computing for Pervasive Healthcare Applications.* ISBN: 3-540-20301-X Seattle, WA, USA, October 12-15, 2003

Merikangas, K.R. & Swanson, S.A. (2010). Comorbidity in anxiety disorders. *Behavioral Neurobiology of Anxiety and its Treatment*, Stein, M. & Steckler, T. (Eds.), pp. 37-59, Springer, e-ISBN: 978-3-642-02911-0

Mitchell, S.; Spiteri, M.; Bates, J. & Coulouris, G. (2000). Context aware multimedia computing in the intelligent hospital. *Proceedings of the 9th ACM SIGOPS European Workshop*, ISBN: 1-23456-789-0, Kolding, Denmark, September 17 - 20, 2000

Niemi, A. "Session Initiation Protocol (SIP) Extension for Event State Publication", RFC 3903, October 2004

Panagiotakopoulos, T.; Lyras, D.; Livaditis, M.; Sgarbas, K.; Anastasopoulos, G. & Lymberopoulos, D. (2010a). A contextual Data Mining Approach Towards Assisting the Treatmnet of Anxiety Disorders. *IEEE Transactions on Information Technology in Biomedicine*, Vol. 14, No. 3, pp. 267-581, ISSN: 1089-7771

Panagiotakopoulos, T.; Malliaris, P.; Fengou, M.A. & Lymberopoulos, D. (2010b). Caregiving Social Networks. Are they adequate to support patients with anxiety disorders and how are they established? *Proceedings of the 10th IEEE International Conference on Information Technology and Applications in Biomedicine (ITAB 2010)*, Corfu, Greece, November 2-5, 2010

Parsons, T. & Rizzo, A. (2008). Affective Outcomes of Virtual Reality Exposure Therapy for Anxiety and Specific Phobias: A Meta-Analysis. *Journal of Behaviour Therapy and Experimental Psychiatry*, Vol. 39, No. 3, pp. 250-261, ISSN: 0005-7916

Pentland, A. (2004). Healthwear: medical technology becomes wearable. *IEEE computer*, Vol. 37, No. 5, pp. 42 – 49, ISSN: 0018-9162

Roach, A. B. (2002). Session Initiation Protocol (SIP)-Specific Event Notification. RFC 3265, June 2002.

Shandley, K.; Austin, D.; Klein, B.; Pier, C.; Schattner, P.; Pierce, D. & Wade, V. (2008). Therapist-Assisted, Internet-Based Treatment for Panic Disorder: Can General Practitioners Achieve Comparable Patient Outcomes to Psychologists? *Journal of Medical Internet Research*, Vol. 10, No. 2, e14, ISSN: 1438-8871

Sung, M.; Marci, C. & Pentland, A. (2005). Wearable feedback systems for rehabilitation. *Journal of NeuroEngineering and Rehabilitation,* 2:17 (June 2005), ISSN: 1743-0003

Weiser, M. (1991). The Computer for the 21st Century. *Scientific American*, Vol. 265, No. 3, pp. 66–75, ISSN: 0036-8733

Wood, D.P.; Murphy, J. A.; Center, K. B.; Russ, C.; McLay, R. N.; Reeves, D.; Pyne, J.; Shilling, R.; Hagan, J. & Wiederhold, B. K. (2008). Combat related post-traumatic stress disorder: a multiple case report using virtual reality graded exposure therapy with physiological monitoring. *Studies in Health Technology and Informatics*, Vol. 132, pp. 556-561, ISSN: 0926-9630

Part 6

Anxiety in Children

17

Separation Anxiety in Children and Adolescents

Malgorzata Dabkowska[1], Aleksander Araszkiewicz[1],
Agnieszka Dabkowska[2] and Monika Wilkosc[3,1]
[1]*Nicolaus Copernicus University, Torun, Collegium Medicum, Bydgoszcz*
[2]*Lord's Transfiguration University Hospital in Poznan*
[3]*Institute of Psychology, Kazimierz Wielki University in Bydgoszcz*
Poland

1. Introduction

Anxiety disorders are among the most common psychological disorders in younger patients, affecting 6% to 20% of developed countries children and adolescents (Walkup et al. 2008). Separation anxiety is the only anxiety disorder restricted to infancy, childhood, or adolescence (APA, 2000). Separation anxiety disorder (SAD) is defined by developmentally inappropriate, excessive, persistent, and unrealistic worry about separation from attachment figures, most commonly parents or other family members. Youths with SAD display distress before separation or during attempts at separation. These children worry excessively about their own or their parents' safety and health when separated, have difficulty sleeping alone, experience nightmares with themes of separation, frequently have somatic complaints, and may exhibit school refusal. Children with separation anxiety disorder exhibit varying degrees of avoidant behaviour that correlate with the severity of their symptoms (Albano et al. 2003). This kind of anxiety in adolescents and schoolchildren significantly interferes with daily activities and developmental tasks. Children with separation anxiety disorder are usually brought to the clinician when SAD results in school refusal or embarrassing somatic symptoms. When analyzing responses to shown images, relative to controls, children with anxiety disorders experience greater negative emotional responses to the presented images, are less successful at applying reappraisals, but show intact ability to reduce their negative emotions following reappraisal. They also may report less frequent use of reappraisal in everyday life (Carthy et al, 2010).

2. The risk factors and background of the separation anxiety

In the aetiology of SAD play a part a complex interplay of biological and genetic vulnerabilities, temperamental qualities, negative environmental influences and negative attachment experiences, parental psychopathology and disadvantageous socio-cultural factors (Pine & Grun, 1999).
Biological risk factors include genetics and child temperament. Studies of environmental risk factors in the development of childhood anxiety disorders have focused on parent-child interactions and parental anxiety.

2.1 Genetic influence

Evidence suggests a genetic link between separation anxiety disorders in children and a history of panic disorder, anxiety, or depression in their parents. Infants with anxious temperaments may have a predisposition toward later development of anxiety disorders. Findings from a number of studies, including Bird et al. (1989), have implicated age of subject and low socioeconomic status as putative risk factors for separation anxiety. Low self-esteem was found to increase risk for the development of anxiety in general. Parental depression played a more important role in the development of anxiety disorders in offspring. Other results of genetic studies of children with separation anxiety (Topolsky et al., 1997) suggested that shared environmental effects are more important than genetic factors in the aetiology of SAD. The liability threshold for SAD is higher for males and increases with age (Tari et al., 1997). Genetic factors seem to play an important role in shaping the co-occurrence of different anxiety dimensions in childhood (Ogliari et al., 2010). Results of a unique 30-year longitudinal study of a group from one town in New Zealand (Gibb et al., 2011) showed that relationship separation is associated with increased rates of depression, suicidal behaviour, and total mental health problems. Parental anxiety disorder has been associated with increased risk of anxiety disorder in offspring. Family aggregation studies suggest that children whose parents have an anxiety disorder are at risk for developing an anxiety disorder themselves. Twin studies also suggest a familial transmission. Separation anxiety disorder in the offspring can be accounted for by the same disorders in the parent (Biederman et al., 2006). Children of anxious parents are likely to have an earlier onset for anxiety disorders than their parents. This phenomenon can be explained as anxious parents can model fear and anxiety, reinforce anxious coping behaviour, and unwittingly maintain avoidance, despite their desire to be of help to their child (Dadds et al., 2001).Lifetime maternal anxiety disorders are related to offspring anxiety disorders. Findings confirm the transmission of anxiety disorders from mother to offspring (Martini et al., 20010).

2.2 Gender

Some studies (Bowen et al. 1990) report a significantly higher prevalence of SAD in girls than boys. In the previously mentioned New Zealand study, an overrepresentation of females was noted among the preadolescent children with separation anxiety disorder (Anderson et al., 1987). Also, higher rates in females than in males were observed among high school students with SAD in Lewinsohn and colleagues (1993) study. It should be noted, however, that there are no reported gender differences in symptomatology (Last et al., 1987). A study including preschool 4-year-old children (Lavigne et al., 2009) showed no gender differences for separation anxiety disorder at any level of impairment, and race or ethnicity differences were not significant. Gender differences have not been observed, although girls do present more often with anxiety disorders in general.

2.3 Temperament

Emotion deregulation is believed to be a key factor in anxiety disorders. Anxious children demonstrate greater intensity and frequency of negative emotional responses relative to controls, deficits in using reappraisal in negative emotional situations and corresponding deficits in reappraisal self-efficacy, and greater reliance on emotion regulation strategies that increase the risk of functional impairment, intense negative emotion, and low emotion regulation self-efficacy (Carthy et al., 2010b). The vigilance-avoidance attention pattern is found in anxious adults and children, who initially gaze more at threatening pictures than non-anxious adults and children (vigilance), but subsequently gaze less at them than non-anxious adults and children (avoidance) (In-Albon et al., 2010). A Korean study (Soo-churl et al., 2009) evaluated temperament and character of children and adolescents with anxiety disorders, in part subjects with separation anxiety, using the Junior Temperament and Character Inventory (JTCI). Separation anxiety disorder was not associated with any temperament and character on the JTCI, opposite to others anxiety diagnosis. Children and adolescents with anxiety disorders could have different temperaments and character profiles in accordance with diagnostic groups, which imply the specific pathophysiological mechanism of each anxiety disorder (Soo-churl et al., 2009).

2.4 Family parent/child attachment

Parenting stress, parental psychopathology, and family functioning are associated with child anxiety (Victor et al., 2007). Separation anxiety would appear to be a core form of anxiety that is associated with anxious attachment. Overprotective, overcontrolling, and overly critical parenting styles that limit the development of autonomy and mastery may also contribute to the development of anxiety disorders in children with temperamental vulnerability. Rejection and control by parents may be positively related to later anxiety and depression (Rapee, 1997). Insecure attachment relationships with caregivers and, specifically, anxious/resistant attachment can increase the risk of childhood anxiety disorders (Manassis & Hood, 1998; Warren et al., 1997). Different attachment patterns (secure, ambivalent, avoidant, and disorganized) may relate to different types of anxiety symptoms, and that behavioural inhibition may moderate these relations. In a sample of 10 - 12-year olds in Brumariu & Kerns study (2010), security attachment was related to lower levels of all types of anxieties, except separation anxiety. Ambivalence attachment was positively related to separation anxiety, although this relation was stronger for boys. Although avoidance attachment was not related to anxiety and disorganization was positively correlated to somatic symptoms, social phobia, and school phobia. Behavioural inhibition moderated the relations of security with social phobia and of disorganization with school phobia (Brumariu & Kerns, 2010).

2.5 Environmental changes

Anxiety states in children can be associated with exposure to negative life events. Separation anxiety disorder is often precipitated by change or stress in the child's life. Symptoms of separation anxiety disorder may be exacerbated by a change in routine, illness, lack of adequate rest, a family move, or change in family structure (such as death, divorce, parent illness, birth of a sibling), starting a new school, a traumatic event, or even a return to school after summer vacation. The child's symptoms may also be affected by a change in caregivers or changes in parents' response to the child in terms of discipline, availability, or daily routine. Even if changes are positive or exciting, the change may feel uncomfortable and precipitate an anxious response in the child.

2.6 Economical factors

Most children with anxiety disorders are from middle to upper-middle class families; however, 50 to 75% of those with SAD come from low socioeconomic status homes (Last et al., 1987; Last et al., 1992; Velez et al., 1989).

3. The prevalence of the disorder

Anxiety disorders as a whole are the most common psychiatric disorders in children and adolescents, with a reported prevalence ranging from 6 to 18%.
Shaffer et al. found that approximately 20% of American children have an impairing anxiety disorder (Shaffer et al., 1995), but even 25% of Dutch children met criteria for an anxiety disorder (Verhulst et al., 1997). When using a higher impairment threshold, a rate of anxiety disorders was closer to 5% (Costello et al. 1996). In a large sample of adolescents, prevalence rates were found at 3.6% of subjects (Bowen et al., 1990). Different epidemiological studies indicate a prevalence of SAD in 4 to 5% children and adolescents. The 12-month prevalence of SAD is generally estimated at around 5%, but there is a significant variation between studies (2-13%)(Costello & Angold, 1995). Among 11-year-old children from the general New Zealand population was found a 1-year rate of 3.5% for SAD (Anderson et al., 1987). In the same population three years later, the prevalence of SAD decreased to 2% (McGee et al., 1990).
In Bird and colleagues' study, diagnosis of SAD in the sample of 4- to 16-year-old Puerto Rican children was made in 4.7% of the children (Bird et al., 1988). The lifetime prevalence of SAD in a randomly selected sample of adolescents was 4.3% (Lewinsohn et al., 1993). A Canadian epidemiological study (1999) found that the 6-month prevalence of SAD was 4.9% in children aged 6 to 8 years and 1.3% in adolescents aged 12 to 14 years (Breton et al., 1999). A study from an Australian community sample of preadolescent children found a rate of 4.2% for SAD (Prior et al., 1999). Self-report interviews with juvenile subjects yield a higher prevalence of SAD than interviews with adult informants, and agreement between informants ranges between low and moderate (Grills & Ollendick, 2003). Little is known about the development of anxiety symptoms from late childhood to late adolescence. In Van Oort and colleagues' (2009) study, anxiety symptoms were assessed in a large community sample of boys and girls at three time-points across a 5-year interval. In that general population, anxiety symptoms first decrease during early adolescence, and subsequently increase from middle to late adolescence (Van Oort et al., 2009). Prevalence estimates of separation anxiety disorder are between 4 and 5% in the population (Masi et al., 2001). Of those diagnosed with separation anxiety disorder, approximately 75% experience school refusal.

4. Classification criteria of the separation anxiety disorder

Separation anxiety disorder represents a more severe and disabling form of a maturational experience that all children normally have. As specified in DSM-IV-TR criteria, separation anxiety disorders are defined largely by the persistence of such symptoms for long enough duration to be considered pathological (APA, 2000). In DSM-IV, disorders that have been long recognized as manifesting during childhood are placed in a separate category, "Disorders usually first diagnosed in infancy, childhood or adolescence." For the anxiety disorders, this includes only separation anxiety disorder (SAD) in DSM-IV. A DSM-IV-TR-based diagnosis of separation anxiety disorder requires that a child exhibits at least three of the following symptoms for at least four weeks (APA, 2000). The characteristic symptoms include three types of distress or worry, three types of behaviours and two physiological symptoms.

DSM-IV-TR diagnostic criteria for separation anxiety disorder (309.21):

a. Developmentally inappropriate and excessive anxiety concerning separation from home or from those to whom the individual is attached, as evidenced by three (or more) of the following:
   1. recurrent excessive distress when separation from home or major attachment figures occurs or is anticipated
   2. persistent and excessive worry about losing, or about possible harm befalling, major attachment figures
   3. persistent and excessive worry that an untoward event will lead to separation from a major attachment figure (e.g., getting lost or being kidnapped)
   4. persistent reluctance or refusal to go to school or elsewhere because of fear of separation
   5. persistently and excessively fearful or reluctant to be alone or without major attachment figures at home or without significant adults in other settings
   6. persistent reluctance or refusal to go to sleep without being near a major attachment figure or to sleep away from home
   7. repeated nightmares involving the theme of separation
   8. repeated complaints of physical symptoms (such as headaches, stomach aches, nausea, or vomiting) when separation from major attachment figures occurs or is anticipated
b. The duration of the disturbance is at least 4 weeks.
c. The onset is before age of 18.
d. The disturbance causes clinically significant distress or impairment in social, academic (occupational), or other important areas of functioning.
e. The disturbance does not occur exclusively during the course of a Pervasive Developmental Disorder, Schizophrenia, or other Psychotic Disorder and, in adolescents and adults, is better not accounted for by Panic Disorder with Agoraphobia.

Specify if:

Early Onset: if onset occurs before age 6 years (APA, 2000).

Diagnostic guidelines of the ICD-10 Classification of Mental and Behavioural Disorders World Health Organization lists similar criteria for separation anxiety disorder (F93.0) (WHO, 1992). The number of studies with clinical samples from zero to 3 year is very limited. The assessments for children zero to 3 years of age are rare and even less common for children aged 0 to 1 year of age. The few prevalence studies in epidemiological samples have concerned preschoolers and reported rates of psychopathology ranging from 7.8 to 50% (Beernink et al., 2007; Skovgaard et al., 2007). In the first study focused on infants younger than 1 year of age, roughly 76% of the infants had an Axis I diagnosis, with anxiety disorders and mixed disorder of emotional expressiveness being the most frequently observed (Viaux-Savelon et al., 2010).

5. Course

The mean age of onset of the disorder is about 7.5 years (Last et al., 1992). Developmental differences have been reported in the presentation of symptoms. Younger children have more symptoms than older children. Children aged 5 to 8 years most commonly report unrealistic worry about harm to attachment figures and school refusal. In children aged 9 to 12 years, the disorder usually manifests as excessive distress at times of separation (Francis et al., 1987). In adolescents, somatic complaints and school refusal are most common. The most frequently observed ages for occurrence of separation anxiety disorder are in children aged five to seven years and again from aged 11 to 14 years. Many studies report a declining prevalence of SAD as children age into adolescence. Separation anxiety in children with severe school refusal evokes often worry about the future with regard to professional career and social integration. In Von Widdern & Lehmkuhl (2011) study, in the group of inpatient treatment because of a separation anxiety disorder assessed at follow up ranged from 4.3 to 11.1 years (average 7.1 years) was found at least one clinical psychiatric diagnosis in one third of all patients at follow-up. Even more of the formerly inpatients reported subthreshold psychiatric symptoms (55%). Estimated remission rate for the separation anxiety disorder was high (89%). The results revealed an important shift of diagnosis to social phobia in one third of cases. The majority of young people considered academic outcome satisfactory but reported pronounced problems in the social integration (Von Widdern & Lehmkuhl, 2011). In Allen and colleagues' (2010) study, among children aged 4-15 years with a primary DSM-IV diagnosis of SAD, the most frequently reported symptoms were separation-related distress, avoidance of being alone/without an adult and sleeping away from caregivers or from home, with nightmares, the least frequently endorsed criterion. Anxiety disorders in childhood are predictors of a range of psychiatric disorders in adolescence. Results come from the Great Smoky Mountains Study indicated that childhood SAD predicted adolescent SAD (Bittner et al., 2007). Among the participants of the Oregon Adolescent Depression Project SAD was a strong risk factor (78.6%) for the development of mental disorders during young adulthood. The major vulnerabilities were for panic disorder and depression (Lewinsohn et al., 2008). The squeals of childhood anxiety disorders include social, family, and academic impairments. Anxiety separation disorders disrupt the normal psychosocial development of a child. Children with SAD may not have the opportunity to develop independence from adults. Social problems include poor problem-solving skills and low self-esteem. Severe separation anxiety can result intra-familial violence.

6. A normative separation anxiety

The separation anxiety disorder (SAD) is qualitatively different from early worries and the normative anxieties. Fear and worry are common in healthy children. Normal, developmentally, fear does not impair a child's functioning. Infants typically experience fear of loud noises, fear of being startled, and later a fear of strangers. Toddlers experience fears of imaginary creatures, fears of darkness, and normative separation anxiety. School-age children commonly have worries about injury and storms. Older children have worries and fears related to school performance, social competence, and health issues. Fears during childhood become problematic, if they do not subside with time and if they impair the child's functioning. Depending on the age, developmental differences are observed in the expression of childhood anxiety symptoms and fears. Results also point toward specific symptoms predominant at certain ages (i.e., separation anxiety symptoms in youths aged 6-9 years, in partial support of predictions (Weems et al., 2005). Normal separation distress usually intensifies during early childhood, then gradually subsides at 3 to 5 years of age, although a percentage of children continue to present closed relation to parents and separation distress into their first school attendance. Separation anxiety diathesis may manifest itself differently over the life span (Deltito & Hahn, 1993).

7. Neurobiology of separation anxiety disorder

Literature still gives very little information on the nature of separation anxiety and evidence based on longitudinal studies. Contemporary knowledge about anxiety is in a prominent part based on animal studies. Up-to-date research has implicated the amygdala and circuits related to these nuclei as being central to several aspects of fear and fear-related behaviors in animals. It can be concluded that in an emotional response, a limbic system holds a key role. Brain structures building this system determinates processing of information from an emotional angle, and because of many projections from other brain regions it leads the best coping method counteracting a threat stimulus (Cummins & Ninan, 2002; Lucey & Corvin, 2005). The amygdala, and its efferent projections, is mainly concerned with a central fear system involved in expression and acquisition of conditioned fear (Cummins & Ninan, 2002; Davis, 1992). One of important functions of the lateral nucleus is to associate conditioned (particularly aversive) and unconditioned stimuli in the course of the anxiety reaction. Because of this network medial nuclei modulates the autonomous and operational components of a defensive reaction. It also coordinates an anxiety response in which a connection with periaqueductal gray activates a freeze reaction to threatening stimulus. Moreover, the connection with paraventricular nuclei of thalamus modulates the activity of endocrine controlled process involved in regulation of autonomous nervous system reaction. Another role of medial nuclei is due to the connection with the compressed monoaminergic neurons in brainstem and cholinergic in Meynert basal nuclei. These structures modulate nonspecific arousal (excitation) and attention mechanisms, which are important in course of anxiety reaction. Due to numerous neuronal pathways with different brain structures, medial nuclei take part in sensorial information reception from all modalities, access to memory modules, regulation of perception and attention mechanisms, and control of cognitive-motivation processes, which play an important role in decision making and choosing the most adaptive coping reaction. The orbitofrontal cortex dysfunction has been implicated in social anxiety disorder and specific phobia as a direct reaction on a phobic object. Dichotomizing the orbitofrontal cortex into medial versus lateral subdivisions according to positive and negative valence, in reward and punishment expectation is well-founded. The limbic system and specified structures play significant role in anxiety reaction and choice of adaptive coping methods in threatening situation. In separation anxiety, its controlling activity does not seem to work properly. Etiopathogenesis of anxiety disorders is multifactorial with a significant role played by neurotransmitters pathways. Anxiety states are considered to be a result of insufficient inhibitory control. In these disorders, a major role is played by the gamma-amino-butyric acid (GABA) system. There are clinical studies proving a decreased GABAergic inhibition in anxiety disorders (Bremner et al., 2000; Domschke & Zwanzger, 2000; Malizia et al. 1998). Deregulation of serotoninergic and noradrenergic functions mediate many symptoms of depression and anxiety disorders. Serotoninergic and noradrenergic dysfunction does not cause directly these disorders. Their role in modulating and being modulated by other neurobiological functions underlies abnormality in mood and anxiety states. Abnormal modulation of cortical-hippocampal-amygdala axis contributes to chronic hypersensitive stress, as well as fear responses. Quite possibly, this mechanism mediates features of anxiety (impaired concentration and memory, uncontrollable worry), anhedonia, aggression, affective discontrol (Ressler & Nemeroff, 2000). Schwartz (2003) et al. longitudinal studies showed that anxiousness correlated with high reactivity of amygdala in response to new stimuli. Among children diagnosed in the age of two as inhibited temperament (timid, anxious, avoidant in new situations) there were more intensive activation of amygdala recorded in contrast to children diagnosed as no inhibited temperament.

7.1 Neuroimaging results in separation anxiety disorder in children

There is very few data about structural and functional neuroimaging in childhood separation anxiety disorder. However, there is an association between separation anxiety disorder and adult panic attacks or panic disorder (Battaglia et al., 1995; Klein, 1995; Pine et al., 1998). Klein and Capps suggested in their investigations that there might be common, heritable biological substrate for both of them (Capps et al., 1996; Klein 1993). The relationship between parental panic disorder or parental depression and childhood separation anxiety disorder is well-defined (Beidel et al., 1997; Capps et al., 1996; Last et al., 1991; Warner et al., 1995; Weissmann et al., 1984). A study by Uchida et al. revealed in adult patients with panic disorder relative increase in gray matter volume in the left insula, in the left superior temporal gyrus, midbrain and pons, as well as relative gray matter deficit in the anterior cingulate cortex of those patients as compared to controls (Uchida et al., 2008). Reduced volume of temporal lobe was detected in other studies (Fontaine et al., 1990; Ontiveros et al., 1989; Vythilingam et al., 2000). However, Massana et al. (2003) didn´t find any changes in temporal lobe (probably because of excluding hippocampus and amygdala in his Region of Interest investigations). There is an evidence of a dysfunction in hippocampus, amygdala, cingulated gyrus revealed in functional magnetic resonance imaging (Bystritsky et al., 2001). Grillon et al. (1997) examined enhanced startle reflex in children of patients with anxiety. According to significance of the amygdala in the startle reflex, this data indicates a potential role of amygdala-based circuits (and hypothetic significance of the bed nucleus of the striaterminalis) in familial risk for anxiety. This report is consistent with a study of increased stratial function to reward in adolescents with temperamental anxiety (Guyer et al., 2006). The meta-analysis of functional magnetic resonance and positron emission tomography studies of post-traumatic stress disorder, social anxiety disorder, and specific phobia in adults showed that all three disorders displayed hyperactivity in amygdala and insula (Etkin & Wager, 2007). In adult patients with social anxiety disorder hyperactivity was seen in the amygdala, parahippocampal gyrus, fusiform gyrus, globus pallidus, insula, inferior frontal gyrus and superior temporal gyrus. Adult patients with specific phobia showed hyperactivity in the amygdala, fusifirm gyrus, substania nigra, insula and mid-cingulate (Etkin & Wager, 2007). Separation anxiety disorder exhibits association with depression in adults. Functional brain changes in early stages of depressive disorder in adults were displayed in three frequency bands of electroencephalography (theta 4-7.5Hz, alpha 7.5-14Hz, beta 14-20Hz, both in Eyes closed and Eyes open conditions). A diffuse enhancement of beta power (correlating with anxiety symptoms) and an increase in theta and alpha activity at parietal occipital sites were revealed (Grin-Yatsenko et al., 2010). The presence of structural and functional abnormalities in the superior temporal gyrus and in the amygdala in children and adults with generalized anxiety disorder was found (De Bellis et al., 2000, 2002; Quirk et al., 1997). Adolescents with anxiety disorder displayed more extreme responses in anterior cingulate cortex, dorsolateral prefrontal cortex, medial and lateral orbitofrontal cortex and ventral striatum than youth with depression (Forbes et al., 2006). A study comparing children with and without anxiety (including separation anxiety disorder) reviewed reduction of the volume of the left amygdala in the morphometric magnetic resonance imaging (Milham et al., 2005). Reduced volume of the brain and of the mediosagittal area of the corpus callosum and increased lateral ventricule (De Bellis et al., 2003), as well as reduced cerebellar volume (De Bellis et al., 2006), but no changes in pituitary gland (Thomas et al., 2004) were found in abused children with post-traumatic stress disorder.

7.2 Cognitive function in separation anxiety disorder

There is a very limited number of data concerning the cognitive functioning of children with a separation anxiety disorder. However, the studies on cognition in anxiety disorders in general, concentrate mainly on biases in attention, information processing, memory and judgment that are considered to underlie them (Bar-Haim et al., 2007). Numerous research studies in adults with anxiety disorders, demonstrating the attentional bias towards threat, are ones of the major findings in this field. They emphasize a role of hyper-vigilance and changes in selective attention in aetiology and maintenance of anxiety (Kindt & van den Hout, 2001). The results of studies performed in anxious children are ambiguous. In the work of Kindt et al. (2003) the processing bias was measured by one of the most often used tools - the emotional Stroop task. It assessed colour-naming latency to threat-relevant and neutral words in children with separation anxiety disorder, social phobia and generalized anxiety disorder and normal controls. It was also controlled whether the bias is domain-specific by monitoring the reactions of children with separation anxiety disorder on words related to separation concerns, social phobia children on words associated with social concerns, and children with generalized anxiety disorder on words linked to physical concerns. They found no evidence for either an anxiety-related bias towards threat or a domain-specificity effect (Kindt et al., 2003). The authors postulate that these discrepancies between adult and children may be connected with age. They suggest that non-anxious children learn with increasing age to inhibit the processing of threat, whereas anxious children do not develop such ability. Thus, only at certain age the differences in processing may be revealed. Moreover, they hypothesize that in adults the content of fear is more stable and represented by domain-specific fear networks, while in children the content of fears changes with the age. It may suggest that representations of fears in children are more flexible and prone to assimilate disconfirming information. In-Albon et al. (2010) performed a study using the eye tracking to identify vigilance-avoidance attention pattern in children with separation anxiety disorder. The model observed in adults with anxiety disorders predicts the initial vigilance for threat stimulus and then its subsequent avoidance. Children were presented with series of pairs of photographs: one with a child separating from an adult woman and the second one with a child reuniting with an adult woman. The results obtained confirmed the vigilance-avoidance model in children with separation anxiety disorder. In the attentional control theory, the influence of anxiety on the main executive functions involving attentional control such as inhibition and shifting is postulated. These changes may affect cognitive performance, e.g. memory. Yet, the effectiveness of performance may not be affected when the compensatory strategies such as e.g. enhanced effort or increased use of processing resources are engaged (Eysenck et al., 2007). The prospective study of Pine et al. (1999) in prepubescent boys aged 7-11 years at risk of delinquency showed verbal and visual memory deficits predicting future anxiety disorders:

social phobia, separation anxiety disorder, overanxious disorder. In addition, the anxiety symptoms were connected more significantly with lower memory ability than with reduced intelligence (Pine et al., 1999). The work of Toren et al. (2000) in a group of children and adolescents aged 6-18 year old presented verbal memory deficits measured by CVLT (California Verbal Learning Test) in separation anxiety and overanxious disorders. Also, the anxiety group performed worse than control group on WCST (Wisconsin Card Sorting Test) measuring working memory, executive function and cognitive flexibility. They found no correlation between anxiety and nonverbal processes (Toren et al., 2000). Vasa et al. (2007) focused on a memory for non-emotional material in offspring with separation anxiety disorder, social phobia and generalized anxiety disorder of parents with panic disorder or major depressive disorder. They presented no relationship between visual memory and verbal memory measured by WRAML (Wide Range Assessment of Memory and Learning) and separation anxiety disorder. The study also indicated that IQ measured using The Kaufman Brief Intelligence Test (K-BIT) is a significant predictor of both visual and verbal memory. What's more, they concluded that anxiety or depressive disorders in parents were unrelated to memory performance in their offspring (Vasa et al., 2007). This finding is in contrary with a study of Merikangas et al. (1999) who found that parental anxiety was connected with visual memory deficits in offspring. They postulated that memory deficits may be considered as a premorbid risk factor for childhood anxiety disorders (Merinkangas et al., 1999). A 2009 study of Mikko et al. concentrated on the executive function of 6– 17 year old children of parents with major depression and/or panic disorder and of controls with neither disorder. Children were diagnosed with generalized anxiety disorder, social phobia, separation anxiety disorder and major depression. A large battery of neuropsychological tests was used to assess cognitive performance. The only significant difference in a group of children with separation anxiety related to their better performance on the CPT (Continuous Performance Task) - False Alarms subtest. The main conclusion of this study was that deficits in executive functioning and processing speed do not serve as trait markers for developing depression or anxiety (Micco et al., 2009). In 2007, Mazzone et al. performed a study, in a sample of children and adolescents attending from elementary to high school, assessing a role of anxiety symptoms in school performance. They concluded that frequency of high self-reported levels of anxiety increased with age and was negatively associated with school performance (Mazzone et al., 2007). Such observation may lead to conclusion that poorer performance at school of children with separation anxiety disorder may be a one of the factor maintaining the increased level of anxiety and also leading to school phobia.

8. Assessment

Separation anxiety disorder is usually under-diagnosed and undertreated. The recognition of this kind of anxiety is important, because if not treated, it may affect the child's normal development. Separation anxiety disorder is generally diagnosed by history, including parental reports; however, a few measures of general anxiety exist that can be used to supplement the history. These include Pediatric Anxiety Rating Scale, Children's Global Assessment Scale, Children's Anxiety Scale, Screen for Child Anxiety Related Emotional Disorders (SCARED-R), Multi-Dimensional Anxiety Scale for Children, and Achenbach's Child Behavior Checklist. Separation anxiety disorder can be predicted by the corresponding subscale of the screening questionnaire - the Anxiety Disorder Interview Schedule (ADIS). Simon and Boegels (2009) rightly concluded that this scale has proved the usefulness of screening for anxiety disorders in primary school children (Simon & Bögels, 2009). A number of simple screening tools have been shown effective in identifying various anxiety disorders in the pediatric population. The Screen for Child Anxiety Related Emotional Disorders (SCARED), a 41-item self-report questionnaire administered to both child and parent, has been shown effective in identifying a pediatric anxiety disorders in both primary care and outpatient settings. The Multidimensional Anxiety Scale for Children (MASC) is a 39-item instrument with both child and parent self-report components available for purchase. The Pediatric Anxiety Rating Scale (PARS) is a clinician-scored instrument that has been used to evaluate the severity of anxiety disorders in children. Researchers conducting a comprehensive review of the most commonly cited and psychometrically valid anxiety scales used in children concluded that the PARS combined with either the SCARED or the MASC, provided an appropriate assessment for pediatric anxiety disorders (Monga et al., 2000). The Separation Anxiety Daily Diary (SADD) assesses the frequency of anxiety-provoking and non-anxiety-provoking separations, along with associated parental anxiety, thoughts, child behaviours, and corresponding parental reactions (Allen et al., 2010). The Revised Child Anxiety and Depression Scale—Parent Version (RCADS-P) is a 47-item parent-report questionnaire of youth anxiety and depression, with scales corresponding to the DSM-IV categories of Separation Anxiety Disorder, Social Phobia, Generalized Anxiety Disorder (GAD), Panic Disorder, Obsessive-Compulsive Disorder, and Major Depressive Disorder (MDD). The RCADS-P demonstrated favourable psychometric properties, including high internal consistency, convergent/divergent validity, as well as strong discriminant validity - evidencing an ability to discriminate between anxiety and depressive disorders, as well as between the targeted anxiety disorders (Ebesutani et al., 2010).

9. Comorbidity

Separation anxiety disorder is closely linked to other anxiety and mood disorders and can also be associated with externalizing psychopathology in children and adolescents. Children and adolescents with anxiety disorders are at risk of developing new anxiety disorders, depression, and substance abuse. Longitudinal studies have suggested that childhood SAD may be a risk factor for other anxiety disorders. It is a question whether this link is specific to, for example, a panic disorder and agoraphobia or whether SAD represents a general factor of vulnerability for a broad range of anxiety disorders (Manicavasagar et al., 1998; Silove et al., 1993). 50 to 75% of children and adolescents with juvenile panic disorder suffer from SAD at the same time (Biederman et al., 1997; Bradley & Hood, 1993; Masi et al., 2000). Some studies confirm the association between separation anxiety in childhood and panic disorder (PD) in adulthood (Capps et al., 1996; Pine et al., 1998). The results from other studies did not confirm a specific link between these two kinds of disorders (Lipsitz et al., 1994; Silove et al., 1996). Some researches consider that a history of SAD identifies a particularly heritable, early-onset form of panic disorder (Battaglia et al., 1995). Fagiolini et al. (1998) hypothesize that childhood SAD cannot transform into panic disorder or other anxiety disorders, but it may simply persist in adulthood, as part of a more comprehensive panic diathesis called panic spectrum. Results from Aschenbrand and colleagues (2003) study argue against the hypothesis that childhood SAD is a specific risk factor for adult panic disorder and agoraphobia. The subjects with a childhood diagnosis of SAD did not display a greater risk for developing panic disorder and agoraphobia in young adulthood than those with other childhood anxiety diagnoses (Aschenbrand et al., 2003). Results of a 4-year, prospective longitudinal Brückl and colleagues (2007) study of a representative cohort of adolescents and young adults aged 14-24 years at baseline showed an increased risk of developing subsequent not only panic disorder with agoraphobia, but also an increased risk of developing subsequent specific phobia, obsessive-compulsive disorder, bipolar disorder, pain disorder, alcohol dependence and generalized anxiety disorder (Brückl et al., 2007; Masi et al., 1999). Similar patterns of vulnerability to carbon dioxide inhalation have been reported in adults with panic disorder (PD) and children with separation anxiety disorder (SAD), suggesting a link between the adult and child conditions. They might be a subtype of SAD at particularly high risk for adult PD (Roberson-Nay et al., 2010). Anxiety disorders in youth often do not present as a single/focused disorder: such disorders in youth overlap in symptoms and are highly comorbid among themselves (Kendall et al., 2010). Anxiety disorders and depression are frequently comorbid in children and adolescents (Axelson & Birmaher, 2001; O'Neil et al., 2010; Pine et al., 1998). Separation anxiety disorder has an association with higher rates of subsequent depression in a limited number of studies (Horn & Wuyek, 2010). Separation anxiety disorders are among the most common comorbid conditions in youth with bipolar disorder (BP) (Sala et al., 2010). A history of separation anxiety disorder is frequently reported by patients with obsessive-compulsive disorder (Mroczkowski et al., 2011). Anxiety disorders in youth increase a risk for later substance use disorders (O'Neil et al., 2011).

10. School phobia

School refusal could be defined as a difficulty attending school associated with emotional distress, especially anxiety and depression. School refusal is considered a symptom rather than a clinical diagnosis and can manifest itself as a sign of many psychiatric disorders, with anxiety disorders predominant. Identified main predictors of school refusal behaviour were in a connection with distinctive feature of community, school and family (Kearney & Hugelshofer, 2000). The behaviour of those children, who stay home from school because of fear or anxiety, has variously been called an anxious school refusal or a school phobia or a variant of separation anxiety disorder (SAD) (King & Bernstein, 2001).

Separation anxiety disorder, generalized anxiety disorder, social phobia, specific phobia, and adjustment disorder with anxiety symptoms are the most common disorders co-occurring with school refusal (King et al., 1995). Mostly severe separation anxiety can result in school refusal. For separation anxiety disorder, the essential feature is excessive anxiety consuming separation from the home or from those to whom the person is attached, an issue that may first surface when a child begins formal schooling. While separation anxiety disorder is associated with school refusal in younger children, other anxiety disorders, especially phobias, are associated with school refusal in adolescents. School phobia has traditionally referred to the youngsters who refuse school with parental knowledge and because of separation anxiety or specific fears. Terms such as separation anxiety and school phobia are often used interchangeably with school refusal. Johnson et al. (1941) coining the term "school phobia", defined it as an anxious fear of school caused by the child's and mother's separation anxieties (Johnson et al., 1941; Kearney & Silverman,1996). Such definitions include the youths who are completely absent from school, who initially attend school but then leave during the school day, who go to school after having behavioural problems such as morning tantrums or psychosomatic complaints, and who display marked distress on school days and plead with their caregivers to allow them to remain home from school. The rates of school absenteeism are much higher in some urban areas. The most common age of onset is 10 to 13 years. Anxious school refuses can be divided into three types: those with separation anxiety, social phobia, and those who are anxious and depressed (King & Bernstein, 2001). The prevalence of school refusal has been reported to be approximately 1% in school-age children and 5% in child psychiatry samples. The prevalence of school refusal is similar among boys and girls. School refusal can occur at any time throughout the child's academic life and at all socio-economic levels. The vulnerabilities associated with pure anxious school refusal include living in a single-parent home, attending a dangerous school, and having a biological or non-biological parent who had been treated for a mental health problem (Egger et al., 2003). Among different kinds of risk factors of school phobia are genetic, biological (obstetric, neonatal), temperament, comorbidity and environmental risk factors such as developmental experience, life events, history of childhood, parent-child relationship (Bernstein et al., 1999; Dabkowska, 1999, 2002; Kearney & Hugelshofer, 2000). The psychiatric disorders are more frequently seen in adult relatives of children with school refusal, which supports a significant role of genetic and environmental factors in the aetiology of school refusal. Approximately 52% of adolescents with school refusal behaviour meet criteria for an anxiety, depressive, conduct-personality, or other psychiatric disorder later in life (Kearney, 2006). Berg et al. (1993) found that a half of the youths with attendance problems had no psychiatric disorder, a third had a disruptive behaviour disorder, and a fifth had an anxiety or mood disorder. School refusal is reported in about 75% of children with SAD, and SAD is reported to occur in up to 80% of children with school refusal (Borchardt et al., 1994; King et al., 1995). Results of studies support the association between anxious school refusal and somatic symptoms (headache, gastrointestinal complaints) occurring mostly in the morning, disturbed sleep, nightmares (Bernstein et al., 1997; Dabkowska, 2006; Egger et al., 2003).The youth with anxiety disorder diagnoses (also separation anxiety disorder) demonstrates significantly lower levels of school functioning than those without anxiety disorders (Mychailyszyn et al., 2010). School refusal behaviour can lead to serious short-term problems, such as distress, academic decline, alienation from peers, family conflict, intrafamilial violence, financial and legal consequences. Long-term consequences may include fewer opportunities to attend facilities of higher education, employment problems, social difficulties, and increased risk for later psychiatric illness (Flakierska-Praquin et al., 1997). Long term follow-up studies of children treated for school refusal due to SAD find that, despite their return to school, many continue to present significant social and affective limitations (Berg & 1985; Flakierska-Praquin et al., 1997). In relation to educational outcomes, about half of school refuses underachieve academically (Flakierska-Praquin et al., 1997; Kearney & Albano, 2000). (Copian et al., 2007; Nelson et al., 2005). Children and adolescents with school refusal are a heterogeneous population and require individualized treatment planning. Variables such as diagnosis and severity at the start of treatment should be taken into consideration when planning treatment. The School Refusal Assessment Scale (revised edition; SRAS-R) is designed to measure the relative strength of the four functional conditions and is given to the child and to both parents. Often children and parents assess basic reasons for school refusal in a different way (Kearney, 2002). Dabkowska study (2007) noticed substantial disagreement between children and parent in identifying the function of school refusal behaviours. The major aim of the treatment is to help the child return to school in the shortest time possible. The treatment should be carried out in cooperation with the child's parents and the school personnel. A widely accepted approach to the treatment of school refusal is one that is concerned with the application of a multi-faceted treatment. Psychosocial and psychopharmacological approaches constitute the crucial parts of the therapeutic process. Today, cognitive behaviour therapy is the most frequently employed approach in the treatment of school refusal (Bahali & Tahiroğlu 2010).The anxious school refusal can be effectively treated with other behavioural interventions, also pharmacotherapy, where mainly selective serotonin reuptake inhibitors could be useful (King & Bernstein, 2001; Last et al., 1998). Finally, it is important to intervene at school to improve the child's comfort and safety.

11. Adult separation anxiety

Adult separation anxiety disorder (ASAD) has only been recognized as a specific mental disorder in the late 90's, with the pioneering work of professor Vijaya Manicavasagar. Adult separation anxiety disorder is likely to be much more common in adults than previously recognized (Manicasavagar & Silove 1997). This anxiety in adulthood has been associated with severe role impairment at work and in social relationships after controlling for potential confounding effect of anxiety comorbidity. In Pini et al. study (2010), some subjects have exhibited adult separation anxiety disorder without a history of childhood separation anxiety and some have had adult separation anxiety disorder with a history of childhood separation anxiety (Pini et al., 2010). Manicavasagar et al. (1998) indicated that adults might experience wide-ranging separation anxiety symptoms, such as extreme anxiety and fear, when separated from major attachment figures; avoidance of being alone; and fears that harm will befall those close to them. Symptomatology of adult separation anxiety disorder usually has a waxing and waning course, with exacerbation in the presence of threats to intimate bonds, which particularly predisposes to severe anxiety symptoms, including panic attacks (Manicavasagar et al., 1998). Separation anxiety disorder may be a neglected diagnosis in adulthood. Only a single research has examined the relationship of attachment styles to adult separation anxiety disorder. Manicavasagar and colleagues (2009) described how the dimensional associations showed strong correlations with scales measuring anxious attachment and separation anxiety in adults. In a 2006 study, Shear at al. found approximately one-third of adults had a childhood case of separation anxiety disorder that persisted into adulthood. However, a significant part of adults with ASAD recorded its first onset of the disorder in adulthood (Shear et al., 2006). More women than men suffer from ASAD. ASAD often occurs along with other psychiatric conditions, especially other anxiety disorders or mood disorders (Manicavasagar et al., 2009). Abelli et al. (2010) concluded that the platelet 18-kDa translocator protein (TSPO) expression may be a useful biological marker of adult separation anxiety co-occurring with other anxiety and mood disorders, including bipolar disorder. In Silove et al. study (2010) adult separation anxiety disorder was associated with PTSD, but not with complicated grief or depression. Results of Silove and colleagues study found that patients with adult separation anxiety disorder (ASAD) may have elevated early separation anxiety scores but this association is unique in females only. Amongst anxiety patients, those with ASAD recorded more severe symptoms of depression, anxiety and stress, higher neuroticism scores, and greater levels of disability (Silove et al., 2010).

12. The therapeutic methods of treating separation anxiety disorder

Children are usually brought to the clinician when SAD results in school refusal or somatic symptoms such as recurrent pain of different parts of body occur. Anxiety disorders can be managed by using non-pharmacological and pharmacological options, or a combination of them. Treatment of the separation anxiety disorder includes behavioural, cognitive, and individual psychotherapies, as well as parent counselling and guiding teachers on how to help the child. The most recent evidence for empirically supported treatments shows that the cognitive-behavioural therapy (CBT) and selective serotonin-reuptake inhibitors (SSRI) are the most efficacious for the improvement of the children health with the separation anxiety disorder (Fisher et al., 2006). Different classes of medications have been used in pediatric anxiety disorders, including benzodiazepines, tricyclics and buspirone. Newer antidepressants (SSRIs and beyond) have had fewer side effects, lower toxicity in overdose and a broader range of indications (Masi et al., 2002). Cognitive behavioural therapies have the best evidence-based support for the treatment of the separation anxiety disorder in children and adolescents (Seligman & Ollendick, 2011). Research findings have supported the efficacy of cognitive behavioural therapy in reducing anxiety symptoms and increasing function in anxious children (Schneider et al., 2011). The outcomes of a randomized clinical trial evaluating an individual cognitive-behavioural, family-based cognitive-behavioural, and family-based education, support and attention treatment for anxious youth, also with diagnosis of separation anxiety disorder showed good efficacy of the psychotherapy (Suveg et al., 2009a). Hirshfeld-Becker et al. (2010) found that developmentally modified parent-child CBT may show a promise in 4 to 7 year-old children. The cognitive-behavioural therapy for the anxious youth, also with separation anxiety disorder could change in emotion regulation. The treated youth exhibited a reduction in anxiety and increased anxiety self-efficacy and emotional awareness at post-treatment (Suveg et al., 2009b). Children's coping skills have been considered to be protective factors in childhood anxiety disorders (Dadds et al., 1999). Learning to use active coping strategies, distraction strategies, and problem-focused rather than avoidant-focused coping have been encouraged in the anxious youths (Ayers et al., 1996). Results of the acute outcomes of the Child/Adolescent Anxiety Multimodal Study (CAMS) trial showed that all active treatments of separation anxiety disorder (cognitive-behaviour therapy or sertraline) were superior to pill placebo, that combination treatment (cognitive-behaviour therapy and SSRI) was superior to the monotherapies, and that the monotherapies were equivalent (Compton et al., 2010). The severity of the anxiety in children was found to be reduced with both cognitive behavioural therapy and sertraline (Walkup et al., 2008). Fluoxetine as others selective serotonin-reuptake inhibitors, seemed useful and well tolerated for the acute treatment of the anxious youths, among others in separation anxiety (Birmaher et al., 2003). Non-pharmacological treatments are the first choice approach in separation anxiety disorder or school refusal. This kind of treatment contains psychoeducational intervention (education of child and parents, collaboration with school personnel, training to increase child's autonomy and competence) and psychotherapeutic approach (behavioural, cognitive-behavioural, psychodynamic or family therapy. Pharmacological management of separation anxiety disorder uses mainly selective serotonin reuptake inhibitors; previously used tricyclic antidepressants, possibly benzodiazepines or buspirone. The use of new drugs (mirtazapine, venlafaxine, nefazodone) needs to be assessed.

13. References

Abelli, M., Chelli, B., Costa, B., Lari, L., Cardini, A., Gesi, C., Muti, M., Lucacchini, A., Martini, C., Cassano, G.B. & Pini, S. (2010) Reductions in Platelet 18-kDa Translocator Protein Density Are Associated with Adult Separation Anxiety in Patients with Bipolar Disorder. *Neuropsychobiology*, Vol. 62, No. 2, pp. 98-103.

Albano, A.M., Chorpita, B.F., & Barlow, D.H. (2003) Childhood anxiety disorders, In: *Child Psychopathology* (2nd ed.), Mash, E.J. & Barkley, R.A. (Eds.), pp. 279-329, Guilford Press, New York.

Allen, J.L., Lavallee, K.L., Herren, C., Ruhe, K., & Schneider, S. (2010) DSM-IV criteria for childhood separation anxiety disorder: Informant, age, and sex differences, *Journal of Anxiety Disorders*, Vol. 24, No. 8, (December 2010), pp. 946-52.

Allen, J.L., Blatter-Meunier, J., Ursprung, A. & Schneider, S. (2010) Maternal Daily Diary Report in the Assessment of Childhood Separation Anxiety. *Journal of Clinical Child & Adolescent Psychology*, Vol. 39, No. 2, pp. 252-259.

American Psychiatric Association (2000) *Diagnostic and Statistical Manual of Mental Disorders* (4th ed., Text Revision) (DMS-IV-TR) American Psychiatric Association, Washington, DC.

Anderson, J.C., Williams, S., McGee, R., et al. (1987) DSM-III disorders in preadolescent children. Prevalence in a large sample from the general population, *Archives of General Psychiatry*, Vol. 44, No. 1, pp. 69-76.

Aschenbrand, S.G., Kendall, P.C., Webb, A., Safford, S.M. & Flannery-Schroeder, E. (2003) Is Childhood Separation Anxiety Disorder a Predictor of Adult Panic Disorder and A goraphobia? A Seven-Year Longitudinal Study. *Journal of the American Academy of Child & Adolescent Psychiatry*. Vol. 42, No.12, pp.1478-1485.

Axelson, D.A. & Birmaher, B.(2001) Relation between anxiety and depressive disorders in childhood and adolescence. *Depression and Anxiety*, Vol.14, pp.67–78, 2001.

Ayers, T. S., Sandler, I. N., West, S. G., & Roosa, M. W. (1996) A dispositional and situational assessment of children's coping: Testing alternative models of coping, *Journal of Personality and Social Psychology*, Vol. 64, pp. 923-958.

Bahali, K., & Tahiroğlu, A.Y. (2010) School Refusal: Clinical Features, Diagnosis and Treatment, *Current Approaches in Psychiatry / Psikiyatride Guncel Yaklasimlar*, Vol. 2, No. 3, pp. 362-383.

Bar-Haim, Y., Lamy, D., Pergamin, L., Bakermans-Kranenburg, M.J. & van IJzendoorn, M.H. (2007) Threat-related attentional bias in anxious and nonanxious individuals: a meta-analytic study. *Psychological Bulletin*, Vol.133, No.1, pp.:1-24.

Battaglia, M., Bertella, S., Politi, E., Bernardeschi, L., Perna, G., Gabriele, A. & Bellodi L. (1995) Age of onset of panic disorder: influence of familial liability to the disease and of childhood separation anxiety disorder. *American Journal of Psychiatry*, Vol. 152, No.9, pp.1362-4.

Beernink, A.C.E., Swinkels, S.H., & Buitelaar, J.K. (2007). Problem behavior in a community sample of 14- and 19-month-old children: Common versus uncommon behaviors, structure, and stability. *European Child and Adolescent Psychiatry*, No.16, pp. 271–280.

Beidel, D.C. & Turner, S.M. (1997). At Risk for Anxiety: I.Psychopathology in the Offspring of Anxious Parents.*Journal of American Academy of Child and Adolescent Psychiatry.* Vol. 36, No.7, pp. 918-924.

Berg, I., Butler, A., Franklin, J., Hayes, H., Lucas, C., & Sims, R. (1993) DSM-III-R Disorders, social factors and management of school attendance problems in the normal population, *The Journal of Child Psychology and Psychiatry*, Vol. 34, pp. 1187–1203.

Berg, I. & Jackson, A. (1985) Teenage school refusers grow-up: a follow up study of 168 subjects, ten years on average after in-patient treatment, *The British Journal of Psychiatry*, Vol. 147, pp. 366-70.

Bernstein, G.A., Warren, S.L., Massie, E.D. & Thuras, P.D. (1999) Family dimensions in anxious-depressed school refusers, *Journal of Anxiety Disorders*, Vol. 13, pp. 513–528.

Bernstein, G.A., Massie, E.D., Thuras, P.D., Perwien, A.R., Borchardt, C.M. & Crosby, R.D. (1997) Somatic symptoms in anxious-depressed school refusers. *Journal of the American Academy of Child and Adolescents Psychiatry*, Vol. 36, pp. 661–668.

Biederman, J., Petty, C., Faraone, S.V., Henin, A., Hirshfeld-Becker, D., Pollack, M.H., de Figueiredo, S., Feeley, R. & Rosenbaum, J.F. (2006) Effects of parental anxiety disorders in children at high risk for panic disorder: A controlled study, *Journal of Affective Disorders*, Vol. 94, No. 1-3, pp. 191-197.

Biederman, J., Faraone, S.V., Marrs, A., Moore, P., Garcia, J., Ablon, S., Mick, E., Gershon, J. & Kearns, M.E. (1997) Panic disorder and agoraphobia in consecutively referred children and adolescents. *Journal of the American Academy of Child and Adolescents Psychiatry*, Vol. 36, No. 2, pp. 214-23.

Bird, H.R., Canino, G., & Rubio-Stipec, M. (1988) Estimates of the prevalence of childhood maladjustment in a community survey in Puerto Rico. The use of combined measures, *Archives of General Psychiatry*, Vol. 45, No. 12, pp. 1120-6.

Bird, H. R., Gould, M. S., Yager, T,, Staghezza, B. & Canino, G. (1989) Risk factors for maladjustment in Puerto Rican children, *Journal of the American Academy of Child and Adolescent Psychiatry*, Vol. 28, pp. 847-850.

Birmaher, B., Axelson, D.A., Monk, K., Kalas, C., Clark, D.B., Ehmann, M., Bridge, J., Heo, J. & Brent, D.A. (2003) Fluoxetine for the treatment of childhood anxiety disorders, *Journal of the American Academy of Child and Adolescent Psychiatry*, Vol. 42, No. 4, (April 2003), pp. 415-432.

Bittner, A., Egger, H.L., Erkanli, A., Jane Costello, E., Foley, D.L. & Angold, A. (2007) What do childhood anxiety disorders predict?, *The Journal of Child Psychology and Psychiatry*, Vol. 48, No. 12, (December 2007), pp. 1174-83.

Borchardt, C.M., Giesler, J., Bernstein, G.A., et al. (1994) A comparison of inpatient and outpatient school refusers, *Child Psychiatry and Human Development*, Vol. 24, No. 4, pp. 255-64.

Bowen, R.C., Offord, D.R. & Boyle, M.H. (1990) The prevalence of overanxious disorder and separation anxiety disorder: results from the Ontario Child Health Study, *Journal of the American Academy of Child and Adolescent Psychiatry*, Vol. 29, No. 5, pp. 753-8.

Bradley, S.J. & Hood, J.(1993) Psychiatrically referred adolescents with panic attacks: presenting symptoms, stressors and comorbidity. *Journal of the American Academy of Child and Adolescent Psychiatry*, Vol. 32, No. 4, pp. 826-9.

Bremner, J.D., Innis, R.B., White, T., Fujita, M., Silbersweig, D., Goddard. A.W., Staib, L., Stern, E., Cappiello, A., Woods, S., Baldwin, R. & Charney, D.S. (2000) SPECT [I-

123]iomazenil measurement of the benzodiazepine receptor in panic disorder. *Biological Psychiatry*, Vol. 47, pp. 96-106.

Breton, J.J., Bergeron, L., Valla, J.P., et al. (1999) Quebec Child Mental Health Survey: prevalence of DSM-III-R mental health disorders, *The Journal of Child Psychology and Psychiatry*, Vol. 40, No. 3, pp. 375-84.

Brumariu, L.E. & Kerns, K.A. (2010) Mother-child attachment patterns and different types of anxiety symptoms: is there specificity of relations? *Child Psychiatry and Human Development*, Vol. 41, No. 6, (December 2010), pp. 663-74.

Brückl, T.M., Wittchen, H-U., Höfler, M., Pfister, H., Schneider, S. & Lieb R. (2007) Childhood Separation Anxiety and the Risk of Subsequent Psychopathology: Results from a Community Study. *Psychotherapy and Psychosomatics*, Vol. 76, pp. 47-56.

Bystritsky, A., Pontillo, D., Powers, M., Sabb, F.W., Craske, M.G. & Bookheimer, S.Y. (2001) Functional MRI changes during panic anticipation and imagery exposure. *Neuroreport*, Vol. 12, No.18, pp. 3953-7.

Capps L, Sigman M, Sena R., Heoker, B. & Whalen C. (1996) Fear, anxiety, and perceived control in children of agoraphobic parents. *The Journal of Child Psychology and Psychiatry*, Vol. 37, No. 4, pp. 445-52.

Carthy, T., Horesh, N., Apter, A., Edge, M.D. & Gross, J.J. (2010a) Emotional reactivity and cognitive regulation in anxious children, *Behaviour Research & Therapy*, Vol. 48, No. 5, (May 2010), pp. 384-393.

Carthy, T., Horesh, N., Apter, A. & Gross, J.J. (2010) Patterns of Emotional Reactivity and Regulation in Children with Anxiety Disorders, *Journal of Psychopathology & Behavioral Assessment*, Vol. 32, No. 1, (March 2010b), pp. 23-36.

Compton, S.N., Walkup, J.T., Albano, A.M., Piacentini, J.C., Birmaher, B., Sherrill, J.T., Ginsburg, G.S., Ryan, M.A., McCracken, J.T., Waslick, B.D., Iyengar, S., Kendall, Ph.C. & March, J.S. (2010) Child/Adolescent Anxiety Multimodal Study (CAMS): rationale, design, and methods. *Child and Adolescent Psychiatry and Mental Health*, Vol. 4, pp. 1-15.

Costello, E.J., Angold, A., Burns, B.J., et al. (1996) The Great Smoky Mountains Study of Youth: goals, design, methods, and the prevalence of DSM-III-R disorders, *Archives of General Psychiatry*, Vol. 53, No. 12, pp. 1129-36.

Costello, E.J. & Angold, A. (1995) Developmental epidemiology, In: *Manual of Developmental Psychopathology*, Cicchetti, D. & Cohen, D. (Eds.), Vol. I, pp. 23-56, Wiley, New York.

Cummins, T.K., Ninan, P.T. (2002). The neurobiology of anxiety in children and adolescents. *International Review of Psychiatry*, Vol. 14; 114-128.

Dabkowska, M. (1999) Risk factors for school phobia. *Lek i Depresja*, Vol. 4, No. 3, pp.186-196.

Dabkowska, M. (2002) School phobia in children with anxiety disorders, *Psychiatria w Praktyce Ogolnolekarskiej*, Vol. 2, No. 3, pp. 167–170.

Dabkowska, M. (2006) The somatic mask of school phobia, *Pediatria Polska*, Vol. 81, No. 11, pp. 839-843.

Dabkowska, M. (2007) Basic reasons for school refusal behaviour by school children and their parents, *Psychiatria i Psychologia Kliniczna*, Vol. 7, No. 2, pp. 76-83.

Dadds, M.R., Holland, D.E., Laurens, KR.., Mullins, M., Barrett, P.M. & Spence, S.H. (1999). Early Intervention and Prevention of Anxiety Disorders in Children: Results at 2-Year Follow-Up. *Journal of Consulting and Clinical Psychology*, Vol. 67, No. 1, 145-150.

Dadds, M.R., Paula, M. & Barrett, P.M. (2001) Practitioner Review: Psychological Management of Anxiety Disorders in Childhood, *The Journal of Child Psychology and Psychiatry*, Vol. 42, No. 8, pp. 999-1011.

Davis M. (1992). The role of the amygdala in conditioned fear. In: Aggleton J.P. (Ed.), The Amygdala: Neurobiological Aspacts of Emotion, Memory and Mental Disfunction (pp.255-305). Wiley-Liss: New York.

De Bellis M.D., Casey, B.J., Dahl, R.E., Birmaher, B., Williamson, D.E., Thomas, K.M., Axelson,

D.A., Frustaci, K., Boring, A.M., Hall, J. & Ryan, N.D. (2000) A pilot study of amygdala volumes in pediatric generalized anxiety disorder. *Biological Psychiatry*, Vol. 48, No.1, pp.51-7.

De Bellis, M.D., Keshavan, M.S., Shifflett, H., Iyengar, S., Dahl, R.E., Axelson, D.A., Birmaher, B., Hall, J., Moritz, G. & Ryan, N.D.(2002) Superior temporal gyrus volumes in pediatric generalized anxiety disorder. *Biological Psychiatry*. Vol. 51, No. 7, pp. 553-62.

De Bellis, M.D. & Keshavar, M.S. (2003) Sex differences in brain maturation in maltreatment-related pediatric PTSD. *Neuroscience & Biobehavioral Reviews*, Vol. 27, No.1-2, pp.103-17.

De Bellis, M.D., Kuchibhatla & M. Cerebellar volumes in pediatric maltreatment-related PTSD. (2006) *Biological Psychiatry*.Vol.60, No. 7, pp. 697-703.

Deltito, J.A. & Hahn, R. (1993) A three-generational presentation of separation anxiety, *Psychopharmacology Bulletin*, Vol. 29, No. 2, pp. 189-93.

Domschke K., Zwanzger P. (2008). GABAergic and Endocannabinoid Dysfunction in Anxiety Future Therapeutic Targets? *Current Pharmaceutical Design*, Vol. 14, pp. 3508-3517.

Ebesutani, Ch, Bernstein, A., Nakamura, B.J., Chorpita, B.F. & Weisz, J.R. (2010) A Psychometric Analysis of the Revised Child Anxiety and Depression Scale—Parent Version in a Clinical Sample. *Journal of Abnormal Child Psychology*, Vol. 38, No.2, pp. 249-260.

Egger, H.L., Costello, E.J. & Angold, A. (2003) School refusal and psychiatric disorders: a community study, *Journal of the American Academy of Child and Adolescent Psychiatry*, Vol. 42, No. 7, (July 2003), pp. 797-807.

Emslie, G.J. (2008) Pediatric anxiety: underrecognized and undertreated, *The New England Journal of Medicine*, Vol. 359, No. 26, pp. 2835-2836.

Etkin, A. & Wager, T.D. (2007) Functional Neuroimaging of Anxiety: A Meta-Analysis of Emotional Processing in PTSD, Social Anxiety Disorder, and Specific Phobia. *American Journal of Psychiatry*, Vol. 164, pp. 1476-1488.

Eysenck, M.W., Derakshan, N., Santos, R. & Calvo, M.G. (2007) Anxiety and cognitive performance: attentional control theory. *Emotion*, Vol.7, No. 2, pp. 336-53.

Fagiolini, A., Shear, M.K., Cassano, G.B. & Frank, E. (1998) Is lifetime separation anxiety a manifestation of a panic spectrum? *CNS Spectrums*, Vol. 3, No.4, pp. 63-72.

Fisher, P.H., Tobkes, J.L., Kotcher, L. & Masia-Warner, C. (2006) Psychosocial and pharmacological treatment for pediatric anxiety disorders, *Expert Review of Neurotherapeutics*, Vol. 6, No. 11, (November 2006), pp. 1707-19.

Flakierska-Praquin, N., Lindstrom, M. & Gillberg, C. (1997) School phobia with separation anxiety disorder: a comparative 20- to 29-year follow-up study of 35 school refusers, *Comprehensive Psychiatry*, Vol. 38, pp. 17–22.

Fontaine, R., Breton, G., Dery, R., Fontaine & Elie, R. (1990) Temporal lobe abnormalities in panic disorder:an MRI study. *Biological Psychiatry*, 27(3):304-10.

Forbes, E.E., May, J.C., Siegle, G.J., Ladouceur, C.D., Ryan, N.D., Carter, C.S., Birmaher, B., Axelson, D.A. & Dahl, R.E. (2006) Reward-related decision -making in pediatric major depressive disorder: an functional magnetic resonance imaging study. *Journal of Child Psychology and Psychiatry*, Vol. 47, No.10, pp. 1031- 1040.

Francis, G., Last, C.G. & Strauss, C.C. (1987) Expression of separation anxiety disorder: the role of age and gender, *Child Psychiatry and Human Development*, Vol.18, No.2, pp. 82-9.

Gibb, S.J., Fergusson, D.M. & Horwood, L.J. (2011) Relationship separation and mental health problems: findings from a 30-year longitudinal study, *Australian and New Zealand Journal of Psychiatry*, Vol. 45, No. 2, (February 2011), pp. 163-169.

Grills, A.E. & Ollendick, T.H. (2003) Multiple informant agreement and the Anxiety Disorders Interview Schedule for Parents and Children, *Journal of the American Academy of Child and Adolescent Psychiatry*, Vol. 42, pp. 30-40.

Grin-Yatsenko, V.A., Baas, I., Ponomarev, V.A. & Kropotov, J.D. (2010) Independent component approach to the analysis of EEG recordings at early stages of depressive disorders. *Clinical Neurophysiology*, Vol. 121, No.3, pp. 281-289.

Grillon, C., Dierker, L. & Merikangas, K.R.(1997) Startle Modulation in Children at Risk for Anxiety Disorders and/or Alcoholism. *Journal of the American Academy of Child and Adolescent* Psychiatry, Vol. 36, No.7, pp. 925-932.

Guyer, A.E., Nelson, E.E., Perez-Edgar, K., Hardin, M.G., Roberson-Nay, R., Monk, C.S., Bjork, J.M., Henderson, H.A., Pine, D.S., Fox, N.A. & Ernst, M. (2006) Striatal functional alteration in adolescents characterized by early childhood behavioral inhibition. *Journal of Neuroscience*, Vol. 26, pp. 6399-6405.

Hirshfeld-Becker, D.R., Masek, B., Henin, A., Blakely, L.R., Pollock-Wurman, R.A., McQuade, J., DePetrillo, L., Briesch, J., Ollendick, T.H., Rosenbaum, J.F. & Biederman, J. (2010) Cognitive Behavioral Therapy for 4- to 7-Year-Old Children With Anxiety Disorders: A Randomized Clinical Trial. *Journal of Consulting & Clinical Psychology*,Vol.78, No. 4, pp. 498-510.

Horn, PJ. & Wuyek, L.A. (2010) Anxiety disorders as a risk factor for subsequent depression. *International Journal of Psychiatry in Clinical Practice*, Vol. 14, No.4, pp. 244-247.

In-Albon, T., Kossowsky, J. & Schneider, S. (2010) Vigilance and Avoidance of Threat in the Eye Movements of Children with Separation Anxiety Disorder, *Journal of Abnormal Child Psychology*, Vol. 38, No. 2, (February 2010), pp. 225-235.

Johnson, A.M., Falstein, E.I. & Szureck, S.A. (1941) School phobia, *American Journal of Orthopsychiatry*, Vol. 11, pp. 702–711.

Kearney, C.A. & Albano, A.M. (2000) When children refuse school: A cognitive-behavioral therapy approach/*Therapist's guide*, The Psychological Corporation, San Antonio, TX.

Kearney, C.A. (2002) Identifying the function of school refusal behavior: A revision of the School Refusal Assessment Scale, *Journal of Psychopathology and Behavioral Assessment*, Vol. 24, pp. 235-245.

Kearney, C.A. (2008) School absenteeism and school refusal behavior in youth: A contemporary review, *Clinical Psychology Review*, Vol. 28, No. 3, pp. 451-471.

Kearney, C.A. (2006) Solutions to school refusal for parents and kids: Pinpoint and address reinforcers of the child's behavior, *Current Psychiatry*, Vol. 5, No. 12, (December 2006), pp. 67-69, 73-76, 78, 83.

Kearney, C.A. & Hugelshofer, D.S. (2000) Systemic and Clinical Strategies for Preventing School Refusal Behavior in Youth, *Journal of Cognitive Psychotherapy*, Vol. 14, No. 1, pp. 51-65.

Kearney, C.A. & Silverman, W.K. (1996) The evolution and reconciliation of taxonomic strategies for school refusal behavior, *Clinical Psychology: Science and Practice*, Vol. 3, pp. 339-354.

Kendall, P.C., Compton, SN., Walkup, JT., Birmaher, B., Albano, A.M., Sherrill, J., Ginsburg, G., Rynn, M., McCracken, J., Gosch, E., Keeton, C., Bergman, L., Sakolsky, D., Suveg, C., Iyengar, S., March, J. & Piacentini, J. (2010) Clinical characteristics of anxiety disordered youth. *Journal of Anxiety Disorders*, Vol. 24, No.3, pp. 360-365.

Kindt, M., & Hout, M. van den (2001) Selective attention and anxiety: A perspective on developmental issues and the causal status. *Journal of Psychopathology and Behavioral Assessment*, 23, 193-2002

Kindt, M., Bogels, S. & Morren, M. (2003) Processing bias in children with separation anxiety disorder, social phobia and generalised anxiety disorder. *Behaviour Change*, Vol. 20, No.3, pp.143-150.

King, N. J. & Bernstein, G. A. (2001): School Refusal in Children and Adolescents: A Review of the past 10 Years. *Journal of the American Academy of Child and Adolescent Psychiatry*, 40:2 197–205.

King, N., Ollendick, T.H. & Tonge, B.J. (1995) *School refusal: assessment and treatment*, Allyn & Bacon, Needham Heights, MA.

Klein, R.G.(1995) Is panic disorder associated with childhood separation anxiety disorder? *Clinical Neuropharmacology*, Vol. 18 (suppl 2), pp. 7-14.

Last, C.G., Francis, G., Hersen, M., et al. (1987) Separation anxiety and school phobia: a comparison using DSM III criteria, *American Journal of Psychiatry*, Vol. 144, No. 5, pp. 653-657.

Last, C.G., Hansen, C. & Franco, N. (1998) Cognitive-behavioral treatment of school phobia, *Journal of the American Academy of Child and Adolescent Psychiatry*, Vol. 37, pp. 404–411.

Last, C.G., Hersen, M., Kazdin, A., Orvaschel, H. & Perrin, S. (1991) Anxiety Disorders in Children and Their Families. *Archives of General Psychiatry*, Vol. 48, No.10, pp.928-93.

Last, C.G., Perrin, S., Hersen, M., et al. (1992) DSM-III-R anxiety disorders in children: sociodemographic and clinical characteristics, *Journal of the American Academy of Child and Adolescent Psychiatry*, Vol. 31, No.6, pp. 1070-6.

Lavigne, J.V., LeBailly, S.A., Hopkins, J., Gouze, K.R. & Binns, H.J. (2009) The Prevalence of ADHD, ODD, Depression, and Anxiety in a Community Sample of 4-Year-Olds,

Journal of Clinical Child and Adolescent Psychology, Vol. 38, No. 3, (May/June 2009), pp. 315-328.

Lewinsohn, P.M., Hops, H., Roberts, R.E., et al. (1993) Adolescent psychopathology: I. Prevalence and incidence of depression and other DSM-III-R disorders in high school students, *Journal of Abnormal Psychology*, Vol. 102, No. 1, pp. 133-44.

Lewinsohn, P.M., Holm-Denoma, J.M., Small, J.W., Seeley, J.R. & Joiner, T.E. Jr. (2008) Separation anxiety disorder in childhood as a risk factor for future mental illness, *Journal of the American Academy of Child and Adolescent Psychiatry*, Vol. 47, No. 5, (May 2008), pp. 548-55.

Lipsitz, J.D., Martin, L.Y., Mannuzza, S., Chapman, T.F., Liebowitz, M.R., Klein, D.F. & Fyer, A.J. (1994) Childhood separation anxiety disorder in patients with adult anxiety disorder. *American Journal of Psychiatry*, Vol. 151, No. 6, pp. 927-9.

Lucey J.A., Corvin A. (2005). *Zaburzenia lękowe. In: Rybakowski J., Rybakowski F. (Ed.), Psychiatria Sedno, tom 1.* Elsevier. Urban and Partner: Wroclaw.

Manassis, K. & Hood, J. (1998) Individual and familial predictors of impairment in childhood anxiety disorders, *Journal of the American Academy of Child and Adolescent Psychiatry*, Vol. 37, pp. 428–434.

Manicavasagar, V. & Silove, D. (1997) Is there an adult form of separation anxiety disorder? brief clinical report, *The Australian and New Zealand Journal of Psychiatry*, Vol. 31, No. 2, (April 1997), pp. 299-303.

Manicavasagar, V., Silove, D., Marnane, C. & Wagner, R. (2009) Adult attachment styles in panic disorder with and without comorbid adult separation anxiety disorder, *The Australian and New Zealand Journal of Psychiatry*, Vol. 43, No. 2, pp. 167-172.

Manicavasagar, V., Silove, D. & Hadzi-Pavlovic D. (1998) Subpopulations of early separation anxiety: relevance to risk of adult anxiety disorder. *Journal of Anxiety Disorders*, Vol. 48, No. 2-3, pp.181-90.

Manicavasagar, V., Silove, D., Marnane, C., Wagner, R. (2009) Adult attachment styles in panic disorder with and without comorbid adult separation anxiety disorder. *Australian & New Zealand Journal of Psychiatry*, Vol. 43, No. 2, pp.167-172.

Malizia, A.L., Cunningham, V.J., Bell, C.J., Liddle, P.F., Jones, T. & Nutt, Q.J. (1998) Decreased brain GABA (A) -benzodiazepine receptor binding in panic disorder: preliminary results from a quantitative PET study. *Archives of General Psychiatry*, Vol. 55, 715-720.

Martini, J., Knappe, S., Beesdo-Baum, K., Lieb, R. & Wittchen, H.U. (2010) Anxiety disorders before birth and self-perceived distress during pregnancy: Associations with maternal depression and obstetric, neonatal and early childhood outcomes, *Early Human Development*, Vol. 86, No. 5, (May 2010), pp. 305-310.

Masi, G., Favilla,. L, Mucci, M. & Millepiedi S. (2000) Depressive comorbidity in children and adolescents with generalized anxiety disorder. *Child Psychiatry & Human Development*, Vol.30, No. 3, pp. 205-15.

Masi, G., Millepiedi, S. & Mucci, M (2002). Efficacy of newer antidepressants for childhood anxiety disorders. *Expert Review of Neurotherapeutics*. Vol. 2, No. 4, pp. 523-31.

Masi, G., Mucci, M., Favilla, L., Romano, R. & Poli P. (1999) Symptomatology and comorbidity of generalized anxiety disorder in children and adolescents. *Comprehensive Psychiatry*, Vol. 40, No.3, pp. 210-5.

Masi, G., Mucci, M. & Millepiedi, M. (2001) Separation Anxiety Disorder in Children and Adolescents. Epidemiology, Diagnosis and Management. *CNS Drugs*, Vol. 15, No. 2, pp. 93-104.

Massana, J., Mercader, J.M., Gomez, B., Tobena, A.& Salamero, M. (2003)Amygdalar atrophy in panic disorder patients detected by volumetric magnetic resonance imaging. *Neuroimage*, Vol. 19, No.1, pp. 80-90.

Mazzone, L,, Ducci, F., Scoto, M.C., Passaniti, E., D'Arrigo, V.G. & Vitiello B.(2007) The role of anxiety symptoms in school performance in a community sample of children and adolescents. *BMC Public Health*, Vol.7, pp. 347.

McGee, R., Feehan, M., Williams, S., et al. (1990) DSM-III disorders in a large sample of adolescents, *Journal of the American Academy of Child and Adolescent Psychiatry*, Vol. 29, No. 40, pp. 611-9.

Merikangas, K.R., Avenevoli, S., Dierker, L. & Grillon, C. (1999) Vulnerability factors among children at risk for anxiety disorders. *Biological Psychiatry*, Vol. 46, pp.1523–1535.

Micco, J.A., Henin, A., Biederman, J., Rosenbaum, J.F., Petty, C., Rindlaub, L.A., Murphy, M. & Hirshfeld-Becker, D.R. (2009) Executive functioning in offspring at risk for depression and anxiety. *Depression and Anxiety*, 26(9):780-90.

Milham, M.P., Nugent, A.C., Drevets, W.C., Dickstein, D.P., Leibenluft, E., Ernst, M., Charney, D. & Pine, D.S.2005. Selective reduction in amygdala volume in pediatric anxiety disorders: a voxel-based morphometry investigations. *Biological Psychiatry*, Vol. 57, No.9, pp.961-6.

Monga, S., Birmaher, B., Chiappetta, L., Brent, D., Kaufman, J., Bridge, J. & Cully M. (2000) Screen for Child Anxiety-Related Emotional Disorders (SCARED): convergent and divergent validity. *Depression & Anxiety*, Vol.12, No. 2, pp. 85-91.

Mroczkowski, M.M., Goes, F.S., Riddle, M.A., Grados, M.A., Joseph, B.O., Greenberg, B.D., Fyer, A.J., McCracken, J.T., Rauch, S.L., Murphy, D.L., Knowles, J.A., Piacentini, J. ,Cullen, B., Rasmussen, S.A., Geller, D.A., Pauls, D.L., Liang, K-Y., Nestadt, G. & Samuels, J.F. (2011) Separation anxiety disorder in OCD. *Depression and Anxiety*, Vol. 28, pp. 256-262.

Mychailyszyn, M.P., Mendez, J.L. & Kendall, P.C. (2010) School functioning in youth with and without anxiety disorders: Comparisons by diagnosis and comorbidity. *School Psychology Review*, Vol. 39, No. 1, pp. 106-121.

Ogliari, A., Spatola, Ch.A., Pesenti-Gritti, P.M., Emanuela, P., Luana, S., Maria, A., Battaglia, M. & Fagnani, C. (2010) The role of genes and environment in shaping co-occurrence of DSM-IV defined anxiety dimensions among Italian twins aged 8–17, *Journal of Anxiety Disorders*, Vol. 24, No. 4, (May 2010), pp. 433-439.

O'Neil, K., Podell, J., Benjamin, C. & Kendall, P. (2010) Comorbid Depressive Disorders in Anxiety-disordered Youth: Demographic, Clinical, and Family Characteristics. *Child Psychiatry & Human Development*, Vol. 41, No.3, pp. 330-341.

O'Neil, K.A., Conner B.T. & Kendall P.C. (2011) Internalizing disorders and substance use disorders in youth: Comorbidity, risk, temporal order, and implications for intervention. *Clinical Psychology Review*, Vol. 31, No. 1, pp.104-112.

Ontiveros, A., Fontaine, R., Breton, G., Elie, R., Fontaine, S.& Dery, R. (1989) Correlation of severity of panic disorder and neuroanatomical changes on MRI. *The Journal of Neuropsychiatry and Clinical Neurosciences*, Vol.1, No. 4, pp. 404-8.

Pine, D.S. & Grun, J. (1999) Childhood anxiety: integrating developmental psychopathology and affective neuroscience, *Journal of Child and Adolescent Psychopharmacology*, Vol. 9, No. 1, pp. 1-12.

Pine, D.S, Wasserman, G.A. & Workman, S.B. (1999) Memory and anxiety in prepubertal boys at risk for delinquency. *Journal of the American Academy of Child and Adolescents Psychiatry,* Vol. 38, pp. 1024–1031.

Pine, D.S., Cohen, P., Gurley, D., Brook, J. & Ma, Y. (1998) The risk for early adulthood anxiety and depressive disorders in adolescents with anxiety and depressive disorders. *Archives of General Psychiatry*, Vol. 55, No.1, pp. 56-64.

Pini, S., Abelli, M., Shear, K.M., Cardini, A., Lari, L., Gesi, C., Muti, M., Calugi, S., Galderisi, S., Troisi, A., Bertolino, A. & Cassano, G.B. (2010) Frequency and clinical correlates of adult separation anxiety in a sample of 508 outpatients with mood and anxiety disorders. *Acta Psychiatrica Scandinavica*, Vol.122, No.1, pp. 40-46.

Prior, M., Sanson, A., Smart, D., et al. (1999) Psychological disorders and their correlates in an Australian community sample of preadolescent children, *The Journal of Child Psychology and Psychiatry*, Vol. 40, No. 4, pp. 563-80.

Quirk, G.J., Armony, J.L. & LeDoux, J.E. (1997) Fear conditioning enhances different temporal components of tone-evoked spike trains in auditory cortex and lateral amygdala. *Neuron,* Vol. 19, No.3, pp. 613-24.

Rapee, R.M. (1997) Potential role of childrearing practices in the development of anxiety and depression, *Clinical Psychology Review,* Vol. 17, No.1, pp. 47-67.

Ressler K.J., Nemeroff C.B. (2000). Research Reviews. Role of serotonergic and noradrenegic systems in the pathophysiology of depression and anxiety disorders. *Depression and Anxiety,* Vol. 12, Suppl. 1, pp.2–19.

Roberson-Nay, R., Klein, D.F., Klein, R.G., Mannuzza, S., Moulton, J.L., Guardino, M. & Pine, D.S. (2010) Carbon Dioxide Hypersensitivity in Separation-Anxious Offspring of Parents with Panic Disorder. *Biological Psychiatry*, Vol. 67, No.12, pp. 1171-1177.

Sala, R., Axelson, D.A., Castro-Fornieles, J., Goldstein, T.R., Ha, W., Liao, F., Gill, M.K., Iyengar, S., Strober, M.A., Goldstein, B.I., Yen, S., Hower, H., Hunt, J., Ryan, N.D., Dickstein, D., Keller, M.B.& Birmaher B.(2010) Comorbid anxiety in children and adolescents with bipolar spectrum disorders: prevalence and clinical correlates. *The Journal of Clinical Psychiatry*, Vol.71, No.10, pp.1344-50.

Schneider, S., Blatter-Meunier, J., Herren, C., Adornetto, C., In-Albon, T., Lavallee, K. (2011) Disorder-Specific Cognitive-Behavioral Therapy for Separation Anxiety Disorder in Young Children: A Randomized Waiting-List-Controlled Trial. *Psychotherapy and Psychosomatics,* Vol.14; 80, No.4, pp.206-215.

Schwartz C.E., Wright C.I., Shin L.M., Kagan J., Rauch S.L. (2003). Inhibited and uninhibited infants „grown up": Adult amygdalar response to novelty. *Science,* Vol. 300, 1952-1953.

Seligman, L.D. & Ollendick, T.H. (2011) Cognitive-behavioral therapy for anxiety disorders in youth, *Child and Adolescent Psychiatric Clinics of North America*, Vol. 20, No. 2, (April 2011), pp. 217-38.

Shaffer, D., Fisher, P., Dulkan, M.K., et al. (1995) The NIMH Diagnostic Interview Schedule for Children Version 2.3 (DISC 2.3): description, acceptability, prevalence rates, and performance in the MACA study, *Journal of the American Academy of Child and Adolescent Psychiatry*, Vol. 35, pp. 865-77.

Shear, K., Jin, R., Meron, R.A., Walters, E. & Kessler, R. (2006) Prevalence and Correlates of Estimated DSM-IV Child and Adult Separation Anxiety Disorder in the National Comorbidity Survey Replication, *American Journal of Psychiatry*, Vol. 163, (June 2006), pp. 1074-1083.

Simon, E. & Bögels, SM. (2009) Screening for anxiety disorders in children. *European Child & Adolescent Psychiatry*, Vol. 18, No. 10, pp. 625-634.

Silove, D., Manicavasaga,r V., O'Connel, D. & Blaszczynski A. (1993) Reported early separation anxiety symptoms in patients with panic and generalized anxiety disorders. *Australian and New Zealand Journal of Psychiatry*, Vol., 27, No.3, pp. 489-94.

Silove, D., Manicavasagar, V., Curti, J. & Blaszczynski, A. (1996) Is early separation anxiety a risk factor for adult panic disorder? a critical review. *Comprehensive Psychiatry*, Vol. 37, No.3, pp. 167-79.

Silove, D.M., Marnane, C.L., Wagner, R., Manicavasagar, V.L. & Rees, S. (2010) The prevalence and correlates of adult separation anxiety disorder in an anxiety clinic. *BMC Psychiatry*,Vol. 10, pp. 21-27.

Skovgaard, A.M., Houmann, T., Christiansen E., Landorph, S.L., Jørgensen, T. (2007) The Prevalence of Mental Health Problems in Children 1½ years of Age - The Copenhagen Child Cohort 2000. *The Journal of Child Psychology and Psychiatry*, Vol. 8, No.1, (January 2007), pp. 62-70.

Soo-churl Cho, Sun-woo Jung, Boong-nyun Kim, Jun-won Hwang, Min-sup Shin, Jae-won Kim, Dong-seon Chungh & Hyo-won Kim (2009) Temperament and character among Korean children and adolescents with anxiety disorders, *European Child and Adolescent Psychiatry*, Vol. 18, No. 1, (January 2009), pp. 60-64.

Suveg, C., Hudson, J.L., Brewer, G., Flannery-Schroeder, E., Gosch, E., Kendall, P.C. (2009a) Cognitive-behavioral therapy for anxiety-disordered youth: Secondary outcomes from a randomized clinical trial evaluating child and family modalities. *Journal of Anxiety Disorders*, Vol. 23, No.3, pp. 341-349.

Suveg, C., Sood, E., Comer, J.S. & Kendall, P.C. (2009b) Changes in Emotion Regulation Following Cognitive-Behavioral Therapy for Anxious Youth. *Journal of Clinical Child & Adolescent Psychology*, Vol. 38, No. 3, pp. 390-401.

Thomas, L.A. & De Bellis, M.D. (2004) Pituitary volumes in pediatric maltreatment- related PTSD. *Biological Psychiatry*, Vol. 55, No.7, pp. 752-8.

Topolski, T.D., Hewitt, J.K., Eaves, L.J., Silberg, J.L., Meyer, J.M., Rutter, R., Pickles, A. & Simonoff, E. (1997) Genetic and Environmental Influences on Child Reports of Manifest Anxiety and Symptoms of Separation Anxiety and Overanxious Disorders: A Community-Based Twin Study, *Behavior Genetics*, Vol. 27, No. I. 1997.

Toren, P., Sadeh, M., Wolmer, L., Eldar, S., Koren, S., Weizman, R. & Laor, N. (2000) Neurocognitive correlates of anxiety disorders in children: A preliminary report. *Journal of Anxiety Disorders* , Vol. 14, pp. ,.239–247.

Uchida, R.R., Del-Ben, CM, Bussato, G.F., Duran, F.L., Guimaraes, F.S., Crippa, J.A., Araujo, D., Santos, A.C. & Graeff, F.G. (2008) Regional gray matter abnormalities in panic disorder: A voxel-based morphometry study. *Psychiatry Research*, Vol. 163, No.1, pp. 21-9.

Van Oort, F.V.A., Greaves-Lord, K., Verhulst, F.C., Ormel, J. & Huizink, A.C. (2009) The developmental course of anxiety symptoms during adolescence: the TRAILS study, *Journal of Child Psychology and Psychiatry*, Vol. 50, No. 10, pp. 1209-1217.

Vasa, R.A., Roberson-Nay, R., Klein, R.G., Mannuzza, S., Moulton, J.L., Guardino, M., Merikangas, A., Carlino, A.R. & Pine, D.S. (2007) Memory deficits in children with and at risk for anxiety disorders. *Depression and Anxiety*, Vol. 24, No. 2, pp. 85-94.

Velez, C.N., Johnson, J. & Cohen, P. (1989) A longitudinal analysis of selected risk factors for childhood psychopathology, *Journal of the American Academy of Child and Adolescent Psychiatry*, Vol. 28, No. 6, pp. 861-4

Verhulst, F.C., van der Ende, J., Ferdinand, R.F., et al. (1997) The prevalence of DSM-III-R diagnoses in a national sample of Dutch adolescents, *Archives of General Psychiatry*, Vol. 54, No. 4, pp. 329-36.

Viaux-Savelon, S., Rabain, D., Aidane, E., Bonnet, P., Montes de Oca, M., Camon-Sénéchal, L., David, M., Couëtoux, F., Wendland, J., Gérardin, P., Mazet, P., Guedeney, A., Keren, M. & Cohen, D. (2010) Phenomenology, psychopathology, and short-term therapeutic outcome of 102 infants aged zero to 12 months consecutively referred to a community-based zero to 3 mental health clinic. *Infant Mental Health Journal*, Vol. 31, No. 2, pp. 242.

Victor, A.M., Bernat, D.H., Bernstein, G.A. & Layne, A.E. (2007) Effects of parent and family characteristics on treatment outcome of anxious children, *Journal of Anxiety Disorders*, Vol. 21, No. 6, pp. 835-48.

von Widdern, S. & Lehmkuhl, G. (2011) How do children with separation anxiety disorder develop after inpatient treatment?, *Praxis Der Kinderpsychologie Und Kinderpsychiatrie*, Vol. 60, No.2, pp.143-57.

Vythilingam, M., Anderson, E.R., Goddard, A., Woods, S.W., Staib, L.H., Charney, D.S. & Bremner, J.D. (2000) Temporal lobe volume in panic disorder- a quantitative MRI study. *Psychiatry* Research, Vol. 99, No. 2, pp. 75-82.

Walkup, J.T., Albano, A.M., Piacentini, J., Birmaher, B., Compton, S.N., Sherrill, J.T., Ginsburg, G.S., Rynn, M.A., McCracken, J., Waslick, B., Iyengar, S., March, J.S. & Kendall, Ph.C. (2008) Cognitive Behavioral Therapy, Sertraline, or a Combination in Childhood Anxiety, *The New England Journal of Medicine*, Vol. 359, No. 26, (December 2008), pp. 2753-2766.

Warner, V., Mufson, L. & Weissman, M.M.(1995) Offspring at High and Low Risk for Depression and Anxiety: Mechanisms of Psychiatric Disorder. *Journal of the American Academy of Child and Adolescent Psychiatry*. Vol. 34, No.6, pp. 786-797.

Warren, S.L., Huston, L., Egeland, B. & Sroufe, L.A. (1997) Child and adolescent anxiety disorders and early attachment, *Journal of the American Academy of Child and Adolescent Psychiatry*, Vol. 36, No. 5, (May 1997), pp. 637-44.

Weems, C.F. & Costa, N. (2005) Developmental differences in the expression of childhood anxiety symptoms and fears, *Journal of the American Academy of Child and Adolescent Psychiatry*, Vol. 44, No. 7, (July 2005), pp. 656-663.

Weissman, M.M; Leckman, J.F., Merikangas, K.R., Gammon, G.D. & Prusoff, B.A. (1984) Depression and Anxiety Disorders in Parents and Children Results From the Yale Family Study. *Archives of General Psychiatry*, Vol. 41, No. 9, pp. 845-852.

World Health Organization (1992) The ICD-10 Classification of Mental and Behavioural Disorders, *World Health Organization*, Geneva.

18

Using Stories to Prevent Anxiety Disorders in a School Context: Dominique's Handy Tricks Program

Jean Gervais[1], Stéphane Bouchard[1,2] and Nadia Gagnier[3]
[1]*Université du Québec en Outaouais,*
[2]*Centre Hospitalier Pierre-Janet*
[3]*Private practice*
Canada

1. Introduction

Several studies have highlighted the significant consequences of anxiety disorders in children (Donovan & Spence 2000; Rapee et al., 2009; Merikangas et al., 2009). These children experience greater difficulties in their social relationships, often suffer from loneliness and are often victims of aggression or rejection from their peers (Last, 1993; March, 1995; Vasey & Dadds, 2001; Morris & March, 2004). Children who suffer from an anxiety disorder can experience fatigue, difficulty concentrating, irritability, and school refusal (Dadds & Barrett, 2001). They are also more susceptible to psychosomatic illnesses and more likely to use health care services (Morris & March, 2004). Along with their distress and their vulnerability to stress, they are more at risk of developing early drug addiction problems or attempting suicide (Morris & March, 2004). Finally, there is a high probability that during adolescence or adulthood they will develop anxiety disorders that will compromise their personal and social lives (Costello et al., 2003; Hirshfield et al., 2008).

The positive results obtained by teaching cognitive-behavioral techniques for anxiety management to young children (Kendall, 1994; Kendall et al., 1997; Barret et al., 2001; Compton et al., 2004; Cartwright-Hatton et al., 2004; Hirshfeld-Becker et al., 2010) militates for the feasibility to develop attitudes and behaviors that could be protective factors for anxiety disorders. Some emotion regulation skills seem to play a key role in the capacity of children to manage their anxiety. These skills include knowledge about physiological reactions to anxiety and stress, the capacity to identify the source of emotion dysregulation and to verbalize their emotions, the ability to restructure dysfunctional thoughts in order to generate emotions that stimulate productive action, the use of problem-solving strategies or of personal support networks, and the capacity to gradually expose oneself to threatening situations (e.g. Miller et al., 2010; Stallard, 2010).

When it comes to developing prevention program, the question arises regarding the relevance of providing prevention interventions to all children or only to children who are at risk (Lowry-Webster et al., 2001). We believe that some cognitive and behavioral characteristics of children who are more vulnerable to anxiety and that are common amongst all anxiety disorders should form the basis and pedagogical strategies of prevention programs. Underlying cognitive characteristics that transcend all anxiety disorders rest on the association between fear and situations that are: perceived as threatening, and / or unexpected, and / or uncontrollable and / or where the child has a poor sense of perceived self-efficacy to cope with the situation. In addition, there is a common transdiagnostic behavioral characteristic that must also be targeted in the prevention of anxiety disorders: avoidance of threatening stimuli (also referred to as safety seeking behaviors). These cognitive and behavioral characteristics are often expressed by children through excessive worries, anxiety sensitivity, avoidance, panic attacks or communicating to adults their feeling that they can't face a problem or a situation (Ollendick & March, 2004).

Learning anxiety management skills could also be of benefit for the majority of children, not only those at risk for a disorder (Hiersfeld-Becker et al., 2002; Lowry-Webster et al., 2001; Stallard, 2010). Anxiety is a normal emotional reaction and most children could benefit from better emotion regulation skills. In addition, many children consider their normal fears as disruptive of their daily activities (Muris et al., 2000). Over the course of their development, all children are faced with various anxiety-producing situations that test their capacity for adaptation (Dacey & Fiore, 2000). These episodes could be related to difficult living conditions (e.g., poverty), a developmental crisis or specific unanticipated events (Becker & Chorpita, 2008). In essence, a universal primary prevention program could be relevant for all children and foster their capacity to adapt to daily problems (Lazarus & Folkman, 1984; Hardy et al., 1993).

2. Using realistic stories to teach coping strategies

Stories and metaphors are already used in treatment programs for anxiety disorders to help adults understand their reactions in order to develop new attitudes and behaviors (Otto, 2000). Using books to teach cognitive-behavioral techniques has also been proven useful with depressed adolescents (Ackerson et al., 1998; Scogin et al., 1990) and with individuals suffering from panic disorders (Gould et al., 1993; Wright et al., 2000). Some books may be self-treatment manuals or simply provide support for the intervention of the therapist. Dominique's Handy Tricks used the latter approach, in which stories about problems in school or at home provide support for a workshop leader to teach relevant anxiety management techniques.

Building a universal and primary prevention program around the use of realistic stories is based on the assumptions that it could: (a) provide meaningful illustrations of key concepts and adaptive behavior, (b) facilitate exchanges with and between participants, (c) normalize emotional reactions to stressors, (d) put into words what the children experiences daily, and (e) offer the opportunity for anxious children to share apprehensions or worries without having to disclose details of events that occurred to them.

The events faced by Dominique and his friends highlight stressors encountered among school-age children, such as having academic problems, being judged by others, being separated from their parents or being ridiculed. Various useful cognitive and behavioral strategies can also be illustrated, such as facing fears, coping with bullying, or confide in adults. The stories also provide non-threatening means of discussing subjects that, if dealt with directly, could embarrass children suffering from an anxiety disorder, induce emotions or reveal confidences that could become detrimental to them (Milich et al., 1992).

In summary, the prevalence of anxiety disorders in children and the fact that all children can benefit from anxiety management techniques lead to the development of a universal prevention program that do not target dysfunctional anxiety up front. The originality of the program rests on the use of storybooks depicting situations that are known stressors for many children, normalize their concerns and set the stage to provide information and exercises to learn the typical cognitive-behavioral techniques used to cope with everyday life stressors as well as anxiety disorders.

3. Description of the program

The program *Dominique's Handy Tricks* (original French title: *Les Trucs de Dominique)* includes 10 illustrated storybooks (on average 50 pages per book) about a little boy named Dominique. In addition to the 10 storybooks, the program uses a children workbook containing the exercises for each of the 10 sessions, a parent's workbook providing information on the program and a workshop leader's guidebook.

3.1 Dominique's stories

Dominique's stories are about situations that are meaningful for elementary school-age children (9 to 12 years old). They were written because they address significant school-age children concerns and worries. Each one explains daily stressors related to the main problem in the book. For example, the book targeting academic problems lead to arguments with parents, worrying about an imminent report card, criticism from the teacher, being made fun of by others, etc. Each of the stories describes typical interactions around the problem, with the adult and child characters adopting attitudes and behaviors that are sometimes appropriate, sometimes not. In the story scenarios, the various characters also express a variety of emotions and ways of thinking as they deal with problems. As part of the program, the aim of these stories is to support the teaching of anxiety prevention and emotion regulation skills by illustrating key concepts or behaviors.

In order to ensure the educational quality of the stories, they were developed by combining deductive and inductive methods. Triangulation of qualitative and quantitative data was performed along the qualitative research methodology proposed by Mayer and Ouellet (1991). For example, the story describing the daily life of a little girl living with an alcoholic mother (used in Session 9) was produced according to the following steps. First, a literature review provided answers to questions such as: What specific everyday problems do children living with alcoholic parents encounter? What are the attitudes and behaviors of peers and adults associated with this family situation? What behaviors are most often associated with resilience? Second, data was collected from about twenty children and their alcoholic parents in order to ensure that the theoretical content was relevant. A draft version of the scenario was then submitted to the same individuals (children and adults), acting as an advisory committee. Focus groups were used to gather primary information on the realism of the narrative, its pertinence, the quality of the information and the accessibility of the language used. Finally, the revised story was submitted to a sample of senior elementary school students. These students filled out a questionnaire of about ten questions aimed at determining the pertinence and educational qualities of the narrative. These questions dealt with how appealing the stories were, their linguistic clarity and the nature of the messages. Once this final verification was complete, the story was illustrated and published. In summary, the qualities of each of the stories (realism, pertinence, accessibility of the language) were subject to field testing prior to their use in the program.

3.2 Children workbook

The general approach for teaching the cognitive-behavioral techniques in this workbook follows a sequence where participants help Dominique or his friends to identify anxiety-producing situations and adopt appropriate strategies to deal with them. Each session highlights one or two specific cognitive or behavioral strategies to reduce or cope with anxiety. These effective coping solutions are called Dominique's handy tricks and homework are given to apply and master these skills at home in stressful situations called "personal challenges".

Many of the exercises in the children's workbook were designed along the same lines as those used in treatment programs for anxiety disorders for children (e.g., Friends and Coping Cat, Kendall, 1992). However, our original approach gives a different angle to these exercises. As universal coping strategies, they are applied in the workshops in reference to a precise section or illustrations in the books. This learning approach is fun and stimulating for children, does not require children to experience an anxiety disorder in order to apply the strategies, as well as favoring instructive interactions between the group and the workshop leader. The core skills addressed in the entire program are (see Table 1): (a) understanding the relationship between stressors, thoughts, emotions/anxiety and actions; (b) detecting early signs of anxiety; (c) cognitive-restructuring; (d) exposure, (e) problem solving and (f) using the social network. Different techniques are used to teach the strategies to children, such as illustrations of key concepts, schematic representation with icons to differentiate stressors, thoughts, emotions and actions, asking children to write in bubbles what a character is thinking or to draw information, etc. The manual and all key concepts are illustrated (see Figure 1).

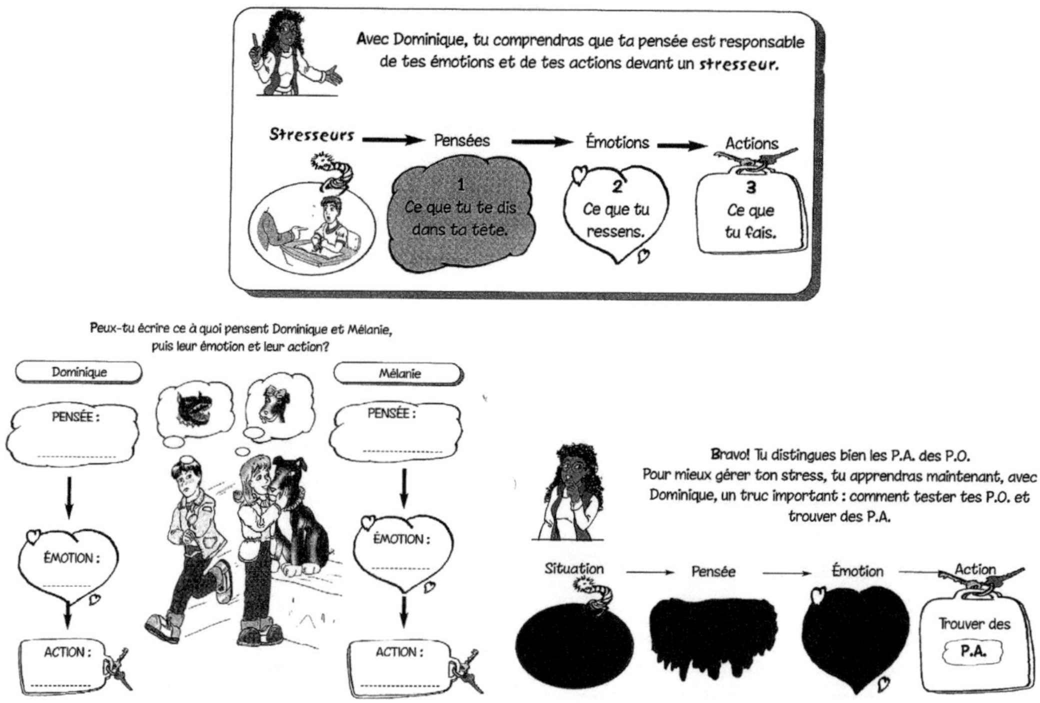

Fig. 1. Excerpts from sections of the children workbook illustrating: (a) key concepts in the program (stressors, thoughts, emotions and actions), (b) the role of appraisal and (c) the introduction of cognitive restructuring to counter dysfunctional thoughts.

Sections of the program	Session#	Learning goals	Stressor illustrated in the book	Dominique's handy tricks
Understanding anxiety	1	The fours components of anxiety: Stressor -> thoughts -> emotions -> actions	Enuresis and children's fear	*Know your stressors!*
	2	Recognizing anxiety symptoms	School situations and academic performance	*Recognize your signs of stress!*
Cognitive restructuring	3	Link thoughts, feeling and actions How to question your thoughts	The opinion of others and self-expectancies	*Find "obstacle thoughts"!*
	4	There are two types of thoughts: worrying-thoughts and reassuring-thoughts.	Divorce	*Find "reassuring thoughts"!*
Introduction to behavioral strategies	5	Avoidance maintains fear	Bullying	*Take the problem in hand!*
Behavioral strategies	6	The basics of exposure	Having a handicapped classmate	*Use small step plan!*
	7	Confide to someone can be helpful Introduction to problem solving	Sexual abuse	*Confide in someone!*
	8	Problem solving	Embarrassment and social rejection	*Apply new solutions!*
	9	Use your social support network	Alcoholism in a parent	*Recharge your batteries!*
Summary and synthesis	10	Integration of the different techniques	Suffering from ADHD	*Remember what you've learned!*

Table 1. Summary of the program's weekly skills, aims and stressors.

3.3 Parent's workbook

This document presents the program and explains different aspects of anxiety, its mechanisms and its consequences. Parents also find information on daily stressors children often meet, children's potential reactions and general recommendations to help their child cope with anxiety-producing situations. The parents also have access to the story books and to supportive recommendations related to the topic addressed in the story. In addition, they are encouraged to follow their child's progress. Some activities requiring the cooperation of the parents are also explained.

3.4 Workshop leader's guidebook

Designed specifically for the workshop leaders, it contains basic notions on the nature of anxiety and the symptoms associated with anxiety management problems. It summarizes the cognitive-behavioral theoretical principles that form the basis of the program and includes explicit details on the aims and activities of each workshop. The general transdiagnostic model for the development of an anxiety disorder proposed that temperamental / genetic risk factors, combined with environmental / familial factors can lead to a greater susceptibility to stressors due to dysfunctional cognitive and behavioral characteristics (see section 1 above). Among susceptible children, various life events could lead to the development of different anxiety disorders, depending on what is associated with threat and avoidance.

3.5 Description of the workshops

Information related to the conduct of the workshops is summarized in Table 1 above. The ten workshops in the program last about seventy-five minutes each. The workshop usually begins with a review of what was learned the week before and the homework exercises done during the week. The reading of the story then follows, lasting about twenty minutes. The learning activities deal first with the identification of everyday stressors related to the workshop themes (e.g., receiving a report card, in the case of academic stress), followed by exercises designed to develop the skills targeted for each session (see Table 1). At this stage, it is important to recall that for the purposes of normalization in the program (as in the text above) the term *stress* is used rather than *anxiety*.

3.5.1 Workshop 1 - Dominique's handy trick: Know your stressors

Supporting story: Dominique still wets his bed at the age of seven. This problem is a great source of stress for him. The same is true for the annoyances that go along with his enuresis: being scolded by his parents, being made fun of by others, not being able to go to summer camp, washing his sheets. Dominique reacts to his stressors in various ways. He thinks he is different from other children and goes through a whole range of emotions, from anger to sadness or shame, which causes him to shut himself off in his room.
In session approach: After being given general information on stress and discussing frequent sources of fear and stress in 8-to-12-year old according to them, the participants attempt to identify the stressors related to Dominique's enuresis. They learn to differentiate his stressors (e.g., the criticisms of his parents) from his reactions to the stress, his thoughts (e.g., I'm a baby!), his emotions (e.g., anger) and his actions (e.g., shutting himself off in his room).
At home approach: The children must each make a list of three "personal" stressors (called *personal challenges*) that will be used to practice *Dominique's handy tricks.* Another exercise asks the children to question their parents about their fears when they were young.

3.5.2 Workshop 2 - Dominique's handy trick: Recognize your signs of stress

Supporting story: School is a great source of stress for Dominique's friend François. His stressors are exams, boredom and recess, as well as arguments with his parents about his poor marks. Specific signs indicate his stress. He is physically tense during exams and obsessed with all kinds of distracting or negative thoughts during classes. His great sadness sometimes turns to despair, making him cry. Fortunately, following a request from his teacher, he presents in class an activity that he finds rewarding. Thanks to this positive experience he thinks, then feels and acts differently; he finds himself more intelligent and recognizes some of his own capacities.

In session approach: The activities during the workshop teach children to distinguish the different signs of anxiety and stress in the character. For example, they note his thoughts, his emotions, his physical reactions and his actions during his exams or following his academic failures.

At home approach: The children identify their own signs of anxiety in accordance with the list of personal challenges produced in the first session.

3.5.3 Workshop 3 - Dominique's handy trick: Find "obstacle thoughts"

Supporting story: For Dominique, Mélanie and their friends, social pressure is an important stressor. They all react to the pressures of competition by making negative judgments about their appearance or their intellectual and athletic capacities. For example, Mélanie is convinced she is fat. Dominique would like to be better at sports and Minh-Thi is unhappy whenever she is not at the top of her class. The judgments of others are such an important source of stress for these grade five students that they forget their own strengths. By chance, a competition organized by the school principal gives Mélanie an opportunity prove her skills against those of other students in her class.

In session approach: The exercises help the children look for and identify obstacle thoughts (dysfunctional beliefs, as opposed to helping thoughts) behind the feelings and behaviors of the characters. By identifying those thoughts (e.g. self-depreciation of the different characters in the story), the children learn how their own thoughts influence both their feelings and their actions.

At home approach: The children review their lists of personal challenges and identify a obstacle thought associated with each of their challenges. In order to firmly establish the idea of a link between thoughts, feelings and actions, they practice their skills in another exercise: finding the logical link between what they thought, felt and did during various situations occurring during the week.

3.5.4 Workshop 4 - Dominique's handy trick: Find "reassuring thoughts"

Supporting story: The separation of Dominique's and his sister Mélanie's parents is accompanied by arguments and frustrations. The reactions of the two children to this major change in their lives are intense and they are afflicted with negative thoughts. Dominique worries in anticipation of the idea of having to move, to leave his friends or to change school. Mélanie feels responsible for the arguments between her parents. Her emotions overwhelm her so much that she is sick to her stomach. Both children are haunted by the fear of losing their parents, of being separated from them or of being abandoned. Over time, the stress experience by the two children diminishes. Mélanie and Dominique finally find a balance and discover a new ways of living happily with their mother and their father.

In session approach: The children work on differentiating in the characters the parts of their internal dialogue that is a source of anxiety from the ones that reassures them. They have to differentiate thoughts that contribute to worrying Dominique (I won't see Mom anymore!) and those that can reassure him (Mom loves us too much to abandon us). The children learn here to test the anxiety-producing thoughts of the characters (obstacle thoughts) and suggest

to the characters *reassuring* (coping) thoughts. Reassuring thoughts are clearly presented as real and grounded thoughts, as opposed to positive thoughts or magical thinking.
At home approach: The take home exercises require the children to identify and note obstacle thoughts and reassuring thoughts related to their personal challenges.

3.5.5 Workshop 5 - Dominique's handy trick: Take the problem in hand

Supporting story: Being persecuted by Simon is a great source of stress for Francis. He is so terrorized when Simon is around that he is unable to concentrate in class. He takes detours to get to school for fear of running into him on the street, convinced he can solve the situation by systematically avoiding his tormentor. What happens is just the opposite: avoidance is a trap, not a solution. In fact, his stress increases every day and he is so obsessed with his fear of Simon that he has nightmares about him. He would like to confront his fear and defend himself, but he does not believe he can solve the problem. He confines himself in the role of victim and his life becomes intolerable. The bullying stopped at last when an incident forces him to disclose the bullying to his parents.
In session approach: The children look for Francis's thoughts that contribute to his avoidance and suggest him new ones to convince him he can solve his problem. They look for alternative behavior to face his fear.
At home approach: As an application exercise, the children report avoidance behaviors in a stress situation experienced during the week by identifying obstacle and reassuring thoughts related to that event.

3.5.6 Workshop 6 - Dominique's handy trick: Use small steps plan

Supporting story: Dominique feels uneasy with persons with disabilities. He reacts with panic and run away when he encounters Benoît, a new student in the class who has cerebral palsy. He is so uncomfortable with Benoît that he is completely disconcerted when he sees him. His presence alone causes him so much stress that all he wants to do is run away. A series of circumstances, however, helps Dominique realize that his concerns are unjustified. Even though he first has difficulty being around the new school mate, progressive and various contacts make Dominique more and more at ease with Benoît. The more he does things with Benoît, the more Dominique becomes able to tame his fears and, finally, he finds he has made a new friend.
In session approach: The activities show to the children how to find the thoughts and progressive exposure steps that help Dominique conquer his fear.
At home approach: With the workshop leader, the children make their own gradual exposure plan called "small steps plan". They divide exposure to a personal challenge into very small stages, planning reassuring thoughts and little rewards to provide encouragement at each small step. They have to carry out their plans one step at a time over a period of two weeks.

3.5.7 Workshop 7 - Dominique's handy trick: Confide in someone

Supporting story: The behavior of Mr. Dubois is a great source of stress and worry for Dominique. He is overwhelmed by contradictory feelings toward Mr Dubois that prevent protecting himself from this abusive neighbour. Dominique feels affection for the man, who has given him privileges. But at the same time, he worries more and more about his physical advances. Gradually, Mr. Dubois' actions become such a source of despair for Dominique that he can no longer sleep and he shuts himself off from his parents and his friends. He has difficulty deciding whom he can share his worries with. Fortunately, he decides to share his secret with his parents.

In session approach: The children have to identify the various thoughts that explain Dominique's contradictory feelings and the ones that prevent him from acting (e.g., I promised to keep it a secret). The identification of obstacle thoughts is followed by looking for reassuring thoughts to encourage Dominique to take action to solve the problem. By helping Dominique evaluate the pros and cons of talking about his concerns, the children are initiated to the basics of problem solving. Finally, the participants propose small steps to Dominique in order to get out of his difficulties.

At home approach: The take home exercise requires participants to identify persons that they could confide in or ask for information in case of problems. They should also complete the last stages of their small steps plan initiated in the previous workshop.

3.5.8 Workshop 8 - Dominique's handy trick: Apply new solutions

Supporting story: Mélissa has no friends at school. To make herself more interesting to students in her class, she tells lies. Far from helping her to make friends, this behavior only makes things worse for her. Moreover, one day she finds herself trapped in a huge lie. She feels foolish and is looking for a solution to avoid facing the ridicule of her peers. She is even considering telling a bigger lie to get herself out of trouble. Fortunately her neighbor Marjorie helps her find a new and more productive solution.

In session approach: The children have to identify the obstacle thoughts that come to Mélissa's mind (e.g., I'm stupid). They suggest to her reassuring thoughts so that she can stop ruminating on feelings of guilt, and stop thinking of herself as foolish and stupid. Helping Mélissa make up for her mistake is an opportunity to learn applying a problem-solving technique that is accessible to children (define the problem, evaluate then choose among alternative solutions, assess the results, etc.).

At home approach: The children apply the problem-solving to a personal challenge.

3.5.9 Workshop 9 - Dominique's handy trick: Recharge your batteries

Supporting story: The story describes problems in the life of Cathou, a girl whose mother is alcoholic and depressed. Cathou finds an outlet for her problems in her passion for gymnastics. Life at home is a source of daily stress for her. She has to take care of herself while supporting her mother. She feels responsible for her mother's problems and is eating her heart out with worries about her. Also, she does not want anyone else to know what is happening with her mother. In order to face the daily problems resulting from her family life, she energizes herself by practicing her favorite activity.

In session approach: After identifying the daily stressors in the life of the main character, the participants suggest to her various actions to charge her batteries, that is, energize herself. The first exercises apply what was learned in the previous workshops: choose for Cathou thoughts that generate energy and help her adopt behaviors that reduce her stress (e.g., seek out information).

At home approach: The children have to find and practice activities that provide them energy, or relaxation, and identify their own personal support networks.

3.5.10 Workshop 10 - Dominique's handy trick: Remember what you've learned

Supporting story: The story recounts the daily problems of Sébastien who suffers from attention-deficit hyperactivity disorder. Sébastien's difficulties are a great source of stress for him. Because of his problems, he is regularly scolded by his teacher and his parents. In the class, he even has to work behind a screen to stop disrupting everyone. He is rejected by his schoolmates. Sébastien's agitation and impulsive behaviors also cause stress for everyone around him. But Sébastien does not understand the reactions of others towards him, whether it comes from father, his sister, his teacher or other students. Sébastien has to learn ways to better manage his situation.

In session approach: This workshop is an opportunity to sum up everything learned in the previous sessions. The participants review the techniques they have learned so far. They have to identify Sébastien's stressors and find his signs of stress. They apply the notions they have learned to explain the reactions of other characters towards him. They have to imagine the thoughts of his teacher or his sister to explain their aggressiveness towards him and suggest to Sébastien solutions to reduce his worries and carry out his tasks (e.g., make a small steps plan).

At home approach: Each child receives a proof of participation in the form of a diploma. The stress management techniques taught in the program are listed on the diploma so that it can be used as a memory aid and a rewarding attestation.

4. Qualitative impressions from the implementation of the program

Dominique handy tricks program has been implemented with 46 children with the hope of improving their feelings of self-efficacy to cope with stressors, reducing anxiety sensitivity and anxiety symptoms and fostering the development of problem-solving skills. After approval from the University of Quebec in Outaouais' Ethics in Research Committee, the program was delivered in the schools according to the manual described in this chapter. For ethical concerns about not providing effective treatment to children that could be screened as potentially severe enough to warrant a treatment, it was decided to exclude and refer to treatment those who would obtain a clinically significant score on the Child Behavior Checklist (global score > 75), on the Screen for Child Anxiety Related Emotional Disorders (global score > 60) or on one of the clinical outcome measure. An initial sample of 59 children were recruited, 55 started the program and 9 did not completed the post-program assessment. Participants were aged between 9 to 12 years old and randomly assigned to a waiting list (and received the program later) or to receive the program. Quantitative analyses of outcome results are being conducted on the Coping Scale for Children and Youth, the Perceived Self-efficacy Towards Problem-solving Scale, the Childhood Anxiety Sensitivity Index, the Multidimensional Anxiety Scale for Children, and the Fear Survey Schedule for Children-Revised and will be the focus of a future article.

To complement the description of the program detailed in this chapter, this section will report on *qualitative* data gathered during a focus group conducted with the seven workshop leaders, during contact with the parents, and through comments from children after their involvement in the implementation and evaluation of the program. These qualitative observations provided important information that is very difficult to obtain in quantitative trials. It also highlights specific challenges experienced during the application of a universal prevention program dedicated to the teaching of cognitive-behavioral techniques for anxiety and stress management.

The program was provided for free and on a voluntary basis. Yet, the research agenda required children and parents to take part in long assessment sessions, which raised worries about the feasibility of a primary prevention program. Our concerns regarding recruitment proved to be unfounded. The program was accepted enthusiastically by those working in the schools, as it was by parents. Both groups expressed on several occasions their enthusiasm to see a program targeting stress experienced by children. In addition, the application of the program took place without any substantial attrition problem (only 4 dropped-out during the program). Very few children missed even one session. Answers from children and the focus group with workshop leaders confirmed that the stories told in each session were an important motivating element for the attendance and participation of the children in the workshops, even for the more delicate topics such as alcoholism and sexual abuse.

Comments from participants confirmed children's interest in the exercises as they appear in the children's workbook. Based on discussions in the focus group, such a program should be applied with some flexibility to adapt the use of these exercises to the characteristics of the participants. In their original form, most of the workshop exercises were designed to be done in discussions or in paper-and-pencil activities. This approach appeared to be particularly well suited to girls but the focus group revealed it may be less suitable for boys, who were more receptive to a presentation of content in the form of interactive activities. These observations supported our impression about the usefulness in the *workshop leader's guidebook* of options to adapt some activities in order to make them more active. After the outcome trial, the guidebook was revised to include several additional suggestions on how to adapt some exercises according to the dynamics of the groups. Distinguishing the thoughts, emotions, physical sensations and actions of a character can, for example, be done either by drawing individually in the workbook or in the form of a group identification game. In the same way, finding reassuring thoughts to convince Francis, victim of bullying, (session 5) to do something to solve his problem could be done in two ways: either by individually writing him a postcard explaining him reasons to act (as suggested in the workbook) or in the form of a group role-play game where participants have to convince Francis to do something and the participant playing the role of Francis expressing which argument he considers most convincing.

Comments from the participants highlighted that planning and carrying out take home activities represented a challenge for the children. Since these exercises are essential for the generalization of recently acquired skills learned learn in session to practical issues occurring in their own lives, compliance with homework deserves to be mentioned. Doing the weekly exercises requires a high level of motivation. However, since the program was not intended for, nor delivered to, a clinical population, the children motivation vanished rapidly once they had left the session. They were not highly motivated to initiate exercises to master their new coping behaviors. This may have contributed to the fact that some of them invested little time in the homework or sometimes failed to complete the exercises in the workbook.

It is reasonable to believe that take home activities could also be perceived as a burden given their already occupied academic agenda and their school homework. Although behavioral changes require involvement and practice, in primary prevention programs it may be more difficult to enroll children to invest in practicing behavior changes if the motivation is extrinsic and rather hypothetical compared to children who want to stop suffering from an anxiety disorder. Even though participants confirmed weekly that the exercises in their workbooks had been completed, it is difficult to ensure that the exercises have not been done hastily or at the last minute. Innovative approaches could be developed to increate adherence to homework, such as on-line contact with the workshop leader during the week (to notify him or her that the exercise has been done) or the use of a buddy system (two children supporting each other in doing the application exercises) as is the case in other programs such as Coping Cat (Kendall, 1992).

The qualitative data also documented a significant and positive impact when parents agreed to get involved and followed weekly the development of the child's exercises in the workbook. Interestingly, we observed that such parental involvement was not without its disadvantages. Many children did not want their parents to look at their exercise workbooks because they felt the contents were personal. This calls into question the relevance and depth of parental involvement in primary prevention program for internalizing disorders. One might posit that parental involvement could just as well create resistance as it could provide positive support to the children's learning.

Participation of at least one of the parents in the three information sessions provided during the program was very low. Family members of less than 15% of the participants attended these information meetings, which were held in the evening to accommodate them. The workshop leaders have, however, reported positive comments from the parents who did attend. Parents reported that the stories facilitated communication with their children and suggested positive attitudes to adopt. The stories also allowed discussing openly about potential anxiety reactions parents had observed in their children following stressful events such as divorce or learning difficulties. Discussions with parents were an opportunity to provide information and alleviate their own worries about children's problems. In spite of these positive observations, the low attendance to the meetings raises the question of the feasibility to involve at least one parent from each family in a primary prevention program. When their child is not suffering from an anxiety disorder, parents may prioritize other family needs instead of attending to meeting in a prevention program. The impact of including or not the parents in the program on children's learning remains however unclear and questionable (Hudson et al., 2008).

The fact that workshops sessions were held in schools facilitated that professionals and teachers put pressure for the inclusion of children with externalized disorders in a universal primary prevention program for anxiety disorders. This reaction was predictable insofar as resources for children in difficulty are scarce. The qualitative data collected confirmed the importance of caution with respect to the inclusion in the groups of children with behavioral disorders, most notably hyperactivity. Many exercises in the program require self-observation by the children and a capacity to identify their feelings or recognize their own reactions to events. Some children who openly claimed to be suffering from attention deficit and hyperactivity disorder appeared to have, in addition to their behavioral problems, difficulties with introspection, which may have complicated their learning and hindered the functioning of the group. In one workshop group, where three children claimed suffering from attention deficit with hyperactivity disorder, the participants became very disruptive in several sessions, requiring the workshop leader to work harder to manage the group.

Although our observations about attention deficit and hyperactivity are based on a small number of cases and were not systematically gathered, they converge with the results of studies showing that learning cognitive techniques is a significant challenge for these children (Abikoff, 1991). This possibility illustrates the importance of careful selection of the children and of the make-up of the groups of children. A universal primary prevention program for anxiety disorders is not a complement for the treatment of ADHD. It is not a free treatment for anxiety disorders either. School staff and sources of referral must understand that primary prevention is meant to be implemented before emotional and behavioral problems occur.

5. Conclusion

The qualitative information collected during and after the implementation of the program should guide further trials of the program. They have raised some shortcomings that will be taken into consideration when revising the program for a new trial. More schools have expressed a desire to implement the program and several pilot projects for new trials are considered. Results of the outcome trial are expected soon, yet some of the less tangible benefits of a universal program have been already observed, such as heightened awareness about anxiety and its consequences, early detection of children at high risk for the development of internalized disorders, and the promotion of psychological services to prevent and treat anxiety disorders. It is hoped that a better understanding of the nature of anxiety and its disorders could contribute to more supportive behaviors from classmates and adults.

The resources allocated for the prevention and treatment of externalized disorders, such as ADHD, are far greater than those allocated for the prevention of internalized disorders. Dominique's handy tricks program can contribute to the promotion of knowledge about anxiety disorders, which are the most prevalent disorders in this age group (Merikangas et al., 2009). Adherence to universal prevention programs and sustained efforts to master new skills may be challenged by motivational issues in children and their parents. New methods that rely on computer technologies (Bouchard, 2011) may increase children's interest toward the use of CBT treatment and prevention tools. In the meantime, it is hoped that by focusing on strategies to cope with various stressors instead of dysfunctional anxiety, Dominique's handy tricks program will stir interests in children.

6. Acknowledgement

This study was funded by a joint research grant from the *Ministère de la Santé et des Services Sociaux and the Régie Régionale de la Santé et des Services Sociaux de l'Outaouais – Programme de subvention en santé publique.* The study was conducted in the Laboratoire de Cyberpsychologie de l'UQO (http://www.uqo.ca/cyberpsy) where the second author now holds the Canada Research Chair in Clinical Cyberpsychology. Corresponding address: Jean Gervais, Département de psychoéducation et de psychologie, Université du Québec en Outaouais, PO Box 1250, Station Hull, Gatineau, Qc, J8X 3X7. e-mail : jean.gervais@uqo.ca. The authors wish to thank Claudie Loranger for her input in the preparation of this chapter.

7. References

Abikoff, H. (1991). Cognitive training in ADHD children: Less to it than meets the eye. *Journal of Learning Disabilities, 24* (4), 205-209.

Ackerson, J., Scogin, F., McKendree-Smith, N., & Lyman, R.D. (1998). Cognitive bibliotherapy for mild and moderate adolescent depressive symptomatology. *Journal of Consulting and Clinical Psychology, 66* (4), 685-690.

Barrett, P.M., Duffy, A.L., Dadds, M.R., & Rapee, R.M. (2001). Cognitive-Behavioral Treatment of Anxiety Disorders in Children: Long-Term (6 year) Follow-Up. *Journal of Consulting and Clinical Psychology, 69* (1), 135-141.

Becker, K.D., & Chorpita, B.F. (2008). *Negative affect*. New York: Guilford Press.

Bouchard, S. (2011). Could virtual reality be effective in treating children with phobias? *Expert Review of Neurotherapeutics, 11*(2), 207-213.

Cartwright-Harton, S., Roberts, C., Chitsabesan, P., Fothergill, C., & Harrington, R. (2004). Systematic review of the efficacy of cognitive behavior therapies for childhood and adolescent anxiety disorders. *British Journal of Clinical Psychology, 40*, 375-384.

Compton, S.N., March, J.S., Brent, D., Albano, A.M., Weersing, V.R., & Curry, J. (2004). Cognitive-behavioral psychotherapy for anxiety and depressive disorders in children and adolescents: An evidence-based medicine review. *Journal of the American Academy of Child and Adolescent Psychiatry, 43*, 930-959.

Costello, E.J., Mustillo, S., Erkanli, A., Keeler, G., & Angold, A. (2003). Prevalence and development of psychiatric disorders in childhood and adolescence. *Archives of General Psychiatry, 60*, 837-844.

Dacey, J.S., & Fiore, L.B. (2000). *Your anxious child: How parents and teachers can relieve anxiety in children*. San Francisco, CA, US: Jossey-Bass.

Dadds, M.R., & Barrett, P.M. (2001). Practitioner Review: Psychological Management of Anxiety Disorders in Childhood. *Journal of Child Psychology and Psychiatry, 42* (8), 999-1011.

Donovan, C.L., & Spence, S.H. (2000). Prevention of childhood anxiety disorders. *Clinical Psychology Review, 20*, 509-531.

Gould, R.A., Clum, G.A., & Shapiro, D. (1993). The use of bibliotherapy in the treatment of panic: A preliminary investigation. *Behavior Therapy, 24* (2), 241-252.

Hardy, D.F., Power, T.G., & Jaedicke, S. (1993) Examining the relation of parenting to children's coping with everyday stress. *Child development, 64* (6), 1829-1841.

Hirshfeld-Becker, D.R., Masek, B., Henin, A., Blakely, L.R., Pollock-Wurman, R.A., McQuade, J., et al. (2010). Cognitive Behavioral Therapy for 4- to 7-Year-Old Children With Anxiety Disorders: A Randomized Clinical Trial. *Journal of Consulting and Clinical Psychology, 78* (4), 498-510.

Hirshfeld, D.R., Micco, J.A., Simoes, N.A., & Henin, A. (2008). High risk studies and developmental antecedents of anxiety disorders. *American Journal of Medical Genetics, Part C: Seminars in Medical Genetics*, 148, 99-117.

Hudson, J.L., Lyneman, H.J., & Rapee, R.M. (2008). Treating childhood behavioral and emotional problems: A step-by-step evidence-based approach. In Eisen, Andrew R. (Ed), *Social Anxiety* (pp. 53-101). New York: Guilford Press.

Kendall, P.C. (1992). *Coping cat workbook*. PA: Wokbook Publishing Inc.

Kendall,P.C. (1994).Treating anxiety disorders in children: Results of a randomized clinical trial. *Journal of Consulting and Clinical Psychology, 62,* 100-110.

Kendall, P. C., Flannery-Schroeder, E., Panichelli-Mindel, S. M., Southam-Gerow, M., Henin, A., & Warman, M. (1997). Therapy for youths with anxiety disorders: A second randomized clinical trial. *Journal of Consulting and Clinical Psychology, 65,* 366-380.

Lazarus, R.S., & Folkman, S. (1984). *Stress, appraisal, and coping*. New York: Springer.

Last, C. (1993). *Anxiety across the lifespan: A developmental perspective*. New York: Springer.

Lowry-Webster, H. M., Barrett, P. M., & Dadds, M. R. (2001). A universal prevention trial of anxiety and depressive symptomatology in childhood: Preliminary data from an Australian study. *Behavior Change, 18,* 36-47.

March, J. S. (1995). Anxiety disorders in children and adolescents. New York: Guilford Press.

Mayer, R. & Ouellet, F. (1991). Méhodologie de recherche pour les intervenants sociaux. Montréal : Gaëtan Morin.

Merikangas, K.R., Nakamura, E.F., Kessler, R.C. (2009). Epidemiology of mental disorders in children and adolescents. *Dialogues in Clinical Neuroscience,* 11 (1), pp. 7-20.

Milich, R., McAnininch, C.B., & Harris M.J. (1992). Effects of stygmatizing information on children's peer relations: Believing is seeing. *School Psychology Review, 21,* 400-409.

Miller, L.D., Short, C., Garland, E.J., & Clark, S. (2010). The ABCs of CBT (Cognitive Behavior Therapy): Evidence-Based Approaches to Child Anxiety in Public School Settings. *Journal of Counselling & Development, 88,* 432-439.

Morris, T. L., & March, J. S. (2004). *Anxiety disorders in children and adolescents* (2nd edition). New York: Guilford Press.

Muris, P., Merckelbach, H., Gadet, B., & Moulaert, V. (2000). Fears, worries, and scary dreams in 4- to 12- year-old children : Their content, developmental pattern, and origins. *Journal of Clinical Child Psychology,* 29 (1), 43-52.

Ollendick T. H., & March, J. S. (2004). Phobic *and anxiety disorders in children and adolescents.* New York: Oxford University Press.

Otto, M.W. (2000). Stories and metaphors in cognitive-behavior therapy. *Cognitive and Behavioral Practice, 7* (2), 166-172.

Rapee, R. M., Schniering, C. A., & Hudson, J. L. (2009). Anxiety disorders during childhood and adolescence: Origins and treatment. *Annual Review of Clinical Psychology, 5,* 311-341.

Scogin, F., Jamison, C., & Davis, N. (1990). Two-year follow-up of bibliotherapy for depression in older adults. *Journal of Consulting and Clinical Psychology, 58* (5), 665-667.

Stallard, P. (2010). Mental health prevention in UK classrooms: the FRIENDS anxiety prevention programme. *Emotional and Behavioural Difficulties, 15* (1), 23-35.

Vasey, M. W., & Dadds, M. R. (2001). *The developmentl psychopathology of anxiety.* Toronto: Oxford University Press.

Wright, J., Clum, G.A., Roodman, A., & Febbraro, G.A.M. (2000). A bibliotherapy approach to relapse prevention in individuals with panic attacks. *Journal of Anxiety Disorders, 14* (5), 483-499.

19

Rational-Emotive and Cognitive-Behavioral Interventions for Children with Anxiety Disorders: A Group Counseling Curriculum

Jerry Wilde
Indiana University East,
USA

1. Introduction

The purpose of this chapter is to provide overview of specific clinical interventions that can be used by rational-emotive and cognitive-behavioral therapists working with children and adolescents who are experiencing difficulties with anxiety. It is worth noting that anxiety disorders are among the most commonly occurring mental and emotional problems in childhood and adolescence. While a majority of publications focus on empirical research, there is still a need for articles that address clinical practices. REBT/CBT is, first and foremost, a system devoted to the *practice* of psychotherapy. Whether it is through articles focused on empirical research or clinical applications, the advancement of REBT/CBT is the ultimate goal. An anxiety management curriculum for group counseling with children is presented. While there is considerable research on the effectiveness of REBT/CBT on the treatment of anxiety, there is significantly less when it comes to the application of these principles in a group setting. The research that is available has generally found positive results for anxiety management conducted in a group counseling setting. Nine discrete lessons are offered in this chapter. The lessons presented start by setting the stage for treatment by helping clients understand that they have the ability to change their thoughts which will lead to a change in their feelings. The connection between thoughts and feelings, which is indispensable in REBT/CBT, is the focus at the beginning of group. Helping clients understand what kinds of thoughts contribute to anxious feelings is also an important component of the process. Several lessons focus on practicing ways of minimizing or managing anxious feelings by using distraction, thought stopping, and rational emotive imagery. A lesson on systematic desensitization, modified for application with children, is also offered.

2. Rational-emotive and cognitive-behavioral interventions for children with anxiety disorders: A group counseling curriculum

Anxiety disorders are among the most common mental and emotional problems to occur during childhood and adolescence. According to the U.S. Department of Health and Human Services (1999), 13% of children and adolescents ages 9 to 17 experienced some type of anxiety disorder. In community samples of adult populations, the range of anxiety disorders was between 5 – 20% with a majority of the estimates lying above 10% (Costello & Angold,

1995). Blanchard, et al., (2006) found that 36% of parents report concerns about the possibility of their children struggling with anxiety.

If left untreated, anxiety disorders can persist into adulthood (Keller, et al., 1992, Pfeffer et al., 1988; Spence, 1988) which may in part explain why the lifetime prevalence rate for anxiety disorders is 28.8%, with a 12-month prevalence of 18.8% (Kessler, & Merikangas, 2004). The same study reported the most common subtypes of anxiety disorders to be specific phobia (12.5%), social anxiety disorder (12.1%), and post-traumatic stress disorder (6.8%).

Rational Emotive Behavior Therapy (REBT) is based on the theory that emotional disturbance is largely the result of illogical and irrational patterns of thinking (Ellis, 1962, 1994). Such ideas date back to the first century A.D. when the Stoic philosopher, Epictetus (1890) wrote, "Men are disturbed not by things but by the views they take of them." In other words, it is not external events alone that cause emotional disturbance, but those events plus a person's perceptions and evaluations about them, as a good many ancient and modern philosphers have stated.

3. The philosophical underpinnings of REBT/CBT

Humans have a powerful predisposition or innate tendency to behave irrationally and self-defeatingly (Ellis, 1979). They have the tendency to avoid thinking things through, to procrastinate, to be overly suggestible, superstitious, and perfectionistic. But they, at the same time, are healthy constructivists, with powerful innate tendencies to solve practical problems of living, to be creative, and to grow and develop.

REBT/CBT theory states that humans also have a strong tendency to be influenced by their environment. This is particularly true during childhood, when their family, peers, and culture have an enormous impact on their beliefs, emotions, and actions.

One of the primary tenets of REBT/CBT is that thoughts, feelings, and behaviors interact and significantly affect each other. Thinking affects, and in some ways creates, an individual's feelings and behaviors; their emotions have a very important effect on their thoughts and actions; and their actions distinctly influence their thoughts and feelings. If one of these processes are somehow altered the others are influenced as well (Ellis, 1962, 1994, 1999, 2000a, 2000b; Ellis & Dryden, 1997; Ellis & MacLaren, 1998).

REBT acknowledges that virtually all humans are basically hedonistic since people are born with a strong tendency to avoid pain, remain alive, and seek happiness. However, it distinguishes between long and short term hedonism in that it does not promote immediate and easy gratification at the expense of future gains.

A cardinal tenet of REBT/CBT is that all humans are fallible and have very many limitations. REBT/CBT encourages people to accept themselves as people that will now and probably forever make continual and numerous mistakes. It is important that they acknowledge their fallibility and still live happily by learning to accept themselves fully despite their limitations.

4. Goals of rational emotive and cognitive behavior therapy

1. To make clients more aware of their self-talk and internal dialogue and particularly of their self-defeating Beliefs, so that they will be able to think more rationally, clearly, logically and self-helpingly.

2. To teach clients to evaluate their thinking, feeling and behavior in order to experience more healthy emotions and fewer dysfunctions.
3. To teach clients the skills to use rational emotive behavioral principles so he or she will act more functionally and be better able to achieve his or her goals in life (Wilde, 1992).

Studies have compared CBT to other forms of treatment and found it to be an effective treatment for adults suffering from various anxiety disorders. Butler et al (1991) compared CBT to behavioral therapy (BT) with results showing a clear advantage for CBT over BT. Borkovec and Costello (1993) examined the efficacy of Nondirective (ND), applied relaxation (AR), and cognitive behavioral (CBT) therapies for generalized anxiety disorder (GAD). Results for AR and CBT were generally equivalent in outcome but superior to ND at post-assessment. A preliminary meta-analysis comparing CBT to pharmacological treatment found both offered efficacy to patients. The authors reported that CBT was associated with significantly greater effects on anxiety severity and was associated with clear maintenance of treatment gains (Gould, et al, 1997).

REBT/CBT has an extensive history of being successfully applied to anxiety problems in children (Brody, 1974; Cangelosi, Gressard, & Mines, 1980; Cristea, Benga, & Opre,2006; DiGiuseppe & Kassinove, 1976; Knaus & Bokor, 1975; Knaus & McKeever, 1977; Meyer, 1981; Micco, et al, 2007; Miller & Kassinove, 1978; Omizo, Lo, & Williams, 1986; Von Pohl, 1982; Warren, Deffenbacher & Brading, 1976; Wilde, 1994, 1995, 1996a). The utility of CBT with anxiety disorders has led mental health officials in the United Kingdom to identify CBT as the first-line approach to treating anxiety disorders (National Institute for Clinical Excellence, 2004).

Rational-emotive and cognitive-behavior interventions have also been found to be beneficial in a host of other commonly occurring childhood problems such as low frustration tolerance (Brody, 1974); impulsivity (Meichenbaum & Goodman, 1971); poor academic performance (Block, 1978; Cangelosi, Gressard, & Mines, 1980), and depression (Wilde, 1994). Research also suggests that CBT is effective in the prevention of depression (Clarke, et al., 2001, Gilliam, et al., 1995) and in the improvement of self-concept and coping capabilities (DeVoge, 1974; DiGiuseppe, 1975; DiGiuseppe & Kassinove, 1976; Katz, 1974; Maultsby, Knipping & Carpenter, 1974; Omizo, Lo & Williams, 1986; Wasserman & Vogrin, 1979). Finally, several studies have established cognitive-behavioral interventions to be effective in increasing rational thinking in children and adolescents (DiGiuseppe & Kassinove, 1976; Harris, 1976; Knaus & Bokor, 1975; Miller & Kassinove, 1978; Ritchie, 1978; Voelm, 1983; Wasserman & Vogrin, 1979; Wilde, 1997a).

5. An anxiety management curriculum for group counseling with children

While there is an abundance of research on the effectiveness of REBT/CBT on the treatment of anxiety, there is significantly less when it comes to the application of these principles in a group setting. The research that is available has generally found positive results for anxiety management conducted in a group counseling setting. Liber et al., (2008) determined that group counseling is an effective means of helping children and adolescents manage feelings of anxiety. There were no outcome differences for anxious children between individual and group treatments. Liber et al. (2004) compared an individual versus a group format in the delivery of a cognitive-behavioral therapy curriculum (FRIENDS) for children with anxiety disorders. Clinically referred children (aged 8 to 12) diagnosed with Separation Anxiety Disorder (n = 52), Generalized Anxiety Disorder (n = 37), Social Phobia (n = 22) or Specific

Phobia (n = 16) were randomly assigned to individual (n = 65) or group (n = 62) treatment. Forty-eight percent of the children in the individual versus 41% in the group treatment were free of any anxiety disorder at post-treatment and 62% versus 54% were free of their primary anxiety disorder. Regression analyses showed no significant difference in outcome between individual and group treatment.

Maes and Heimann (1970) examined the relative effectiveness of client-centered, rational-emotive, and desensitization therapies in reducing test anxiety among high school students. Thirty-three subjects with high State anxiety but average or low Trait anxiety were selected. Each student was counseled from seven to eleven times during a five-week period by advanced graduate students. There were no significant differences between the four groups in the Spielberger State-Trait Anxiety Inventory (STAI); but significant differences at <.05 level were found in the predicted direction between group treatments and controls on criteria of galvanic skin response (GSR) and heart rate (HR). Post hoc analyses disclosed significance for the desensitization treatment group on GSR, and the rational-emotive treatment group on HR. Final analysis revealed differences only with the rational-emotive treatment group and controls on HR.

Wessel and Mersch (1994) examined the effectiveness of REBT and exposure in vivo on test-anxious adolescents. The treatment was more effective than a control waiting-list period in reducing test and social anxiety, the degree of anxiety experienced in individual anxiety-provoking situations, and the degree of avoidance of these situations.

6. The group counseling lessons

6.1 Lesson 1: Setting the stage

What follows are descriptions of a series of lessons to be used in a group setting with children experiencing difficulties with anxiety. These lessons were designed to be used in small groups of 6-10 clients but the ideas can easily be adapted for individual sessions.

Initially it is important to set the stage by helping clients accept that improvement is only possible if they take ownership over their progress. What follows is an excerpt from the book *Hot Stuff to Help Kids Worry Less.*

We're ready to get started except for one thing...the hard part. Are you ready to hear about the hard part? You had to know there had to be a catch, didn't you? There's always a catch. Okay, here it is.

Since there really isn't any magic in the world, you won't feel differently if you don't think and act differently. Your friends, parents, teachers, dogs, cats, and gerbils can't make you feel better. We certainly can't magically fix your life with a book, but we can help you learn some ideas and activities that have been proven to work. To feel better you're going to have to actually do some of the things that will be suggested in this book. Your life won't suddenly be perfect, but you'll have the opportunity to learn some skills that will put you in charge of your feelings.

Over the years, I have worked with hundreds of students and they've had a lot of luck with the ideas I'm going to teach you. You can learn to have a happier life, but it will not be easy. If you work hard at the things in this book, you'll probably feel better. If you don't work hard, you probably won't feel any differently. The choice is totally up to you. But keep in mind, you are also free to experience all the worries and unhappiness your heart can bear.

Learning to control your anxieties is like learning any new skill. It takes a lot of hard work and practice. There are absolutely no shortcuts, but the rewards are worth the effort. (Wilde, 2008, p. 14-15).

Sometime during the first session some type of anxiety instrument should be administered as a means of assessing the severity of the symptoms. A simple screening tool can also be introduced as a pre- and post-test to determine improvement. Below is a short screening instrument that can be used as such. It is not statistically validated and should only be used as a pre- and post-test measure.

6.1.1 The anxiety survey

Strongly Disagree — Strongly Agree

1. If something bad might happen, I have to worry about it.
   1 2 3 4 5 6
2. I have no control over my worrying.
   1 2 3 4 5 6
3. Worrying about something can keep it from happening.
   1 2 3 4 5 6
4. If what I worry about *did* happen, it would be the worst thing in the world.
   1 2 3 4 5 6
5. My worries have a "mind of their own" and can't be managed.
   1 2 3 4 5 6
6. If what I worry about *did* happen, I couldn't stand it.
   1 2 3 4 5 6
7. Because I worry about things, it proves I'm worthless and weak.
   1 2 3 4 5 6
8. Worries never seem to go away. Once you've got them, you're stuck with them.
   1 2 3 4 5 6

TOTAL___________

6.2 Lesson 2: Thoughts and feelings

From an REBT model, it is vitally important that clients understand the connection between thoughts and feelings. The next activity is designed to help clients learn that thoughts influence, and largely control, feelings.

What follows is the story if "the blind student in the hall." It is a commonly used story in REBT circles designed to illustrate the connection between thoughts and feelings.

Let's pretend you were walking down the hall at school and somebody came up behind you and knocked all your books out of your hands. How would you feel? You'd start whistling a happy tune, right? No, seriously, how would you feel? If you're like most people, you'd probably be angry or anxious or maybe both.

But when you turned around to see who hit your books, you realized it was a blind student who accidentally bumped into you. He couldn't see where he was going and he bumped into you. Now how would you feel? Would you still feel angry and/or anxious? Probably not.

Here's the important part. You still got your books knocked out of your hands so this event (having your books scattered) can't make you feel anything. People would have different reactions to having their books knocked around. Some would feel angry, some would get anxious, and others would laugh it off along with everyone else. If events caused feelings, then everyone would feel the same way after the same events. But people don't feel the same way about things. People tend to feel differently about events so the experiences don't cause emotions. It must be something else.

That "something else" is your thoughts. Your thoughts, beliefs, and ideas determine your feelings…not the events. (Wilde, 2008, p. 31-32.)

The second part of the lesson is designed to provide clients with additional practice making the connection between thoughts and feelings.

Below is a list of thoughts. Your job is to match the feeling that would go with each thought. You'll probably be able to do this pretty easily. Why? Because thoughts influence feelings. If they didn't, your answers would be totally different from your friends but I'll bet they'll be mostly the same. Give this a try and see how it goes.

6.2.1 Thoughts and feelings

What type of feeling would you have if you thought:

"Oh, no...I didn't know there was a test today."

*Feeling*______________________________

"What do you mean I'm grounded?"

*Feeling*______________________________

"I'm worthless. Everyone hates me."

*Feeling*______________________________

"Life stinks."

*Feeling*______________________________

"I hope my parents won't forget to pick me up after basketball practice."

*Feeling*______________________________

"It's snowing hard right now. We might have a day off of school tomorrow."

*Feeling*______________________________

"My mom and dad are having an argument."

*Feeling*______________________________

(Wilde, 2008, p. 36-37).

6.3 Lesson 3: Focus on anxiety

At this point it is time to start the examination of a client's anxieties. The following activity provides information about specific anxiety provoking situations as well as the intensity of the feelings related to that event or situation.

Below is a list of things that some kids worry about. Next to each item, check either "yes, I worry about it" or "no, I don't worry about it." If you checked yes, there's another column where you can record your rating from 1 to 100. This rating is called a SUDs scale, which stands for "Subjective Units of Discomfort." Scores closer to 1 mean you have less worries and scores nearer to 100 mean you have more worries. Your lowest score should be the item you have the least worries about and your highest score would be the event that you worry about the most.

6.3.1 My worry list

	Yes	*No*	*SUDs Score*
Ghosts/Monsters	____	____	____
Thunderstorms	____	____	____
Spiders or other bugs	____	____	____
Being away from my parents	____	____	____
Doctors/Dentists	____	____	____
Being made fun of	____	____	____

Feeling left out by my friends	____	____	____
Getting hurt	____	____	____
A terrorist attack	____	____	____
Something happening to my parents	____	____	____
Tests at school	____	____	____
Doing poorly at school	____	____	____
Shots/Injections	____	____	____
Snakes	____	____	____
Feeling Pain	____	____	____
Fires	____	____	____
Burglars/robbers	____	____	____
Getting in trouble	____	____	____
The dark	____	____	____
Elevators	____	____	____
Escalators	____	____	____
Choking	____	____	____

(Wilde, 2008, p. 39-40).

6.4 Lesson 4: Where do worries come from?

This lesson is designed to help students understand how situations turn from a concern to an anxiety.

As we explained a little bit earlier, worries (and all other feelings) come from thoughts. But worries don't come from just any thought. If you had the thought, "I love ice cream," you wouldn't feel anxious. Worries come from certain types of thoughts that are usually related to the possibility of something bad happening. Look over your "My Worries" list. Each item on the list could lead to something bad happening. For example, some kids are afraid of dogs because dogs could bite them. Others are afraid of being away from their parents because they're worried something might happen to their moms and dads. So most worries have at least one thing in common. There is the potential for something bad happening.

But think about this, is there any event that doesn't at least have the possibility of something bad happening? Wouldn't it be possible to win the lottery and then get a really bad paper cut from the check? Couldn't you get the bike you've always wanted and then wipe out? If your parents would let you eat all the ice cream in the world, you could get a severe case of "brain freeze."

So where do worries really come from? They come from exaggerating the "badness" of the bad outcome. I know that's not the correct way to say it but it seems to make sense to the kids I've worked with over the years. It's making the badness even badder! It's taking a bad event making it ten times worse by letting your imagination run away with you.

Now it's time to apply this idea to your worries. If you have a # 1 worry, write it down here. Think of a # 1 worry as the thing that you worry the most about.

My # 1 worry is:

____

____

Okay, time for the same drill. What are three things worse than your # 1 worry?

1. ____
2. ____
3. ____

The point of this exercise is to try to help you gain some perspective. Sometimes we get ourselves so worked up worrying about the possibility of a bad event that worrying about it is worse than when it actually happens! (Wilde, 2008, p. 42-43).

It is also important to acknowledge that some clients have anxieties related to events that, if they did transpire, would have a profound impact on their lives. The treatment of these anxieties must be addressed differently. Previously the goal was to help clients gain some perspective on the negative consequences of the event (it it were to occur). When the anxiety provoking event actually has the potential to be life-threatening, it is better to focus on the statistical improbability of the event actually occurring.

But for some of you, your # 1 worry is something that would change your life forever like something bad happening to a parent or maybe a terrorist attack or a natural disaster. You probably won't be able to list three things worse than your # 1 (but try anyway). If this is you, your worries are coming from an entirely different place. ***Your worries are coming from exaggerating the possibility of the bad event really happening.***

Let's say your worries are related to another terrorist attack like the one that took place on 9/11. While a terrorist attack is always possible, the odds of you personally being harmed are incredibly slim. That's because your brain gets stuck on a certain worries and completely ignores other potential dangers. For example, I'll bet you didn't know that there have been more than 50 people killed by falling vending machines since 1978. Yet, I've never met a single person who constantly worries about being crushed to death by a pop machine.

That's sort of like people who are afraid to fly on planes. They know that they are much safer traveling by plane than by car but they are still worried. And you know why? Knowing something in your brain is much different than feeling it in your "gut." When your brain and your "gut" get into a disagreement, your "gut" usually wins. At least for a few rounds until the brains gets better prepared (Wilde, 2008, p. 44-45).

6.5 Lesson 5: Distraction

The cardinal tenet of REBT is that emotions are not caused directly by events but are primarily the result of the thoughts and beliefs an individual has *about* the event. Therefore, if children are able to modify their thoughts about an event, they will change their feelings as well. One of the simplest and most effective techniques designed to bring about a change in thinking involves the use of a distraction technique (Wilde, 1997b; Wilde 1996b; Wilde 1995).

Distraction is not an "elegant solution" as Ellis would say. It does not involve a change in assessment of the event and, therefore, it would not be considered to be bringing about cognitive restructuring. Distraction, as the name implies, merely attempts to help children think of something other than their current situation. This is more difficult than it sounds because when children are getting anxious, the only thing they seem to be able to think about is the situation at hand. That is why clients need to decide what to think about *before* they start becoming anxious.

Encourage clients to pick "a scene" to use before they encounter the event they become anxious about. This memory should be either the happiest, funniest, or most relaxing scene they can remember. For example:

- A memorable day at the beach or on vacation
- The time they won a game
- A hysterically funny event from their past
- A memorable birthday party

Have clients take a few minutes and think about the distraction scene. You may need to help clients select the scene that fits their individual needs. Now they need to practice imagining this scene several times daily for the next few days or weeks. When clients have some free time have them close their eyes and picture their distraction scene. Clients should be advised to bring in all the details that they can possibly remember to make the scene vivid.
What were the people wearing?
What were the sounds they can remember?
Were there any smells in the air?
Encourage clients to create scenes in their minds just like watching a videotape of the event. It can also be helpful to have them draw their distraction scene and then explain it to the therapist.
The idea is to switch to this distraction scene when the clients find themselves getting anxious. Instead of focusing on the situation they are getting anxious about, they are to concentrate on their distraction scene. Instead of getting anxious before an important examination in school, they are to concentrate on the distraction scene until the feelings start to subside. Whenever they feel themselves getting anxious, they are to switch to their scene.
It is impossible for clients to think of a distraction scene and still become anxious. Since anxiety is produced by beliefs, thinking about a funny or happy memory will keep them from getting upset or minimize the intensity of the emotions.

6.6 Lesson 6: Rational emotive imagery

What follows is an example of how the imagination game or rational-emotive imagery (REI) can be used with children and adolescents who have anxiety problems. Ellis (1994; 1979) and Wilde (1995; 1996a; 1997b) have used REI extensively in the treatment of anxiety and anger problems. This technique is most effective if there is a particular situation (i.e., certain social situations, public speaking, separation from parents) in which anxiety is likely to occur.
Start by having the child vividly describe the troublesome scenario. Get as many details as possible about the sights, sounds, and events in this situation. Then have the child get as relaxed as possible in his or her chair with both feet on the floor. Spend several minutes describing relaxing images until you can see the behavioral manifestations of relaxations starting to appear. The use progressive relaxation techniques with the successive contracting and relaxing of various muscle groups can be very helpful. After the client appears to be sufficiently relaxed, start with the following dialogue.
Therapist: Anna, I want you to listen very closely to what I'm going to tell you. I want you to be aware only of my voice and focus on what I say. Try to block everything else out of your mind for the time being.
Imagine you are back in your classroom and students are taking turns reading aloud. Picture the room in your mind. See all the posters on the walls and everything else that is in your class. Now go ahead and let yourself feel like you do when it's reading time. Feel all the anxiety you felt back then. Stay with that scene and try to feel just like you felt in the class. When you feel that way, wiggle your finger and let me know you're there.
(Author's note - It's a good idea to look for behavioral signs confirming that the child is actually feeling anxious. The jaw may tighten, eyebrows furrow and many children will shift or squirm in their seats.)
Stay with that feeling. Keep imagining that you are in your classroom.

(Author's note - Allow the child to stay in this state for approximately 20 to 40 seconds. Remind him or her to mentally stay in the situation.)
Now I want you to keep thinking you are in the class but I want you to calm yourself down. Stay in the classroom in your mind but try to calm down. Instead of being very upset, try to get calmer. Instead of being really anxious, try to work toward feeling calmer. Keep working at it until you can calm yourself down. When you can make yourself calm, wiggle your finger again.
Usually students can reach a state of relative calm within a fairly short period of time. Once a child has wiggled his or her finger, it is time to bring him or her back to the here and now. Simply say something like, "Okay, now open your eyes." Next ask, "*What did you say to yourself to calm yourself down?*" If the child was able to calm down, he or she had to be thinking some type of rational coping statement. The only other way to calm down would be to mentally leave the situation (i.e., no longer visualize the classroom). This usually doesn't happen but if it does, try the exercise over encouraging the child to keep imagining the scene but working to calm down.
After completing the imagination game students should then be able to state the thought that allowed them to calm down. A typical calming thought that might have been produced from the above scenario would be, "Even though I don't read well, it's not that big of a deal. It doesn't mean I'm a bad person. Other students have problems reading aloud."
Once the child has produced a rational coping statement, write it down. Now he or she can practice this mental imagery several times a day and use this same calming thought each time. In effect, this technique allows kids to mentally practice dealing with a difficult situation in a new, more productive way. It's very important that they practice REI on a regular basis if they are going to learn to handle their anxiety in a more productive fashion.
Usually children can learn to do the Imagination Game by themselves after having been led through the technique a few times by the therapist. It is also possible to make a tape recording of this intervention for the child to use at home as some students like using the tape rather than leading themselves through this technique. Both can be effective if used regularly.

6.7 Lesson 7: Thought stopping

Ever since Joseph Wolpe (1958) first published descriptions of thought-stopping techniques, clinicians have been applying these types of interventions. There has been a plethora of case studies published over the years claiming reductions in anxiety symptoms with both adults and children. However, the results of experimental investigations have been inconsistent. Several of these studies have suffered from methodological shortcomings such as the lack of a control group or no follow-up analysis to determine if results have been maintained.
The general framework for teaching clients to use thought-stopping techniques follows a progression that begins with the therapist being more overtly involved and gradually diminishing involvement until the client is able to use the intervention independently. This interventions starts by having clients imagine the anxiety-provoking situation and vocalizing their thoughts. When clients first utter an irrational anxiety-producing thought such as, "If I did a bad job of reading in front of the class, I'd die," the therapist shouts, "Stop." Practice this first step until clients report that the therapist shouting, "Stop" interrupted their irrational thinking. The second step involves having clients merely *think* of the anxiety-provoking situation and signal the therapist whenever they were thinking an irrational thought. Upon observing the signal, the therapist again shouts, "Stop."

The problem with most thought stopping interventions is that they stop at this point. Clients can learn how to stop a disturbing thought but unless they can replace the anxiety-producing thought with a rational cognition, the original thought will quickly return. The next important step involves having clients think about positive, rational and/or calming thoughts that could substitute for the anxiety producing thought. Clients are taught to imagine the anxiety-provoking situation and when they began to think irrational thought they are to say their rational coping statement aloud. Once again, practice this until clients report that they are able to consistently reduce their anxiety to a manageable level. The use of a self-report scale (such as the subjective units of discomfort scale) with a range from 1-10 can be helpful to quantify the intensity of their emotions. The final step involves having clients practice transferring the rational coping statement from an overt statement to internal dialogue. Now they are to merely think their rational coping statement whenever they notice they are beginning to feel anxious.

6.8 Lesson 8: Systematic desensitization

This lesson teaches the clients how to use gradual exposure and relaxation as a means of learning to manage specific phobias.

One of the most common ways to get over a specific anxiety is to start by approaching the problem slowly. You know, taking small steps toward your goal until you are better able to manage the anxiety. Mental health professionals call this systematic desensitization and it is used a lot with kids and adults who have difficulties with anxiety.

If you were afraid of the water, there are a number of ways you could try to conquer your anxiety. You could get in a boat, drive out into the middle of a lake, and jump in. That would be one approach but probably not the best one. You could also start by using a pool. At first, you might need to stand on the deck of the pool and not actually go near the water. After you were able to stand on the deck without being too anxious, maybe you could slowly wade into the water. Maybe you'd have to start the wading in the baby pool. Each day you could go a couple of inches deeper and stay there until you were able to relax. With enough time and plenty of support, you'd eventually be able to go all the way into the water. That's the way systematic desensitization works and we're going to try to help you understand how to apply it to your worries.

One of the first things to do is create a "Fear Thermometer" which is kind of like the SUDs scale. You start by listing the things that you get a little anxious about (like standing on the side of the pool), and you keep going up the thermometer until you list the things you are very anxious about (jumping in the deep end of the pool). The thermometer goes from 1 to 100 so for each event you have to give it a score (or temperature).

Using the pool example, a Fear Thermometer might look like this:

Event	*Temperature*
Jumping into deep end without life jacket	*99*
Jumping into deep end with life jacket	*90*
Wading in chest deep water	*75*
Wading in waist deep water	*65*
Wading in knee deep water	*50*
Walking into the water at a pool	*40*
Walking into the water at the baby pool	*35*
Standing on the deck of a pool	*20*

Looking at a pool 10
Seeing people swimming on video 5

So the plan would be to start at the bottom with video of people swimming. While watching the video, you would repeat a self-calming statement while doing rational-emotive imagery just like we practiced a few pages ago. It might be a self-calming statement like, "I am safe. Nothing bad is going to happen to me in the water" or something like that. Some people use a mental picture of a relaxing event (like clouds floating across the sky) and when they start to feel anxious, they switch to that image. Feel free to experiment to determine which one works best for you. When you can look at that video of someone swimming without feeling overwhelmed by worries, it is time to move to the next event on the Fear Thermometer. You keep using the same set of procedures until you can reach the top of the Fear Thermometer.

Now, it's time for you to make your own Fear Thermometer. I used eight lines but if you need more, feel free to take out a separate sheet of paper.

	Event	*Temperature*
1.	______________________________	
	______________________________	*Temp.*__________
2	______________________________	
	______________________________	*Temp.*__________
3.	______________________________	
	______________________________	Temp.__________
4.	______________________________	
	______________________________	Temp.__________
5.	______________________________	
	______________________________	Temp.__________
6.	______________________________	
	______________________________	Temp.__________
7.	______________________________	
	______________________________	Temp.__________
8.	______________________________	
	______________________________	Temp.__________

Write down your self-calming statement or calming mental image you will use to relax here.

____

____

____

Remember, start at the bottom and when you are able to "manage" that situation without feeling too much anxiety, move up the list. This will take time so be patient. Sometimes it will take weeks and even months to work through your list. Don't expect to master the list overnight
Wilde, 2008, p. 58-62).

6.9 Lesson 9: Worry brain vs. calm brain

This lesson is to determine if clients have mastered the skill of understanding the difference between 1) a rational thought and 2) an irrational exaggeration. Clients are challenged to come up with both for this lesson.

I call this "Worry Brain vs. Calm Brain." It can be used with any situation you get anxious about but it's a good idea to use it with the one you've been having the most trouble with. Below are two

sets of brains. Your job is to write a "Worry Brain" thought and a "Calm Brain" thought in the lines provided.
Let's use the example of being afraid of storms to illustrate what you are supposed to do. In this scenario, you have just seen that the sky is turning dark. The worry brain thinks, "Oh no, it might thunder and lightning and that would be terrible." The calm brain thinks, "Well, there might be a storm but that wouldn't be the worst thing in the world. I'm safe here inside." Next, the worry brain thinks, "It could turn into a tornado and come right at the house." The calm brain thinks, "It could turn into a tornado but it never has before. In fact, in the history of our town, there's never been a single house hit by a tornado. The odds are that I'll be safe." Do you see how it works? This will give your calm brain a chance to practice overpowering your worry brain. Select a situation you get anxious about and practice writing both "Worry Brain" thoughts and then countering that with a "Calm Brain" answers. Give it a shot! Feel free to take out a blank piece of paper and practice this "Worry Brain vs. Calm Brain" all you want. It's easy once you get the hang of it.

1. *Worry Brain Thought*______________________________

____

1.a. *Calm Brain Thought* ______________________________

____

2. *Worry Brain Thought* ______________________________

____

2.a. *Calm Brain Thought* ______________________________

____

(Wilde, 2008, p. 66-67)

7. Summary

Anxiety problems are among the most commonly diagnosed mental and emotional problems to occur during childhood and adolescence. Research suggests that if left untreated, many children will struggle with anxiety later in life. The interventions discussed in this article are relatively brief and are designed to be used in a group counseling setting. While there is an abundance of research on the effectiveness of REBT and CBT on the treatment of anxiety, there is significantly less when it comes to the application of these principles in a group setting. The research that is available has generally found positive results for anxiety management conducted in a group counseling setting. The lessons presented in this chapter start by setting the stage by helping clients understand that they have the ability to change their thoughts and thus, change their feelings. The connection between thoughts and feeling—essential when using REBT/CBT—is stressed in the beginning of group. Helping clients understand what kinds of thoughts contribute to anxious feelings is also an important component of the process. Several lessons focus on clients practicing ways of minimizing and managing anxiety are also presented (distraction, thought stopping, rational emotive imagery). Finally, a lesson designed to allow clients to practice using systematic desensitization is offered.

8. References

Blanchard L.T., Gukra, M., Blackman, J. (2004). Emotional, developmental, and behavioral health of American *children* and their families: A report from the 2003 National Survey of *Children's* Health. *Pediatrics, 117,* 6, 1202-12.

Block, J. (1978). Effects of rational-emotive mental health program on poorly achieving, disruptive high school students. *Journal of Counseling Psychology, 25,* 61-65.

Borkovec, T, and Costello, E. (1993). Efficacy of applied relaxation and cognitive-behavioral therapy in the treatment of generalized anxiety disorder. *Journal of Consulting and Clinical Psychology, 61,* 611-619.

Brody, M. (1974). *The effects of rational-emotive affective education on anxiety, self-esteem, and frustration tolerance.* Unpublished doctoral dissertation, Temple University, Philadelphia.

Butler, G. Fennell, M., Robson, P., Gelder, M. (1991). Comparison of behavior therapy and cognitive behavior therapy in the treatment of generalized anxiety disorder. *Journal of Consulting and Clinical Psychology, 59,* 167-175.

Cangelosi, A., Gressard, C., & Mines, R. (1980). The effects of rational thinking groups on self-concepts in adolescents. *The School Counselor, 14,* 357-361.

Clarke, G. N., Hornbrook, M., Lynch, F., Polen, M., Gale, J., & Beardslee, W., (2001). A randomized trial of a group *cognitive* intervention for preventing depression in adolescent offspring of depressed parents. *Archives of General Psychiatry, 58,* 1127–1134.

Costello, E.J. & Angold, A. (1995). Epidemiology. In J.S. March (ed.), *Anxiety disorders in children and adolescents.* New York, Guildford.

Cristea, I. A. ; Benga, O. & Opre, A. (2006). The comparative efficiency of a rational-emotive education intervention for anxiety in 3rd grade children: An analysis of relevant developmental constraints. *Cognitie, Creier, Comportament/Cognition, Brain, Behavior, 10,* 637-657.

DeVoge, C. (1974). A behavioral approach to RET with children. *Rational Living, 9,* 23-26.

DiGiuseppe, R. (1975) *A developmental study on the efficacy of rational-emotive education.* Unpublished doctoral dissertation, Hofstra University.

DiGiuseppe, R., & Kassinove, H. (1976). Effects of a rational-emotive school mental health program in children's emotional adjustment. *Journal of Community Psychology, 4,* 382-387.

Ellis, A. (1962). *Reason and emotion in psychotherapy.* Philadelphia: Citadel Press.

Ellis, A. (1979). The theory of rational-emotive therapy. In A. Ellis & J. Whiteley (Eds.), *Theoretical and empirical foundations of rational-emotive therapy.* (p. 9 - 26). Monterey, CA: Brooks/Cole.

Ellis, A. (1994). *Reason and emotion in psychotherapy: Revised edition.* Philadelphia: Citadel Press.

Ellis, A. (1999). *How to be happy and remarkably less disturbable.* Atascadero, CA: Impact Publishers.

Ellis, A. (2001) *Feeling better, getting better, staying better.* Atascadero, CA: Impact Publishers.

Ellis, A. (2000b) *Rational emotive self-help techniques.* New York, NY: Guilford Press.

Ellis, A. & Dryden, W. (1997). *The practice of rational emotive behavior therapy.* New York, NY: Springer Publishing.

Ellis, A., & Harper, R. (1975). *The new guide to rational living.* Los Angeles: Wilshire.

Ellis, A., & Harper, R. (1997). *A guide to rational living.* North Hollywood: Wilshire.

Ellis, A. & MacLaren, C. (1998). *Rational emotive behavior therapy: A therapist's guide.* Atascadero, CA: Impact Publishers.

Gillham, J. E., Reivich, K. J., Jaycox, L. H., & Seligman, M. P. E. (1995). Prevention of depressive symptoms in schoolchildren: Two-year follow-up. *Psychological Science, 6,* 343–351.

Gould, M., Otto, M., Pollack, M., and Yap, L. (1997). Cognitive behavioral and pharmacological treatment of generalized anxiety disorder: A preliminary meta-analysis. *Behavior Therapy, 28,* 285-305.

Katz, S. (1974). *The effect of emotional education on locus of control and self-concept.* Unpublished doctoral dissertation, Hofstra University.

Keller, M. B., Lavori, P., Wunder, J., Beardslee, W. R., Schwarts, C. E., & Roth, J. (1992). Chronic course of *anxiety* disorders in *children* and adolescents. *Journal of the American Academy of Child and Adolescent Psychiatry, 31,* 595–599.

Kessler, R. & Merikangas, K. (2004). The national comorbidity survey replication (NCS-R): Background and aims. *International Journal of Methods in Psychiatric Research, 13,* 2, 60-68.

Knaus, W., & Bokor, S. (1975). The effects of rational-emotive education on anxiety and self-concept. *Rational Living, 10,* 7-10.

Knaus, W., & McKeever, C. (1977). Rational-emotive education on anxiety and self-concept. *Journal of Rational Living, 10,* 7-10.

Liber, J., Van Widenfelt, B. Utens, E., Ferdinand, R. Van Der Leeden, A., Van Gastel, W., & Treffers, P. (2008). No differences between group versus individual treatment of childhood anxiety disorders in a randomised clinical trial. *Journal of Child Psychology and Psychiatry, 49,* 886-893.

Maes, W., & Heimann, R. (1970). *The comparison of three approaches to the reduction of test anxiety in high school students.* U.S. Department of Health, Education and Welfare, Washington, D.C., 1-73.

Maultsby, M., Knipping, P., & Carpenter, L. (1974). Teaching self-help in the classroom with rational self-counseling. *Journal of School Health, 44,* 445-448.

Meichenbaum, D., & Goodman, J. (1971). Training impulsive children to talk to themselves. *Journal of Abnormal Psychology, 77,* 115-126.

Meyer, D. (1981). *Effects of rational-emotive therapy upon anxiety and self-esteem of learning disabled children.* Ann Arbor, MI: University of Michigan.

Micco, J.; Choate-Summers, M.; Ehrenreich, J.; Pincus, D.& Mattis, S. (2007). Identifying efficacious *treatment* components of panic control *treatment* for adolescents: A preliminary examination. *Child & Family Behavior Therapy, 29, 1-23.*

Miller, N., & Kassinove, H. (1978). Effects of behavioral rehearsal, written homework, and level of intelligence on the efficacy of rational-emotive education in elementary school children. *Journal of Community Psychology, 6,* 366-373.

National Institute for Clinical Excellence (2004). *Anxiety: Management of anxiety (panic disorder, with or without agoraphobia, and generalized anxiety disorder) in adults in primary, secondary and community care.* Retrieved October 7, 2007 from www.nice.org.uk/CG022quickrefguide.

Omizo, M., Lo, F., & William, R. (1986). Rational-emotive education, self-concept, and locus of control among learning disabled students. *Journal of Humanistic Education and Development, 25,* 59-69.

Pfeffer, C., Lipkins, R., Plutchik, R. & Mizruchi, M. (1988). Normal children at risk for suicidal behavior: A two-year follow-up study. *Journal of the American Academy of Child and Adolescent Psychiatry, 27,* 34-41.

Ritchie, B. (1978). *The effects of rational-emotive education on irrational beliefs, assertiveness, and/or locus of control in fifth grade students.* Unpublished doctoral dissertation, Virginia Polytechnic University.

Spence, S. (1998). A measure of anxiety symptoms among children. *Behavior and Research Therapy. 36,* 545-566.

U.S. Department of Health and Human Services. (1999). *Mental Health: A Report of the Surgeon General*. Rockville, MD: U.S. Department of Health and Human Services.

Voelm, C. (1983). *The efficacy of teaching rational-emotive education to acting-out and socially withdrawn adolescents.* Unpublished doctoral dissertation, California School of Professional Psychology.

Von Pohl, R. (1982). *A study to assess the effects of rational-emotive therapy with a selected group of emotionally disturbed children in day and residential treatment.* Unpublished doctoral dissertation, University of Alabama, Birmingham.

Wasserman T., & Vogrin D. (1979). Relationship of endorsement of rational beliefs, age, months treatment and intelligence to overt behavior of emotionally disturbed children. *Psychological Reports, 44,* 911-917.

Warren, R., Deffenbacher, J., & Brading, P. (1976). Rational-emotive therapy and the reduction of test anxiety in elementary school students. *Rational Living, 11,* 28-29.

Wessel, I. & Mersch, P. (1994). A cognitive-behavioural group treatment for test-anxious adolescents. *Anxiety, Stress & Coping: An International Journal,* Vol.7(2), 149-160.

Wilde, J. (1992). *Rational counseling with school aged populations: A practical guide.* Muncie, IN: Accelerated Development.

Wilde, J. (1994). The effects of the let's get rational board game on rational thinking, depression, and self-acceptance in adolescents. *The Journal of Rational-Emotive and Cognitive-Behavior Therapy, 12,* 189-196.

Wilde, J. (1995). *Anger management in schools: Alternatives to student violence.* Lancaster, PA: Technomic Publishing Company, Inc.

Wilde, J. (1996a). Rational-emotive behavior therapy and the treatment of phobias in children. *Anxiety Disorders Practice Journal,* 2 (2), 189-195.

Wilde, J. (1996b). *Treating anger, anxiety, and depression in children and adolescents: A cognitive-behavioral perspective.* Muncie, IN: Accelerated Development.

Wilde, J. (1997a). The efficacy of short-term rational-emotive education with fourth grade students. *Elementary School Guidance and Counseling, 31,* 131-138.

Wilde, J. (1997b) *Hot stuff to help kids chill out: The anger management book.* East Troy, WI: LGR Publishing.

Wilde, J. (2008) *Hot stuff to help kids worry less: The anxiety management book.* Richmond, IN: LGR Publishing.

Wolpe, J. (1958). *Psychotherapy by reciprocal inhibition.* Stanford University Press, Berkley, CA.